ESSENTIALS OF
NURSING
RESEARCH

Methods, Appraisal, and Utilization

ESSENTIALS OF
NURSING RESEARCH

Methods, Appraisal, and Utilization

Denise F. Polit, PhD
President
Humanalysis, Inc.
Saratoga Springs, New York

Cheryl Tatano Beck, DNSc, CNM, FAAN
Professor
University of Connecticut School of Nursing
Storrs, Connecticut

SIXTH EDITION

LIPPINCOTT WILLIAMS & WILKINS
A **Wolters Kluwer** Company

Philadelphia • Baltimore • New York • London
Buenos Aires • Hong Kong • Sydney • Tokyo

Acquisitions Editor: Margaret Zuccarini
Managing Editor: Joseph Morita
Editorial Assistant: Delema Caldwell-Jordan
Senior Production Manager: Helen Ewan
Managing Editor / Production: Erika Kors
Art Director: Carolyn O'Brien
Design Coordinator: Brett MacNaughton
Manufacturing Manager: William Alberti
Compositor: TechBooks
Printer: R. R. Donnelley, Crawfordsville

Sixth Edition

9 8 7 6 5 4 3

Library of Congress Cataloging-in-Publication Data

Polit, Denise F.
  Essentials of nursing research : methods, appraisal, and utilization / Denise F. Polit,
Cheryl Tatano Beck.—6th ed.
    p. ; cm.
  Includes bibliographical references and index.
  ISBN 0-7817-4972-7 (alk. paper)
  1. Nursing—Research.
  [DNLM: 1. Nursing Research. WY 20.5 P769e 2006]   I. Beck, Cheryl Tatano.   II. Title.

  RT81.5.P63 2006
  610.73'072—dc22   2004027850

Care has been taken to confirm the accuracy of the information presented and to describe generally accepted practices. However, the authors, editors, and publisher are not responsible for errors or omissions or for any consequences from application of the information in this book and make no warranty, express or implied, with respect to the content of the publication.
  The authors, editors, and publisher have exerted every effort to ensure that drug selection and dosage set forth in this text are in accordance with the current recommendations and practice at the time of publication. However, in view of ongoing research, changes in government regulations, and the constant flow of information relating to drug therapy and drug reactions, the reader is urged to check the package insert for each drug for any change in indications and dosage and for added warnings and precautions. This is particularly important when the recommended agent is a new or infrequently employed drug.
  Some drugs and medical devices presented in this publication have Food and Drug Administration (FDA) clearance for limited use in restricted research settings. It is the responsibility of the health care provider to ascertain the FDA status of each drug or device planned for use in his or her clinical practice.

To our families:

Alan, Nate, Alaine, Lauren, Norah
and
Chuck, Lisa, Curt

Reviewers

PREFACE

Writing this sixth edition of *Essentials of Nursing Research: Methods, Appraisal, and Utilization* has been exhilarating! We have never been so enthusiastic about any of the earlier editions of this book, despite the fact that, edition after edition, it has been an award-winning and top-ranking textbook used around the world.

    This edition retains all of the features that have made the text popular in the past, while introducing important innovations that we think will make it more useful to nurses and students who are learning to critically appraise research reports (and easier for instructors to use). These innovations are designed to make the textbook more relevant in an environment that is increasingly focused on evidence-based nursing practice. There is a growing expectation that nurses will base their practice on sound evidence—in particular on the findings from disciplined research. A major purpose of this book is to assist consumers of nursing research in evaluating the adequacy of research findings in terms of their merit and potential for utilization.

NEW TO THIS EDITION

Enhanced Assistance in Critiquing Studies

This edition is more focused on the art—and science—of research critiques than ever before. Each chapter offers specific opportunities for critiquing aspects of a study or research report that were discussed in the chapter. In most chapters, students are invited to answer critiquing questions for up to four studies (usually two quantitative and two qualitative). Some exercises are based on studies that are included in their entirety in the appendices of the book (four full studies are included in this edition; two in the book and two on the Student Resource CD-ROM), while others are based on

studies that are summarized at the end of the chapters. Students can then consult the accompanying CD-ROM or a website (connection.lww.com/go/polit) to find our thoughts about each critiquing exercise, so that students can get immediate feedback about their grasp of material in the chapter. This edition also includes full critiques of the two studies on the CD-ROM, which students can use as models for a comprehensive research critique. Many more critiquing opportunities are available in the Study Guide, which includes seven studies in their entirety in the appendices.

More Emphasis on Evidence-Based Practice Implications

We have made several changes to ensure that this textbook will better help to prepare students for evidence-based practice (EBP). We remind readers to think about the implications of research for EBP throughout the book, and emphasize that EBP relies on strong evidence from high-quality research. Some examples of how research evidence has affected nursing practice are introduced in the first chapter. We have also substantially revised the concluding chapter on research utilization and EBP. One particularly important addition is a discussion about how to critique integrative reviews (including meta-analyses and metasyntheses), which have become a cornerstone of EBP. Two integrative reviews are presented in their entirety in appendices of the Study Guide.

Better Coverage of Qualitative Research

Every new edition of this textbook has improved on the quality and quantity of information provided to students about qualitative research. This edition is no exception. In particular, we describe the three main qualitative research traditions (ethnography, phenomenology, grounded theory) early in this book (Chapter 3) and then point out differences and similarities among them in subsequent chapters.

Greater Facilitation in Learning the Basics

This textbook has been widely hailed for its clear, concise, and "user-friendly" presentation. In this edition, however, we have gone to great lengths to write in an even simpler, more straightforward fashion—it is designed to help consumers progress fairly slowly into the complexities of disciplined research. In addition to our consumer "tips" that have become a feature of previous editions, we have added new "How-to-Tell" tips in many chapters that specifically help students learn how to identify fundamental features—for example, how to tell if a study is experimental or nonexperimental—or how to tell if a journal article is a *study* or something else.

Enhanced Support for Instructors

In this edition we have put more effort than ever before on facilitating learning, including the development of additional supports for instructors. One important addition is PowerPoint slides, which students often find useful as well. The instructors' resource materials have been greatly expanded, with some suggestions for class projects that we think will prove stimulating

Greater Acknowledgment of International Contributions

This edition gives better recognition to the contributions of nurse researchers from around the globe. Research examples have been selected to reflect the diversity of interests and approaches of nurse researchers worldwide.

ORGANIZATION OF THE TEXT

The content of this edition is organized into six main parts.

Part 1—Overview of Nursing Research serves as the overall introduction to fundamental concepts in nursing research. Chapter 1 introduces and summarizes the history and future of nursing research, discusses the philosophical underpinnings of qualitative research versus quantitative research, and describes the major purposes of nursing research. Chapter 2 introduces readers to key terms, with new emphasis on terms related to the quality of research evidence. Chapter 3 presents an overview of the steps in the research process for both qualitative and quantitative studies. Chapter 4 provides an introduction to research reports—what they are and how to read them. Chapter 5 is devoted to a discussion of ethics in research studies.

Part 2—Preliminary Steps in the Research Process includes three chapters and focuses on the steps that are taken in getting started on a research project. Chapter 6 focuses on the development of research questions and the formulation of research hypotheses. Chapter 7 discusses how to prepare and critique literature reviews. Chapter 8 presents information about theoretical and conceptual frameworks.

Part 3—Designs for Nursing Research presents material relating to the design of qualitative and quantitative nursing studies. Chapter 9 describes some fundamental design principles and discusses many specific aspects of quantitative research design. Chapter 10 addresses the various research traditions that have contributed to the growth of naturalistic inquiry and qualitative research. Chapter 11 provides an introduction to some specific types of research (e.g., evaluations, surveys, secondary analyses, case studies), and also describes integrated qualitative/quantitative designs. Chapter 12 presents various designs for sampling of study participants.

Part 4—Data Collection deals with the collection of research data. Chapter 13 discusses the full range of data collection options available to researchers, including both qualitative and quantitative approaches. Chapter 14, an especially important chapter for critiquing qualitative studies, explains methods of assessing data quality.

Part 5—Data Analysis is devoted to the organization and analysis of research data. Chapter 15 reviews methods of quantitative analysis. The chapter assumes no prior instruction in statistics and focuses primarily on helping readers to understand why statistics are needed, what tests might be appropriate in a given research situation, and what statistical information in a research report means. Chapter 16 presents a discussion of qualitative analysis, greatly expanded and improved in this edition.

Part 6—Critical Appraisal and Utilization of Nursing Research is intended to sharpen the critical awareness of consumers with respect to several key issues. Chapter 17 discusses the interpretation and appraisal of research reports. An important new feature is the inclusion of two critiques in their entirety, which can be found on the Student Resource CD-ROM. Chapter 18, the final chapter, offers guidance for research utilization and EBP.

KEY FEATURES

We have retained many of the features that were successfully used in previous editions to assist consumers of nursing research.

Research Examples: Each chapter concludes with critical thinking exercises that include summaries of two or more actual research examples. (In this edition, we summarize the studies in an "abstract style" that we think will be more compelling.) Students are asked to evaluate features of these studies using the chapter's critiquing guidelines, with some supplementary questions targeted specifically to the selected study. As noted previously, our suggested "answers" have been made available to students both on the accompanying Student Resource CD-ROM and online. In addition, we used many actual recent nursing studies to illustrate key concepts in the text. The use of relevant examples is crucial to the development of both an understanding of and an interest in the research process.

Tips for Consumers of Nursing Research: Each chapter contains numerous tips on what to expect in research reports vis-à-vis the topics that have been discussed in the chapter. In these tips, we have paid special attention to helping students *read* research reports, which are often daunting to those without specialized research training. This feature will enable students to translate the material presented in the textbook into meaningful concepts as they approach the research literature.

Guidelines for Critiquing Research Reports: Each chapter has a section devoted to guidelines for conducting a critique. These sections provide a list of questions that walk students through a study, drawing attention to aspects of the study that are amenable to appraisal by research consumers.

FEATURES FOR STUDENT LEARNING

To enhance and reinforce learning, we have used several features to guide students' attention:

Chapter Objectives: Learning objectives are identified on the chapter opener to focus students' attention on critical content.

Key New Terms: Each chapter includes a list of new terms, which are defined in context (and bolded) when used for the first time in the text. In this edition, we have made the list less daunting by including only *key* new terms.

Chapter Summary Points: A succinct list of summary points that focus on salient chapter content is included in each chapter.

Suggested Readings: Two lists of suggested readings, methodologic and substantive resources, are provided in each chapter to direct the student's further inquiry.

Full-Length Research Examples: This edition includes four recent full-length examples of research studies—two quantitative and two qualitative—that students can read, analyze, and critique. Two appear in the appendices of the text, and two in the CD-ROM packaged with the book.

Critical Thinking Activities: Each chapter of the textbook includes activities designed to reinforce student learning and provide opportunities to practice critiquing skills.

TEACHING-LEARNING PACKAGE

Essentials of Nursing Research: Methods, Appraisal, and Utilization, Sixth Edition has an ancillary package designed with both students and instructors in mind.

The Study Guide augments the text and provides students with application exercises for each text chapter. Critiquing skills are emphasized, but there are also activities to support the learning of fundamental research terms. This edition offers exercises designed to reinforce learning while at the same time being "fun"—specifically, crossword puzzles with new terms have been developed for each chapter. Seven recent studies are included in the appendices, and many chapter exercises are based on these studies.

Free CD-ROM: The study guide also includes a CD-ROM providing 290 review questions to assist students in self-testing. This review program provides the rationale for both correct and incorrect answers, helping students to identify areas of strength and areas needing further study.

The Instructor's Resource CD-ROM includes a chapter for every chapter in the textbook.

Each chapter of the instructor's manual contains the following: Statement of Intent, Special Class Projects, Answers to Selected Study Guide Exercises, and Test Questions and Answers. In the special class projects, we offer opportunities (new in this edition) for students to develop a quantitative and (or) qualitative data set. With regard to test questions to evaluate student learning, we offer in this edition multiple choice and true/false questions (as in previous editions), but we have added questions specifically designed to test students' comprehension of research reports.

It is our hope and expectation that the content, style, and organization of this sixth edition of *Essentials of Nursing Research* will be helpful to those students desiring to become intelligent and thoughtful readers of nursing research studies and to those wishing to improve their clinical performance based on research findings. We also hope that this textbook will help to develop an enthusiasm for the kinds of discoveries and knowledge that research can produce.

Denise F. Polit, PhD
Cheryl Tatano Beck, DNSc, CNM, FAAN

Acknowledgments

This sixth edition, like the previous five editions, depended on the contribution of many individuals. We are deeply appreciative of those who made all six editions possible, including the many faculty and students who used the text during the past 25 years and have made invaluable suggestions for its improvement. In addition to all those who assisted us with earlier editions, there are some who deserve special mention for this new work.

In this edition, we must pay special tribute to the nine reviewers of the previous edition, who were anonymous to us when we read their comments in 2003. We heard a very clear message that inspired us to make exciting pedagogical changes: Provide better support for students learning to critique research reports. These reviewers were seminal in our thinking about how to restructure this sixth edition, and we are quite confident that the resulting text is the best we have ever produced. We cannot thank these reviewers enough.

Inspiration came from another source as well: Eileen J. Porter and Tamam B. Mansour published an analysis of methods instructors use to teach nursing research to undergraduates in the journal *Research in Nursing & Health*.[1] This article, which was published just as we were planning this sixth edition, helped to further refine our ideas about how best to help students develop research skills. One further source of broad inspiration: Ruth Griffith, who was eye-opening as well as deeply supportive.

Other individuals made more specific contributions. Although it would be impossible to mention all, we note with thanks the nurse researchers who shared their work with us as we developed examples, including work that in some cases was not yet published. We are also grateful for the insights of Dr. Robert Gable regarding data quality issues in Chapter 14. Finally, we worked closely with authors of the reports that appear in the appendices. We shared with them our "answers" to the critiquing exercises to make sure that we had not misread or misinterpreted their reports, and they gave generously of their time in reviewing our material. Special thanks to Sandy Motzer, Tish Knobf, Jon Seskevich, James Lane, and Donna Clemmens.

We also extend our warmest thanks to those who helped to turn the manuscript into a finished product. The staff at Lippincott Williams & Wilkins has been of tremendous assistance in the support they have given us over the years. We are indebted to Joe Morita, Margaret Zuccarini, Helen Kogut, Erika Kors, Doris Wray, and all the others behind the scenes for their fine contributions.

Finally, we thank our family, our loved ones, and our friends, who provided ongoing support and encouragement throughout this endeavor.

[1] Porter, E. J., & Mansour, T. B. (2003). Teaching nursing research to undergraduates: A text analysis of instructors' intentions. *Research in Nursing & Health, 26,* 128–142.

Contents

Overview of Nursing Research

Introducing Research and Its Use in Nursing Practice

STUDENT OBJECTIVES

On completing this chapter, you will be able to:

▶ Describe why research is important in the nursing profession and discuss why evidence-based practice is needed
▶ Describe historical trends and future directions in nursing research
▶ Describe alternative sources of evidence for nursing practice
▶ Describe major characteristics of the positivist and naturalistic paradigms, and discuss similarities and differences between the traditional scientific method (quantitative research) and naturalistic methods (qualitative research)
▶ Identify several purposes of qualitative and quantitative research
▶ Define new terms in the chapter

AN INTRODUCTION TO NURSING RESEARCH

It is an exciting—and challenging—time to be a nurse. Nurses are managing their clinical responsibilities at a time when the nursing profession and the larger health care system require an extraordinary range of skills and talents of them. Nurses are expected to deliver the highest-possible quality care in a compassionate manner, while also being mindful of costs. To accomplish these diverse (and sometimes conflicting) goals, nurses continually need to access and evaluate new information, and incorporate it into their clinical decision making. In today's world, *nurses must become lifelong learners,* capable of reflecting on, evaluating, and modifying their clinical practice based on emerging knowledge from systematic nursing and health care research.

What Is Nursing Research?

Research is systematic inquiry that uses disciplined methods to answer questions or solve problems. The ultimate goal of research is to develop, refine, and expand a base of knowledge.

Nurses are increasingly engaged in disciplined studies that benefit the profession and its patients. **Nursing research** is systematic inquiry designed to develop knowledge about issues of importance to nurses, including nursing practice, nursing education, and nursing administration.

In this book, we emphasize clinical nursing research, that is, research designed to generate evidence to guide nursing practice and to improve the care and quality of life of clients. Clinical nursing research typically begins with questions stemming from practice-related problems—problems such as ones you may have already encountered.

 Examples of nursing research questions

▶ How intense is fatigue in HIV-positive individuals, and what psychological and physiological factors affect or are associated with such fatigue? (Barroso, Carlson, & Meynell, 2003)
▶ What does having a positive attitude mean for patients undergoing treatment for cancer? (Wilkes, O'Baugh, Luke, & George, 2003)

The Importance of Research in Nursing

Nurses increasingly are expected to adopt an **evidence-based practice (EBP)**, which is broadly defined as the use of the best clinical evidence in making patient care decisions. Evidence for EBP can come from various sources, but there is general agreement that research findings from rigorous studies constitute the best type of evidence for informing nurses' decisions, actions, and interactions with clients. Nurses are accepting the need to base specific nursing actions and decisions on evidence indicating that the actions are clinically appropriate and cost-effective, and result in positive outcomes for clients. Nurses who incorporate high-quality research evidence into their clinical decisions and advice are being professionally accountable to their clients. Research-based evidence for clinical nursing decisions comes from both nursing studies and studies in a broad array of other disciplines.

Example of evidence-based practice

Numerous clinical practice changes over the past 2 decades reflect the impact of research. For example, a recent nursing study documented that "kangaroo care" (the holding of diaper-clad preterm infants skin-to-skin, chest-to-chest by parents) is now widely practiced in neonatal intensive care units (NICUs) in the United States (Engler et al., 2002), but this is a new trend. As recently as the early 1990s, only a minority of NICUs offered kangaroo care options. The adoption of this practice reflects the accumulating evidence that early skin-to-skin contact has clinical benefits without any apparent negative side effects (Anderson et al., 2003). Some of that accumulated evidence was developed in rigorous studies by nurse researchers in the United States, Australia, Canada, Taiwan, and other countries (Chwo et al., 2002).

Another reason for nurses to engage in research involves the spiraling costs of health care and the cost-containment practices being instituted in health care facilities. Now, more than ever, nurses need to document the effectiveness of their practice not only to the profession but also to nursing care consumers, health care administrators, third-party payers (e.g., insurance companies), and government agencies. Some research findings will help eliminate nursing actions that do not achieve desired outcomes. Other findings will help nurses identify the practices that improve health care outcomes and contain costs as well.

Nursing research can help in a broad array of problem-solving situations. Research enables nurses to understand a particular nursing situation about which little is known, assess the need for an intervention, identify factors that must be considered in planning nursing care, predict the probable outcomes of certain nursing decisions, control the occurrence of undesired outcomes, provide advice to enhance client health, and initiate activities to promote appropriate client behavior. These are all activities that nurses already undertake; research findings can enhance the likelihood that the activities will have the desired results.

CONSUMER TIP

Every time you make a clinical decision or undertake a procedure, your action is based on something—perhaps what you learned in school, what you read in a book or journal, what you were told to do by a supervisor, or what your "intuition" tells you is appropriate. It is a professional responsibility to ask: How do I *know* this is really the most effective decision or action? Some practices that are based on tradition rather than on research are simply *not* the best way to do things.

Roles of Nurses in Research

With the current emphasis on EBP, it has become *every* nurse's responsibility to engage in one or more research activity along a continuum of research participation. At one end of the continuum are those nurses whose involvement in research is indirect. Users (consumers) of nursing research read research reports to develop new skills and to keep up-to-date on relevant findings that may affect their practice. Nurses are expected to maintain this level of involvement with research, at a minimum. **Research utilization**—the use of findings from research in a practice setting—depends on intelligent nursing research consumers.

At the other end of the continuum are nurses who design and undertake research. At one time, most nurse researchers were academics who taught in schools of nursing, but research is increasingly being conducted by practicing nurses who want to find what works best for their clients.

Example of research by hospital-based nurses

Tranmer and three other nurses (2003) who worked at the Kingston General Hospital in Ontario undertook a study to better understand the sleep experience of medical and surgical patients during a hospital stay. They found that a number of personal factors and environmental factors in the unit, many of which were amenable to interventions, strongly influenced the sleep experience.

Between these two end points on the continuum lies a rich variety of research-related activities in which nurses engage to improve their effectiveness and enhance their professional lives. Even if you never conduct a study, you may well do one or more of the following:

▶ Participate in a **journal club** in a practice setting, which involves regular meetings among nurses to discuss and critique research articles
▶ Attend research presentations at professional conferences
▶ Evaluate completed research for its possible use in practice
▶ Help to develop an idea for a clinical study
▶ Review a proposed research plan and offer clinical expertise to improve the plan
▶ Assist researchers in collecting information for a study (e.g., distributing questionnaires to clients)
▶ Provide information and advice to clients who are participating in studies
▶ Discuss the implications and relevance of research findings with clients

CONSUMER TIP

Here is a headline about a study of over 13,000 nurses that appeared in newspapers throughout the United States in July 2004: "Study: Vegetables are good brain food. Broccoli, spinach shown to have effects on mental sharpness." What would you say if clients asked you about this study? Would you be able to comment on the believability of the findings, based on your assessment of how rigorously the study was conducted? You should be able to do this after you have completed this course. ▪

In all these possible research-related activities, nurses who have some research skills are in a better position to make a contribution to nursing and to EBP than those who do not. A knowledge of nursing research can improve the depth and breadth of every nurse's professional practice. Learning about research methods allows you to evaluate and synthesize new information (i.e., become an intelligent research consumer), develop knowledge that can be used in practice, and engage meaningfully in various research-related roles.

NURSING RESEARCH: PAST, PRESENT, AND FUTURE

Although nursing research has not always had the prominence and importance it enjoys today, its long and interesting history portends a distinguished future. Table 1-1 summarizes some of the key events in the historical evolution of nursing research.

TABLE 1.1	Historical Landmarks Affecting Nursing Research

YEAR	EVENT
1859	Nightingale's *Notes on Nursing* published
1900	*American Nursing Journal* begins publication
1923	Columbia University establishes first doctoral program for nurses
	Goldmark Report with recommendations for nursing education published
1930s	*American Journal of Nursing* publishes clinical cases studies
1948	Brown publishes report on inadequacies of nursing education
1952	The journal *Nursing Research* begins publication
1955	Inception of the American Nurses' Foundation to sponsor nursing research
1957	Establishment of nursing research center at Walter Reed Army Institute of Research
1963	*International Journal of Nursing Studies* begins publication
1965	American Nurses' Association (ANA) begins sponsoring nursing research conferences
1966	Nursing history archive established at Mugar Library, Boston University
1969	*Canadian Journal of Nursing Research* begins publication
1971	ANA establishes a Commission on Research
1972	ANA establishes its Council of Nurse Researchers
1976	Stetler and Marram publish guidelines on assessing research for use in practice
1978	The journals *Research in Nursing & Health* and *Advances in Nursing Science* begin publication
1979	*Western Journal of Nursing Research* begins publication
1982	The Conduct and Utilization of Research in Nursing (CURN) project publishes report
1983	*Annual Review of Nursing Research* begins publication
1985	ANA Cabinet on Nursing Research establishes research priorities
1986	National Center for Nursing Research (NCNR) established within U.S. National Institutes of Health
1987	The journal *Scholarly Inquiry for Nursing Practice* begins publication
1988	The journals *Applied Nursing Research* and *Nursing Science Quarterly* begin publication
	Conference on Research Priorities (CORP #1) is convened by NCNR
1989	U.S. Agency for Health Care Policy and Research (AHCPR) is established
1992	The journal *Clinical Nursing Research* begins publication
1993	NCNR becomes a full institute, the National Institute of Nursing Research (NINR)
	CORP #2 is convened to establish priorities for 1995–1999
	The Cochrane Collaboration is established
	Journal of Nursing Measurement begins publication
1994	The journal *Qualitative Health Research* begins publication
1997	Canadian Health Services Research Foundation is established with federal funding
1999	AHCPR is renamed Agency for Healthcare Research and Quality (AHRQ)
2000	NINR issues funding priorities for 2000–2004; annual funding exceeds $100 million
	The Canadian Institute of Health Research is launched
	The journal *Biological Research for Nursing* begins publication
2004	The journal *Worldviews on Evidence-Based Nursing* begins publication

The Early Years: From Nightingale to the 1960s

Most people would agree that nursing research began with Florence Nightingale. Based on her skillful analyses of factors affecting soldier mortality and morbidity during the Crimean War, she was successful in effecting some changes in nursing care—and, more generally, in public health. Her landmark publication, *Notes on Nursing* (1859), describes her early research interest in environmental factors that promote physical and emotional well-being—an interest of nurses that continues nearly 150 years later.

For many years after Nightingale's work, the nursing literature contained little research. Some attribute this absence to the apprenticeship nature of nursing. The pattern of nursing research that eventually emerged at the turn of the century was closely aligned to the problems confronting nurses. For example, most studies conducted between 1900 and 1940 concerned nursing education. As more nurses received university-based education, studies concerning students—their problems, characteristics, and satisfactions—became more numerous. When hospital staffing patterns changed, fewer students were available over a 24-hour period. As a consequence, researchers focused their investigations not only on the supply and demand of nurses but also on the amount of time required to perform certain nursing activities. During these years, nursing struggled with its professional identity, and nursing research took a twist toward studying nurses: who they were, what they did, how other groups perceived them, and what type of person entered the profession.

In the 1950s, a number of forces combined to put nursing research on the rapidly accelerating upswing it is on today. More nurses with baccalaureate and advanced academic preparation, the establishment of the journal *Nursing Research*, government funding to support nursing research in the United States, and upgraded research skills among nursing faculty are a few of the forces propelling nursing research. In the late 1950s, the need for studies addressing clinical nursing problems was recognized.

During the 1960s, clinical nursing research began in earnest as practice-oriented research on various clinical topics emerged in the literature. Nursing research advanced worldwide: The *International Journal of Nursing Studies* began publication in 1963, and the *Canadian Journal of Nursing Research* appeared in 1969.

Example of a nursing research breakthrough in the 1960s

Jeanne Quint Benoliel began a program of research that had a major impact on medicine, medical sociology, and nursing. She explored the subjective experiences of patients following diagnosis with a life-threatening illness (1967). Physicians in the early 1960s usually did not advise women that they had breast cancer, even following a mastectomy. Quint's (1962, 1963) seminal study of the personal experiences of women following radical mastectomy contributed to changes in communication and information control by physicians and nurses.

Nursing Research Since 1970

By the 1970s, the growing number of studies and the increased discussion of theoretical and contextual issues relating to nursing research created the need for additional communication outlets. Several additional journals that focus on nursing research were established in the 1970s, including

Advances in Nursing Science, Research in Nursing & Health, the *Western Journal of Nursing Research*, and the *Journal of Advanced Nursing*. During that decade, there was a decided shift in emphasis from areas such as teaching, administration, and nurses themselves to the improvement of client care. Nurses also began to pay more attention to the utilization of research findings in nursing practice. A seminal article by Stetler and Marram (1976) offered guidance on assessing research for application in practice settings.

Example of a nursing research breakthrough in the 1970s

Kathryn Barnard's research led to breakthroughs in the area of neonatal and child development. Her research program focused on the identification and assessment of children at risk of developmental and health problems, such as abused and neglected children and failure-to-thrive children (Barnard, 1973, 1976; Barnard & Collar, 1973; Barnard et al., 1977). Her research contributed to work on early interventions for children with disabilities, and to the field of developmental psychology.

Several events in the 1980s provided impetus for nursing research. For example, the first volume of the *Annual Review of Nursing Research* was published in 1983. These annual reviews include summaries of current research knowledge on selected areas of nursing practice and encourage utilization of research findings. Of particular importance in the United States during the 1980s was the establishment in 1986 of the National Center for Nursing Research (NCNR) within the National Institutes of Health (NIH). The purpose of NCNR was to promote—and financially support—research training and clinical research focused on patient care. Additionally, the Center for Research for Nursing was created in 1983 by the American Nurses Association. The Center's mission is to develop and coordinate a research program to serve as the source of national information for the profession. In Canada, federal funding for nursing research also became available in the late 1980s through the National Health Research Development Program.

Also in the 1980s, nurses began to conduct formal research utilization projects, and an important new journal was established: *Applied Nursing Research*. This journal includes research reports on studies of special relevance to practicing nurses. In Australia, the *Australian Journal of Nursing Research* was launched in the 1980s.

Several forces outside of nursing in the late 1980s helped to shape today's nursing research landscape. A group from the McMaster Medical School in Canada designed a clinical learning strategy that was called evidence-based medicine (EBM). EBM, which promulgated the view that research findings were far superior to the opinions of authorities as a basis for clinical decisions, constituted a profound shift for medical practice and has had a major effect on all health care professions.

In 1989, the U.S. government established the Agency for Health Care Policy and Research (AHCPR). AHCPR (renamed the Agency for Healthcare Research and Quality, or AHRQ, in 1999) is the federal agency that has been charged with supporting research specifically designed to improve the quality of health care, reduce health costs, and enhance patient safety, and thus plays a pivotal role in the promulgation of EBP in the United States, as well as in Canada.

Example of a nursing research breakthrough in the 1980s

A team of researchers headed by Dorothy Brooten engaged in studies that led to the development and testing of a model of site transitional care. Brooten and her colleagues (1986, 1988, 1989), for example, conducted studies of nurse specialist–managed home follow-up services for very-low-birth-weight infants who were discharged early from the hospital, and later expanded to other high-risk patients (1994). The site transitional care model, developed in anticipation of government cost-cutting measures in the 1980s, has been used as a framework for patients who are at health risk as a result of early discharge from hospitals, and has been recognized by numerous health care disciplines.

After a long crusade by nursing organizations in the United States, nursing research was strengthened and given more visibility in 1993 when NCNR was promoted to full institute status within NIH. The birth of the National Institute of Nursing Research (NINR) helped to put nursing research into the mainstream of research activities enjoyed by other health disciplines in the United States. Funding for nursing research has also grown. In 1986, the NCNR had a budget of $16.2 million, whereas in fiscal year 2004, the budget for NINR was over $130 million.

Funding opportunities for nursing research expanded in Canada as well during the 1990s. The Canadian Health Services Research Foundation (CHSRF) was established in 1997 with an endowment from federal funds, and plans for the Canadian Institutes of Health Research were underway. Beginning in 1999, the CHSRF allocated $25 million for nursing research through the establishment of a series of research chairs and related programs specific to nursing with a health services orientation.

In addition to growth in funding opportunities, the 1990s witnessed the birth of several more journals for nurse researchers, including *Qualitative Health Research*, *Clinical Nursing Research*, and *Clinical Effectiveness*. These journals emerged in response to the growth in clinically oriented and in-depth research among nurses, and interest in EBP. Another major contribution to EBP was inaugurated in 1993: the Cochrane Collaboration, an international network of institutions and individuals that maintains and updates systematic reviews of hundreds of clinical interventions to facilitate EBP.

Example of a nursing research breakthrough in the 1990s

Many studies that have been identified as breakthroughs in nursing research (Donaldson, 2000) were conducted in the 1990s. As but one example, several nurse researchers had breakthroughs in the area of psychoneuroimmunology (PNI). Barbara Swanson and Janice Zeller, for example, conducted several studies relating to HIV infection and neuropsychological function (1993, 1998) that have led to discoveries in environmental management as a means of improving immune system status.

Nursing research in the 1990s was partially guided by priorities established by prominent nurse researchers, who were brought together by NCNR for two Conferences on Research Priorities (CORP). The priorities established by the first CORP included such topics as low birth weight, HIV infection, long-term care, symptom management, and health promotion. In 1993, the second CORP established research emphases for a portion of NINR funding from 1995 through 1999 on topics such as community-based nursing models, approaches to remediating cognitive impairment, coping with chronic illness, and interventions to promote immunocompetence.

Directions for Nursing Research in the New Millennium

Nursing research continues to develop at a rapid pace and will undoubtedly flourish in the 21st century. Broadly speaking, the priority for nursing research in the future will be the promotion of excellence in nursing science. Toward this end, nurse researchers and practicing nurses will be sharpening their research skills and using those skills to address emerging issues of importance to the profession and its clientele.

Certain trends for the beginning of the 21st century are evident from developments that were taking shape at the turn of the millennium:

▸ *Heightened focus on evidence-based practice.* Efforts to translate research findings into practice are sure to continue, and nurses at all levels will be encouraged to engage in evidence-based patient care. In turn, improvements will be needed both in the quality of nursing studies and in nurses' skills in understanding, critiquing, and utilizing study results.

▸ *Stronger knowledge base through multiple confirmatory strategies.* Practicing nurses cannot be expected to change a procedure or adopt an innovation on the basis of a single, isolated study. Confirmation is usually needed through the deliberate **replication**, that is, the repeating of studies with different clients, in different clinical settings, and at different times to ensure that findings are robust.

▸ *Greater stress on integrative reviews.* **Integrative reviews** of nursing knowledge, which are considered a cornerstone of EBP, will take on increased importance. The emphasis in an integrative review is on amassing comprehensive research information on the topic, weighing pieces of evidence, and integrating information to draw conclusions about the state of knowledge.

▸ *Increased emphasis on multidisciplinary collaboration.* Interdisciplinary collaboration of nurses with researchers in related fields (as well as intradisciplinary collaboration among nurse researchers) is likely to continue to expand in the 21st century as researchers address fundamental problems at the biobehavioral and psychobiologic interface. In turn, such collaborative efforts could lead to nurse researchers playing a more prominent role in national and international health care policies.

▸ *Expanded dissemination of research findings.* The Internet and other modes of electronic communication have a big impact on the dissemination of research information, which in turn may help to promote EBP. Through online publishing (e.g., the *Online Journal of Knowledge Synthesis for Nursing* and the *Online Journal of Clinical Innovation*); online resources such as Lippincott's NursingCenter.com; electronic document retrieval and delivery; e-mail; and electronic mailing lists, information about innovations can be communicated more widely and more quickly than ever before.

▸ *Increased interest in outcomes research.* **Outcomes research** is designed to assess and document the effectiveness of health care services. The growing number of studies that can be characterized as outcomes research has been stimulated by the need for cost-effective care that achieves positive outcomes without compromising quality. Nurses are increasingly engaging in outcomes research that is focused both on patients and on the overall delivery system.

▸ *Emphasis on the visibility of nursing research.* Efforts to increase the visibility of nursing research will likely expand, with the onus falling on the shoulders of nurse researchers themselves. Most people are unaware that nurses are scholars and researchers. Nurse researchers must market themselves and their research to professional organizations, consumer organizations, and the corporate world to increase support for their research. As Baldwin and Nail (2000) have noted, nurse researchers are one of the best-qualified groups to meet the need in today's world for clinical outcomes research, but they are not recognized for their expertise.

In terms of substantive areas, research priorities and goals for the future are also under discussion. Groups of experts, convened by NINR in meetings held over a yearlong period, helped to formulate five research themes that are part of NINR planning for the future. In a statement issued in 2003, NINR announced that the themes are: (1) Changing lifestyle behaviors for better health; (2) Managing the effects of chronic illness to improve quality of life; (3) Identifying effective strategies to reduce health disparities; (4) Harnessing advanced technologies to serve human needs; and (5) Enhancing the end-of-life experience for patients and their families.

SOURCES OF EVIDENCE FOR NURSING PRACTICE

As a nursing student, you are being taught how to practice nursing, but it is important to recognize that learning about best-practice nursing will continue throughout your career. Some of what you have learned thus far is based on systematic research, but much of it is not. In fact, Millenson (1997) estimated that 85% of health care practice has not been scientifically validated. Clinical nursing practice relies on a collage of information sources that vary in dependability and validity. Increasingly there are discussions of evidence hierarchies that acknowledge that certain types of evidence and knowledge are superior to others. A brief discussion of some alternative sources of evidence shows how research-based information is different.

Tradition and Authority

Within Western culture and within the nursing profession, certain beliefs are accepted as truths—and certain practices are accepted as effective—simply based on custom. However, tradition may undermine effective problem solving. That is, traditions may be so entrenched that their validity or usefulness is not questioned or evaluated. There is growing concern that many nursing interventions are based on tradition, customs, and "unit culture" rather than on sound evidence.

Another common source of knowledge is an authority, a person with specialized expertise and recognition for that expertise. Reliance on nursing authorities (such as nursing faculty) is to some degree unavoidable; however, like tradition, authorities as a source of information have limitations. Authorities are not infallible (particularly if their expertise is based primarily on personal experience), yet their knowledge often goes unchallenged.

Clinical Experience and Intuition

Our own clinical experience is a familiar and functional source of knowledge. The ability to recognize regularities, to generalize, and to make predictions based on observations is a hallmark of the human mind. Nevertheless, personal experience has limitations as a source of evidence for practice because each person's experience is too narrow to be useful in general terms, and personal experiences are often colored by biases.

Nurses sometimes rely on "intuition" in their practice. Intuition is a type of knowledge that cannot be explained on the basis of reasoning or prior instruction. Although intuition and hunches undoubtedly play a role in nursing practice—as they do in the conduct of research—it is inappropriate to use intuition as a source of evidence in developing policies and practices for nurses.

Trial and Error

Sometimes we tackle problems by successively trying out alternative solutions. This approach may in some cases be practical, but it is often fallible and inefficient. The method tends to be haphazard, and the solutions are, in many instances, idiosyncratic.

Assembled Information

In making clinical decisions, health care professionals use information that has been assembled for various purposes. For example, local, national, and international *bench-marking data* provide information on such issues as the rates of using various procedures (e.g., rates of cesarean deliveries) or rates of infection (e.g., nosocomial pneumonia rates), and can help in evaluating clinical practices. *Quality improvement and risk data,* such as medication error reports, can be used to assess practices and determine the need for practice changes. Such sources, while offering information that can be used in practice, provide no mechanism for determining whether improvements in patient outcomes result from their use.

Disciplined Research

Research conducted within a disciplined format is the most sophisticated method of acquiring evidence that humans have developed. Nursing research combines aspects of logical reasoning with other features to create systems of problem solving that, although fallible, tend to be more reliable than other methods of acquiring knowledge.

The current emphasis on evidence-based health care requires nurses to base their clinical practice to the extent possible on research-based findings rather than on tradition, intuition, or personal experience—although nursing will always remain a rich blend of art and science.

PARADIGMS AND METHODS FOR NURSING RESEARCH

A **paradigm** is a world view, a general perspective on the complexities of reality. Disciplined inquiry in the field of nursing is being conducted mainly (although not exclusively, as we discuss in Chapter 10) within two broad paradigms, both of which have legitimacy for nursing research. This section describes the two paradigms and broadly outlines the research methods associated with them.

The Positivist/Postpositivism Paradigm

A paradigm that dominated thinking about disciplined inquiry for decades is known as *positivism*. Positivism is rooted in 19th-century thought, guided by such philosophers as Comte, Newton, and Locke. Positivism is a reflection of a broader cultural phenomenon (*modernism*) that emphasizes the rational and scientific.

TABLE 1.2	Major Assumptions of the Positivist and Naturalistic Paradigms	
TYPE OF ASSUMPTION	**POSITIVIST PARADIGM**	**NATURALISTIC PARADIGM**
The nature of reality	Reality exists; there is a real world driven by real natural causes	Reality is multiple, subjective, and mentally constructed by individuals
The relationship between the researcher and those being studied	The researcher is independent from those being researched	The researcher interacts with those being researched and findings are the creation of the interaction
The role of values in the inquiry	Values are to be held in check; objectivity is sought	Subjectivity and values are inevitable and desirable
Best methods for obtaining evidence/ knowledge	▶ Seeks generalizations ▶ Emphasis on discrete concepts ▶ Fixed design ▶ Focus on the objective and quantifiable ▶ Measured, quantitative information; statistical analysis ▶ Control over context; decontextualized ▶ Outsider knowledge—researcher as external ▶ Verification of researcher's hunches ▶ Focus on the product	▶ Seeks patterns ▶ Emphasis on the whole ▶ Flexible design ▶ Focus on the subjective and nonquantifiable ▶ Narrative information; qualitative analysis ▶ Context-bound; contextualized ▶ Insider knowledge—researcher as internal ▶ Emerging interpretations grounded in participants' experiences ▶ Focus on product and process

As shown in Table 1-2, a fundamental assumption of positivists is that there is a reality *out there* that can be studied and known. Adherents of the positivist approach assume that nature is basically ordered and regular and that an objective reality exists independent of human observation, awaiting discovery. In other words, the world is assumed not to be merely a creation of the human mind. The related assumption of **determinism** refers to the positivists' belief that *phenomena* (observable facts and events) are not haphazard or random, but rather have antecedent causes. If a person develops lung cancer, the scientist in a positivist tradition assumes that there must be one or more reasons that can be potentially identified. Within the **positivist paradigm**, much research activity is directed at understanding the underlying causes of natural phenomena.

Because of their belief in an objective reality, positivists seek to be **objective** in their pursuit of knowledge. Their approach calls for orderly, disciplined procedures with tight controls over the research situation to test researchers' hunches about the nature of the phenomena being studied and relationships among them.

Strict positivist thinking has been challenged and undermined, and few researchers adhere to the tenets of pure positivism. In the **postpositivist paradigm**, there is still a belief in reality and a desire to understand it, but postpositivists recognize the impossibility of total objectivity. They do, however, see objectivity as a goal and strive to be as neutral as possible. Postpositivists also appreciate the impediments to knowing reality with certainty and therefore seek *probabalistic* evidence—i.e., of learning what the true state of a phenomenon *probably* is, with a high and ascertainable degree of likelihood. This modified positivist position remains a dominant force in scientific research. For the sake of simplicity, we refer to it as positivism.

The Naturalistic Paradigm

The **naturalistic paradigm** (also referred to as the *constructivist paradigm*) began as a counter-movement to positivism with writers such as Weber and Kant. The naturalistic paradigm represents a major alternative system for conducting disciplined inquiry. Table 1-2 compares four major assumptions of the positivist and naturalistic paradigms.

For the naturalistic inquirer, reality is not a fixed entity but rather a construction of the individuals participating in the research; reality exists within a context, and many constructions are possible. Naturalists thus take the position of relativism: If there are always multiple interpretations of reality that exist in people's minds, then there is no process by which the ultimate truth or falsity of the constructions can be determined.

The naturalistic paradigm assumes that knowledge is maximized when the distance between the inquirer and the participants in the study is minimized. The voices and interpretations of those under study are key to understanding the phenomenon of interest, and subjective interactions are the primary way to access them. The findings from a naturalistic inquiry are the product of the interaction between the inquirer and the participants.

Paradigms and Methods: Quantitative and Qualitative Research

Broadly speaking, **research methods** are the techniques researchers use to structure a study and to gather and analyze information relevant to a research question. The two alternative paradigms have strong implications for the research methods to be used to develop evidence. The methodologic distinction typically focuses on differences between **quantitative research**, which is most closely allied with the positivist tradition, and **qualitative research**, which is most often associated with naturalistic inquiry—although positivists sometimes undertake qualitative studies, and naturalistic researchers sometimes collect quantitative information. It is important to recognize that the use of different approaches does not exclusively reflect philosophical disagreements about the nature of reality—different approaches are used to answer different types of questions about that reality, as we discuss later in this chapter.

THE SCIENTIFIC METHOD AND QUANTITATIVE RESEARCH

The traditional, positivist **scientific method** is a general set of orderly, disciplined procedures used to acquire information. Quantitative researchers typically move in a systematic fashion from the definition of a problem and the selection of concepts on which to focus, to the solution of the problem. By *systematic* we mean that the investigator progresses logically through a series of steps, according to a prespecified plan of action. The researcher uses, to the extent possible, mechanisms designed to control the study, which involves imposing conditions on the research situation so that biases are minimized and precision and validity are maximized.

Quantitative researchers gather **empirical evidence**—evidence that is rooted in objective reality and gathered directly or indirectly through the senses rather than through personal beliefs or hunches. Evidence for a study in the positivist paradigm is gathered systematically, using formal instruments to collect needed information. Usually (but not always) the information gathered is quantitative, that is, numeric information that results from formal measurement and that is analyzed with statistical procedures. Scientists strive to go beyond the specifics of a research situation; the degree to which research findings can be generalized is a widely used criterion for assessing the quality and importance of quantitative studies.

The traditional scientific method used by quantitative researchers has enjoyed considerable stature as a method of inquiry, and it has been used productively by nurse researchers studying a wide range of nursing problems. This is not to say, however, that this approach can solve all nursing problems. One important limitation—common to both quantitative and qualitative research—is that research methods cannot be used to address moral or ethical questions. Many persistent and intriguing questions fall into this area (e.g., Should euthanasia be practiced? Should abortion be legal?). Given the many moral issues that are linked to health care, it is inevitable that the nursing process will never rely exclusively on scientific information.

The scientific method also must contend with *problems of measurement*. In studying a phenomenon, a scientist attempts to measure it, that is, to attach numeric values that express quantity. For example, if the phenomenon of interest were patient morale, a researcher may want to know if a patient's morale is high or low, or higher under certain conditions than under others. Although physiologic phenomena such as blood pressure and cardiac activity can be measured with considerable accuracy and precision, the same cannot be said of psychological phenomena, such as hope or self-esteem.

A final issue is that nursing research tends to focus on human beings, who are inherently complex and diverse. Within any given study, the scientific method typically focuses on a relatively small portion of the human experience (e.g., weight gain, depression, chemical dependency). Complexities tend to be controlled and, insofar as possible, eliminated in scientific studies rather than studied directly. Sometimes this narrow focus obscures insights. Finally and relatedly, quantitative research conducted in the positivist paradigm has sometimes been accused of a narrowness and inflexibility of vision, a problem that has been called a *sedimented view* of the world that does not fully capture the reality of experiences.

NATURALISTIC METHODS AND QUALITATIVE RESEARCH

Naturalistic methods of inquiry deal with the issue of human complexity by exploring it directly. Researchers in the naturalistic tradition stress the inherent depth of humans, the ability of humans to shape and create their own experiences, and the idea that truth is a composite of realities. Consequently, naturalistic investigations emphasize *understanding* the human experience as it is lived, usually through the collection and analysis of qualitative materials that are narrative and subjective.

Researchers who reject the traditional scientific method believe that a major limitation of the classical model is that it is *reductionist*—that is, that it reduces human experience to the few concepts under investigation, and those concepts are defined in advance by the researcher rather than emerging from the experience of those under study. Naturalistic researchers tend to focus on the dynamic, holistic, and individual aspects of phenomena and attempt to capture those aspects in their entirety, within the context of those who are experiencing them.

Flexible, evolving procedures are used to capitalize on findings that emerge in the course of the study. Naturalistic inquiry always takes place in naturalistic settings, frequently over an extended period of time. The collection of information and its analysis typically progress concurrently. As the researcher sifts through the existing information and gains insight, new questions emerge, calling for additional evidence to amplify or confirm the insights. Through an inductive process, the researcher integrates the evidence to develop a theory or framework that helps explain the processes under observation.

Naturalistic studies yield rich, in-depth information that can potentially clarify the multiple dimensions of a complicated phenomenon (e.g., the process by which cancer patients cope with their illness). The findings from in-depth qualitative research are typically grounded in the real-life experiences of people with first-hand knowledge of a phenomenon. However, the approach has several limitations. Human beings are the direct instruments through which qualitative information is gathered, and humans are intelligent and sensitive—but fallible—tools. The highly personal approach that enriches the analytic insights of skillful researchers can sometimes result in petty and trivial "findings" among less competent ones.

Another potential limitation involves the subjective nature of the inquiry, which can raise questions about the idiosyncratic nature of the conclusions. Would two naturalistic researchers studying the same phenomenon in the same setting arrive at the same results? Moreover, most naturalistic studies involve a relatively small group of participants. Thus, the generalizability of findings from naturalistic inquiries can sometimes be challenged.

CONSUMER TIP

Researchers usually do not discuss the underlying paradigm of their studies in their reports. Qualitative researchers are more likely to explicitly mention the naturalistic paradigm (or to say they have undertaken a naturalistic inquiry) than are quantitative researchers to mention positivism. ▬

Multiple Paradigms and Nursing Research

Paradigms are lenses that help us to sharpen our focus on a phenomenon of interest; they are not blinders that limit our intellectual curiosity. The emergence of alternative paradigms for studying nursing problems is, in our view, a healthy and desirable trend in the pursuit of new evidence for practice. Nursing knowledge would be meager, indeed, without a rich array of approaches and methods available within the two paradigms—methods that are often complementary in their strengths and limitations.

We have emphasized the differences between the positivist and naturalistic paradigms and their associated methods so that their distinctions would be easy to understand. Despite their differences, however, the alternative paradigms have many features in common. A few are mentioned below:

- *Ultimate goals*. The ultimate aim of disciplined inquiry, regardless of the paradigm, is to gain understanding. Both quantitative and qualitative researchers seek the truth about an aspect of the world in which they are interested, and both can make significant—and mutually beneficial—contributions. Moreover, qualitative studies often serve as a crucial starting point for more controlled quantitative studies.
- *External evidence*. Although the word *empiricism* has come to be allied with the classic scientific method, researchers in both traditions gather and analyze external evidence empirically, that is, through their senses. Neither qualitative nor quantitative researchers are "armchair" analysts, relying on their own beliefs and world views to generate their evidence.
- *Reliance on human cooperation*. Because evidence for nursing research comes primarily from humans, the need for human cooperation is essential. To understand people's characteristics and experiences, researchers must persuade them to participate in the investigation *and* to act

and speak candidly. The need for candor and cooperation can be a challenging requirement—for researchers in either tradition.

▸ *Ethical constraints.* Research with human beings is guided by ethical principles that sometimes interfere with the researcher's ultimate goal. For example, if a researcher's aim is to test a potentially beneficial intervention, is it ethical to withhold the treatment from some people to see what happens? As discussed in Chapter 5, ethical dilemmas often confront researchers, regardless of paradigms or methods.

▸ *Fallibility of disciplined research.* Virtually all studies—in either paradigm—have limitations. Every research question can be addressed in many different ways, and inevitably there are tradeoffs. Financial constraints are often an issue, but limitations may exist even when resources are abundant. This does not mean that small, simple studies intrinsically have no value. It means that no single study can ever definitively answer a research question. Completed studies add to a body of accumulated evidence. If several researchers pose the same question and if each obtains the same or similar results, increased confidence can be placed in the answer to the question. The fallibility of any single study makes it important for you as a consumer of research to understand and critique the researchers' decisions when evaluating the quality of their evidence.

Thus, despite philosophical and methodologic differences, researchers using the traditional scientific method or naturalistic methods share overall goals and face many similar constraints and challenges. The selection of an appropriate method depends to some degree on the researcher's personal taste and philosophy but largely on the nature of the research question. If a researcher asks, "What are the effects of surgery on circadian rhythms (biologic cycles)?" the researcher needs to express the effects through the careful quantitative measurement of various bodily processes subject to rhythmic variation. On the other hand, if a researcher asks, "What is the process by which parents learn to cope with the death of a child?" the researcher would be hard pressed to quantify the process. Researchers' personal world views help to shape the types of question they ask.

In reading about the alternative paradigms for nursing research, you were probably more attracted to one of the two paradigms—the paradigm that corresponds most closely to your view of the world and of reality. However, learning about and respecting both approaches to disciplined inquiry and recognizing the strengths and limitations of each are important. In this textbook, we provide an overview of the methods associated with both qualitative and quantitative research and offer guidance on how to understand, critique, and use findings from both.

HOW-TO-TELL TIP

How can you tell if a study is qualitative or quantitative? As you progress through this book, you should be able to identify most studies as qualitative versus quantitative based simply on the title, or based on terms appearing in the abstract at the beginning of the report. At this point, though, it may be easiest to distinguish the two types of studies based on how many numbers appear in the report, especially in tables. Qualitative studies may have no tables with quantitative information, or only a single table with numbers describing participants' characteristics (e.g., the percentage who were male or female). Quantitative studies typically have several tables with numbers and statistical information. Qualitative studies, by contrast, may have "word tables" or diagrams and figures illustrating processes inferred from the narrative information gathered.

PURPOSES OF NURSING RESEARCH

The general purpose of nursing research is to answer questions or solve problems of relevance to the nursing profession. Sometimes a distinction is made between basic and applied nursing research. As traditionally defined, *basic research* is undertaken to extend the base of knowledge in a discipline, or to formulate or refine a theory. For example, a researcher may do a study to better understand normal grieving processes, without having *explicit* nursing applications in mind. *Applied research* focuses on finding solutions to existing problems. For example, a study to determine the effectiveness of a nursing intervention to ease grieving would be applied research. Basic research is appropriate for discovering general principles of human behavior and biophysiology; applied research is designed to show how these principles can be used to solve problems in nursing practice. In nursing, the findings from applied research may pose questions for basic research, and the results of basic research often suggest clinical applications.

CONSUMER TIP

Researchers rarely specify whether their intent is to address a pragmatic problem or to generate basic knowledge. The study's intent generally has to be inferred and, in some cases, may be ambiguous. ▬

The specific purposes of nursing research include identification, description, exploration, explanation, prediction, and control. Within each purpose, various types of question are addressed by nurse researchers; certain questions are more amenable to qualitative than to quantitative inquiry and vice versa.

Identification and Description

Many qualitative studies focus on phenomena about which little is known. In some cases, so little is known that the phenomenon has yet to be clearly identified or named—or it has been inadequately defined or conceptualized. The in-depth, probing nature of qualitative research is well suited to the task of answering such questions as "What is this phenomenon?" and "What is its name?" (Table 1-3). In quantitative research, by contrast, the researcher begins with a phenomenon that has been studied or defined previously, sometimes in a qualitative study. Thus, in quantitative research, identification typically precedes the inquiry.

Qualitative example of identification

Dewar (2003) conducted an in-depth study in Canada to determine how individuals were able to live with catastrophic illnesses and injuries. She called one of the strategies they used *boosting*—people's efforts to improve their self-esteem, which helped them endure their circumstances.

| | TYPES OF QUESTIONS: | TYPES OF QUESTIONS: |
PURPOSE	QUANTITATIVE RESEARCH	QUALITATIVE RESEARCH
Identification		What is this phenomenon? What is its name?
Description	How prevalent is the phenomenon? How often does the phenomenon occur? What are the characteristics of the phenomenon?	What are the dimensions of the phenomenon? What variations exist? What is important about the phenomenon?
Exploration	What factors are related to the phenomenon? What are the antecedents of the phenomenon?	What is the full nature of the phenomenon? What is really going on here? What is the process by which the phenomenon evolves or is experienced?
Explanation	What are the measurable associations between phenomena? What factors cause the phenomenon? Does the theory explain the phenomenon?	How does the phenomenon work? Why does the phenomenon exist? What is the meaning of the phenomenon? How did the phenomenon occur?
Prediction and control	What will happen if we alter a phenomenon or introduce an intervention? If phenomenon X occurs, will phenomenon Y follow? How can we make the phenomenon happen, or alter its nature or prevalence? Can the occurrence of the phenomenon be controlled?	

TABLE 1.3 Research Purposes and Research Questions

Description of phenomena is another important purpose of research. In a descriptive study, researchers observe, count, delineate, elucidate, and classify. Nurse researchers have described a wide variety of phenomena. Examples include patients' stress and coping, adaptation processes, health beliefs, and time patterns of temperature readings.

Description can be a major purpose for both qualitative and quantitative researchers. Quantitative description focuses on the prevalence, incidence, size, and measurable attributes of a phenomenon. Qualitative researchers, on the other hand, use in-depth methods to describe the dimensions, variations, and importance of phenomena. Table 1-3 compares descriptive questions posed by quantitative and qualitative researchers.

Quantitative example of description

Lierh, Mehl, Summers, and Pennebaker (2004) performed a study to describe some of the experiences and physiologic changes that people went through in the midst of stressful upheaval on September 11, 2001.

Qualitative example of description

Zakrzewski and Hector (2004) undertook an in-depth study to describe the experience of alcohol addiction among male members of Alcoholics Anonymous.

Exploration

Like descriptive research, exploratory research begins with some phenomenon of interest; however, rather than simply observing and describing it, exploratory research investigates the full nature of the phenomenon and other factors to which it is related. For example, a descriptive quantitative study of patients' preoperative stress might seek to document the degree of stress patients experience before surgery and the percentage of patients who actually experience it. An exploratory study might ask the following: What factors are related to a patient's stress level? Is a patient's stress related to behaviors of the nursing staff? Does a patient's behavior change in relation to the level of stress experienced?

Exploratory studies are undertaken when a new area or topic is being investigated, and qualitative methods are especially useful for exploring a little-understood phenomenon. Exploratory qualitative research is designed to shed light on the various ways in which a phenomenon is manifested and on underlying processes.

Quantitative example of exploration

Reynolds and Neidig (2002) studied the incidence and severity of nausea accompanying combinative antiretroviral therapies among HIV-infected patients, and explored patterns of nausea in relation to patient characteristics.

Qualitative example of exploration

Through interviews with and observations of eight critical care nurses, Currey, Botti, and Browne (2003) explored the variability of critical care nurses' hemodynamic decision-making in the 2-hour period after cardiac surgery.

Explanation

The goals of explanatory research are to understand the underpinnings of specific natural phenomena and to explain systematic relationships among phenomena. Explanatory research is often linked to a *theory*, which represents a method of deriving, organizing, and integrating ideas about the manner in which phenomena are manifested or interrelated. Whereas descriptive research provides new information and exploratory research provides promising insights, explanatory research focuses on understanding the causes or full nature of a phenomenon.

In quantitative research, theories or prior findings are used deductively as the basis for generating explanations that are then tested empirically. That is, based on existing theory or a body of evidence, researchers make specific predictions that, if upheld by the findings, lend credibility to the explanation. In qualitative studies, researchers may search for explanations about how or why a phenomenon exists or what a phenomenon means as a basis for developing a theory that is grounded in rich, in-depth, experiential evidence.

Quantitative example of explanation

McGinley (2004) undertook a study designed to explain women's use of hormone replacement therapy on the basis of their health beliefs and views about menopause.

Qualitative example of explanation

Kidner and Flanders-Stepans (2004) undertook a study designed to develop an explanatory model of the experience of mothers whose pregnancies were complicated with HELLP syndrome (hemolysis, elevated liver enzyme, and low platelets).

Prediction and Control

Many research problems defy absolute comprehension and explanation. Yet, it is possible to predict and control phenomena based on research findings, even without complete understanding. For example, research has shown that the incidence of Down syndrome in infants increases with the age of the mother. Therefore, we can predict that a woman aged 40 years is at higher risk of bearing a child with Down syndrome than a woman aged 25 years. The incidence of Down syndrome may be partially controlled by educating women about the risks and offering amniocentesis to women older than 35 years of age. Note, however, that the ability to predict and control in this example does not depend on an explanation of *why* older women are at a higher risk for having an abnormal child. There are many examples of nursing and health-related studies—typically, quantitative ones—in which prediction and control are key objectives. For example, studies designed to test health-care effectiveness are typically concerned with controlling patient outcomes or the costs of care.

Quantitative example of prediction

The main purpose of a study by Lambert, Lambert, and Ito (2004) was to identify the workplace stressors and demographic characteristics that were the best predictors of physical and mental health of Japanese hospital nurses.

CONSUMER TIP

It is the researcher's responsibility to explain the purpose of the study, and this usually happens fairly early in a research report. Most nursing studies have multiple aims. Almost all studies have some descriptive intent. Some exploratory studies are undertaken with the expectation that the results will serve a predictive or control function. Truly explanatory studies are the least common in nursing literature.

ASSISTANCE TO CONSUMERS OF NURSING RESEARCH

This book is designed to help you develop skills that will allow you to read, evaluate, and use nursing studies (i.e., to become intelligent consumers and users of nursing research). In each chapter of this book, we present information relating to the methods used by nurse researchers and provide specific guidance to consumers in several ways. First, interspersed throughout the chapters, we offer tips on what you can expect to find in actual research reports with regard to the content in the chapter. These include special "how-to-tell" tips that help you find concepts discussed in this book in research reports. These tips are identified with this icon: 📖. Second, we include guidelines for critiquing those aspects of a study covered in each chapter. The questions in Box 1-1 are designed to assist you in using the information in this chapter in an overall preliminary assessment of a research report.

And third, we offer opportunities to apply your newly acquired skills. The critical activities at the end of each chapter guide you through appraisals of real research examples of both qualitative and quantitative studies (some of which are presented in their entirety in the

---

BOX 1.1   Questions for a Preliminary Overview of a Research Report

1. How relevant is the research problem to the actual practice of nursing? Does the study focus on a topic that is considered a priority area for nursing research?
2. Is the research quantitative or qualitative?
3. What is the underlying purpose (or purposes) of the study—identification, description, exploration, explanation, or prediction and control?
4. What might be some clinical implications of this research? To what type of people and settings is the research most relevant? If the findings are accurate, how might the results of this study be used by *me*?

appendices to this book or to the accompanying *Study Guide*, or in the Research Articles section of the Student Resource CD-ROM). These activities also challenge you to think about how the findings from these studies could be used in nursing practice. A discussion of these critical thinking activities with suggested answers to the questions can be found on the Student Resource CD-ROM.

CONSUMER TIP

Tip: The following websites are useful starting points for further information about nursing research and EBP:
- *National Institutes of Health's National Institute of Nursing Research: http://ninr.nih.gov/ninr*
- *Agency for Healthcare Research and Quality: www.ahrq.gov*
- *Sigma Theta Tau International: www.nursingsociety.org*
- *Cochrane Collaboration: www.cochrane.org*
- *Lippincott's Nursing Center: www.nursingcenter.com*

CHAPTER REVIEW

Key new terms introduced in the chapter, together with a summary of major points, are presented in this section. In addition, Chapter 1 of the *Study Guide to Accompany Essentials of Nursing Research,* 6th edition offers various exercises and study suggestions for reinforcing the concepts presented in this chapter. For additional review, see the Student Self-Study Review Questions section of the Student Resource CD-ROM provided with this book.

KEY NEW TERMS

Determinism
Empirical evidence
Evidence-based practice (EBP)
Evidence hierarchy
Integrative review
Journal club
National Institute of Nursing Research
Naturalistic paradigm
Nursing research
Outcomes research

Paradigm
Positivist paradigm
Postpositivist paradigm
Qualitative research
Quantitative research
Replication
Research
Research methods
Research utilization
Scientific method

SUMMARY POINTS

- **Nursing research** is systematic inquiry to develop knowledge about issues of importance to nurses and serves to establish a scientific base of knowledge for nursing practice.
- Nurses in various settings are adopting an **evidence-based practice (EBP)** that incorporates research findings into their decisions and their interactions with clients.
- Knowledge of nursing research enhances the professional practice of all nurses, including both consumers of research (who read, evaluate, and use studies) and producers of research (who design and undertake studies).

▷ Nursing research began with Florence Nightingale but developed slowly until its rapid acceleration in the 1950s. Since the 1970s, nursing research has focused on problems relating to clinical practice.

▷ The **National Institute of Nursing Research** (NINR), established at the U.S. National Institutes of Health in 1993, affirms the stature of nursing research.

▷ Future emphases of nursing research are likely to include EBP and research utilization projects, **replications** of research, **integrative reviews**, multidisciplinary studies, expanded dissemination efforts, and **outcomes research**.

▷ Disciplined research is widely considered superior to other sources of evidence for nursing practice, such as tradition, authority, clinical experience, trial and error, intuition, and assembled information (e.g., quality improvement data).

▷ Disciplined inquiry in nursing is conducted mainly within two broad **paradigms**, or world views with underlying assumptions about the complexities of reality: the positivist paradigm and the naturalistic paradigm.

▷ In the **positivist paradigm**, it is assumed that there is an objective reality and that natural *phenomena* (observable facts and events) are regular and orderly. The related assumption of **determinism** refers to the belief that events are not haphazard but rather the result of prior causes. Pure positivism has been replaced with a *postpositivist* perspective that acknowledges the difficulty of objective observation and the inability to know reality with certainty.

▷ In the **naturalistic paradigm**, it is assumed that reality is not a fixed entity but is rather a construction of human minds, and thus "truth" is a composite of multiple constructions of reality.

▷ The positivist paradigm is associated with **quantitative research**—the collection and analysis of numeric information. Quantitative research is typically conducted within the traditional **scientific method**, which is a systematic and controlled process. Quantitative researchers base their findings on **empirical evidence** (evidence collected by way of the human senses) and strive for generalizability of their findings beyond a single setting or situation.

▷ Researchers within the naturalistic paradigm emphasize understanding the human experience as it is lived through the collection and analysis of subjective, narrative materials using flexible procedures that evolve in the field; this paradigm is associated with **qualitative research**.

▷ Nursing research can be either *basic* (designed to provide information for the sake of knowledge) or *applied* (designed to solve specific problems). Specific research purposes include identification, description, exploration, explanation, prediction, and control.

RESEARCH EXAMPLES | **Critical Thinking Activities**

 EXAMPLE 1: Quantitative Research

Aspects of a quantitative nursing study, featuring terms and concepts discussed in this chapter, are presented below, followed by some questions to guide critical thinking. (The full research report is available in *Research in Nursing & Health, 26,* 40–52).

Study

"Effects of Tellington touch in healthy adults awaiting venipuncture" (Wendler, 2003)

research examples continue on page 26

RESEARCH EXAMPLES *Continued*

Study Purpose

Wendler designed a study to test the safety and effectiveness of a nursing intervention during a routine procedure. The intervention was Tellington touch (TTouch), a form of gentle physical touch originally developed for the calming of horses.

Study Procedures

Ninety-three healthy men and women soldiers undergoing a routine physical examination were recruited for the study. Half the soldiers, at random, were put in a group that received 5 minutes of TTouch with a trained nurse prior to venipuncture, while the other half were put in a group that received a 5-minute social visit with a medic. Research staff who measured outcomes did not know which group the soldiers were in.

Patient Outcomes

The two groups were compared in terms of mean blood pressure (MBP) and heart rate (HR) duing and after the 5-minute intervention, as well as anxiety and pain before and after venipuncture.

Key Findings

▶ There were clinically significant differences between the two groups in terms of MBP and HR: Those in the TTouch group had lower MBP and HR during the intervention than those in the other group, although the groups were similar just before and after the venipuncture.
▶ There were no differences between the two groups in terms of anxiety and pain.

Conclusions

Wendler concluded that TTouch may provide a noninvasive alternative for the temporary control of MBP and HR in stressful, transient situations. She noted that further study is needed to explore the utility and safety of TTouch in acutely or critically ill persons.

Critical Thinking Suggestions*

*See the Student Resource CD-ROM for a discussion of these questions.
1. Answer the questions in Box 1-1 regarding this study.
2. Also consider the following targeted questions, which may assist you in assessing aspects of the study's merit:
   a. Why do you think Wendler decided to have a group of soldiers who did not get TTouch?
   b. Why do you think Wendler had a medic talk to the second group of soldiers for 5 minutes?
   c. If you wanted to replicate this study to see if the findings could be confirmed, what might you want to change to maximize the utility of the replication? For example, what type of people would you recruit to participate?
   d. Could this study have been undertaken as a qualitative study? Why or why not?

RESEARCH EXAMPLES *Continued*

 EXAMPLE 2: Qualitative Research

Aspects of a qualitative nursing study, featuring key terms and concepts discussed in this chapter, are presented below, followed by some questions to guide critical thinking. (The full research report is available in *Qualitative Health Research, 11,* 221–237.)

Study

"Moving them on and in: The process of searching for and selecting an aged care facility" (Cheek & Ballantyne, 2001)

Study Purpose

Cheek and Ballantyne did a study to describe the search and selection process for an aged care facility following discharge of a family member from acute hospital settings in Australia, and to explore the effects the process had on the individuals and their families.

Study Procedures

Twelve elders who were recently admitted to an aged care facility and 20 family members participated in the study. Face-to-face in-depth interviews were conducted with residents in the aged care facilities and with family members in their homes. They were all asked to talk about their personal experiences of the search and selection process and its effect on their well-being. These interviews were audiotaped and then transcribed.

Key Findings

The transcripts of these interviews were read by at least two members of the research team, who individually identified themes from each interview. Five themes were identified; for example:

▶ One theme was labeled "Dealing with the system—cutting through the maze," which involved the perception of being in the middle of a war zone. This sense of battle was related to confusion, lack of control, and the feeling of being at the system's mercy.

▶ A second major theme was labeled "Urgency—moving them on and in." Family members felt a sense of urgency in finding a suitable facility to have the elder transferred to. Sponsors felt pressured to make on-the-spot decisions to accept or reject a place in a facility once it had become available.

Conclusions

The researchers concluded that the decision to institutionalize a family member is a stressful experience and should be viewed as a family crisis.

Critical Thinking Suggestions

1. Answer the questions in Box 1-1 regarding this study.

research examples continue on page 28

RESEARCH EXAMPLES *Continued*

2. Also consider the following targeted questions, which may assist you in assessing aspects of the study's merit:
   a. Why do you think Cheek and Ballantyne collected data from elders *and* their family members?
   b. Why do you think the researchers audiotaped and transcribed their in-depth interviews with study participants?
   c. Do you think it would have been appropriate for the researchers to conduct this study using quantitative research methods? Why or why not?

 EXAMPLE 3: Quantitative Research

1. Read the abstract and the introduction from Motzer et al.'s study ("Sense of Coherence") in Appendix A of this book, and then answer the questions in Box 1-1.
2. Also consider the following targeted questions, which may further sharpen your critical thinking skills and assist you in assessing aspects of the study's merit:
   a. What gap in the existing research was the study designed to fill?
   b. Would you describe this study as applied or basic, based on information in the abstract?
   c. Could this study have been undertaken as a qualitative study? Why or why not?

 EXAMPLE 4: Qualitative Research

1. Read the abstract and the introduction from Beck's (2004) study ("Birth Trauma") in Appendix B of this book, and then answer the questions in Box 1-1.
2. Also consider the following targeted questions, which may further sharpen your critical thinking skills and assist you in assessing aspects of the study's merit:
   a. What gap in the existing research was the study designed to fill?
   b. Was Beck's study conducted within the positivist paradigm or the naturalistic paradigm? Provide a rationale for your choice.

SUGGESTED READINGS

Methodologic and Theoretical References

Baldwin, K. M., & Nail, L. M. (2000). Opportunities and challenges in clinical nursing research. *Journal of Nursing Scholarship, 32*, 163–166.

Donaldson, S. K. (2000). Breakthroughs in scientific research: The discipline of nursing, 1960–1999. *Annual Review of Nursing Research, 18*, 247–311.

Guba, E. G. (Ed.). (1990). *The paradigm dialog.* Newbury Park, CA: Sage Publications.

Lincoln, Y. S., & Guba, E. G. (1985). *Naturalistic inquiry.* Beverly Hills: Sage Publications.

Millenson, M. L. (1997). *Demanding medical evidence.* Chicago: University of Chicago Press.

Nightingale, F. (1859). *Notes on nursing: What it is and what it is not.* Philadelphia: J.B. Lippincott.

Stetler, C. B., & Marram, G. (1976). Evaluating research findings for applicability in practice. *Nursing Outlook, 24,* 559–563.

Studies Cited in Chapter 1

Anderson, G. C., Moore, E., Hepworth, J., & Bergman, N. (2003). Early skin-to-skin contact for mothers and their healthy newborn infants. *Cochrane Database Systematic Reviews*, (2), CD003519.

Barnard, K. E. (1973). The effects of stimulation on the sleep behavior of the premature infant. In M. Batey (Ed.), *Communicating nursing research* (vol. 6, pp. 12–33). Boulder, CO: WICHE.

Barnard, K. E. (1976). The state of the art: Nursing and early intervention with handicapped infants. In T. Tjossem (Ed.), *Proceedings of the 1974 President's Committee on Mental Retardation*. Baltimore, MD: University Park Press.

Barnard, K. E., & Collar, B. S. (1973). Early diagnosis, interpretation, and intervention. *Annals of the New York Academy of Sciences, 205,* 373–382.

Barnard, K. E., Wenner, W., Weber, B., Gray, C., & Peterson, A. (1977). Premature infant refocus. In P. Miller (Ed.), *Research to practice in mental retardation: Vol. 3, Biomedical aspects*. Baltimore, MD: University Park Press.

Barroso, J. E., Carlson, J. R., & Meynell, J. (2003). Physiological and psychological markers associated with HIV-related fatigue. *Clinical Nursing Research, 12,* 49–68.

Brooten, D., Brown, L. P., Munro, B. H., York, R., Cohen, S., Roncoli, M., et al. (1988). Early discharge and specialist transitional care. *Image: Journal of Nursing Scholarship, 20,* 64–68.

Brooten, D., Gennaro, S., Knapp, H., Brown, L. P., & York, R. (1989). Clinical specialist pre- and post-discharge teaching of parents of very low birthweight infants. *Journal of Obstetric, Gynecologic, & Neonatal Nursing, 18,* 316–322.

Brooten, D., Kumar, S., Brown, L. P., Butts, P., Finkler, S., Bakewell-Sachs, S., et al. (1986). A randomized clinical trial of early hospital discharge and home follow-up of very low birthweight infants. *New England Journal of Medicine, 315,* 934–939.

Brooten, D., Roncoli, M., Finkler, S., Arnold, L., Cohen, A., & Mennuti, M. (1994). A randomized clinical trial of early hospital discharge and home follow-up of women having cesarean birth. *Obstetrics and Gynecology, 84,* 832–838.

Cheek, J., & Ballantyne, A. (2001). Moving them on and in: The process of searching for and selecting an aged care facility. *Qualitative Health Research, 11,* 221–237.

Chwo, M. J., Anderson, G. C., Good, M., Dowling, D. A., Shiau, S. H., & Chu, D. M. (2002). A randomized controlled trial of early kangaroo care for preterm infants: Effects on temperature, weight, behavior, and acuity. *Journal of Nursing Research, 10,* 129–142.

Currey, J., Botti, M., & Browne, J. (2003). Hemodynamic team decision making in the cardiac surgical intensive care context. *Heart & Lung, 32,* 181–189.

Dewar, A. (2003). Boosting strategies: Enhancing the self-esteem of individuals with catastrophic illnesses and injuries. *Journal of Psychosocial Nursing & Mental Health Services, 41,* 24–32.

Engler, A. J., Ludington-Hoe, S. M., Cusson, R. M., Adams, R., Bahnsen, M., Brumbaugh, E., et al. (2002). Kangaroo care: National survey of practice, knowledge, barriers, and perceptions. *MCN: The American Journal of Maternal/Child Nursing, 27,* 146–153.

Kidner, M. C., & Flanders-Stepans, M. B. (2004). A model for the HELLP syndrome: The maternal experience. *Journal of Obstetric, Gynecologic, & Neonatal Nursing, 33,* 44–53.

Lambert, V. A., Lambert, C. E., & Ito, M. (2004). Workplace stressors, ways of coping, and demographic characteristics as predictors of physical and mental health of Japanese hospital nurses. *International Journal of Nursing Studies, 41,* 85–97.

Liehr, P., Mehl, M. R., Summers, L. C., & Pennebaker, J. W. (2004). Connecting with others in the midst of stressful upheaval on September 11, 2001. *Applied Nursing Research, 17,* 2–9.

McGinley, A. M. (2004). Health beliefs and women's use of hormone replacement therapy. *Holistic Nursing Practice, 18,* 18–25.

Quint, J. C. (1962). Delineation of qualitative aspects of nursing care. *Nursing Research, 11,* 204–206.

Quint, J. C. (1963). The impact of mastectomy. *American Journal of Nursing, 63,* 88–91.

Quint, J. C. (1967). *The nurse and the dying patient*. New York: Macmillan Co.

Reynolds, N. R., & Neidig, J. L. (2002). Characteristics of nausea reported by HIV-infected patients initiating combination antiretroviral regimens. *Clinical Nursing Research, 11,* 71–88.

Swanson, B., Cronin-Stubbs, D., Zeller, J. M., Kessler, H. A., & Bielauskas, L. A. (1993). Characterizing the neuropsychological functioning of persons with human immunodeficiency virus infection. *Archives of Psychiatric Nursing, 7,* 82–90.

Swanson, B., Zeller, J. M., & Spear, G. (1998). Cortisol upregulates HIV p24 antigen in cultured human monocyte-derived macrophages. *Journal of the Association of Nurses in AIDS Care, 9,* 78–83.

Tranmer, J. E., Minard, J., Fox, L. A., & Rebelo, L. (2003). The sleep experience of medical and surgical patients. *Clinical Nursing Research, 12,* 159–173.

Wendler, M. C. (2003). Effects of Tellington touch in healthy adults awaiting venipuncture. *Research in Nursing & Health, 26,* 40–52.

Wilkes, L. M., O'Baugh, J., Luke, S., & George, A. (2003). Positive attitudes in cancer: Patients' perspectives. *Oncology Nursing Forum, 30,* 412–416.

Zakrzewski, R. F., & Hector, M. A. (2004). The lived experiences of alcohol addiction: Men of Alcoholics Anonymous. *Issues in Mental Health Nursing, 25,* 61–77.

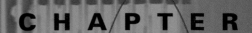

CHAPTER 2

Comprehending Key Concepts in Qualitative and Quantitative Research

STUDENT OBJECTIVES

On completing this chapter, you will be able to:

▶ Define new terms presented in the chapter
▶ Distinguish terms associated with quantitative and qualitative research
▶ Discuss some of the major challenges faced by qualitative and quantitative researchers in doing rigorous research

THE BUILDING BLOCKS OF RESEARCH

Research, like nursing or any other discipline, has its own language and terminology—its own *jargon*. Some terms are used by both qualitative and quantitative researchers, but other terms are used mainly with one or the other approach.

The Places and Faces of Research

When researchers address a problem or answer a question through disciplined research—regardless of whether it is qualitative or quantitative—they are doing a **study** (or an *investigation* or a *research project*). **Clinical studies** are specifically designed to generate knowledge to guide clinical practice. **Collaborative studies**, involving a research team with a mixture of clinical, theoretical, and methodologic skills, are increasingly common in health care research.

Example of a collaborative study

McCain and an interdisciplinary team of colleagues (2003)—including nurses, an immunologist, a pathologist, an infectious disease physician, a molecular diagnostician, and a biostatistician—underdertook a collaborative study to test the effects of two stress management interventions on a battery of psychoneuroimmunologic outcomes in persons with HIV disease.

HOW-TO-TELL TIP

How can you tell if an article appearing in a nursing journal is a *study*? In journals that specialize in research (e.g., the journal *Nursing Research*), most articles are original research reports, but in specialty journals there is usually a mix of research and nonresearch articles. Sometimes you can tell by the title, but sometimes you cannot. For example, Schaefer (2003) wrote an article entitled "Sleep disturbances linked to fibromyalgia" in *Holistic Nursing Practice*. This article discusses research findings, but it is not a study. Look at the major headings of an article, and if there is no heading called "Method" or "Methodology" (the section that describes what a researcher *did*) and no heading called "Findings" or "Results" (the section that describes what a researcher *learned*), then it is probably not an original study.

Studies with humans involve two sets of people: those who conduct the study and those who provide the information. In a quantitative study, the people being studied are called **subjects** or **study participants**, as shown in Table 2-1. (When subjects provide information by answering questions, as in an interview, they may be called **respondents**.) In a qualitative study, the individuals cooperating in the study play an active rather than a passive role and are therefore referred to as **informants**, **key informants**, or study participants. The person who conducts a study is called the **researcher** or *investigator* (or sometimes—more often in quantitative studies—the *scientist*). Studies are sometimes undertaken by a single researcher, but more often involve a research team.

Research can be undertaken in a variety of *settings* (the specific places where information is gathered), and in one or more *sites*. Some studies take place in **naturalistic settings**—in the **field**—(e.g., in people's homes); at the other extreme, some studies are done in highly

TABLE 2.1	Key Terms Used in Quantitative and Qualitative Research	
CONCEPT	**QUANTITATIVE TERM**	**QUALITATIVE TERM**
Person contributing information	Subject Study participant Respondent	Study participant Informant, key informant
Person undertaking the study	Researcher, investigator	Researcher, investigator
That which is being studied	Concepts Constructs Variables	Phenomena Concepts Constructs
Information gathered	Data (numerical values)	Data (narrative descriptions)
Links between concepts	Relationships (causal, functional)	Patterns of association
Logical reasoning processes	Deductive reasoning	Inductive reasoning
Quality of evidence	Reliability, validity, generalizability	Trustworthiness

controlled **laboratory settings**. Qualitative researchers, especially, are likely to engage in **field-work** in natural settings because they are interested in the contexts of people's lives and experiences. A site is the overall location for the research—it could be an entire community (e.g., a Haitian neighborhood in Miami) or an institution within a community (e.g., a clinic in Boston). Researchers sometimes engage in **multisite studies** because the use of multiple sites usually offers a larger or more diverse group of study participants.

Example of a multisite study in naturalistic settings

Rossen and Knafl (2003) studied older women's response to relocation from their homes to institutional congregate living facilities (CLFs). The researchers interviewed participants first in their homes prior to the move, and then about 4 months later in the CLF to which they had relocated. Women from 12 CLFs of varying sizes and characteristics were included.

Phenomena, Concepts, and Constructs

Research focuses on abstract rather than tangible phenomena. For example, the terms *pain, coping, resilience,* and *grief* are all abstractions of particular aspects of human behavior and characteristics. These abstractions are often referred to as **concepts** (or, in qualitative research, **phenomena**).

Researchers also use the term *construct*. Kerlinger and Lee (2000) distinguish concepts from constructs by noting that **constructs** are abstractions that are deliberately and systematically invented (or constructed) by researchers or theorists for a specific purpose. For example, *self-care* in Orem's model of health maintenance is a construct. The terms *construct* and *concept* may be used interchangeably although, by convention, a construct often refers to a slightly more complex abstraction than a concept.

Theories, Models, and Frameworks

A **theory** is a systematic, abstract explanation of some aspect of reality. In a theory, concepts are knitted together into a coherent system to explain some aspect of the world. Theories play a role in both qualitative and quantitative research.

In a quantitative study, researchers may start with a theory or a **conceptual model** or **framework** (the distinction is discussed in Chapter 8) and, using deductive reasoning, make predictions about how phenomena would behave *if the theory were true*. The specific predictions are then tested through research, and the results are used to reject, modify, or lend credence to the theory.

In qualitative research, theories may be used in various ways. Sometimes frameworks derived from various disciplines or qualitative research traditions (which we describe in the next chapter) offer an orienting world view with clear conceptual underpinnings. In many qualitative studies, however, theory is the *product* of the research. Information from participants is the starting point for the researcher's conceptualization that seeks to explain patterns and commonalities emerging from researcher–participant interactions. The goal is to develop a theory that explains phenomena as they exist, not as they are preconceived. Theories generated in a qualitative study are sometimes subjected to more controlled confirmation through quantitative research.

Variables

In a quantitative study, concepts are usually referred to as **variables**. A variable, as the name implies, is something that varies. Weight, anxiety level, and body temperature are all variables (i.e., each of these properties varies from one person to another). In fact, nearly all aspects of human beings and their environment are variables. For example, if everyone weighed 150 pounds, weight would not be a variable; it would be a *constant*. But it is precisely because people and conditions *do* vary that research is conducted. Most quantitative researchers seek to understand how or why things vary and to learn how differences in one variable are related to differences in another. For example, lung cancer research is concerned with the variable of lung cancer. It is a variable because not everybody has the disease. Researchers have studied what variables might be linked to lung cancer and have identified cigarette smoking. Smoking is also a variable because not everyone smokes. A variable, then, is any quality of a person, group, or situation that varies or takes on different values—typically, numeric values.

CONSUMER TIP

TIP: Every study focuses on one or more phenomena, concepts, or variables, but these terms *per se* are not necessarily used in research reports. For example, a report might say: "The purpose of this study is to examine the effect of primary nursing on patient satisfaction." Although the researcher has not explicitly labeled anything a concept, the concepts (variables) under study are *type of nursing* and *patient satisfaction*. Key concepts or variables are often indicated right in the study title. ▬

Variables are often inherent characteristics of people, such as age, blood type, or height. Sometimes, however, researchers *create* a variable. For example, if a researcher is testing the effectiveness of patient-controlled analgesia compared with intramuscular analgesia in relieving pain after surgery, some patients would be given patient-controlled analgesia and others would receive intramuscular analgesia. In the context of this study, method of pain management has become a variable because different patients are given different analgesic methods.

Sometimes a variable can take on a range of different values that can be represented on a continuum (e.g., height or weight). Other variables take on only a few values; sometimes such variables convey quantitative information (e.g., number of children) but others simply involve placing people into categories (e.g., male, female, or blood type A, B, AB, or O).

DEPENDENT VARIABLES AND INDEPENDENT VARIABLES

Many quantitative studies seek to determine the causes of phenomena. Does a nursing intervention *cause* improved patient outcomes? Does a certain procedure *cause* stress? The presumed cause is called the **independent variable**, and the presumed effect is called the **dependent variable**.

Variation in the dependent variable is presumed to *depend on* variation in the independent variable. For example, researchers investigate the extent to which lung cancer (the dependent variable) depends on or is caused by smoking (the independent variable). Or, researchers might examine the effect of tactile stimulation (the independent variable) on weight gain in premature infants (the dependent variable). The dependent variable (sometimes called the **outcome variable**) is the variable researchers want to understand, explain, or predict. In lung cancer/smoking research, it is the cancer that researchers are trying to explain and predict, not smoking.

Frequently, the terms *independent variable* and *dependent variable* are used to designate the *direction of influence* between variables rather than cause and effect. For example, suppose a researcher studied the mental health of caretakers caring for spouses with Alzheimer's disease and found better mental health outcomes for wives than for husbands. The researcher might be unwilling to take the position that the spouse's mental health was *caused* by gender. Yet the direction of influence clearly runs from gender to mental health: It makes *no* sense to suggest that mental health status influenced the spouse's gender! Although in this example the researcher does not infer a cause-and-effect connection, it is appropriate to conceptualize mental health as the dependent variable and gender as the independent variable.

Many dependent variables studied by nurse researchers have multiple causes or antecedents. If we were interested in studying influences on people's weight, for example, we might consider age, height, physical activity, and eating habits as the independent variables. Two or more *dependent* variables also may be of interest to the researcher. For example, suppose we wanted to compare the effectiveness of two methods of nursing care for children with cystic fibrosis. Several dependent variables could be designated as measures of treatment effectiveness, such as length of hospital stay, number of recurrent respiratory infections, presence of cough, and so forth. In short, it is common to design studies with multiple independent and dependent variables.

Variables are not *inherently* dependent or independent. A dependent variable in one study may be an independent variable in another study. For example, a study might examine the effect of nurses' contraceptive counseling (the independent variable) on unwanted births (the dependent variable). Another study might investigate the effect of unwanted births (the independent variable) on the incidence of child abuse (the dependent variable). The role that a variable plays in a particular study determines whether it is an independent or a dependent variable.

The distinction between dependent and independent variables is often difficult for students. Don't be discouraged—it is something that will become a lot easier with practice.

CONSUMER TIP

TIP: Few research reports *explicitly* label variables as dependent and independent, despite the importance of this distinction. Moreover, variables (especially independent variables) are sometimes not fully spelled out. Take the following research question: What is the effect of exercise on heart rate? In this example, heart rate is the dependent variable. Exercise, however, is not in itself a variable. Rather, exercise versus something else (e.g., no exercise) is a variable; "something else" is implied rather than stated in the research question. Note that if exercise were not compared to something else, such as no exercise or different amounts of exercise, then exercise would not be a variable.

Example of independent and dependent variables

Research question: Does the type of health care provider (physician versus physician-nurse team) affect hypertension in adult women? (Scisney-Matlock, Makos, Saunders, Jackson, & Steigerwalt, 2004)
Independent variable: Type of health care provider
Dependent variable: 24-hour systolic and diastolic blood pressure readings

Conceptual and Operational Definitions

Concepts in a study need to be defined and explicated, and dictionary definitions are almost never adequate. Two types of definitions are of particular relevance in a study—conceptual and operational.

The concepts in which researchers are interested are abstractions of observable phenomena, and researchers' world view shapes how those concepts are defined. A **conceptual definition** is the abstract or theoretical meaning of the concepts being studied. Even seemingly straightforward terms need to be conceptually defined by researchers. The classic example of this is the concept of *caring*. Morse and her colleagues (1990) scrutinized the writings of nurse theorists to determine how *caring* was defined, and identified five different types of conceptual definitions—as a human trait; a moral imperative; an affect; an interpersonal relationship; and a therapeutic intervention. Researchers undertaking studies of caring need to make clear which conceptual definition of caring they have adopted. In qualitative studies, conceptual definitions of key phenomena may be a major end product, reflecting an intent to have the meaning of concepts defined by those being studied.

In quantitative studies, however, researchers need to clarify and define research concepts at the outset, because they must indicate how variables will be observed and measured. An **operational definition** of a variable specifies the operations that researchers must perform to collect the required information. Operational definitions should correspond to conceptual definitions.

Variables differ in the ease with which they can be operationalized. The variable weight, for example, is easy to define and measure. We might operationally define weight as follows: the amount that an object weighs in pounds, to the nearest full pound. Note that this definition designates that weight will be determined with one measuring system (pounds) rather than another (grams). The operational definition might also specify that subjects' weight will be measured to the nearest pound using a spring scale with subjects fully undressed after 10 hours of fasting. This operational definition clearly indicates what is meant by the variable *weight.*

Unfortunately, few variables of interest in nursing research are operationalized as easily as weight. There are multiple methods of measuring most variables, and researchers must choose the method that best captures the variables as they conceptualize them. Take, for example, *anxiety,* which can be defined in terms of either physiologic or psychological functioning. For researchers choosing to emphasize physiologic aspects of anxiety, the operational definition might involve a measure such as the Palmar Sweat Index. If, on the other hand, researchers conceptualize anxiety as primarily a psychological state, the operational definition might involve a paper-and-pencil measure such as the State Anxiety Scale. Readers of research reports may not agree with how investigators conceptualized and operationalized variables, but precision in defining terms has the advantage of communicating exactly what terms mean within the context of the study.

Example of conceptual and operational definitions

Beck and Gable (2001) conceptually defined various aspects of *postpartum depression* and then described how the definitions were linked operationally to a measure Beck had developed, the Postpartum Depression Screening Scale (PDSS). For example, one aspect of postpartum depression is *cognitive impairment,* conceptually defined as "a mother's loss of control over her thought processes [that] leaves her frightened she may be losing her mind." Operationally, the PDSS captured this conceptual dimension by having women indicate their level of agreement with such statements as "I could not stop the thoughts that kept racing in my mind."

CONSUMER TIP

Most research reports never use the term *operational definition* explicitly. Quantitative research reports do, however, provide information on how key variables were measured (i.e., they specify the operational definitions even if they do not use this label). This information is generally included in a section of the research report called "Research Measures" or "Instruments."

Data

Research **data** (singular, datum) are the pieces of information obtained in a study. All the pieces of data that researchers gather for a study comprise their **data set**.

In quantitative studies, researchers identify the variables of interest, develop operational definitions of those variables, and then collect relevant data from subjects. The actual values of the study variables constitute the study data. In quantitative studies, researchers collect primarily **quantitative data** (i.e., numeric information). As an example, suppose we were conducting a quantitative study in which a key variable was *depression.* In such a study, we would try to

---

BOX 2.1   Example of Quantitative Data

Question

Thinking about the past week, how depressed would you say you have been on a scale from 0 to 10, where 0 means "not at all" and 10 means "the most possible"?

Data

Subject 1: 9
Subject 2: 0
Subject 3: 4

---

measure how depressed different study participants were. We might ask, "Thinking about the past week, how depressed would you say you have been on a scale from 0 to 10, where 0 means 'not at all' and 10 means 'the most possible'?" Box 2-1 presents some quantitative data from three fictitious respondents. The subjects have provided a number corresponding to their degree of depression: 9 for subject 1 (a high level of depression), 0 for subject 2 (no depression), and 4 for subject 3 (very mild depression). The numeric values for all subjects in the study, collectively, would comprise the data on the variable depression.

In qualitative studies, researchers collect primarily **qualitative data,** which are narrative descriptions. Narrative information can be obtained by having conversations with participants, by making notes about how participants behave in naturalistic settings, or by obtaining narrative records, such as diaries. Suppose we were studying depression qualitatively. Box 2-2 presents some qualitative data from three participants responding conversationally to the question, "Tell me about how you've been feeling lately. Have you felt sad or depressed at all, or have you generally been in good spirits?" Here, the data consist of rich narrative descriptions of participants' emotional state. The analysis of such qualitative data is a particularly labor-intensive process.

BOX 2.2   Example of Qualitative Data

Question

Tell me about how you've been feeling lately—have you felt sad or depressed at all, or have you generally been in good spirits?

Data

Participant 1: "I've been pretty depressed lately, to tell you the truth. I wake up each morning and I can't seem to think of anything to look forward to. I mope around the house all day, kind of in despair. I just can't seem to shake the blues, and I've begun to think I need to go see a shrink."
Participant 2: "I can't remember ever feeling better in my life. I just got promoted to a new job that makes me feel like I can really get ahead in my company. And I've just gotten engaged to a really great guy who is very special."
Participant 3: "I've had a few ups and downs the past week, but basically things are on a pretty even keel. I don't have too many complaints."

Relationships

Researchers usually study phenomena in relation to other phenomena—they examine relationships. A **relationship** is a bond or connection between two or more phenomena; for example, researchers repeatedly have found that there is a *relationship* between cigarette smoking and lung cancer. Both qualitative and quantitative studies examine relationships, but in different ways.

In quantitative studies, researchers are primarily interested in the relationship between independent variables and dependent variables. Variation in the dependent variable is presumed to be systematically related to variation in the independent variable. Relationships are often explicitly expressed in quantitative terms, such as *more than*, *less than*, and so on. For example, let us consider as a possible dependent variable a person's body weight. What variables are related to (associated with) a person's weight? Some possibilities include height, caloric intake, and exercise. For each of these three independent variables, we can make a prediction about the nature of its relationship to the dependent variable:

> *Height: Taller people weigh more than shorter people.*
> *Caloric intake: People with higher caloric intake are heavier than those with lower caloric intake.*
> *Exercise: The lower the amount of exercise, the greater the person's weight.*

Each of these statements expresses a presumed relationship between weight (the dependent variable) and a measurable independent variable. Most quantitative research is conducted to determine whether relationships do or do not exist among variables, and often to quantify how strong the relationship is.

CONSUMER TIP

Relationships are expressed in two basic forms, depending on what the variables are like. First, relationships can be expressed as "if more of Variable X, then more of (or less of) Variable Y." For example, there is a relationship between height and weight: With more height, there tends to be more weight; i.e., taller people tend to weigh more than shorter people. The second form is sometimes confusing to students because there is no explicit relational statement. The second form involves relationships expressed as group differences. For example, there is a *relationship* between gender and height: Men tend to be taller than women. ■

Variables can be related to one another in different ways. One type of relationship is a **cause-and-effect** (or **causal**) **relationship**. Within the positivist paradigm, natural phenomena are assumed not to be haphazard; they have antecedent causes that are presumably discoverable. In our example about a person's weight, we might speculate that there is a causal relationship between caloric intake and weight: All else being equal, eating more calories causes weight gain.

Example of a study focusing on a causal relationship

Schoenfelder and Rubenstein (2004) studied whether a 3-month ankle-strengthening and walking program would casuse improvements in nursing home residents' balance, ankle strength, walking speed, and risk of falling.

Not all relationships between variables can be interpreted as cause-and-effect relationships. There is a relationship, for example, between a person's pulmonary artery and tympanic temperatures: People with high readings on one have high readings on the other. We cannot say, however, that pulmonary artery temperature caused tympanic temperature, nor that tympanic temperature caused pulmonary artery temperature, despite the relationship that exists between the two variables. This type of relationship is sometimes referred to as a *functional* (or *associative*) *relationship* rather than a causal one.

Example of a study focusing on a functional relationship

Pressler and Hepworth (2002) examined the relationship between a preterm neonate's behavioral competence on the one hand, and the infant's gender and race on the other. Race and gender were not assumed to cause behavioral competence.

HOW-TO-TELL TIP

How can you tell if a researcher is testing a causal relationship? The researcher is likely to ask whether the outcome variable is *caused by, affected by, resulted from,* or *influenced by* the independent variable. If the researcher is not seeking to establish a causal relationship, he or she is more likely to ask whether the outcome variable is *related to, linked to,* or *associated with* the independent variable. ▬

Qualitative researchers are not concerned with quantifying relationships, nor in testing and confirming causal relationships. Rather, qualitative researchers seek patterns of association as a way of illuminating the underlying meaning and dimensionality of phenomena of interest. Patterns of interconnected themes and processes are identified as a means of understanding the whole.

Example of a qualitative study of patterns

Lam and Mackenzie (2002) explored Chinese parents' experiences in parenting a child with Down syndrome. One major theme that emerged from the in-depth interviews was parental acceptance of the child. Although the researchers had not specifically sought to examine differences between mothers and fathers, they noted that mothers and fathers did not accept their child at the same pace.

Logical Reasoning

Logical reasoning plays an important role in both qualitative and quantitative research. Two intellectual mechanisms are used in reasoning. **Inductive reasoning** is the process of developing conclusions from specific observations. For example, a nurse may observe a constellation of anxious behaviors and comments of (specific) hospitalized children and conclude that (in general) children's separation from their parents is stressful. Inductive reasoning is an important tool in disciplined research and plays an especially important role in qualitative research, where the emphasis is on weaving together pieces of information into a coherent and cohesive pattern.

Deductive reasoning is the process of developing specific predictions from general principles. For example, if we assume that separation anxiety occurs in hospitalized children (in general), we might predict that the (specific) children in Memorial Hospital whose parents do not room in would manifest symptoms of stress. Quantitative studies would examine the validity of the prediction—that is, they would test **hypotheses** about how variables are related. In our example, the hypothesized relationship would be between *rooming in* (i.e., rooming in versus not rooming in) and *stress levels* in hospitalized children.

Logical reasoning can be used to solve problems even in the absence of systematic research. However, reasoning in and of itself is limited because the validity of reasoning depends on the accuracy of the information (or premises) with which one starts. Systematic research can be structured to provide maximally useful information, the accuracy of which can be evaluated.

CRITICAL CHALLENGES OF CONDUCTING RESEARCH

Researchers face numerous challenges in conducting research. For example, there are conceptual challenges (e.g., How should key concepts be defined?); financial challenges (How will the study be paid for?); ethical challenges (Can the study achieve its goals without infringing on human rights?); and methodologic challenges (Will the adopted methods yield results that can be trusted and applied to other settings?). Most of this book provides guidance relating to the last question, and this section highlights key methodologic challenges as a way of introducing important terms and concepts and illustrating key differences between qualitative and quantitative research. In reading this section, it is important for you to remember that the worth of a study's evidence for EBP is based on how well researchers deal with these challenges and communicate their decisions.

Reliability, Validity, and Trustworthiness

Researchers want their findings to reflect the *truth*. Research cannot contribute evidence to guide clinical practice if the findings are inaccurate, biased, or fail to adequately represent the experiences of the target group. Research users need to assess the quality of evidence offered in a study by evaluating the conceptual and methodologic decisions researchers made, and researchers need to strive to make good decisions to produce evidence of the highest possible quality.

Quantitative researchers use several criteria to assess the quality of a study, sometimes referred to as its **scientific merit**. Two of the most important criteria are reliability and validity. **Reliability** refers to the accuracy and consistency of information obtained in a study. The term is most often associated with the methods used to measure research variables. For example, if a thermometer measured Bob's temperature as 98.1°F one minute and as 102.5°F the next minute, the reliability of the thermometer would be highly suspect. The concept of reliability is also important in interpreting statistical analyses. Statistical reliability refers to the probability that the same results would be obtained with a completely new sample of subjects—that is, that the results accurately reflect the outcomes of a wider group than just the particular people who participated in the study.

Validity is a more complex concept that concerns the *soundness* of the study's evidence—that is, whether the findings are cogent, convincing, and well-grounded. Like reliability, validity is an important criterion for assessing the methods of measuring variables. In this context, the validity question is whether there is evidence to support the assertion that the methods are really measuring the abstract concepts that they purport to measure. Is a paper-and-pencil measure of depression *really* measuring depression? Or is it measuring something else, such as loneliness, low self-esteem, or stress? The validity criterion underscores the importance of having solid conceptual definitions of research variables—as well as high-quality methods to operationalize them.

Another aspect of validity concerns the quality of the researcher's evidence regarding the link between the independent variable and the dependent variable. Did a nursing intervention *really* bring about improvements in patients' outcomes—or were other factors responsible for patients' progress? Researchers make numerous methodologic decisions that can influence this type of study validity.

Qualitative researchers use somewhat different criteria (and different terminology) in evaluating a study's quality. Generally, qualitative researchers discuss methods of enhancing the **trustworthiness** of the study's results (Lincoln & Guba, 1985). Trustworthiness encompasses several different dimensions, one of which is credibility.

Credibility, an especially important aspect of trustworthiness, is achieved to the extent that the research methods engender confidence in the truth of the data and in the researchers' interpretations of the data. Credibility can be enhanced through various strategies (Chapter 14), but one in particular merits early discussion because it has implications for the design of all studies, including quantitative ones. **Triangulation** is the use of multiple sources or referents to draw conclusions about what constitutes the truth. In a quantitative study, this might mean having alternative operational definitions of a dependent variable to determine if results are consistent across the two. In a qualitative study, triangulation might involve trying to understand the full complexity of a poorly understood phenomenon by using multiple means of data collection to converge on the truth (e.g., having in-depth conversations with study participants, as well as observing them in natural settings). Nurse researchers are also beginning to triangulate across paradigms—that is, to integrate both qualitative and quantitative data in a single study to offset the limitations of each approach.

 Example of triangulation

Tarzian (2000) used triangulation in her qualitative study on caring for dying patients with air hunger. Tarzian interviewed 10 nurses who had cared for air-hungry patients and, to complement the nurses' accounts, two family members who witnessed spouses suffering from air hunger. Trustworthiness of the study findings was enhanced because family members confirmed important themes. For example, nurses disclosed that air hunger evoked a physical effect, such as feeling out of breath just watching patients struggling to breathe. Family members supported this theme. One husband recalled, "My chest hurt just watching her, breathing like that all day long" (p. 139).

Nurse researchers need to design their studies in such a way that threats to the reliability, validity, and trustworthiness of their studies are minimized, and users of research must evaluate the extent to which they were successful.

CONSUMER TIP

In reading and evaluating research reports, it is appropriate to assume a "show me" attitude—that is, to expect researchers to build and present a solid case for the merit of their findings. They do this by presenting evidence that the findings are reliable and valid or trustworthy.

■

Bias

Bias is a major concern in research because it can threaten the study's validity and trustworthiness. In general, a **bias** is an influence that produces a distortion in the study results. Biases can affect the quality of evidence in both qualitative and quantitative studies. Bias can result from a number of factors, including study participants' lack of candor or desire to please, researchers' preconceptions, or faulty methods of collecting data.

To some extent, bias can never be avoided totally because the potential for its occurrence is so pervasive. Some bias is haphazard and affects only small segments of the data. As an example of such random bias, a handful of study participants might fail to provide accurate information because they were tired at the time of data collection. Systematic bias results when the bias is consistent or uniform. For example, if a spring scale consistently measured people's weight as being 2 pounds heavier than their true weight, there would be systematic bias in the data on weight. Rigorous research methods aim to eliminate or minimize bias—or, at least, to detect its presence so it can be taken into account in interpreting the data.

Researchers adopt a variety of strategies to address bias. Triangulation is one such approach, the idea being that multiple sources of information or points of view help to counterbalance biases and offer avenues to identify them. In quantitative research, methods to combat bias often entail research control.

Research Control

Quantitative studies typically involve efforts to tightly control various aspects of the research. **Research control** involves holding constant other influences on the dependent variable so that the true relationship between the independent and dependent variables can be understood. In other words, research control attempts to eliminate contaminating factors that might cloud the relationship between the variables that are of central interest.

The issue of contaminating factors—or **extraneous variables** as they are called—can best be illustrated with an example. Suppose we were interested in answering the question, Does young maternal age affect infant birth weight? Existing studies have shown that teenagers have a higher rate of low-birth-weight babies than women in their 20s or 30s; the question here is whether maternal age itself (the independent variable) causes differences in birth weight (the dependent variable) or whether there are other mechanisms that account for or mediate the relationship between age and birth weight. We need to design a study that controls other influences on the dependent variable to clarify the effect of the independent variable.

Two possible extraneous variables are the women's nutritional habits and their prenatal care. Teenagers tend to be less careful than older women about their eating patterns during pregnancy, and are also less likely to obtain adequate prenatal care. Both nutrition and the amount of care could, in turn, affect birth weight. Thus, if these two factors are not controlled, then any observed relationship between the mother's age and her baby's weight at birth could be caused by the mother's age itself, her diet, or her prenatal care. It would be impossible to know what the underlying cause really is.

These three possible explanations might be portrayed schematically as follows:

1. Mother's age → infant birth weight
2. Mother's age → adequacy of prenatal care → infant birth weight
3. Mother's age → nutritional adequacy → infant birth weight

The arrows here symbolize a causal mechanism or an influence. In explanations 2 and 3, the effect of maternal age on infant birth weight is mediated by prenatal care and nutrition, respectively; these variables would be considered **mediating variables** in these last two models. Some research is specifically designed to test paths of mediation, but in the present example these variables are extraneous to the research question. Our task is to design a study so that the first explanation can be tested. Both nutrition and prenatal care must be controlled if we want to learn if explanation 1 is valid. If they are not controlled, they will confound the results. How can we impose such control? There are a number of ways, as discussed in Chapter 9, but the general principle underlying each alternative is the same: *the extraneous variables of the study must be held constant*. The extraneous variables must be handled so that, *in the context of the study*, they are not related to the independent or dependent variable.

Research control is a fundamental feature of quantitative studies. The world is complex, and variables are interrelated in complicated ways. In quantitative studies, it is difficult to examine this complexity directly. Researchers analyze a few relationships at a time and put the pieces together like a jigsaw puzzle. That is why even modest quantitative studies can make contributions to knowledge. The extent of the contribution, however, is often related to how well a researcher controls contaminating influences. In reading reports of quantitative studies, you will need to consider whether the researcher has, in fact, appropriately controlled extraneous variables.

Although research control in quantitative studies is viewed as a critical tool for managing bias and enhancing validity, there are situations in which too much control can introduce bias. For example, if researchers tightly control the ways in which key study variables can manifest themselves, it is possible that the true nature of those variables will be obscured. When key concepts are phenomena that are poorly understood or whose dimensions have not been clarified, then an approach that allows some flexibility (as in a qualitative study) is better suited to the study aims. Research rooted in the naturalistic paradigm does not impose controls. With their emphasis on holism and the individuality of human experience, qualitative researchers typically adhere to the view that to impose controls on a research setting is to remove irrevocably some of the meaning of reality.

Randomness and Reflexivity

For quantitative researchers, a powerful tool for eliminating bias involves the concept of **randomness**—having certain features of the study established by chance rather than by design or personal preference. When people in a community are selected at random to participate in a study, for example, each person in the community has an equal chance of being selected. This in turn means that there are no systematic biases in the make-up of the study group. Men are as likely to be selected as women, for example.

Qualitative researchers do not consider randomness a useful tool for understanding phenomena. Qualitative researchers tend to use information obtained early in the study in a purposeful (nonrandom) fashion to guide their inquiry and to pursue information-rich sources that can help them refine their conceptualizations. Researchers' judgments are viewed as indispensable vehicles for uncovering the complexities of the phenomenon of interest. However, qualitative researchers often rely on reflexivity to guard against personal bias in making judgments. **Reflexivity** is the process of reflecting critically on the self and of analyzing and making note of personal values that could affect data collection and interpretation.

Generalizability and Transferability

Nurses increasingly rely on evidence from disciplined research as a guide in their clinical practice. If study findings are totally unique to the people, places, or circumstances of the original research, can they be used as a basis for changes in practice? The answer, clearly, is no.

As noted in Chapter 1, **generalizability** is the criterion used in a quantitative study to assess the extent to which study findings can be applied to other groups and settings. How do researchers enhance the generalizability of a study? First, they must design studies strong in reliability and validity. There is little point in wondering whether results are generalizable if they are not accurate or valid. In selecting subjects, researchers must also give thought to the types of people to whom the results might be generalized—and then select them in such a way that an appropriate sample is obtained. If a study is intended to have implications for male and female patients, then men and women should be included as participants. If an intervention is intended to benefit patients in urban and rural hospitals, then perhaps a multisite study is needed.

Qualitative researchers do not specifically seek to make their findings generalizable. Nevertheless, qualitative researchers often seek understandings that might prove useful in other situations. Lincoln and Guba (1985), in their highly influential book on naturalistic inquiry, discuss the concept of **transferability**—the extent to which qualitative findings can be transferred to other settings—as an aspect of a study's trustworthiness. An important mechanism for promoting transferability is the amount of information qualitative researchers provide about the contexts of their studies. **Thick description**, a widely used term among qualitative researchers, refers to a rich and thorough description of the research setting and of observed transactions and processes. Quantitative researchers, like qualitative researchers, need to thoroughly describe their study participants and their research settings so that the utility of the evidence for nursing practice can be assessed.

GENERAL QUESTIONS IN REVIEWING A RESEARCH STUDY

Most of the remaining chapters of this book contain guidelines to help you evaluate different aspects of a research report critically, focusing primarily on the methodologic decisions that the researcher made in conducting the study. Box 2-3 presents some further suggestions for performing a preliminary overview of a research report, drawing on concepts explained in this chapter. These guidelines supplement those presented in Box 1-1 in Chapter 1.

BOX 2.3   Additional Questions for a Preliminary Overview of a Study

1. What is the study all about? What are the main phenomena, concepts, or constructs under investigation?
2. If the study is quantitative, what are the independent and dependent variables?
3. Do the researchers examine relationships or patterns of association among variables or concepts? Does the report imply the possibility of a causal relationship?
4. Are key concepts clearly defined, both conceptually and operationally?
5. Are you able to discern any steps the researcher took to enhance the study's reliability, validity, and generalizability (quantitative research) or trustworthiness (qualitative research)?

CHAPTER REVIEW

Key new terms introduced in the chapter, together with a summary of major points, are presented in this section. In addition, Chapter 2 of the *Study Guide to Accompany Essentials of Nursing Research*, 6th edition offers various exercises and study suggestions for reinforcing the concepts presented in this chapter. For additional review, see the Student Self-Study Review Questions section of the Student Resource CD-ROM provided with this book.

KEY NEW TERMS

Bias
Cause-and-effect (causal) relationship
Concept
Conceptual definition
Construct
Credibility
Data
Data set
Deductive reasoning
Dependent variable
Extraneous variable
Fieldwork
Generalizability
Hypothesis
Independent variable
Inductive reasoning
Mediating variable
Operational definition

Outcome variable
Qualitative data
Quantitative data
Phenomena
Randomness
Reflexivity
Relationship
Reliability
Research control
Study participant
Subject
Theory
Thick description
Transferability
Triangulation
Trustworthiness
Validity
Variable

SUMMARY POINTS

▷ A **study** (or an **investigation** or a **research project**) is undertaken by one or more **researchers** (or **investigators** or scientists). The people who provide information in a study are called **subjects** or **study participants** (in quantitative research) or study participants or **informants** (in qualitative research).

▷ **Collaborative studies** involving a research team with both clinical and methodologic expertise is increasingly common in addressing problems of clinical relevance.

▷ The site is the overall location for the research; researchers sometimes engage in **multisite studies**. Settings—the more specific places where data collection occurs—range from **naturalistic settings** (in the **field**) to formal laboratories.

▷ Researchers investigate phenomena or **concepts** (or **constructs**), which are abstractions or mental representations inferred from behavior or events.

▷ Concepts are the building blocks of **theories,** which are systematic explanations of some aspect of the real world.

▷ In quantitative studies, concepts are called variables. A **variable** is a characteristic or quality that takes on different values (i.e., varies from one person to another).

▷ The **dependent** (or **outcome**) **variable** is the behavior, characteristic, or outcome the researcher is interested in explaining, predicting, or affecting. The **independent variable** is the presumed cause of, antecedent to, or influence on the dependent variable.

▷ A **conceptual definition** clarifies the abstract or theoretical meaning of a concept being studied. An **operational definition** specifies the procedures and tools required to measure a variable.

▷ **Data**—the information collected during the course of a study—may take the form of narrative information (**qualitative data**) or numeric values (**quantitative data**).

▷ Researchers often focus on the relationship between two concepts. A **relationship** is a bond or connection (or pattern of association) between two phenomena; when the independent variable causes or determines the dependent variable, it is a **cause-and-effect** (or **causal**) **relationship**.

▷ **Inductive reasoning** is the process of developing conclusions from specific observations, while **deductive reasoning** is the process of developing specific predictions from general principles.

▷ Researchers face numerous conceptual, practical, ethical, and methodologic challenges. The major methodologic challenge is designing studies that are reliable and valid (quantitative studies) or trustworthy (qualitative studies).

▷ **Reliability** refers to the accuracy and consistency of information obtained in a study. **Validity** is a more complex concept that broadly concerns the *soundness* of the study's evidence—that is, whether the findings are cogent, convincing, and well-grounded.

▷ **Trustworthiness** in qualitative research encompasses several different dimensions, including credibility. **Credibility** is achieved to the extent that the research methods engender confidence in the truth of the data and in the researchers' interpretations. **Triangulation**, the use of multiple sources or referents to draw conclusions about what constitutes the truth, is one approach to establishing credibility.

▷ A **bias** is an influence that distorts study results. In quantitative research, a powerful tool to eliminate bias concerns **randomness**—having features of the study established by chance rather than by design or preference.

▷ Qualitative researchers often keep personal biases in check through **reflexivity**, the process of reflecting critically on the self and noting personal values that could affect data collection and interpretation.

▷ Quantitative researchers use various methods of **research control** to hold constant outside influences on the dependent variable so that its relationship to the independent variable can be better understood. The external influences are **extraneous variables**—extraneous to the purpose of the study.

▷ **Generalizability** is the criterion used in a quantitative study to assess the extent to which the findings can be applied to other groups and settings.

▷ A similar concept in qualitative studies is **transferability**, the extent to which qualitative findings can be transferred to other settings. A mechanism for promoting transferability is **thick description**, the rich, thorough description of the research context so that others can make inferences about contextual similarities.

RESEARCH EXAMPLES | Critical Thinking Activities

 ### EXAMPLE 1: Quantitative Research

Aspects of a quantitative nursing study, featuring key terms and concepts discussed in this chapter, are presented below, followed by some questions to guide critical thinking. (The full research report is available in *Research in Nursing & Health, 25,* 3–13.)

Study

"A randomized trial of behavioral management for continence with older rural women" (Dougherty et al., 2002)

Study Purpose

The researchers designed a study to test the effectivness of a behavioral management for continence (BMC) intervention for older women with urinary incontinence (UI) in seven rural counties in north Florida. The in-home intervention involved self-monitoring, bladder training, and pelvic muscle exercise with biofeedback.

Study Procedures

Two hundred and eighteen women aged 55 and older who had regular involuntary urine loss were recruited for the study. Half the subjects, at random, were put in a group that received the BMC intervention, while the other half were put in a group that did not. Outcome data were gathered through follow-up visits to both groups every 6 months for up to 2 years.

Outcome Variables

The primary outcome variable was urine loss, operationalized as the amount of urine lost in grams per 24 hours (determined by the change in weight of incontinence pads). Secondary outcomes included measures obtained from 3-day bladder diaries that subjects maintained (e.g., micturition frequency and episodes of urine loss). Additionally, the researchers assessed the effect of the intervention on subjects' quality of life, operationalized with a paper-and-pencil measure known as the Incontinence Impact Questionnaire (IIQ). The IIQ, which asks 26 questions about the extent to which incontinence affects functioning in various areas (e.g., daily living, social interactions, self-perception), previously had been shown to be a reliable and valid indicator of quality of life.

Key Findings

▷ Over the 2 years in which the women were followed, the BMC group sustained UI improvement, while those in the other group experienced worsening severity in urine loss.

research examples continue on page 48

RESEARCH EXAMPLES *Continued*

▷ The two groups also differed at follow-up with regard to episodes of urine loss and quality of life.

Critical Thinking Suggestions*

*See the Student Resource CD-ROM for a discussion of these questions.

1. Answer questions 1, 2, 3, and 5 from Box 2-3 regarding this study.
2. Also consider the following targeted questions, which may assist you in assessing aspects of the study's merit:
   a. What is your perception of the validity of the outcome measures?
   b. How did the researchers reduce bias in forming the two groups that were compared?
   c. What might be some of the extraneous variables the researchers would have needed to control—what factors other than the intervention could have affected the outcomes?
   d. What was one thing the researchers did to enhance the generalizability of the study findings? What might be some constraints on generalizability?
   e. Would it have been appropriate for the researchers to address the research question using qualitative research methods? Why or why not?
3. If the results of this study are valid and generalizable, what are some of the uses to which the research evidence might be put in clinical practice?

 EXAMPLE 2: Qualitative Research

Aspects of a qualitative nursing study, featuring key terms and concepts discussed in this chapter, are presented below, followed by some questions to guide critical thinking. (The full research report is available in *Qualitative Health Research, 12,* 74–90.)

Study

"In their own words: The lived experience of pediatric liver transplantation" (Wise, 2002)

Study Purpose

Wise sought to understand and thoroughly describe the experience of children who received liver transplants, from the time before transplantation through the surgery and after.

Study Procedures

Wise conducted interviews with nine children between the ages of 7 and 15. She interviewed the children herself either in their homes or in an outpatient setting, in conversations ranging in length from 20 to 40 minutes. The interviews were audiotaped and transcribed. Before the interviews, Wise asked the children to draw two pictures of themselves, one before the transplantation and one that reflected their present status. The artwork helped the children to relax and also provided rich information and an opening for the interviews. An art therapist interpreted the children's artwork. Wise maintained a journal in which she documented her ongoing observations and decisions.

RESEARCH EXAMPLES *Continued*

Key Findings

Wise used thick description in reporting her results. Four themes described the essence of the phenomenon of pediatric liver transplantation:

▶ A search for connections with peers prior to and after the transplant, and also for connections with the donor;
▶ Ordinary and extraordinary experiences of hospitalization;
▶ Painful responses and being out of control; and
▶ Parents' responses to the illness. The following quote illustrates this fourth theme: "I will never tell my Mom how I feel about anything. I don't think I would ever tell the truth because I would never want to upset her. I can just see the expression on her face. I know how she feels...she has been through so much stuff with me. I basically worry if she is all right instead of me" (p. 86).

Critical Thinking Suggestions

1. Answers questions 1, 3, and 5 from Box 2-3 regarding this study.
2. Also consider the following targeted questions, which may assist you in assessing aspects of the study's merit:
   a. Identify at least one thing the researcher did to enhance the credibility of the study.
   b. Which activity described in the summary indicates an effort to reduce bias?
   c. Wise did not control extraneous variables, nor did she use randomness in this study. Would these decisions affect the quality of the study?
   d. Some actual data are presented in the summary—indicate what the data are.
   e. What did Wise do to improve the transferability of her findings?
   f. Would it have been appropriate for Wise to address the research question using quantitative research methods? Why or why not?
3. If the results of this study are trustworthy, what are some of the uses to which the findings might be put in clinical practice?

 EXAMPLE 3: Quantitative Research

1. Read the abstract and the introduction from Motzer et al.'s study ("Sense of Coherence") in Appendix A of this book, and then answer the relevant questions in Box 2-3.
2. Also consider the following targeted questions, which may further sharpen your critical thinking skills and assist you in assessing aspects of the study's merit:
   a. What is the name of the theory that the researchers used as a basis for their inquiry?
   b. Did the researchers randomly assign subjects to groups in this study?
   c. The researchers compared women with and without IBS in terms of sense of coherence and quality of life. What are some of the extraneous variables that the researchers would have wanted to control?

research examples continue on page 50

RESEARCH EXAMPLES · *Continued*

 EXAMPLE 4: Qualitative Research

1. Read the abstract, introduction, and literature review section of Beck's study ("Birth Trauma") in Appendix B of this book, and then answer the relevant questions in Box 2-3.
2. Also consider the following targeted questions, which may further sharpen your critical thinking skills and assist you in assessing aspects of the study's merit:
   a. Find an example of actual *data* in this study. (You will need to look at the first few paragraphs of the "Results" section of the report.)
   b. Does Beck's report discuss reflexivity?
   c. Would it have been appropriate for Beck to conduct her study of birth trauma using quantitative research methods? Why or why not?

SUGGESTED READINGS

Methodologic References

Kerlinger, F. N., & Lee, H. B. (2000). *Foundations of behavioral research* (4th ed.). Orlando, FL: Harcourt College Publishers.

Lincoln, Y. S., & Guba, E. G. (1985). *Naturalistic inquiry.* Newbury Park, CA: Sage Publications.

Morse, J. M., Solberg, S. M., Neander, W. L., Bottorff, J. L., & Johnson, J. L. (1990). Concepts of caring and caring as a concept. *Advances in Nursing Science, 13,* 1–14.

Morse, J. M., & Field, P. A. (1995). *Qualitative research methods for health professionals* (2nd ed.). Thousand Oaks, CA: Sage Publications.

Studies Cited in Chapter 2

Beck, C. T., & Gable, R. K. (2001). Ensuring content validity: An illustration of the process. *Journal of Nursing Measurement, 9,* 201–215.

Dougherty, M., Dwyer, J., Pendergast, J., Boyington, A., Tomlinson, B., Coward, R., Duncan, R. P., Vogel, B., & Rooks, L. (2002). A randomized trial of behavioral management for continence with older rural women. *Research in Nursing & Health, 25,* 3–13.

Lam, L. W., & Mackenzie, A. E. (2002). Coping with a child with Down syndrome: The experiences of mothers in Hong Kong. *Qualitative Health Research, 12,* 223–37.

McCain, N. L., Munjas, B. A., Munro, C. L., Elswick, R. K. Jr., Robins, J. L., Ferreira-Gonzalez, A., Baliko, B., Kaplowitz, L. G., Fisher, E. J., Garrett, C. T., Brigle, K. E., Kendall, L. C., Lucas, V., & Cochran, K. L. (2003). Effects of stress management on PNI-based outcomes in persons with HIV disease. *Research in Nursing & Health, 26,* 102–117.

Pressler, J. L., & Hepworth, J. T. (2002). A quantitative use of the NIDCAP® tool. *Clinical Nursing Research, 11,* 89–102.

Rossen, E. K., & Knafl, K. A. (2003). Older women's response to residential relocation: Description of transition styles. *Qualitative Health Research, 13,* 20–36.

Schaefer, K. M. (2003). Sleep disturbances linked to fibromyalgia. *Holistic Nursing Practice, 17,* 120–127.

Schoenfelder, D. P., & Rubenstein, L. M. (2004). An exercise program to improve fall-related outcomes in elderly nursing home residents. *Applied Nursing Research, 17,* 21–31.

Scisney-Matlock, M., Makos, G., Saunders, T., Jackson, F., & Steigerwalt, S. (2004). Comparison of quality-of-hypertension care indicators for groups treated by physician versus groups treated by physician-nurse team. *Journal of the American Academy of Nurse Practitioners, 16,* 17–23.

Tarzian, A. J. (2000). Caring for dying patients who have air hunger. *Journal of Nursing Scholarship, 32,* 137–143.

Wise, B. (2002). In their own words: The lived experience of pediatric liver transplantation. *Qualitative Health Research, 12,* 74–90.

Understanding the Research Process in Qualitative and Quantitative Studies

STUDENT OBJECTIVES

On completing this chapter, you will be able to:

▶ Distinguish experimental and nonexperimental research
▶ Identify the three main disciplinary traditions for qualitative nursing research
▶ Describe the flow and sequence of activities in quantitative and qualitative research, and disucss why they differ
▶ Define new terms persented in the chapter

Researchers usually decide early on whether to conduct a quantitative or qualitative study; they typically work within a paradigm that is consistent with their world view and that gives rise to the types of question that excite their curiosity. After selecting a paradigm, researchers proceed to design and implement their study, but the progression of activities differs in qualitative and quantitative research. In this chapter, we discuss the flow of both types of study.

CONSUMER TIP

The flow of a research project is not transparent to those reading a research report. Researchers rarely articulate the progression of steps they took in completing a study. This chapter is not, therefore, designed to help you to critique a report (i.e., you will not have to evaluate whether researchers followed an appropriate sequence of steps), but will help you better understand the research process. It is also intended to heighten your awareness of the many decisions that researchers make—decisions that have a strong bearing on study quality.

MAJOR CLASSES OF QUANTITATIVE AND QUALITATIVE RESEARCH

Before describing the evolution of a research project, we briefly describe broad categories of quantitative and qualitative research.

Quantitative Research: Experimental and Nonexperimental Studies

A basic distinction in quantitative studies is between experimental and nonexperimental research. In **experimental research**, researchers actively introduce an intervention or treatment. In **nonexperimental research**, on the other hand, researchers collect data without making changes or introducing treatments. For example, if a researcher gave bran flakes to one group of subjects and prune juice to another to evaluate which method facilitated elimination more effectively, the study would be experimental because the researcher intervened in the normal course of things. If, on the other hand, a researcher compared elimination patterns of two groups of people whose regular eating patterns differed—for example, some normally took foods that stimulated bowel elimination and others did not—there is no intervention. Such a study, which focuses on existing attributes, is nonexperimental.

Example of experimental research

Norr and colleagues (2003) tested the effectiveness of a home-visit intervention that was designed to reduce infant mortality and improve infant development in low-income minority families. Mothers who received the home-visit intervention by a nurse–health advocate team were compared to mothers who did not receive it in terms of various health, parenting, and child development outcomes (e.g., infant immunizations, quality of the home environment) at 2, 6, and 12 months after birth.

Experimental studies are explicitly designed to test causal relationships. Sometimes nonexperimental studies also seek to elucidate or detect causal relationships, but doing so is tricky and less conclusive. Experimental studies offer the possibility of greater control over extraneous variables than nonexperimental studies.

In this example, the researchers intervened by designating that some families would receive the home visit intervention and others would not. In other words, the researcher had control over the independent variable, which in this case was receipt or nonreceipt of the intervention.

Example of nonexperimental research

Turner, Boyle, and O'Rourke (2003) searched for maternal factors associated with the receipt of age-appropriate vaccinations for infants in Australia. They found that women who were experiencing mental health problems such as anxiety or depression were significantly less likely than other women to have maintained an age-appropriate vaccination schedule.

In this nonexperimental study, which was also concerned with infant outcomes, the researchers did not intervene in any way. They merely observed and measured the study participants' characteristics and behavior. The independent variable was the mothers' postpartum mental health, a variable over which the researchers did not have control (i.e., they could not *assign* some women to be depressed and others to not be depressed—their level of depression was a "given"). Yet the researchers *were* interested in the possibility that the mothers' emotional state affected their parenting behavior. We will see in Chapter 9 why making such a causal inference in nonexperimental studies is a thorny issue.

Qualitative Research: Disciplinary Traditions

Qualitative studies (which are almost invariably nonexperimental) are often rooted in research traditions that originate in the disciplines of anthropology, sociology, and psychology. Three such traditions have had especially strong influences on qualitative nursing research and are briefly described here so that we can better explain their similarities and differences throughout the book. Chapter 10 provides a fuller discussion of alternative research traditions and the methods associated with them.

The **grounded theory** tradition, which was developed in the 1960s by two sociologists, Glaser and Strauss (1967), seeks to describe and understand the key social psychological and structural processes that occur in a social setting. Most grounded theory studies focus on an evolving social experience—the social and psychological stages and phases that characterize a particular event or episode. A major component of grounded theory is the discovery of a *core variable* (or *core category*) that is central in explaining what is going on in that social scene.

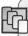

Example of a grounded theory study

Bonner and Walker (2004) conducted a grounded theory study to examine the process of "blurring the boundaries" between nursing and medicine among expert nephrology nurses in Australia.

Grounded theory researchers strive to generate comprehensive explanations of phenomena that are grounded in reality.

Phenomenology, which has its disciplinary roots in both philosophy and psychology, is concerned with the lived experiences of humans. Phenomenology is an approach to thinking about what life experiences of people are like and what they mean. The phenomenological researcher asks the questions, What is the *essence* of this phenomenon as experienced by these people? or, What is the meaning of the phenomenon to those who experience it?

Example of a phenomenological study

Ironside (2003) and 5 other nurses—who were graduate students in a research course—conducted a phenomenological study designed to describe the common experiences and shared meanings of living with a chronic illness.

Ethnography is the primary research tradition within anthropology, and provides a framework for studying the patterns and experiences of a defined cultural group in a holistic fashion. Ethnographers typically engage in extensive fieldwork, often participating to the extent possible in the life of the culture under study. The aim of ethnographers is to learn from (rather than to "study") members of a cultural group to understand their world view as they perceive and live it.

Example of an ethnographic study

DeVera (2003) used ethnographic methods to study the cultural beliefs of Yaqui Native Americans with diabetes regarding medical and traditional methods for healing foot ulcers.

MAJOR STEPS IN A QUANTITATIVE STUDY

In quantitative studies, researchers move from the beginning point of a study (posing a question) to the end point (getting an answer) in a fairly linear sequence of steps. This section describes the progression of activities that is typical in a quantitative study; the next section describes how qualitative studies differ.

Phase 1: The Conceptual Phase

The early steps in a quantitative study typically involve activities with a strong conceptual or intellectual element. During this phase, researchers call on such skills as creativity, deductive reasoning, insight, and a firm grounding in previous research on the topic of interest.

STEP 1: FORMULATING AND DELIMITING THE PROBLEM

The first step is to identify an interesting, significant research problem and to develop research questions. In developing research questions, nurse researchers need to consider substantive issues (Is the research question significant?); clinical issues (Could the findings be useful in practice?); methodologic issues (How can this study be designed to yield high-quality evidence?); practical issues (Are adequate resources available to do the study?); and ethical issues (Can this question be rigorously addressed without committing ethical transgressions?).

STEP 2: REVIEWING THE RELATED RESEARCH LITERATURE

Quantitative research is typically conducted within the context of previous knowledge. Quantitative researchers typically strive to understand what is already known about a topic by conducting a thorough **literature review** before any data are collected.

STEP 3: UNDERTAKING CLINICAL FIELDWORK

Researchers embarking on a clinical nursing study often benefit from spending time in appropriate clinical settings, discussing the topic with clinicians and health care administrators and observing current practices. Such clinical fieldwork can provide perspectives on recent clinical trends, current diagnostic procedures, and relevant health care delivery models; it can also help researchers better understand affected clients and the settings in which care is provided.

STEP 4: DEFINING THE FRAMEWORK AND DEVELOPING CONCEPTUAL DEFINITIONS

When quantitative research is performed within the context of a theoretical framework (i.e., when previous theory is used as a basis for generating predictions that can be tested), the findings may have broader significance and utility. Even when the research question is not embedded in a theory, researchers must have a clear sense of the concepts under study. Thus, an important task in the initial phase of a project is the development of conceptual definitions.

STEP 5: FORMULATING HYPOTHESES

As noted in Chapter 2, hypotheses state researchers' expecations about relationships between study variables. The research question identifies the variables and asks how they might be related; a hypothesis is the predicted answer. For example, the research question might be: Is preeclamptic toxemia in pregnant women related to stress factors present during pregnancy? This might lead to the following hypothesis: Pregnant women who report high levels of stress during pregnancy will be more likely than women with lower levels of stress to experience preeclamptic toxemia. Most quantitative studies are designed to test hypotheses.

Phase 2: The Design and Planning Phase

In the second major phase of a quantitative study, researchers make decisions about the methods to use to address the research question, and plan for the actual collection of data. As a consumer, you should be aware that the methodologic decisions that researchers make during this phase affect the integrity, interpretability, and clinical utility of the results. Thus, you must be able to evaluate the decisions so that you can determine how much faith to put in the evidence. A major objective of this book is to help you evaluate methodologic decisions.

STEP 6: SELECTING A RESEARCH DESIGN

The **research design** is the overall plan for obtaining answers to the research questions and for addressing the challenges we described in Chapter 2. In quantitative studies, research designs tend to be highly structured and to include controls to reduce the effects of contaminating influences. There is a wide variety of experimental and nonexperimental research designs.

STEP 7: DEVELOPING PROTOCOLS FOR THE INTERVENTION

In experimental research, researchers create the independent variable, which means that participants are exposed to two or more different treatments or conditions. An **intervention protocol** must be developed, specifying exactly what the intervention will entail (e.g., what it is, who will administer it, how frequently and over how long a period it will last, and so on) *and* what the alternative condition will be. The goal of well-articulated protocols is to have all subjects in each group treated the same way. In nonexperimental research, of course, this step would not be necessary.

STEP 8: IDENTIFYING THE POPULATION TO BE STUDIED

Quantitative researchers need to specify a population, indicate what attributes subjects should possess, and clarify the group to which study results can be generalized. A **population** is *all* the individuals or objects with common, defining characteristics. For example, a researcher might specify that the study population consists of all licensed nurses residing in New York State.

STEP 9: DESIGNING THE SAMPLING PLAN

Researchers typically collect data from a **sample**, which is a subset of the population. Using samples is practical, but the risk is that the sample will not adequately reflect the population's traits. In a quantitative study, a sample's adequacy is assessed by the criterion of *representativeness*; that is, the quality of the sample is a function of how typical, or representative, the sample is of the population. The **sampling plan** specifies in advance *how* the sample will be selected and *how many* subjects there will be.

STEP 10: SPECIFYING METHODS TO MEASURE VARIABLES

Quantitative researchers must develop or borrow methods to measure the study variables as accurately as possible. Based on the conceptual definitions, researchers select or design methods to operationalize the variables (i.e., to collect the data). A variety of quantitative data collection approaches exist; the primary methods are self-reports (e.g., interviews), observations, and biophysiologic measurements.

STEP 11: DEVELOPING METHODS TO PROTECT HUMAN/ANIMAL RIGHTS

Most nursing studies involve human subjects, although some involve animals. In either case, procedures need to be developed to ensure that the study adheres to ethical principles. Each aspect of the study plan needs to be reviewed to determine whether the rights of subjects have been adequately protected.

STEP 12: FINALIZING AND REVIEWING THE RESEARCH PLAN

Before collecting any data, researchers often seek feedback from colleagues or advisers and perform a number of "tests" to ensure that plans will work smoothly. For example, they may evaluate the *readability* of any written materials to determine if participants with low reading skills can comprehend them, or they might *pretest* their measuring instruments to assess their adequacy. If researchers have concerns about their study plans, they may undertake a **pilot study**, which is a small-scale version or trial run of the major study.

Phase 3: The Empirical Phase

The empirical portion of a quantitative study involves collecting research data and preparing those data for analysis. The empirical phase is often the most time-consuming part of the investigation.

STEP 13: COLLECTING THE DATA

Data collection in a quantitative study normally proceeds according to a preestablished plan. The *data collection plan* typically specifies procedures for actually collecting the data (e.g., where, when, and how the data will be gathered), for recruiting the sample, and for training those who will collect the data.

STEP 14: PREPARING DATA FOR ANALYSIS

The data collected in a quantitative study are rarely amenable to direct analysis. Preliminary steps are needed before the analysis can proceed. One such step is **coding**, which is the process of translating data into numeric form. For example, patients' responses to a question about their gender might be coded (1) for females and (2) for males. Another preliminary step involves transferring data from written forms to computer files for analysis.

Phase 4: The Analytic Phase

The quantitative data gathered in the empirical phase are not reported in *raw* form (i.e., as a mass of numbers). They are subjected to analysis and interpretation, which occurs in the fourth major phase of the project.

STEP 15: ANALYZING THE DATA

Research data must be processed and analyzed in an orderly fashion so that patterns and relationships can be discerned and validated, and hypotheses can be tested. Quantitative data are analyzed through **statistical analyses**, which include some simple procedures as well as complex and sophisticated methods.

STEP 16: INTERPRETING THE RESULTS

Interpretation is the process of making sense of the results and examining their implications within a broader context. In quantitative studies, researchers attempt to interpret study results in light of prior evidence and theory and in light of the adequacy of the methods used in the study. Interpretation also involves determining how the findings can best be used in clinical practice, or what further research is needed before utilization can be recommended.

Phase 5: The Dissemination Phase

In the analytic phase, the researcher comes full circle: the questions posed at the outset are answered. The researcher's job is not completed, however, until the study results are disseminated.

STEP 17: COMMUNICATING THE FINDINGS

A study cannot contribute evidence to nursing pracice if the results are not communicated. Another—and often final—task of a research project, therefore, is the preparation of a **research report** that can be shared with others. We discuss research reports in the next chapter.

STEP 18: UTILIZING RESEARCH EVIDENCE IN PRACTICE

Many studies have little effect on nursing practice. Ideally, the concluding step of a high-quality study is to plan for its use in practice settings. Although nurse researchers may not always be able to implement a plan for utilizing research findings, they can contribute to the process by developing recommendations regarding how study findings could be incorporated into nursing practice and by vigorously pursuing opportunities to disseminate their findings to practicing nurses.

ACTIVITIES IN A QUALITATIVE STUDY

Quantitative research involves a fairly linear progression of tasks (i.e., researchers lay out in advance the steps to be taken to maximize the integrity of the study and then follow them as faithfully as possible). In a qualitative study, by contrast, the progression is closer to a circle than to a straight line—qualitative researchers are continually examining and interpreting data and making decisions about how to proceed based on what has already been discovered.

Because qualitative researchers have a flexible approach to collecting and analyzing data, it is impossible to define the flow of activities precisely—the flow varies from one study to another, and researchers themselves do not know ahead of time exactly how the study will unfold. We try to provide a sense of how a qualitative study is conducted, however, by describing some major activities and indicating how and when they might be performed.

Conceptualizing and Planning a Qualitative Study

IDENTIFYING A RESEARCH PROBLEM

Qualitative researchers generally begin with a general topic area, often focussing on an aspect of a topic that is poorly understood and about which little is known. They therefore do not develop hypotheses or pose refined research questions at the outset. Qualitative researchers often proceed with a fairly broad research question that allows the focus to be sharpened and delineated more clearly once they are in the field.

DOING A LITERATURE REVIEW

Qualitative researchers do not all agree about the value of doing an upfront literature review. Some believe that the literature should not be consulted before collecting new data. Their concern is that prior studies might unduly influence their conceptualization of the phenomenon under study. According to this view, the phenomenon should be elucidated based on participants' viewpoints rather than on prior information. Others believe that researchers should conduct at least a cursory literature review at the outset. In any event, qualitative researchers typically find a relatively small body of relevant literature because of the type of questions they ask.

SELECTING AND GAINING ENTRÉE INTO RESEARCH SITES

Before going into the field, qualitative researchers must identify a site that is consistent with the research topic. For example, if the topic is the health care beliefs of the urban poor, an inner-city neighborhood with a concentration of low-income residents must be identified. In many cases, researchers need to make preliminary contacts with key actors in the site to ensure cooperation and access to informants (i.e., researchers need to **gain entrée** into the site). Gaining entrée typically involves negotiations with *gatekeepers* who have the authority to permit entry into their world.

DESIGNING QUALITATIVE STUDIES

Quantitative researchers do not collect data before finalizing the research design. Qualitative researchers, by contrast, use an **emergent design**—a design that emerges during the course of data collection. Certain design features are guided by the study's qualitative tradition, but qualitative studies do not have a rigid structure that prohibits changes in the field.

ADDRESSING ETHICAL ISSUES

Qualitative researchers, like quantitative researchers, must also develop plans for addressing ethical issues—and, indeed, there are special concerns in qualitative studies because of the more intimate nature of the relationship that typically develops between researchers and study participants.

Conducting a Qualitative Study

In qualitative studies, the activities of sampling, data collection, data analysis, and interpretation typically take place iteratively. Qualitative researchers begin by talking with or observing people who have first-hand experience with the phenomenon under study. The discussions and observations are loosely structured, allowing participants to express a full range of beliefs, feelings, and behaviors. Analysis and interpretation are ongoing, concurrent activities, used to guide decisions about whom to sample next and what questions to ask or observations to make. The actual process of data analysis involves clustering together related types of narrative information into a coherent scheme.

As analysis and interpretation progress, the researcher begins to identify *themes* and categories, which are used to build a descriptive theory of the phenomenon. The kinds of data obtained become increasingly focused and purposeful as a theory emerges. Theory development and verification shape the sampling and data gathering process—as the theory develops, the researcher seeks participants who can confirm and enrich the theoretical understandings as well as participants who can potentially challenge them and lead to further theoretical development.

Quantitative researchers decide in advance how many subjects to include in the study, but qualitative researchers' sampling decisions are guided by the data themselves. Many qualitative researchers use the principle of **saturation**, which occurs when themes and categories in the data become repetitive and redundant, such that no new information can be gleaned by further data collection.

Quantitative researchers seek to collect high-quality data by using measuring instruments with demonstrated reliability and validity. Qualitative researchers, by contrast, *are* the main data collection instrument and must take steps to ensure the trustworthiness of the data while in the field. The central feature of these efforts is to confirm that the findings accurately reflect the experiences and viewpoints of the participants, rather than the researchers' perceptions. For example, one confirmatory activity involves going back to participants and sharing preliminary interpretations with them so that they can evaluate whether the researcher's thematic analysis is consistent with their experiences.

Disseminating Qualitative Findings

Both qualitative and quantitative nurse researchers strive to share their findings with other nurses and health care specialists. Qualitative research reports are increasingly being published in the nursing literature.

Quantitative reports almost never contain any **raw data**—data exactly in the form they were collected, which are numeric values. Qualitative reports, by contrast, are generally filled with rich verbatim passages directly from study participants. The excerpts are used in an evidential fashion to support or illustrate researchers' interpretations and thematic construction.

Example of raw data in a qualitative report:

Stewart (2003) conducted a grounded theory study to examine uncertainty experienced by children with cancer. The children's uncertainty was sometimes a reflection of not being sure about what things meant, as illustrated by the following quote:

Well, I thought like something was going on when I was first sick because two doctors would come into the room with like five nurses and I'd be worried. It scared me...I thought they would have to wheel me away or something [laughs] and do some experiments on me or something (p. 400).

Like quantitative researchers, qualitative nurse researchers want to see their findings used by others. Qualitative findings often are the basis for formulating hypotheses that are tested by quantitative researchers, and for developing measuring instruments used for both research and clinical purposes. Qualitative findings can also provide a foundation for designing effective nursing interventions. Qualitative studies help to shape nurses' perceptions of a problem or situation, their conceptualization of potential solutions, and their understanding of patients' concerns and experiences.

CHAPTER REVIEW

Key new terms introduced in the chapter, together with a summary of major points, are presented in this section. In addition, Chapter 3 of the *Study Guide to Accompany Essentials of Nursing Research,* 6th edition offers various exercises and study suggestions for reinforcing the concepts presented in this chapter. For additional review, see the Student Self-Study Review Questions section of the Student Resource CD-ROM provided with this book.

KEY NEW TERMS

Coding
Emergent design
Ethnography
Experimental research
Gaining entrée
Grounded theory
Intervention protocol
Literature review
Nonexperimental research
Phenomenology

Pilot study
Population
Raw data
Research design
Research report
Sample
Sampling plan
Saturation
Statistical analyses

S U M M A R Y   P O I N T S

- Quantitative studies are either experimental or nonexperimental. In **experimental research**, researchers actively intervene or introduce a treatment, while in **nonexperimental research**, researchers make observations of existing characteristics and behavior without intervening.

- Qualitative nursing research often is rooted in research traditions that originate in the disciplines of anthropology, sociology, and psychology. Three such traditions are ethnography, grounded theory, and phenomenology.

- **Grounded theory** seeks to describe and understand key social psychological and structural processes that occur in a social setting.

- **Phenomenology** is concerned with lived experiences and is an approach to learning about what people's life experiences are like and what they mean.

- **Ethnography** provides a framework for studying the meanings, patterns, and experiences of a defined cultural group in a holistic fashion.

- In a quantitative study, researchers progress in a linear fashion from posing a research question to answering it in fairly standard steps.

- The main phases in a quantitative study are the conceptual, planning, empirical, analytic, and dissemination phases.

- The conceptual phase involves: defining the problem to be studied, doing a **literature review**, engaging in clinical fieldwork for clinical studies, developing a framework and conceptual definitions, and formulating hypotheses to be tested.

- The design and planning phase entails selecting a **research design**; formulating the **intervention protocol**; specifying the **population**; developing a **sampling plan**; specifying methods to measure the research variables; designing procedures to protect subjects' rights, and finalizing the research plan (and, in some cases, conducting a **pilot study**).

- The empirical phase involves collecting the data and preparing the data for analysis (e.g., **coding** the data).

- The analytic phase involves analyzing the data through **statistical analysis** and interpreting the results.

- The dissemination phase entails communicating the findings and promoting their utilization.

- The flow of activities in a qualitative study is more flexible and less linear than in a quantitative study.

- Qualitative researchers begin with a broad question that is narrowed through the actual process of data collection and analysis.

- In the early phase of a qualitative study, researchers select a site and then take steps to **gain entrée** into it; gaining entrée typically involves enlisting the cooperation of *gatekeepers* within the site.

- Qualitative studies typically involve an **emergent design**: researchers select informants, collect data, and then analyze and interpret the data in an ongoing fashion. Field experiences help to shape the design of the study.

- Early analysis leads to refinements in sampling and data collection, until **saturation** (redundancy of information) is achieved.

- Qualitative researchers conclude by disseminating findings that can subsequently be used to inform the direction of further studies, to guide the development of structured measuring tools, and to influence nurses' perceptions of a problem or situation and their conceptualizations of potential solutions.

RESEARCH EXAMPLES   Critical Thinking Activities

EXAMPLE 1: Quantitative Research

The progression of activities in a quantitative study by one of this book's authors (Beck) is summarized below, followed by some questions to guide critical thinking. (The full research report is available in *Nursing Research, 25,* 155–164.)

Study

"Further validation of the Postpartum Depression Screening Scale" (Beck & Gable, 2001)

Study Purpose

Beck and Gable undertook a study to evaluate the Postpartum Depression Screening Scale (PDSS), an instrument designed for use by clinicians and researchers to screen mothers for postpartum depression (PPD).

Phase 1. Conceptual Phase, 1 Month: This phase was the shortest, because most of the conceptual work had been done earlier in developing the screeening instrument (Beck & Gable, 2000). The literature had already been reviewed, so all that was needed was to update the review. The same framework and conceptual definitions that had been used in the first study were used in the new study.

Phase 2. Design and Planning Phase, 6 Months: The second phase involved fine-tuning the research design, gaining entrée into the hospital where subjects were recruited, and obtaining approval from the hospital's ethics review committee. During this period Beck met with statistical consultants and an instrument development consultant numerous times to finalize the study design.

Phase 3. Empirical Phase, 11 Months: The design called for administering the PDSS to 150 mothers who were 6 weeks postpartum, and then scheduling a psychiatric diagnostic interview for them to determine if they were suffering from PPD. Recruitment of subjects and data collection took nearly a year before the desired sample size was achieved.

Phase 4. Analytic Phase, 3 Months: Statistical tests were performed to determine a cut-off score on the PDSS above which mothers would be identified as having screened positive for PPD. Data analysis also was undertaken to determine the accuracy of the PDSS in predicting diagnosed PPD.

Phase 5. Dissemination Phase, 18 Months: The researchers prepared a research report and submitted it to the journal *Nursing Research* for possible publication. It was accepted for publication within 4 months, but it was "in press" (awaiting publication) for 14 months. During this period, the authors presented their findings at regional and international conferences, and prepared a summary report for the agency that funded the research.

Key Findings

Beck and Gable found that the PDSS was a reliable and valid tool for screening mothers and considered that the scale was ready for routine use.

RESEARCH EXAMPLES *Continued*

Critical Thinking Suggestions*

*See the Student Resource CD-ROM for a discussion of these questions.

1. Answers questions 1 and 3 from Box 1-1 (Chapter 1) regarding this study.

2. Also consider the following targeted questions, which may further sharpen your critical thinking skills and assist you in understanding this study:

    a. Was the study experimental or nonexperimental?

    b. What do you think the *population* for this study was?

    c. How would you evaluate Beck and Gable's dissemination plan?

    d. What are your thoughts about how time was allocated in this study, i.e., how much time was spent in each phase?

    e. Would it have been appropriate for the researchers to address the research question using qualitative research methods? Why or why not?

3. If the results of this study are valid and generalizable, what are some of the uses to which the findings might be put in clinical practice?

 EXAMPLE 2: Qualitative Research

The progression of activities in a qualitative study by one of this book's authors (Beck) is summarized below, followed by some questions to guide critical thinking. (The full research report is available in *Qualitative Health Research, 12,* 593–608.)

Study

"Releasing the pause button: Mothering twins during the first year of life" (Beck, 2002)

Study Purpose

The researcher undertook a grounded theory study to explore the phenomenon of mothering twins during the first year after delivery.

Phase 1. Conceptual Phase, 3 Months: Beck became interested in mothers of multiples as a result of her quantitative studies on postpartum depression (PPD). These studies had revealed a much higher prevalence of PPD among mothers of multiples than among those of singletons. Beck had never studied multiple births before, and so she carefully reviewed that literature. Gaining entrée into the research site (a hospital) did not take long because she had previously conducted a study there and was known to the hospital's gatekeepers.

Phase 2. Design and Planning Phase, 4 Months: After reviewing the literature in the conceptual phase, a grounded theory design was selected because Beck wanted to (1) discover the basic problem mothers with twins experience and (2) describe the process these mothers used to cope with this problem during the first year of their twins' lives. The researcher met with the nurse who headed a support group to plan the best approach for recruiting mothers of twins into the study. Plans were also made for Beck to attend the monthly meetings of the support group. Once the design was finalized, the research proposal was submitted to ethics review committees.

research examples continue on page 64

| **RESEARCH EXAMPLES** | *Continued* |

Phase 3. Empirical/Analytic Phase, 10 Months: Data collection and data analysis occurred simultaneously in this study. Beck attended the "parents of multiples" support group for 10 months. During that period, she conducted in-depth interviews with 16 mothers of twins in their homes, and analyzed her rich and extensive data. Some steps Beck used to enhance the trustworthiness of her findings included (1) audiotaping all the interviews so that she would have verbatim transcripts to use for data analysis and (2) validating her developing grounded theory with mothers of twins who attended one of the multiple birth parent meetings at the hospital.

Phase 4. Dissemination Phase, 23 Months: A manuscript was written describing this study and submitted for publication to *Qualitative Health Research*, which published the report in 2002. Beck also presented the findings at a regional nursing research conference and a neonatal/perinatal symposium in the midwest.

Key Findings

Beck's analysis indicated that "life on hold" was the basic problem mothers of twins experienced during the first year of their twins' lives. As mothers attempted to resume their own lives, they progressed through a four-stage process that Beck called "releasing the pause button."

Critical Thinking Suggestions

1. Answer questions 1 and 3 from Box 1-1 (Chapter 1) regarding this study.
2. Also consider the following targeted questions, which may further sharpen your critical thinking skills and assist you in understanding this study:
    a. What are your thoughts about how time was allocated in this study, that is, how much time was spent in each phase?
    b. Given the focus of the study, do you think that grounded theory was the appropriate research design to use?
    c. Who was one of the gatekeepers in the hospital who helped Beck recruit her sample?
    d. Would it have been appropriate for the researchers to address the research question using quantitative research methods? Why or why not?
3. If the results of this study are valid and generalizable, what are some of the uses to which the findings might be put in clinical practice?

 EXAMPLE 3: Quantitative Research

The progression of activities in the Motzer et al. study ("Sense of Coherence") in Appendix A is not spelled out in detail in the report (this is normal), but there are a few clues that provide some insights about scheduling. Answer the following questions regarding the timeframes of the study:

1. Over how long a period were the data for this study collected? (See the subsection labeled "Sample.") Why do you think it took this long to collect the data?
2. When do you think the investigators wrote a research proposal to apply for financial support from NINR, given when the data were collected?
3. When was the study accepted for publication? (See the end of the report, prior to the references.) What does this suggest about when the data were analyzed and the report was written?

RESEARCH EXAMPLES | *Continued*

4. How long did it take between when the report was accepted for publication and when it was published?

5. What is your estimate of how long the study took, from the time it was conceptualized until the time when the report was published?

 EXAMPLE 4: Qualitative Research

The progression of activities in Beck's study ("Birth Trauma") in Appendix B is not spelled out in detail in the report, but there are a few clues that provide some insights about scheduling. Answer the following questions regarding the timeframes of the study:

1. Over how long a period were the data for this study collected? (See the subsection labeled "Procedure.") Why do you think it took this long to collect the data?

2. Did Beck receive funding to complete her study? (Information regarding funding is usually found at the end of a report, just prior to references, or in a footnote on the first page of a report.)

3. When was the study accepted for publication? (See the end of the report, prior to the references.) What does this suggest about when the data were analyzed and the report was written?

4. How long did it take between when the report was accepted for publication and when it was published?

5. What is your estimate of how long the study took, from the time it was conceptualized until the time when the report was published?

SUGGESTED READINGS

Methodologic References

Creswell, J. W. (1998). *Qualitative inquiry and research design: Choosing among five traditions*. Thousand Oaks, CA: Sage Publications.

Glaser, B. G., & Strauss, A. L. (1967). *The discovery of grounded theory: Strategies for qualitative research*. Chicago: Aldine.

Kerlinger, F. N., & Lee, H. B. (2000). *Foundations of behavioral research*. (4th ed.). Orlando, FL: Harcourt College Publishers.

Studies Cited in Chapter 3

Beck, C. T. (2002). Releasing the pause button: Mothering twins during the first year of life. *Qualitative Health Research, 12,* 593–608.

Beck, C. T., & Gable, R. K. (2000). Postpartum Depression Screening Scale: Development and psychometric testing. *Nursing Research, 49,* 272–282.

Beck, C. T., & Gable, R. K. (2001). Further validation of the Postpartum Depression Screening Scale. *Nursing Research, 50,* 155–164.

Bonner, A., & Walker, A. (2004). Nephrology nursing: Blurring the boundaries—the reality of expert practice. *Journal of Clinical Nursing, 13,* 210–218.

deVera, N. (2003). Perspectives on healing foot ulcers by Yaquis with diabetes. *Journal of Transcultural Nursing, 14,* 39–47.

Ironside, P. M., Scheckel, M., Wessels, C., Bailey, M. E., Powers, S., & Seeley, D. K. (2003). Experiencing chronic illness: Cocreating new understandings. *Qualitative Health Research, 13,* 171–183.

Norr, K. F., Crittendon, K. S., Lehrer, E. L., Reyes, O., Boyd, C. B., Nacion, K. W., Watanabe, K. et al. (2003). Maternal and infant outcomes at one year for a nurse-health advocate home visiting program serving African American and Mexican Americans. *Public Health Nursing, 20,* 190–203.

Stewart, J. L. (2003). "Getting used to it": Children finding the ordinary and routine in the uncertain context of cancer. *Qualitative Health Research, 13,* 394–407.

Turner, C., Boyle, F., & O'Rourke, P. (2003). Mothers' health post-partum and their patterns of seeking vaccination for their infants. *International Journal of Nursing Practice, 9,* 120–126.

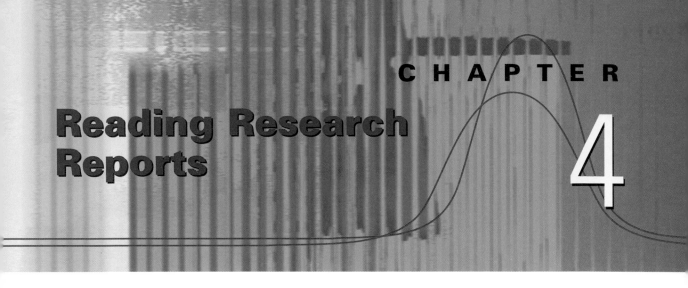

Reading Research Reports

CHAPTER 4

STUDENT OBJECTIVES

On completing this chapter, you will be able to:

▶ Name major types of research reports
▶ Identify and describe the major sections in a research journal article
▶ Characterize the style used in quantitative and qualitative research reports
▶ Distinguish research summaries and research critiques
▶ Define new terms in the chapter

TYPES OF RESEARCH REPORTS

Evidence from nursing studies is communicated through *research reports* that describe what was studied, how it was studied, and what was found. Research reports—especially reports for a quantitative study—are often daunting to readers without research training. This chapter is designed to help make research reports more accessible even before you become familiar with research methods.

Researchers communicate information about their studies in various ways. The most common types of research reports are theses and dissertations, books, presentations at conferences, and journal articles. Nurses are most likely to be exposed to research results at professional conferences or in journals.

Presentations at Professional Conferences

Research findings are presented at conferences as oral presentations or poster sessions.

▶ *Oral presentations* follow a format similar to that used in journal articles, which we discuss later in this chapter. The presenter of an oral report is typically allotted 10 to 20 minutes to describe the most important aspects of the study.

▶ In **poster sessions**, many researchers simultaneously present visual displays summarizing their studies, and conference attendees circulate around the room perusing these displays.

Conference presentations are an important avenue for communicating research information. One attractive feature is that less time may elapse between the completion of a study and the dissemination of findings than is the case with journal articles. Conferences also offer an opportunity for dialogue between researchers and conference attendees. The listeners at oral presentations and viewers of poster displays can ask questions to help them better understand how the study was conducted or what the findings mean; moreover, they can offer the researchers suggestions relating to the clinical implications of the study. Thus, professional conferences offer a particularly valuable forum for a clinical audience.

Research Journal Articles

Research **journal articles** are reports that summarize studies in professional journals. Because competition for journal space is keen, the typical research article is brief—generally only 10 to 25 double-spaced manuscript pages. This means that researchers must condense a lot of information about the study purpose, research methods, findings, interpretation, and clinical significance into a short report.

Journals accept research reports on a competitive basis. Usually, research articles are reviewed by two or more **peer reviewers** (other researchers doing work in the field) who make recommendations about whether the article should be accepted, rejected, or revised and re-reviewed. These are usually **"blind" reviews**—reviewers are not told researchers' names, and researchers are not told reviewers' names.

In major nursing research journals, the rate of acceptance is low—it can be as low as 5% of submitted articles. Thus, consumers of research journal articles have some assurance that the reports have already been scrutinized for their merit by other nurse researchers. Nevertheless, the publication of an article does not mean that the findings can be uncritically accepted. The validity of the findings and their utility for clinical practice depend on how the study was conducted. Research methods courses help consumers to evaluate the quality of research evidence reported in journal articles.

THE CONTENT OF RESEARCH JOURNAL ARTICLES

Research reports in journals tend to follow a certain format and to be written in a particular style. Research reports begin with a title that succinctly conveys (typically in 15 or fewer words) the nature of the study. In qualitative studies, the title normally includes the central phenomenon and group under investigation; in quantitative studies, the title generally indicates the independent and dependent variables and the population.

Quantitative reports—and many qualitative reports—typically follow a conventional format for organizing content referred to as the **IMRAD format**. This format involves organizing material into four sections—Introduction, Methods, Results, and Discussion. The main text of the report is usually preceded by an abstract and followed by references.

The Abstract

The **abstract** is a brief description of the study placed at the beginning of the journal article. The abstract answers, in about 100 to 200 words, the following questions: What were the research questions? What methods did the researcher use to address those questions? What did the researcher find? and What are the implications for nursing practice? Readers can review an abstract to assess whether the entire report should be read.

Some journals have moved from having traditional abstracts—which are single paragraphs summarizing the main features of the study—to slightly longer and more informative abstracts with specific headings. For example, abstracts in *Nursing Research* after 1997 present information about the study organized under the following headings: Background, Objectives, Method, Results, Conclusions, and Key Words.

Box 4-1 presents abstracts from two actual studies. The first is a "new style" abstract for a quantitative study entitled "Predictors of infectious disease symptoms in inner city households" (Larson, Lin, & Gomez-Pichardo, 2004). The second is a more traditional abstract for a qualitative study entitled "Families of origin of homeless and never-homeless women" (Anderson & Imle, 2001). These two studies are used as illustrations throughout this chapter.

The Introduction

The introduction acquaints readers with the research problem and its context. The introduction usually describes the following:

▶ *The central phenomena, concepts, or variables under study.* The problem area under investigation is identified.
▶ *The statement of purpose, research questions, and/or hypotheses to be tested.* Readers are told what the researcher set out to accomplish by conducting the study.

BOX 4.1   **Examples of Abstracts From Published Research**

Quantitative Study

Background: Despite the fact that hygienic practices have been associated with reduced risk of infection for decades, the potential role of specific home hygiene and cleaning practices in reducing risk has not been explicated.

Objective: This study aimed to determine the incidence and predictors of infectious disease symptoms over a 48-week period in inner city households.

Methods: Cleaning and hygiene practices and the incidence of infectious disease symptoms were closely monitored prospectively for 48 months in 238 households. Each household was contacted by trained interviewers weekly via telephone, was visited monthly, and underwent an extensive home interview quarterly.

Results: The incidence of new symptoms in the month before quarterly home visits ranged from 8.9% to 12.4% for individuals and from 32% to 39.7% for households. Four factors were significantly associated with infection. Drinking only bottled water increased risk (relative risk [RR], 2.1; 95% confidence interval [CI], 1.2-3.7). Using hot water (RR, 0.7; 95% CI, .5-.9) and bleach (RR, 0.29; 95% CI, .23-.66) for laundry and reporting that germs were most likely to be picked up in the kitchen (RR, 0.5; 95% CI, .3-.8) were protective. No other hygiene practices, including hand washing, were associated with infection risk.

Conclusions: Further studies of a potential role for bottled water in infections are warranted, as is a renewed appreciation for the potential protective role of laundry practices such as using bleach and hot water (Larson, Lin, & Gomez-Pichardo, 2004).

Qualitative Study

Naturalistic inquiry was used to compare the characteristics of families of origin of homeless women with never-homeless women. The women's experiences in their families of origin were explored during in-depth interviews using Lofland and Lofland's conceptions of meanings, practices, episodes, roles, and relationships to guide the analysis. The two groups were similar with respect to family abuse history, transience, and loss. The never-homeless women had support from an extended family member who provided unconditional love, protection, a sense of connection, and age-appropriate expectations, as contrasted with homeless women who described themselves as being without, disconnected, and having to be little adults in their families of origin. The experiences of family love and connection seemed to protect never-homeless women from the effects of traumatic life events in childhood. These findings provide support for the influence of a woman's family of origin as a precursor to homelessness (Anderson & Imle, 2001).

▶ *A review of the related literature.* Current knowledge relating to the study problem is briefly described so readers can understand how the study fits in with previous findings and can assess the contribution of the new study.

▶ *The theoretical framework.* In theoretically driven studies, the framework is usually presented in the introduction.

▶ *The significance of and need for the study.* Most research reports include an explanation of why the study is important to nursing.

Thus, the introduction sets the stage for a description of what the researcher did and what was learned. The information in the introduction corresponds roughly to the activities undertaken in the conceptual phase of the project, as described in Chapter 3.

Example of an introductory paragraph

The homeless in the United States continue to increase in numbers and in diversity.... An estimated 760,000 people experience homelessness at some time during a 1-year period.... Women and families make up the fastest-growing segment of the homeless population, and women head an estimated 90% of homeless families. The purpose of this study was to compare the characteristics of families of origin of homeless women with the families of origin of never-homeless women whose childhood experiences placed them at risk for homelessness (Anderson & Imle, 2001, p. 394).

In this paragraph, the researchers described the background of the problem, the population of primary interest (homeless women), and the study purpose.

CONSUMER TIP

The introduction section of many reports are not specifically labeled "Introduction." The report's introduction immediately follows the abstract.

■

The Method Section

The method section describes the methods the researcher used to answer the research questions. The method section tells readers about major methodologic decisions and may offer rationales for those decisions. For example, a report for a qualitative study often explains why a qualitative approach was considered to be especially appropriate and fruitful.

In a report for a quantitative study, the method section usually describes the following, which may be in specifically labeled subsections:

▶ *The research design.* A description of the research design focuses on the overall plan for structuring the study, often including the steps the researcher took to minimize biases and control extraneous variables.
▶ *The sample.* Quantitative research reports usually describe the population under study, specifying the criteria by which the researcher decided whether a person would be eligible for the study. The method section also describes the actual sample, indicating how people were selected and the number of subjects in the sample.
▶ *Measures and data collection.* In the method section, researchers describe the methods and procedures used to collect the data, including how the critical research variables were operationalized; they also present information concerning the quality of the measuring tools.
▶ *Study procedures.* The method section contains a description of the procedures used to conduct the study, including a description of any intervention. The researcher's efforts to protect the rights of human subjects may also be documented in this section.

Table 4-1 presents excerpts from the method section of the quantitative study by Larson and her colleagues (2004), describing aspects of their research design, sample, data collection strategies, and procedures.

Qualitative researchers discuss many of the same issues, but with different emphases. For example, reports for a qualitative study often provide more information about the research

TABLE 4.1	Excerpts From Method Section, Quantitative Report
METHODOLOGIC ELEMENT	**EXCERPT FROM LARSON et al.'s STUDY, 2004***
Research design	This descriptive correlational study was a component of a larger double-blinded clinical trial in which households were randomly assigned to use personal and household cleaning products with and without antimicrobial ingredients (p. 190).
Sample	The study was conducted in an inner city community in northern Manhattan composed of Hispanics (>90%) living primarily in large, multiunit apartment buildings....Potential households were recruited by experienced bilingual interviewers through posters and flyers written in English and Spanish and placed at local churches, preschools, clinics, WIC offices, and elementary schools....The study enrolled 238 households....(pp. 190–191).
Data collection	The Home Hygiene Assessment Form was designed specifically for this study and was tested extensively for validity and reliability in pilot work....This form is a 31-page interview booklet including demographic factors and illness information for each household member (and) detailed information (54 items) about home hygiene practices....(p. 191).
Procedures	Households recruited over a 3-month period received a baseline visit and then four additional home visits (quarterly) for the subsequent 48 weeks, between October 2000 and February 2002 (p. 191).

* From Larson, E. L., Lin, S. X., & Gomez-Pichardo, C. (2004). Predictors of infectious disease symptoms in inner-city households. *Nursing Research, 53*, 190–197.

setting and the study context and less information on sampling. Also, because formal instruments are not used to collect qualitative data, there is little discussion about data collection methods, but there may be more information on data collection procedures. Increasingly, reports of qualitative studies are including descriptions of the researchers' efforts to ensure the trustworthiness of the data. Some qualitative reports also have a subsection on data analysis. There are fairly standard ways of analyzing quantitative data, but such standardization does not exist for qualitative data, so qualitative researchers may describe their analytic approach. Table 4-2 presents excerpts from the method section of the qualitative study by Anderson and Imle (2001), describing aspects of their design, sample, data collection, and data analysis.

In quantitative studies, the method section describes decisions made during the design and planning phase of the study and implemented during the empirical phase (see Chapter 3). In qualitative studies, the methodologic decisions are made during the planning stage and also during the course of fieldwork.

CONSUMER TIP

The method section is sometimes called "Method" and sometimes called "Methods" (plural). Either is acceptable, although the manual of style used by many nursing journals (from the American Psychological Association) says "Method."

TABLE 4.2 **Excerpts From Method Section, Qualitative Report**

METHODOLOGIC ELEMENT	EXCERPT FROM ANDERSON & IMLE'S STUDY, 2001*
Design	Naturalistic inquiry was used to explore the families of origin of homeless and never-homeless women from their perspectives (p. 397).
Sample	The criteria for inclusion in the study were that the women had never been homeless, had experienced traumatic childhoods, were at least 18 years of age and spoke English.... The inclusion criteria for the study of homeless women were that the women had experienced homelessness, had taken steps toward moving away from life on the streets, were age 18 or over, and spoke English. The homeless ($n = 12$) and never-homeless ($n = 16$) women were similar in age, number of persons in the family of origin... education, ethnicity, and abuse histories (p. 398).
Data collection	One to three in-depth interviews, lasting 45 minutes to 2 hours, were conducted with both homeless and never-homeless women. Intensive interviewing is especially well suited to a retrospective study that relies on the participant to recall their memories because the setting described no longer exists.... All interviews were conducted by the author (p. 397).
Data analysis	Social units of analysis... were used to organize and assist in the coding and analysis of the interview data. The five social units that emerged during the interviews with the homeless sample were analyzed in the sample of never-homeless women and themes were identified (p. 400)

* From Anderson, D. G., & Imle, M. A. (2001). Families of origin of homeless and never-homeless women. *Western Journal of Nursing Research*, *23*, 394–413.

The Results Section

The results section presents the research **findings** (i.e., the results obtained in the analyses of the data). The text presents a narrative summary of the findings, often accompanied by tables or figures that highlight the most noteworthy results.

Virtually all results sections contain basic descriptive information, including a description of the study participants (e.g., their average age). In quantitative studies, the researcher provides descriptive information about key variables, using simple statistics. For example, in a study of the effect of prenatal drug exposure on the birth outcomes of infants, the results section might begin by describing the average birth weights and Apgar scores of the infants, or the percentage who were of low birth weight (under 2500 g).

In quantitative studies, the results section also reports the following information relating to the statistical analyses performed:

▶ *The name of statistical tests used.* A **statistical test** is a procedure for testing hypotheses and evaluating the believability of the findings. For example, if the percentage of low-birth-weight infants in the sample of drug-exposed infants is computed, how probable is it that the percentage is accurate? If the researcher finds that the average birth weight of drug-exposed infants in the sample is lower than the birth weight of infants who were not exposed to drugs, how probable is it that the same would be true for other infants not in the sample? That is, is the relationship between prenatal drug exposure and infant birth weight *real* and likely to be replicated with a new sample of infants from the same population? Statistical tests answer such questions. Statistical tests are based on common principles; you do not have to know the names of all statistical tests (there are dozens of them) to comprehend the findings.

▶ *The value of the calculated statistic.* Computers are used to compute a numeric value for the particular statistical test used. The value allows the researchers to draw conclusions about the meaning of the results. The *actual* numeric value of the statistic, however, is not inherently meaningful and need not concern you.

▶ *The significance.* The most important information is whether the results of the statistical tests were significant (not to be confused with important or clinically relevant). If a researcher reports that the results were **statistically significant**, it means that, based on the statistical test, the findings are probably reliable and replicable with a new group of people. Research reports also indicate the **level of significance**, which is an index of how probable it is that the findings are reliable. For example, if a report indicates that a finding was significant at the .05 level, this means that only 5 times out of 100 ($5 \div 100 = .05$) would the obtained results be spurious. In other words, 95 times out of 100, similar results would be obtained with other samples from the same population. Readers can therefore have a high degree of confidence—but not total assurance—that the findings are accurate.

Example from the results section of a quantitative study

Only 49.2% of the households in which bleach was used reported infectious disease symptoms, as compared with 76.7% of the households in which bleach was not used (relative risk [RR], .29, 95% confidence interval [CI], .23–.66; $p = .001$) (Larson et al., 2004, p. 192).

In this excerpt, the authors indicated that the rate of infectious disease symptoms was different in households that differed with regard to the use of bleach for laundry. The use of bleach was *significantly* protective, with over 50 percent more households reporting a symptom if bleach was not used. The difference of nearly 28 percentage points in rates of experiencing symptoms was unlikely to have been a fluke of this sample, and would likely be replicated with a new sample. The probability (*p*) that the difference between "bleach" and "no bleach" households is spurious is less than 1 in 1000 ($1 \div 1000 = .001$). Thus, the finding is highly reliable. Note that to comprehend this finding, you do not need to understand what the RR statistic is or what a confidence interval is, nor do you need to concern yourself with the actual value of the statistic, .29.

CONSUMER TIP

Be especially alert to the *p* values (probabilities) when reading statistical results. If a *p* value is greater than .05 (e.g., $p = .08$), the results are considered *not* to be statistically significant by conventional standards. Nonsignificant results are sometimes abbreviated NS. Also, be aware that the results are *more* reliable if the *p* value is smaller. For example, there is a higher probability that the results are accurate when $p = .01$ (only 1 in 100 chance of a spurious result) than when $p = .05$ (5 in 100 chances of a spurious result). Researchers sometimes report an exact probability estimate (e.g., $p = .03$) or a probability below conventional thresholds (e.g., $p < .05$—less than 5 in 100).

■

In qualitative reports, the researcher often organizes findings according to the major *themes*, processes, or categories that were identified in the data. The results section of qualitative reports sometimes has several subsections, the headings of which correspond to the researcher's labels for the themes. Excerpts from the raw data are presented to support and provide a rich description of the thematic analysis. The results section of qualitative studies may also present the researcher's emerging theory about the phenomenon under study, although this may appear in the concluding section of the report.

Example from the results section of a qualitative study

The homeless people interviewed did not have a sense of connectedness.... In contrast, the never-homeless women had connections to family and friends, and to larger social systems that lasted into adulthood and the foreseeable future.... Many of the never-homeless also described tangible links to their past. Robin, for example, described her dining room set that had belonged to her adopted grandparents:

> *I was always told that this table came with them on a covered wagon.... They paid $35 for this set; that includes the chairs and buffet.... There are places on here that have [her brother's] teeth marks. I used to play house under here (Anderson & Imle, 2001, p. 409).*

In this excerpt, the researchers illustrate their finding that never-homeless women maintained rich connections with their past with a direct quote from a study participant.

The Discussion

In the discussion section, the researcher draws conclusions about the meaning and implications of the findings. This section tries to unravel what the results mean, why things turned out the way they did, and how the results can be used in practice. The discussion in both qualitative and quantitative reports may incorporate the following elements:

▶ *An interpretation of the results.* The interpretation involves the translation of findings into practical, conceptual, or theoretical meaning.
▶ *Implications.* Researchers often offer suggestions for how their findings could be used to improve nursing, and they may also make recommendations on how best to advance knowledge in the area through additional research.
▶ *Study limitations.* The researcher is in the best position possible to discuss study limitations, such as sample deficiencies, design problems, and so forth. Reports that identify these limitations indicate to readers that the author was aware of these limitations and probably took them into account in interpreting the findings.

Example from a discussion section of a quantitative report

It might be expected that if bleach and hot water had an important protective effect against infections, this would have been described previously....The microbicidal efficacy of bleach is well established..., and therefore a protective effect of hypochlorites is plausible. To the authors' knowledge, however, this is the first study to identify a protective effect of home laundry practices against infectious disease symptoms (Larson et al., 2004, p. 195).

As this example illustrates, researchers may speculate in the discussion section about *why* certain findings turned out the way they did.

References

Research journal articles conclude with a list of the books, reports, and journal articles that were referenced in the report. If you are interested in pursuing additional reading on a substantive topic, the reference list of a recent study is an excellent place to begin.

THE STYLE OF RESEARCH JOURNAL ARTICLES

Research reports tell a story. However, the style in which many research journal articles are written—especially reports of quantitative studies—makes it difficult for beginning research consumers to become interested in the story. To unaccustomed audiences, research reports may seem pedantic or bewildering. Four factors contribute to this impression:

- *Compactness.* Journal space is limited, so authors compress many ideas and concepts into a short space. Interesting, personalized aspects of the investigation often cannot be reported. And, in qualitative studies, only a handful of supporting quotes can be included.
- *Jargon.* The authors of both qualitative and quantitative reports use research terms that are assumed to be part of readers' vocabulary but that may seem esoteric.
- *Objectivity.* Quantitative researchers normally avoid any impression of subjectivity, and so their research stories are told in a way that makes them sound impersonal. For example, most quantitative research reports are written in the passive voice (i.e., personal pronouns are avoided). Use of the passive voice tends to make a report less inviting and lively than use of the active voice, and it tends to give the impression that the researcher did not play an active role in conducting the study. (Qualitative reports, by contrast, are more subjective and personal and are written in a more conversational style.)
- *Statistical information.* In quantitative reports, numbers and statistical symbols may intimidate readers who do not have strong mathematic interest or training. Most nursing studies are quantitative; thus, most research reports summarize the results of statistical analyses.

A goal of this textbook is to assist you in understanding the content of research reports and in overcoming anxieties about jargon and statistical information.

READING, SUMMARIZING, AND CRITIQUING RESEARCH REPORTS

Nurses who want to develop an evidence-based practice must be able to read and critically appraise research reports. This section offers some general guidance on reading and evaluating nursing research reports.

Reading and Summarizing Research Reports

The skills involved in critical appraisal take time to develop. The first step in being able to use research findings in clinical practice is to comprehend research reports. Your first few attempts to read a research report might be overwhelming, and you may wonder whether being able to understand, let alone appraise, research reports is a realistic goal. As you progress through this textbook, you will acquire skills to help you evaluate various aspects of research reports. Some preliminary tips on digesting research reports follow:

▶ Grow accustomed to the style of research reports by reading them frequently, even though you may not yet understand all the technical points. Try to keep the underlying rationale for the style of research reports in mind as you read.

▶ Read from a report that has been photocopied so that you can use a highlighter, underline material, write notes in the margins, and so on.

▶ Read journal articles slowly. It may be useful to skim the article first to get the major points and then to read the article more carefully a second time.

▶ On the second or later reading of a journal article, train yourself to become an *active* reader. Reading actively involves constantly monitoring yourself to determine whether you understand what you are reading. If you have comprehension problems, go back and re-read difficult passages or make notes about your confusion so that you can ask someone for clarification. In most cases, that "someone" will be your research instructor or another faculty member, but also consider contacting the researchers themselves. The postal and e-mail addresses of the researchers are usually included in the journal article, and researchers are generally more than willing to discuss their research with others.

▶ Keep this textbook with you as a reference while you read articles initially, so that you can look up unfamiliar terms in the glossary at the end of the book or in the index.

▶ Try not to get bogged down in (or scared away by) the statistical information. Try to grasp the gist of the story without letting formulas and numbers frustrate you.

▶ Until you become accustomed to the style and jargon of research journal articles, you may want to "translate" them mentally or in writing. You can do this by expanding compact paragraphs into looser constructions, by translating jargon into more familiar terms, by recasting sentences into an active voice, and by summarizing findings with words rather than with numbers. As an example, Box 4-2 presents a summary of a fictitious study about the psychological consequences of having an abortion, written in the style typically found in research journal articles. Terms that can be looked up in the glossary of this book are underlined, and bolded marginal notes indicate the type of information the author is communicating. Box 4-3 presents a "translation" of this summary, recasting the research information into language that is more digestible. Note that it is not just the jargon specific to research methods that makes the original version complicated (e.g., "sequelae" is more obscure than "consequences"). Thus, a dictionary may also be needed when reading research reports.

When you attain a reasonable level of comprehension of a research report, a useful next step is to write a brief (one- to two-page) synopsis of the study. A synopsis summarizes the study's purpose, research questions, methods, findings, interpretation of the findings, and implications for practice. You do not need to be concerned at this point about critiquing the study's strengths and weaknesses, but rather about succinctly and objectively presenting a summary of what was done and what was learned. By preparing a synopsis, you will become more aware of aspects of the study that you did not comprehend.

Critiquing Research Reports

A written research **critique** is different from a research summary or synopsis. A research critique is a careful, critical appraisal of a study's strengths and limitations. Critiques usually conclude

BOX 4.2   Summary of a Fictitious Study for Translation

Purpose of the study	The potentially negative sequelae of having an abortion on the psychological adjustment of adolescents have not been adequately studied. The present study sought to determine whether alternative pregnancy resolution decisions have different long-term effects on the psychological functioning of young women.	**Need for the study**
Research design	Three groups of low-income pregnant teenagers attending an inner-city clinic were the <u>subjects</u> in this study: those who delivered and kept the baby; those who delivered and relinquished the baby for adoption; and those who had an abortion.	**Study population**
Research instruments	There were 25 subjects in each group. The study <u>instruments</u> included a self-administered <u>questionnaire</u> and a battery of psychological tests measuring depression, anxiety, and psychosomatic symptoms. The instruments were administered upon entry into the study (when the subjects first came to the clinic) and then 1 year after termination of the pregnancy.	**Research sample**
Data analysis procedure	The <u>data</u> were analyzed using <u>analysis of variance (ANOVA)</u>. The ANOVA tests indicated that the three groups did not differ significantly in terms of depression, anxiety, or psychosomatic symptoms at the initial testing. At the <u>post-test</u>, however, the abortion group had significantly higher scores on the depression scale, and these girls were significantly more likely than the two delivery groups to report severe tension headaches. There were no <u>significant</u> differences on any of the <u>dependent variables</u> for the two delivery groups.	**Results**
Implications	The results of this study suggest that young women who elect to have an abortion may experience a number of long-term negative consequences. It would appear that appropriate efforts should be made to follow up abortion patients to determine their need for suitable treatment.	**Interpretation**

BOX 4.3   Translated Version of Fictitious Research Study

As researchers, we wondered whether young women who had an abortion had any emotional problems in the long run. It seemed to us that not enough research had been done to know whether any psychological harm resulted from an abortion.

We decided to study this question ourselves by comparing the experiences of three types of teenagers who became pregnant—first, girls who delivered and kept their babies; second, those who delivered the babies but gave them up for adoption; and third, those who elected to have an abortion. All teenagers in our sample were poor, and all were patients at an inner-city clinic. Altogether, we studied 75 girls—25 in each of the three groups. We evaluated the teenagers' emotional states by asking them to fill out a questionnaire and to take several psychological tests. These tests allowed us to assess things such as the girls' degree of depression and anxiety and whether they had any complaints of a psychosomatic nature. We asked them to fill out the forms twice: once when they came into the clinic, and then again a year after the abortion or the delivery.

We learned that the three groups of teenagers looked pretty much alike in terms of their emotional states when they first filled out the forms. But when we compared how the three groups looked a year later, we found that the teenagers who had abortions were more depressed and were more likely to say they had severe tension headaches than teenagers in the other two groups. The teenagers who kept their babies and those who gave their babies up for adoption looked pretty similar 1 year after their babies were born, at least in terms of depression, anxiety, and psychosomatic complaints.

Thus, it seems that we might be right in having some concerns about the emotional effects of having an abortion. Nurses should be aware of these long-term emotional effects, and it even may be advisable to institute some type of follow-up procedure to find out if these young women need additional help.

---

with the reviewer's summary of the study's merits, recommendations regarding the value of the evidence, and suggestions about improving the study or the report itself.

Research critiques of individual studies are prepared for various reasons, and they differ in scope, depending on their purpose. Peer reviewers who are asked to prepare a written critique for a journal considering publication of the report generally critique the following aspects of the study:

▶ *Substantive*—Was the research problem significant to nursing? Can the study make an important contribution?
▶ *Theoretical*—Were the conceptual or theoretical underpinnings sound?
▶ *Methodologic*—Were the methods appropriate? Are the resulting findings believable?
▶ *Interpretive*—Did the researcher properly interpret data and develop reasonable conclusions?
▶ *Ethical*—Were the rights of study participants protected?
▶ *Stylistic*—Is the report clearly written, grammatical, and well organized?

In short, peer reviewers do a comprehensive review to provide feedback to the researchers and to journal editors about the merit of both the study and the report, and typically offer suggestions for improvements (e.g., for redoing some analyses).

By contrast, a critique of a study that is designed to inform decisions about nursing practice need not be as comprehensive. For example, it is of little significance to practicing nurses that a research report is ungrammatical. A critique on the clinical utility of a study focuses on whether the findings are accurate, believable, and clinically meaningful. If the findings cannot be trusted, it makes little sense to incorporate them into nursing practice.

By understanding research methods, you will be in a position to critique the scientific merit of studies, and this is a primary aim of this book. Most chapters in this book offer guidelines for evaluating various research decisions that will help you to make an overall appraisal of a research study.

Competent consumers of research must be able to critique not only single, independent studies, but also a body of studies on a topic of clinical interest. We discuss literature reviews in Chapter 7, and we further explore the role of integrative reviews in the final chapter.

CHAPTER REVIEW

Key new terms introduced in the chapter, together with a summary of major points, are presented in this section. In addition, Chapter 4 of the *Study Guide to Accompany Essentials of Nursing Research,* 6th edition offers various exercises and study suggestions for reinforcing the concepts presented in this chapter. For additional review, see the Student Self-Study Review Questions section of the Student Resource CD-ROM provided with this book.

KEY NEW TERMS

Abstract	Level of significance
Blind review	p
Critique	Peer reviewer
Findings	Poster session
IMRAD format	Statistical significance
Journal article	Statistical test

SUMMARY POINTS

▷ The most common types of research reports are theses and dissertations, books, conference presentations (including oral reports and **poster sessions**), and, especially, journal articles.

▷ Research **journal articles** provide brief descriptions of research studies and are designed to communicate the contribution the study has made to knowledge.

▷ Quantitative journal articles (and many qualitative ones) typically follow the **IMRAD format** with the following sections: **I**ntroduction (explanation of the study problem and its context); **M**ethods (the strategies used to address the research problem); **R**esults (the actual study **findings**); **and D**iscussion (the interpretation of the findings).

▷ Journal articles typically begin with an **abstract** (a brief synopsis of the study) and conclude with references (a list of works cited in the report).

▷ Research reports are often difficult to read because they are dense, concise, and contain a lot of jargon.

▷ Qualitative research reports are written in a more inviting and conversational style than quantitative ones, which are more impersonal and include information on statistical tests.

▷ **Statistical tests** are procedures for testing research hypotheses and evaluating the believability of the findings. Findings that are **statistically significant** are ones that have a high probability (p) of being accurate.

▷ The ultimate goal of this book is to help students to prepare a research **critique**, which is a careful, critical appraisal of the strengths and limitations of a piece of research, often for the purpose of considering the worth of its evidence for nursing practice.

RESEARCH EXAMPLES Critical Thinking Activities

EXAMPLE 1: Quantitative Research

An abstract for a quantitative nursing study is presented below, followed by some questions to guide critical thinking. (The full research report is available in *Journal of Cardiovasular Nursing, 18,* 197–206.)

Study

"Compliance behaviors of elderly patients with advanced heart failure" (Evangelista, Doering, Dracup, Westlake, Hamilton, & Fonarow, 2003)

Abstract

Although compliance behaviors of heart failure (HF) patients have become the focus of increasing scrutiny in the last decade, the prevalence of noncompliance among elderly patients with HF is poorly understood. We conducted this study to describe and compare the compliance behaviors of elderly patients ($\geq$65 years) and younger patients ($<$65 years) with HF on six prescribed activities: medical appointments, medications, diet, exercise, smoking cessation, and alcohol abstinence. Data from a sample of 140 older (50%) and younger (50%) HF patients matched for gender and disease severity were collected with the HF Compliance Questionnaire and analyzed via descriptive statistics, chi-square, paired *t*-tests, and Pearson correlations. We found that elderly patients were more compliant with diet (77% versus 65%, $p = .001$) and exercise (67% versus 55%, $p = .021$) than were their younger counterparts. There was no difference in the other health care behaviors. Of the 70 elderly patients, 51% reported some degree of difficulty complying with exercise while 37%, 24%, and 23% had difficulty following diet, keeping follow-up appointments, and taking medications, respectively. A smaller percentage of elders continued to smoke (9%) and drink alcohol (18%). Patients were asked why they had difficulty following their health care regimens; responses varied by prescribed activity. Lastly, we found inverse relationships between perceived difficulty following and compliance with all of the six behaviors measured ($p < .001$); as difficulty increased, compliance decreased. Strategies to help older patients minimize perceived difficulties associated with health care regimens may improve compliance and long-term morbidity and mortality from HF. Assumptions about older age being related to noncompliance appear invalid in patients with HF.

Critical Thinking Suggestions*

*See the Student Resource CD-ROM for a discussion of these questions.
1. "Translate" the abstract into a summary that is more consumer-friendly. (Underline any technical terms and look them up in the glossary.)
2. Also consider the following targeted questions:
    a. What was the independent variable in this study? How was it operationalized?
    b. What was the dependent variable in this study? How was it operationalized?
    c. Was the study experimental or nonexperimental?
    d. The abstract specifically mentions that the researchers controlled for two extraneous variables. Can you identify what those two variables were?

RESEARCH EXAMPLES *Continued*

> **e.** Would it have been appropriate for the researchers to address the research question using qualitative research methods? Why or why not?

3. If the results of this study are valid and generalizable, what are some of the uses to which the research evidence might be put in clinical practice?

 EXAMPLE 2: Qualitative Research

An abstract for a qualitative nursing study is presented below, followed by some questions to guide critical thinking. (The full research report is available in *Qualitative Health Research, 13,* 319–332.)

Study

"Prenatal care use among women of low income: A matter of 'taking care of self'" (Sword, 2003)

Abstract

The grounded theory study discussed in this article provides a theoretical explanation of prenatal care use among women of low income. The author recruited 26 women from two communities in Ontario, Canada, to participate in an individual or focus group interview and analyzed data using descriptive coding, interpretive coding, and constant comparison. Perceptions of the health care system were identified as important influences on usage behavior. This broad theme included two subthemes: (a) program and service attributes and (b) service provider characteristics. Within each subtheme, both barriers to and facilitative factors for prenatal care became apparent. The author examined relationships among categories to identify a unifying construct. Taking care of self emerged as the central phenomenon that explained usage behavior. Women weigh the pros and cons when deciding whether to access prenatal care, and then take charge, ultimately making a decision in terms of its meaning for self.

Critical Thinking Suggestions

1. "Translate" the abstract into a summary that is more consumer-friendly. (Underline any technical terms and look them up in the glossary.)

2. Also consider the following targeted questions:
   a. What was the phenomenon under investigation in this study?
   b. What qualitative research tradition was used in this study? Based on what you've learned thus far about qualitative research traditions, does the selected tradition appear to be appropriate to address the research question?
   c. In this traditional abstract what main features of the study were summarized?
   d. Would it have been appropriate for the researchers to address the research question using quantitative research methods? Why or why not?

3. If the results of this study are trustworthy, what are some of the uses to which the research evidence might be put in clinical practice?

research examples continue on page 92

RESEARCH EXAMPLES   *Continued*

 EXAMPLE 3: Quantitative Research

Read the abstract for the study by Seskevich and colleagues, "Beneficial Effects of Noetic Therapies," which can be found in the Research Articles section of the Student Resource CD-ROM. "Translate" the abstract into a summary that is more consumer-friendly.

 EXAMPLE 4: Qualitative Research

Read the abstract for Knobf's study ("Carrying On"), also on the Student Resource CD-ROM. "Translate" the abstract into a summary that is more consumer-friendly.

SUGGESTED READINGS

Methodologic References

Downs, F. S. (1999). How to cozy up to a research report. *Applied Nursing Research, 12,* 215–216.

Rankin, M., & Esteves, M. D. (1996). How to assess a research study. *American Journal of Nursing, 96,* 32–37.

Sandelowski, M., & Barroso, J. (2002). Finding the findings in qualitative studies. *Journal of Nursing Scholarship,* 34, 213–219.

Tornquist, E. M., Funk, S. G., Champagne, M. T., & Wiese, R. A. (1993). Advice on reading research: Overcoming the barriers. *Applied Nursing Research, 6,* 177–183.

Studies Cited in Chapter 4

Anderson, D. G., & Imle, M. A. (2001). Families of origin of homeless and never-homeless women. *Western Journal of Nursing Research, 23,* 394–413.

Evangelista, L., Doering, L. V., Dracup, K., Westlake, C., Hamilton, M., & Fonarow, G. C. (2003). Compliance behaviors of elderly patients with advanced heart failure. *Journal of Cardiovascular Nursing, 18,* 197–206.

Larson, E. L., Lin, S. X., & Gomez-Pichardo, C. (2004). Predictors of infectious disease symptoms in inner-city households. *Nursing Research, 53,* 190–197.

Sword, W. (2003). Prenatal care use among women of low income: A matter of "taking care of self." *Qualitative Health Research, 13,* 319–332.

Reviewing the Ethical Aspects of a Nursing Study

STUDENT OBJECTIVES

On completing this chapter, you will be able to:

▶ Discuss the historical background that led to the creation of various codes of ethics
▶ Understand the potential for ethical dilemmas stemming from conflicts between ethics and requirements for high quality research evidence
▶ Identify the three primary ethical principles articulated in the *Belmont Report* and the important dimensions encompassed by each
▶ Identify procedures for adhering to ethical principles and protecting study participants
▶ Understand the issues relating to research misconduct
▶ Given sufficient information, evaluate the ethical dimensions of a research report
▶ Define new terms in the chapter

ETHICS AND RESEARCH

Nurses face many ethical issues in their practice. The prolongation of life by artificial means, the institution of tube feedings when patients are unable to sustain oral nourishment, and the testing of new products with critically ill patients are but a few examples. Situations such as these have led to numerous discussions about ethics in nursing practice. Similarly, increased research with humans has led to ethical concerns about the rights of study participants. Ethics can create particular challenges to nurse researchers because ethical requirements sometimes conflict with the need to produce the highest possible quality evidence for practice. This chapter discusses some of the major ethical principles that should be considered in reviewing studies.

Historical Background

As modern, civilized people, we might like to think that systematic violations of moral principles within a research context occurred centuries ago rather than in recent times, but this is not the case. The Nazi medical experiments of the 1930s and 1940s are the most famous example of recent disregard for ethical conduct. The Nazi program of research involved the use of prisoners of war and racial "enemies" in experiments designed to test the limits of human endurance and human reaction to diseases and untested drugs. The studies were unethical not only because they exposed these people to permanent physical harm and even death, but also because the participants could not refuse participation.

There are recent examples from the United States and other western countries. For instance, between 1932 and 1972, a study known as the Tuskegee Syphilis Study, sponsored by the U. S. Public Health Service, investigated the effects of syphilis on 400 men from a poor Black community. Medical treatment was deliberately withheld to study the course of the untreated disease. Similarly, Dr. Herbert Green of the National Women's Hospital in Auckland, New Zealand studied women with cervical cancer in the 1980s; patients with carcinoma *in situ* were not given treatment so that researchers could study the natural progression of the disease. Another well-known case of unethical research involved the injection of live cancer cells into elderly patients at the Jewish Chronic Disease Hospital in Brooklyn in the 1960s without the consent of those patients. At about the same time, Dr. Saul Krugman was conducting research on hepatitis in the Willowbrook Study in nearby Staten Island. At Willowbrook, an institution for the mentally retarded, children were deliberately infected with the hepatitis virus. Even more recently, it was revealed in 1993 that U. S. federal agencies had sponsored radiation experiments since the 1940s on hundreds of people, many of them prisoners or elderly hospital patients. Many other examples of studies with ethical transgressions—often less obvious than these examples—have emerged to give ethical concerns the high visibility they have today.

Codes of Ethics

In response to human rights violations, various codes of ethics have been developed. One of the first internationally recognized sets of ethical standards is the Nuremberg Code, developed in 1949 after the Nazi atrocities were made public in the Nuremberg trials. Another notable set of international standards is the Declaration of Helsinki, which was adopted in 1964 by the World Medical Assembly and most recently revised in 2000. The ethical principles of the Declaration of Helsinki can be viewed at the World Medical Association website, www.wma.net/e/policy/b3.htm.

Most disciplines have established their own **code of ethics**. For example, guidelines for psychologists were published by the American Psychological Association (2002) in *Ethical Principles of Psychologist and Code of Conduct*. The American Sociological Association published the most recent version of its *Code of Ethics* in 1997. The American Medical Association regularly updates its *Code of Medical Ethics*. There is considerable overlap in the research-related principles articulated in these documents, but each deals with problems of particular concern to their respective disciplines.

Nurses have developed their own ethical guidelines. In the United States, the American Nurses Association (ANA) issued a statement in 1968 entitled "The Nurse in Research: ANA Guidelines on Ethical Values," and then in 1975 published *Human Rights Guidelines for Nurses in Clinical and Other Research*. In 1995 the ANA issued *Ethical Guidelines in the Conduct, Dissemination, and Implementation of Nursing Research* (Silva, 1995). Box 5-1 presents the nine ethical principles outlined in that document. Finally, in 2001 the ANA published a revised *Code of Ethics for Nurses With Interpretive Statements*, a document that covers primarily ethical issues for practicing nurses but that also includes principles that apply to nurse researchers. In Canada, the Canadian Nurses Association first published a document entitled *Ethical Guidelines for Nurses in Research Involving Human Participants* in 1983, which was revised most recently in 2002.

Some nurse ethicists have called for an international code of ethics for nursing research, but nurses in most countries have developed their own professional codes or follow the codes established by their governments. The International Council of Nurses, however, has developed a *Code for Nurses*, which was most recently updated in 2000.

BOX 5.1   Ethical Principles in Nursing Research

The investigator . . .

1. Respects autonomous research participants' capacity to consent to participate in research and to determine the degree and duration of that participation without negative consequences.
2. Prevents harm, minimizes harm, and/or promotes good to all research participants, including vulnerable groups and others affected by the research.
3. Respects the personhood of research participants, their families, and significant others, valuing their diversity.
4. Ensures that the benefits and burdens of research are equitably distributed in the selection of research participants.
5. Protects the privacy of research participants to the maximum degree possible.
6. Ensures the ethical integrity of the research process by use of appropriate checks and balances throughout the conduct, dissemination, and implementation of the research.
7. Reports suspected, alleged, or known incidents of scientific misconduct in research to appropriate institutional officials for investigation.
8. Maintains competency in the subject matter and methodologies of his or her research, as well as in other professional and societal issues that affect nursing research and the public good.
9. Involved in animal research maximizes the benefits of the research with the least possible harm or suffering to the animals.

From Silva, M. C. (1995). *Ethical guidelines in the conduct, dissemination, and implementation of nursing research* (pp. v–vi). Washington, DC: American Nurses Association.

Federal Regulations for Protecting Study Participants

In the United States, an especially important code of ethics was adopted by the National Commission for the Protection of Human Subjects of Biomedical and Behavioral Research (1978). The Commission, established by the National Research Act (Public Law 93-348), issued a report in 1978 (sometimes referred to as the ***Belmont Report***), which has been a model for many of the guidelines adopted by specific disciplines.

The *Belmont Report* also served as the basis for regulations affecting research sponsored by the federal government, including studies supported by NINR. The U.S. Department of Health and Human Services (DHHS) has issued ethical regulations that have been codified at Title 45 Part 46 of the Code of Federal Regulations. These regulations, revised most recently in 2001, are among the most widely used guidelines in the United States for evaluating the ethical aspects of studies in most disciplines.

CONSUMER TIP

The following websites offer information about various professional codes of ethics and ethical requirements for government-sponsored research:
▶ U.S. federal policy for the protection of human subjects in health research, from the Office of Human Subjects Research of NIH: http://ohsr.od.nih.gov
▶ American Nurses Association: www.ana.org/ethics
▶ International Council of Nurses: www.icn.ch/icncode.pdf
▶ American Psychological Association: www.apa.org/ethics/code.html
▶ American Sociological Association: www.asanet.org/members/ecoderev.html

Ethical Dilemmas in Conducting Research

Research that violates ethical principles is rarely done to be cruel but more typically occurs out of a conviction that knowledge is important and beneficial in the long run. There are situations in which the rights of participants and the demands of the research project are put in direct conflict, creating **ethical dilemmas** for researchers. In reading research reports, you need to be aware of such dilemmas. Here are some examples of research questions in which the desire for strong evidence conflicts with ethical considerations:

1. *Research question:* Are nurses equally empathic in their treatment of male and female patients in intensive care units?
   Ethical dilemma: Ethics require that participants be cognizant of their role in a study. Yet if the researcher informs the nurses in this study that their empathy in treating male and female patients will be scrutinized, will their behavior be "normal"? If the nurses alter their behavior because they know research observers are watching, the findings will not be valid.
2. *Research question:* What are the coping mechanisms of parents whose children have a terminal illness?
   Ethical dilemma: To answer this question, the researcher may need to probe into the psychological state of the parents at a vulnerable time in their lives; such probing could be painful and disturbing. Yet knowledge of the parents' coping mechanisms might help to design more effective ways of dealing with parents' grief and anger.

3. *Research question:* Does a new medication prolong life in cancer patients?
   Ethical dilemma: The best way to test the effectiveness of an intervention is to administer the intervention to some participants but withhold it from others to see whether differences between the groups emerge. However, if a new drug is untested, the group receiving it may be exposed to potentially hazardous side effects. On the other hand, the group *not* receiving the drug may be denied a beneficial treatment.
4. *Research question:* What is the process by which adult children adapt to the day-to-day stresses of caring for a parent with Alzheimer's disease?
   Ethical dilemma: In a qualitative study, which would be appropriate for this research question, the researcher sometimes becomes so closely involved with participants that they become willing to share "secrets" and privileged information. Interviews can become confessions—sometimes of unseemly or even illegal or immoral behavior. In this example, suppose a woman admitted to abusing her mother physically—how does the researcher respond to that information without undermining a pledge of confidentiality? And, if the researcher divulges the information to appropriate authorities, how can a pledge of confidentiality be given in good faith to other participants?

As these examples suggest, researchers are sometimes in a bind: Their goal is to advance knowledge, using the best methods possible, but they must also adhere to the dictates of ethical rules that have been developed to protect the rights of study participants.

ETHICAL PRINCIPLES FOR PROTECTING STUDY PARTICIPANTS

The *Belmont Report* articulates three primary ethical principles on which standards of ethical conduct in research are based: beneficence, respect for human dignity, and justice. We briefly discuss these principles and then describe procedures researchers adopt to comply with these principles.

Beneficence

One of the most fundamental ethical principles in research is that of **beneficence**, which imposes a duty on researchers to minimize harm and to maximize benefits. Human research should be intended to produce benefits for subjects themselves or—a situation that is more common—for other individuals or society as a whole. Ethical Principle 2 of the ANA guidelines (Box 5-1) addresses beneficence. This principle covers multiple dimensions.

THE RIGHT TO PROTECTION FROM HARM AND DISCOMFORT

A principle related to beneficence is **nonmaleficence**—researchers' duty to avoid, prevent, or minimize harm to study participants. Participants must not be subjected to unnecessary risks of harm or discomfort, and their participation in research must be essential to achieving scientifically and societally important aims that could not otherwise be realized. In research with humans, *harm* and *discomfort* can take many forms: they can be physical, emotional, social, or financial. Ethical researchers must use strategies to minimize all types of harms and discomforts, even ones that are temporary.

Exposing study participants to experiences that result in serious or permanent harm clearly is unacceptable. Ethical researchers must be prepared to terminate their research if they suspect that continuation would result in injury, death, or undue distress to study participants. Although protecting human beings from physical harm may be reasonably straightforward, the psychological consequences of participating in a study are generally subtle and thus require close attention and sensitivity. For example, participants may be asked questions about their personal views, weaknesses, or fears. Such queries might lead people to reveal sensitive personal information. The point is not that researchers should refrain from asking questions but rather that they need to analyze the nature of the intrusion on people's psyches.

The need for sensitivity may be even greater in qualitative studies, which often involve in-depth exploration into highly personal areas. In-depth probing may expose deep-seated worries and anxieties that study participants had previously repressed. Qualitative researchers, regardless of the underlying research tradition, must thus be especially vigilant in anticipating such problems.

THE RIGHT TO PROTECTION FROM EXPLOITATION

Involvement in a study should not place participants at a disadvantage or expose them to situations for which they have not been prepared. Participants need to be assured that their participation, or information they might provide, will not be used against them. For example, a woman divulging her income should not fear losing public health benefits; a person reporting drug abuse should not fear exposure to criminal authorities.

Study participants enter into a special relationship with researchers, and this relationship should not be exploited. Exploitation might be overt and malicious (e.g., sexual exploitation, use of participants' identification to create a mailing list, use of donated blood to develop a commercial product), but it might also be less flagrant (e.g., getting participants to provide additional information in a 1-year follow-up interview, without having warned them of this possibility at the outset).

Because nurse researchers may have a nurse–client (in addition to a researcher–participant) relationship, special care may be needed to avoid exploiting that bond. Patients' consent to participate in a study may result from their understanding of the researcher's role as *nurse,* not as *researcher.*

In qualitative research, the risk of exploitation may be especially acute because the psychological distance between investigators and participants typically declines as the study progresses. The emergence of a pseudotherapeutic relationship between researchers and participants is not uncommon, and this imposes additional responsibilities on researchers—and additional risks that exploitation could inadvertently occur. On the other hand, qualitative researchers are typically in a better position than quantitative researchers to do good, rather than just to avoid doing any harm, because of the close relationships they often develop with participants.

Respect for Human Dignity

Respect for the human dignity of participants is the second ethical principle articulated in the *Belmont Report.* This principle, which includes the right to self-determination and the right to full disclosure, is covered in the ANA guidelines under principles 1 and 3 (Box 5-1).

THE RIGHT TO SELF-DETERMINATION

Humans should be treated as autonomous agents, capable of controlling their own activities. The principle of *self-determination* means that prospective participants have the right to decide voluntarily whether to participate in a study, without the risk of incurring adverse consequences. It also means that participants have the right to ask questions, to refuse to give information, or to withdraw from the study.

A person's right to self-determination includes freedom from coercion of any type. *Coercion* involves explicit or implicit threats of penalty for failing to participate in a study or excessive rewards from agreeing to participate. The obligation to protect potential participants from coercion requires careful consideration when researchers are in a position of authority, control, or influence, as might be the case in a nurse–patient relationship. The issue of coercion may also require scrutiny even when there is not a preestablished relationship. For example, a generous monetary incentive (or **stipend**) offered to encourage the participation of an economically disadvantaged group (e.g., the homeless) might be mildly coercive because such incentives could place undue pressure on prospective participants.

In certain circumstances, participants' right to self-determination poses challenges. An important issue concerns some people's inability to make well-informed judgments about the costs and benefits of participation (e.g., children). We discuss the issue of special classes of research participants later in this chapter.

THE RIGHT TO FULL DISCLOSURE
The principle of respect for human dignity includes people's right to make informed, voluntary decisions about study participation, which requires full disclosure. **Full disclosure** means that the researcher has fully described the nature of the study, the person's right to refuse participation, the researcher's responsibilities, and the likely risks and benefits that would be incurred. The right to self-determination and the right to full disclosure are the two major elements on which informed consent—discussed later in this chapter—is based.

Adherence to the guideline for full disclosure is not, unfortunately, always straightforward. Full disclosure can sometimes result in two types of biases: (1) biases resulting from inaccurate data and (2) biases resulting from sample recruitment problems. Suppose we were testing the hypothesis that high school students with a high rate of absenteeism are more likely to be substance abusers than students with good attendance. If we approached potential participants and fully explained the study purpose, some students likely would refuse to participate. Nonparticipation would be selective; in fact, we would expect that those least likely to volunteer would be students who are substance abusers—the group of primary interest. Moreover, by knowing the specific research question, those who do participate might not give candid responses. It could be argued that full disclosure would totally undermine the study.

One technique that researchers sometimes use in such situations is **covert data collection**, or *concealment*—the collection of information without participants' knowledge and thus without their consent. This might happen, for example, if a researcher wanted to observe people's behavior in a real-world setting and was concerned that doing so openly would change the very behavior of interest. Researchers might choose to obtain information through concealed methods, such as by observing through a one-way mirror, videotaping participants through hidden equipment, or observing while pretending to be engaged in other activities.

A second, and more controversial, technique is the use of deception. *Deception* can involve either deliberately withholding information about the study or providing participants with false information. For example, we might describe the study of high school students' use of drugs as research on students' health practices, which is a mild form of misinformation.

Deception and concealment are problematic ethically because they interfere with the participants' right to make a truly informed decision about the personal costs and benefits of participation. Some people argue that the use of deception or concealment is never justified. Others, however, believe that if the study involves low risk to participants and if there are anticipated benefits to science and society, deception or concealment may be justified to enhance the validity of the findings. The ANA guidelines offer this advice about deception and concealment:

> *The investigator . . . understands that before concealment or deception is used, certain criteria must be met: (1) The study must be of such small risk to the research participant and of such great significance to the advancement of the public good that concealment or deception can be morally justified. . . . (2) The acceptability of concealment or deception is related to the degree of risks to research participants. . . . (3) Concealment or deception are used only as last resorts, when no other approach can ensure the validity of the study's findings. . . . (4) The investigator has a moral responsibility to inform research participants of any concealment or deception as soon as possible and to explain the rationale for its use (Silva, 1995, p. 10, Section 4.2).*

Another issue relating to full disclosure has emerged recently concerning the collection of data from people over the Internet (e.g., analyzing the content of messages posted to chat rooms or on listserves). The issue is whether such messages can be used as data without the authors' consent. Some researchers believe that anything posted electronically is in the public domain and therefore can be used without consent for purposes of research. Others, however, feel that the same ethical standards must apply in cyberspace research and that electronic researchers must carefully protect the rights of individuals who are involved in "virtual" communities. Schrum (1995) has developed some ethical guidelines for such researchers. As one example, she advocates that researchers negotiate their entry into an electronic community (e.g., a chat room) with the list owner prior to collecting electronic data.

Justice

The third broad principle articulated in the *Belmont Report* concerns justice. This principle includes participants' right to fair treatment and their right to privacy.

THE RIGHT TO FAIR TREATMENT
Justice connotes fairness and equity, and so one aspect of the justice principle concerns the equitable distribution of benefits and burdens of research. The selection of study participants should be based on research requirements and not on the vulnerability or compromised position of certain people. Historically, subject selection has been a key ethical concern, with many researchers selecting groups deemed to have lower social standing (e.g., poor people, prisoners, slaves, the mentally retarded) as study participants. The principle of justice imposes particular obligations toward individuals who are unable to protect their own interests (e.g., dying patients) to ensure that they are not exploited for the advancement of knowledge.

Distributive justice also imposes duties to neither neglect nor discriminate against individuals and groups who may benefit from advances in research. During the 1980s and early 1990s, there was growing evidence that women and minorities were being unfairly excluded from many clinical studies. This led to the promulgation of regulations requiring that researchers who sought funding from the National Institutes of Health (including NINR) include women and minorities as study participants. The regulations also required researchers to examine whether clinical interventions had any differential effects (e.g., whether benefits were different for men than for women).

The principle of fair treatment covers issues other than subject selection. For example, the right to fair treatment means that researchers must treat people who decline to participate in a study (or who withdraw from the study after agreeing to participate) in a nonprejudicial manner; that they must honor all agreements made with participants (including the payment of any promised stipends); that they demonstrate sensitivity to and respect for the beliefs, habits, and lifestyles of people from different cultures; and that they afford participants courteous and tactful treatment at all times.

THE RIGHT TO PRIVACY

Virtually all research with humans constitutes an intrusion into personal lives. Researchers should ensure that their research is not more intrusive than it needs to be and that the participants' privacy is maintained throughout the study. Participants have the right to expect that any data they provide will be kept in strictest confidence. Privacy issues have become even more salient in the U.S. health care community since the passage of the Health Insurance Portability and Accountability Act of 1996 (HIPAA), which articulates federal standards to protect patients' medical records and other health information.

CONSUMER TIP

The following websites provide advice about the effect of HIPAA on research: http://privacyruleandresearch.nih.gov and www.hhs.gov/ocr/hipaa/guidelines/ research.pdf. Olson (2003) also describes HIPAA privacy regulations and nursing research. ■

PROCEDURES FOR PROTECTING STUDY PARTICIPANTS

Now that you are familiar with fundamental ethical principles for conducting research, you need to understand the procedures researchers follow to adhere to them. It is these procedures that should be evaluated in critiquing the ethical aspects of a study.

CONSUMER TIP

When information about ethical considerations is presented in research reports, it almost always appears in the method section, typically in the subsection devoted to data collection procedures but sometimes in the subsection describing the sample. ■

Risk/Benefit Assessments

One of the strategies that researchers use to protect study participants—and that you as a reviewer can use to assess the ethical aspects of a study—is to conduct a **risk/benefit assessment**. Such an assessment is designed to determine whether the benefits of participating in a

BOX 5.2   Potential Benefits and Risks of Research to Participants

Major Potential Benefits to Participants

- Access to an intervention that might otherwise be unavailable to them
- Comfort in being able to discuss their situation or problem with a friendly, objective person
- Increased knowledge about themselves or their conditions, either through opportunity for introspection and self-reflection or through direct interaction with researchers
- Escape from a normal routine, excitement of being part of a study
- Satisfaction that information they provide may help others with similar problems or conditions
- Direct monetary or material gain through stipends or other incentives

Major Potential Risks to Participants

- Physical harm, including unanticipated side effects
- Physical discomfort, fatigue, or boredom
- Psychological or emotional distress resulting from self-disclosure, introspection, fear of the unknown, discomfort with strangers, fear of eventual repercussions, anger or embarrassment at the type of questions being asked
- Social risks, such as the risk of stigma, adverse effects on personal relationships, loss of status
- Loss of privacy
- Loss of time
- Monetary costs (e.g., for transportation, child care, time lost from work)

study are in line with the costs, be they financial, physical, emotional, or social—i.e., whether the *risk/benefit ratio* is acceptable. Box 5-2 summarizes major costs and benefits of research participation.

CONSUMER TIP

In your evaluation of the risk/benefit ratio of a study, you might consider whether you yourself would have felt comfortable being a study participant.

The risk/benefit ratio should also be considered in terms of whether the risks to research participants are commensurate with the benefit to society and the nursing profession. The degree of risk to be taken by those participating in the research should never exceed the potential humanitarian benefits of the knowledge to be gained. Thus, an important question in assessing the overall risk/benefit ratio is whether the study focuses on a significant topic that has the potential to improve patient care.

All research involves some risks, but in many cases, the risk is minimal. **Minimal risk** is defined as risks anticipated to be no greater than those ordinarily encountered in daily life or during routine physical or psychological tests or procedures. When the risks are not minimal, researchers must proceed with caution, taking every step possible to reduce risks and maximize benefits.

Example of risk/benefit assessment

Hentz (2002) studied the phenomenon of *body memory* following the loss of a loved one. Here is how she described risks and benefits: "One of the benefits for the participants was the ability to share experiences with someone interested and concerned. The other benefit was in knowing that the participants' stories may help others facing similar experiences. The actual interview often evoked strong emotions; however, many of the participants commented that they felt better having told their stroies. Having their stories heard and acknowledged was experienced by participants as therapeutic" (p. 165).

Informed Consent

One particularly important procedure for safeguarding human subjects and protecting their right to self-determination involves obtaining their informed consent. **Informed consent** means that participants have adequate information regarding the research; comprehend the information; and have the power of free choice, enabling them to consent voluntarily to participate in the research or decline participation. Researchers usually document the informed consent process by having participants sign a **consent form**, an example of which is presented in Figure 5-1. This form includes information about the study purpose, specific expectations regarding participation (e.g., how much time will be involved), the voluntary nature of participation, and potential costs and benefits.

Researchers rarely obtain written informed consent when the primary means of data collection is through self-administered questionnaires. Researchers generally assume **implied consent** (i.e., that the return of the completed questionnaire reflects the respondent's voluntary consent to participate). This assumption, however, is not always warranted (e.g., if patients feel that their treatment might be affected by failure to cooperate).

In some qualitative studies, especially those requiring repeated contact with participants, it is difficult to obtain a meaningful informed consent at the outset. Qualitative researchers do not always know in advance how the study will evolve. Because the research design emerges during the data collection and analysis process, researchers may not know the exact nature of the data to be collected, what the risks and benefits to participants will be, or how much of a time commitment will be required. Thus, in a qualitative study, consent may be viewed as an ongoing, transactional process, referred to as **process consent**. In process consent, researchers continuously renegotiate the consent, allowing participants to play a collaborative role in the decision-making process regarding their ongoing participation.

Example of informed consent in a quantitative study

Wilbur, Miller, Chandler, and McDevitt (2003) studied the factors that predicted women's adherence to a 24-week home-based walking program. Potential participants were screened for eligibility (e.g., no symptoms of cardiovascular disease). At the health assessment, the study was explained to the women; those who were eligible were asked to sign an informed consent form.

I understand that I am being asked to participate in a research study at Saint Francis Hospital and Medical Center. This research study will evaluate: What it is like being a mother of multiples during the first year of the infants' lives. If I agree to participate in the study, I will be interviewed for approximately 30 to 60 minutes about my experience as a mother of multiple infants. The interview will be tape-recorded and take place in a private office at St. Francis Hospital. No identifying information will be included when the interview is transcribed. I understand I will receive $25.00 for participating in the study. There are no known risks associated with this study.

I realize that I may not participate in the study if I am younger than 18 years of age or I cannot speak English.

I realize that the knowledge gained from this study may help either me or other mothers of multiple infants in the future.

I realize that my participation in this study is entirely voluntary, and I may withdraw from the study at any time I wish. If I decide to discontinue my participation in this study, I will continue to be treated in the usual and customary fashion.

I understand that all study data will be kept confidential. However, this information may be used in nursing publications or presentations.

I understand that if I sustain injuries from my participation in this research project, I will not be automatically compensated by Saint Francis Hospital and Medical Center.

If I need to, I can contact Dr. Cheryl Beck, University of Connecticut, School of Nursing, any time during the study.

The study has been explained to me. I have read and understand this consent form, all of my questions have been answered, and I agree to participate. I understand that I will be given a copy of this signed consent form.

_____   _____
Signature of Subject   Date

_____   _____
Signature of Witness   Date

_____   _____
Signature of Investigator   Date

FIGURE 5.1 Example of an informed consent form.

Example of process consent

Wuest, Ford-Gilboe, Merritt-Gray, and Berman (2003) studied the health promotion processes of single-parent families after leaving abusive partners/fathers. Tape-recorded interviews were conducted with 36 mothers in a location of their choice; each woman gave informed consent prior to participation. As data analysis proceeded, the researchers conducted second interviews with each family. On repeat interviews, consent was reconfirmed.

Confidentiality Procedures

Participants' right to privacy is protected either through anonymity or through other confidentiality procedures. **Anonymity** occurs when even the researcher cannot link a participant with his or her data. For example, if a researcher distributed questionnaires to a group of nursing home residents and asked that they be returned without any identifying information, the responses would be anonymous. As another example, if a researcher reviewed hospital records from which all identifying information (e.g., name, address, Social Security number, and so forth) had been expunged, anonymity would again protect people's right to privacy.

Example of anonymity

McKenna, Smith, Poole, and Coverdale (2003) studied interpersonal conflict ("horizontal violence") among nurses in New Zealand. An anonymous questionnaire was mailed to over 1000 newly registered nurses, asking them about the type and frequency of any interpersonal conflict they had experienced in their jobs.

In situations in which anonymity is impossible, researchers implement other confidentiality procedures. A promise of **confidentiality** to participants is a pledge that any information they provide will not be publicly reported or made accessible to parties not involved in the research.

Researchers generally develop elaborate confidentiality procedures. These include securing individual confidentiality assurances from everyone involved in collecting or analyzing research data; maintaining identifying information in locked files to which few people have access; substituting **identification (ID) numbers** for participants' names on study records and computer files to prevent any accidental *breach of confidentiality*; and reporting only aggregate data for groups of participants or taking steps to disguise a person's identity in a research report.

Extra precautions are often needed to safeguard participants' privacy in qualitative studies. Anonymity is rarely possible in qualitative research because researchers become thoroughly involved with participants. Moreover, because of the in-depth nature of many qualitative studies, there may be a greater invasion of privacy than in quantitative research. Researchers who spend time in participants' homes may, for example, have difficulty segregating the public behaviors participants are willing to share from the private behaviors that unfold unwittingly during data collection. A final thorny issue many qualitative researchers face is adequately disguising participants in their research reports to avoid a breach of confidentiality. Because the number of respondents is small and because rich descriptive information is presented in research reports, qualitative researchers need to take extra precautions to safeguard participants' identity. This may mean more than simply using a fictitious name—it may also mean withholding information about the characteristics of the informant, such as age and occupation.

Example of confidentiality procedures

Spiers (2002) described interpersonal contexts in which care was negotiated between home care nurses and their patients. Her qualitative study was based on an analysis of 31 videotaped home visits. The video portion of the tapes was not altered, inasmuch as the researcher wanted to analyze facial expressions. However, any audio containing names or other identifying information was removed in dubbed tapes. Pseudonyms were used in the transcripts.

CONSUMER TIP

As a means of enhancing both personal and institutional privacy, research reports frequently avoid giving explicit information about the locale of the study. For example, the report might state that data were collected in a 200-bed, private, for-profit nursing home, without mentioning its name or location.

                                                                                            ■.

Debriefings and Referrals

Researchers can often show their respect for study participants—and proactively minimize emotional risks—by carefully attending to the nature of the interactions they have with them. For example, researchers should always be gracious and polite, should phrase questions tactfully, and should be sensitive to cultural and linguistic diversity.

There are also more formal strategies that researchers can use to communicate their respect and concern for participants' well-being. For example, it is sometimes advisable to offer **debriefing** sessions after data collection is completed to permit participants to ask questions or air complaints. Debriefing is especially important when the data collection has been stressful or when ethical guidelines had to be "bent" (e.g., if any deception was used in explaining the study). Researchers can also demonstrate their interest in study participants by offering to share study findings with them once the data have been analyzed (e.g., by mailing them a summary or advising them of an appropriate website). Finally, in some situations, researchers may need to assist study participants by making referrals to appropriate health, social, or psychological services.

Example of referrals

In a study of the health of nearly 4000 poor women, Polit and co-researchers (2001) conducted 90-minute interviews covering such sensitive topics as substance abuse, depression, parenting stress, and domestic violence. Each interviewer had an information sheet with contact information for local service providers who could assist with any issue about which participants mentioned a need for help.

Treatment of Vulnerable Groups

Adherence to ethical standards is often straightforward. The rights of special vulnerable groups, however, may need to be protected through additional procedures and heightened sensitivity. **Vulnerable subjects** (the term used in federal guidelines) may be incapable of giving informed consent (e.g., comatose patients), may have *diminished autonomy* (e.g., prisoners), or may be at high risk of unintended side effects because of their circumstances (e.g., pregnant women). You should pay particular attention to the ethical dimensions of a study when people who are vulnerable are involved. Vulnerable groups include the following:

▶ *Children.* Legally and ethically, children do not have the competence to give their informed consent; therefore, the informed consent of children's parents or legal guardians should be obtained. However, it is advisable—especially if the child is at least 7 years old—to obtain the child's assent as well. **Assent** refers to the child's affirmative agreement to participate. If the child is developmentally mature enough to understand the basic information involved in informed consent (e.g., a 13-year-old), researchers should obtain written consent from the child as well, as evidence of respect for the child's right to self-determination.

▶ *Mentally or emotionally disabled people.* People whose disability makes it impossible for them to weigh the risks and benefits of participation and make an informed decision (e.g., people affected by cognitive impairment, mental illness, coma, and so on) also cannot legally or ethically provide informed consent. In such cases, researchers obtain written consent from the person's legal guardian. To the extent possible, informed consent from prospective participants should be sought as a supplement to consent from guardians.

▶ *Physically disabled people.* For certain physical disabilities, special procedures for obtaining consent may be required. For example, with deaf people, the entire consent process may need to be in writing. For people who cannot read or write or who have a physical impairment preventing them from writing, alternative procedures for documenting informed consent (e.g., videotaping the consent proceedings) can be used.

▶ *The terminally ill.* Terminally ill people who participate in a study can seldom expect to benefit personally from the research, and thus the risk/benefit ratio needs to be carefully assessed. Researchers must also take steps to ensure that if the terminally ill participate in the study, their health care and comfort are not compromised.

▶ *Institutionalized people.* Nurses often conduct studies with hospitalized or institutionalized people, and such people may feel pressured into participating or may believe that their treatment would be jeopardized by failure to cooperate. Inmates of prisons and other

---

Example of research with a vulnerable group

Anderson, Nyamathi, McAvoy, Conde, and Casey (2001) explored the perceptions of risk for HIV/AIDS among adolescents in juvenile detention. The researchers obtained approval to conduct the study from the presiding judge, the detention facility, and a human subjects committee at their own institution. They structured their protocols to assure teens that their participation would be voluntary and would influence neither the duration of their detention nor their adjudication process. Prospective participants received verbal and written explanations about the study. The explanations included directions about how to notify the researchers about their participation decision, which ensured the privacy of their decision from each other and from probation staff. After informed consent was obtained, the data were collected in spaces that provided privacy for sound and afforded visual surveillance by probation staff.

correctional facilities, who have lost their autonomy in many spheres of activity, may similarly feel constrained in their ability to give free consent. Researchers studying institutionalized groups need to emphasize the voluntary nature of participation.

▶ *Pregnant women.* The U.S. government has issued stringent requirements governing research with pregnant women. These requirements reflect a desire to safeguard both the pregnant woman, who may be at heightened physical and psychological risk, and the fetus, who cannot give informed consent. The regulations stipulate that pregnant women cannot be involved in a study unless risks to them and the fetus are minimal or unless the purpose of the research is to meet the women's health needs.

CONSUMER TIP

Some terms introduced in this chapter rarely are used explicitly in research reports. For example, a report almost never calls to the readers' attention that the study participants were *vulnerable subjects*. You need to be sensitive to the special needs of groups that may be unable to act as their own advocates or to assess adequately the costs and benefits of participating in a study.

Institutional Review Boards and External Reviews

It is sometimes difficult for researchers to be objective in doing risk-benefit assessments or in developing procedures to protect participants' rights. Biases may arise as a result of researchers' commitment to an area of knowledge and their desire to conduct a valid study. Because of the risk of a biased evaluation, the ethical dimensions of a study are usually subjected to external review.

Most hospitals, universities, and other institutions where research is conducted have established formal committees for reviewing research plans. These committees are sometimes called *human subjects committees* or (in Canada) *Research Ethics Boards*. If the researcher received funding from the U. S. government to help pay for the research, the committee likely will be called an **Institutional Review Board (IRB)**.

Studies supported with federal funds are subject to strict guidelines regarding the treatment of study participants, and the IRB's duty is to ensure that proposed procedures adhere to these guidelines. Before undertaking their study, researchers must submit research plans to the IRB, and must also undergo formal IRB training. An IRB can approve the proposed plans, require modifications, or disapprove them.

Example of IRB approval

Suen, Morris, and McDougall (2004) studied memory functions of older Taiwanese American adults. The researchers obtained approval from the IRB of their university, and also from the Taiwan Center (a community center) from which study participants were recruited.

Not all research is subject to federal guidelines, and not all studies are reviewed by IRBs or other formal committees. Nevertheless, researchers have a responsibility to ensure that their research plans are ethically acceptable, and it is a good practice for researchers to solicit external advice even when they are not required to do so.

CONSUMER TIP

Detailed information about the IRB process for NIH grants is available at http://ohrs.nih.gov/irb/irb.html.

OTHER ETHICAL ISSUES

When critiquing the ethical dimensions of a study, a prime consideration is the researchers' treatment of human study participants. Two other ethical issues also deserve mention: the treatment of animals in research and research misconduct.

Ethical Issues in Using Animals in Research

A small but growing number of nurse researchers use animals rather than human beings as their subjects, typically focusing on biophysiologic phenomena. Despite some opposition to such research by animal rights activists, it seems likely that researchers in health fields will continue to use animals to explore basic physiologic mechanisms and to test experimental interventions that could pose risks (as well as offer benefits) to humans.

Ethical considerations are clearly different for animals and humans; for example, the concept of *informed consent* is not relevant for animal subjects. Specific guidelines have been developed governing humane treatment of animal subjects. In the United States, the Public Health Service issued a "Policy on Humane Care and Use of Laboratory Animals," most recently amended in 2002 (http://grants.nih.gov/grants/olaw/references/phspol.htm). The guidelines articulate nine principles for the proper care and treatment of animals used in biomedical and behavioral research. These principles cover such issues as the transport of research animals, alternatives to using animals, pain and distress in animal subjects, researcher qualifications, the use of appropriate anesthesia, and euthanizing animals under certain conditions during or after the study.

Holtzclaw and Hanneman (2002), in discussing the use of animals in nursing research, noted several important considerations. First, there must be a compelling reason to use an animal model—not simply convenience or novelty. Second, the study procedures should be humane, well planned, and well funded. They noted that animal studies are not necessarily less costly than those with human participants, and they require serious ethical and scientific consideration to justify their use.

Example of animal research

Bartfay and Bartfay (2002) conducted a study to explore the link between iron overload and heart failure using a murine model. Twenty mice were housed in cages (five per cage) in a temperature- and humidity-controlled room with 12-hour light–dark cycles and given access to food and water. Half the mice were assigned to an iron-overload condition and the other half got a placebo. The researchers specifically noted that the study had institutional approval and that it conformed to the standards for animal treatment issued by the Canadian Council on Animal Care and by the Province of Ontario.

Research Misconduct

Millions of movie-goers watched breathlessly as Dr. Richard Kimble (Harrison Ford) exposed the fraudulent scheme of a medical researcher in the film *The Fugitive*. The film reminds us that ethics in research involves not only the protection of the rights of human and animal subjects, but also protection of the public trust.

The issue of **research misconduct** (also referred to as *scientific misconduct)* has received increasing attention in recent years as incidents of researcher fraud and misrepresentation have come to light. Currently, the federal agency responsible for overseeing efforts to improve research integrity in the United States and for handling allegations of research misconduct is the Office of Research Integrity (ORI) within the Department of Health and Human Services (http://ori.dhhs.gov), established in 1992.

The official definition of research misconduct is being revised, but the Public Health Service regulation (42 CFR Part 50, Subpart A) currently defines scientific misconduct as "fabrication, falsification, plagiarism, or other practices that seriously deviate from those that are commonly accepted within the scientific community for proposing, conducting, or reporting research. It does not include honest error or honest differences in interpretation or judgments of data." *Fabrication* involves making up study results and reporting them. *Falsification* involves manipulating research materials, equipment, or processes; it also involves changing or omitting data, or distorting results such that the research is not accurately represented in research reports. *Plagiarism* involves the appropriation of someone's ideas, results, or words without giving due credit, including information obtained through the confidential review of research proposals or manuscripts. Although the official definition focuses on only these three types of misconduct, there is widespread agreement that research misconduct covers many other issues including improprieties of authorship, poor data management, conflicts of interest, inappropriate financial arrangements, failure to comply with governmental regulations, and unauthorized use of confidential information.

Research dishonesty and fraud are major concerns in nursing—although examples of publicly exposed misconduct by nurse researchers are rare. Rankin and Esteves (1997), however, asked a sample of nursing research coordinators and deans about their experience with research misconduct; nearly half perceived that plagiarism occasionally occurred among faculty in their institutions, and about a third perceived that other offenses such as misrepresentation of findings or protocol violations sometimes occurred. Interest in the issue has not subsided. In May 2003, NINR and other institutes within NIH teamed with ORI to offer grants for researchers to study the factors that affect, both positively and negatively, integrity in research. The announcement indicated that NINR was particularly interested in research done by nurses in this area of interest.

In reading research reports, you are not likely to be able to detect research misconduct. Awareness of this issue is, however, critical to being an intelligent consumer of research.

CRITIQUING THE ETHICS OF RESEARCH STUDIES

Guidelines for critiquing the ethical aspects of a study are presented in Box 5-3. A person serving on an IRB or human subjects committee should be provided with sufficient information to answer all these questions. Research reports, however, do not always include detailed information

| BOX 5.3 | Questions for Critiquing the Ethical Aspects of a Study |

1. Was the study approved and monitored by an Institutional Review Board or other similar ethics review committee?
2. Were study participants subjected to any physical harm, discomfort, or psychological distress? Did the researchers take appropriate steps to remove or prevent harm?
3. Did the benefits to participants outweigh any potential risks or actual discomfort they experienced? Did the benefits to society outweigh the costs to participants?
4. Was any type of coercion or undue influence used to recruit participants? Did they have the right to refuse to participate or to withdraw without penalty?
5. Were participants deceived in any way? Were they fully aware of participating in a study and did they understand the purpose and nature of the research?
6. Were appropriate informed consent procedures used with all participants? If not, were there valid and justifiable reasons?
7. Were adequate steps taken to safeguard the privacy of participants? How were data kept anonymous or confidential?
8. Were vulnerable groups involved in the research? If yes, were special precautions instituted because of their vulnerable status?
9. Were groups omitted from the inquiry without a justifiable rationale (e.g., women, minorities)?

about ethical procedures because of space constraints in journals. Thus, it may not always be possible to critique researchers' adherence to ethical guidelines. Nevertheless, we offer a few suggestions for considering the ethical aspects of a study.

Many research reports do acknowledge that the study procedures were reviewed by an IRB or human subjects committee of the institution with which the researchers are affiliated. When a research report specifically mentions a formal external review, it is generally safe to assume that a panel of concerned people thoroughly reviewed the ethical issues raised by the study.

You can also come to some conclusions based on a description of the study methods. There may be sufficient information to judge, for example, whether study participants were subjected to physical or psychological harm or discomfort. Reports do not always specifically state whether informed consent was secured, but you should be alert to situations in which the data could not have been gathered as described if participation were purely voluntary (e.g., if data were gathered unobtrusively).

In thinking about the ethical aspects of a study, you should also consider who the study participants were. For example, if the study involved vulnerable groups, there should be more information about protective procedures. You might also need to attend to whom the study participants were *not*. For example, there has been considerable concern about the omission of certain groups (e.g., minorities) from clinical research.

It is often especially difficult to determine by reading research reports whether the privacy of the participants was safeguarded unless the researcher specifically mentions pledges of confidentiality or anonymity. A situation requiring special scrutiny arises when data are collected from two people simultaneously (e.g., a husband and wife who are jointly interviewed); in such situations, the absence of privacy raises not only ethical concerns but also questions regarding participants' candor.

CONSUMER TIP

Consumers, like researchers, must deal with ethical dilemmas. As a reviewer assessing the quality of research evidence for nursing practice, you must be critical of methodologic weaknesses—yet some weaknesses may reflect the researcher's need to conduct research ethically. ■

CHAPTER REVIEW

Key new terms introduced in the chapter, together with a summary of major points, are presented in this section. In addition, Chapter 5 of the *Study Guide to Accompany Essentials of Nursing Research,* 6th edition offers various exercises and study suggestions for reinforcing the concepts presented in this chapter. For additional review, see the Student Self-Study Review Questions section of the Student Resource CD-ROM provided with this book.

KEY NEW TERMS

Anonymity	Implied consent
Assent	Informed consent
Belmont Report	Institutional Review Board (IRB)
Beneficence	Minimal risk
Code of ethics	Nonmaleficence
Consent form	Process consent
Confidentiality	Research misconduct
Covert data collection	Risk/benefit assessment
Debriefing	Stipend
Ethical dilemma	Vulnerable subjects
Full disclosure	

SUMMARY POINTS

▷ Because research has not always been conducted ethically, and because of the genuine **ethical dilemmas** researchers often face in designing studies that are both ethical and methodologically rigorous, **codes of ethics** have been developed to guide researchers.

▷ The three major ethical principles incorporated into most guidelines are beneficence, respect for human dignity, and justice.

▷ **Beneficence** involves the performance of some good, and the protection of participants from physical and psychological harm and exploitation (**nonmaleficence**).

▷ *Respect for human dignity* includes the participants' right to **self-determination**, which means participants have the freedom to control their own activities, including their voluntary participation in the study.

▷ **Full disclosure** means researchers have fully described the study, including risks and benefits, to prospective participants. When full disclosure poses the risk of biased results, researchers sometimes use **covert data collection** or *concealment* (the collection of information without the participants' knowledge or consent) or *deception* (either withholding information from participants or providing false information).

▷ The principle of *justice* includes the right to fair and equitable treatment and to privacy.

▷ Various procedures have been developed to safeguard study participants' rights, including the performance of a risk/benefit assessment, the implementation of informed consent procedures, and taking steps to safeguard participants' confidentiality.

▷ In a **risk/benefit assessment**, the individual benefits of participation in a study (and societal benefits of the research) are weighed against the costs to individuals.

▷ **Informed consent** procedures, which provide prospective participants with information needed to make a reasoned decision about participation, normally involve the signing of a **consent form** to document voluntary and informed participation. In qualitative studies, consent may need to be continually renegotiated with participants as the study evolves, through **process consent** procedures.

▷ Privacy can be maintained through **anonymity** (wherein not even researchers know the participants' identity) or through formal **confidentiality** procedures that safeguard the information participants provide.

▷ Researchers sometimes offer **debriefing** sessions after data colllection to provide participants with more information or an opportunity to air complaints.

▷ **Vulnerable subjects** require additional protection as participants. They may be vulnerable because they are not able to make a truly informed decision about study participation (e.g., children), because of dimished autonomy (e.g., prisoners), or because their circumstances heighten the risk of physical or psychological harm (e.g., pregnant women).

▷ External review of the ethical aspects of a study by an **Institutional Review Board (IRB)** or other human subjects committee is highly desirable and may be required by either the agency funding the research or the organization from which participants are recruited.

▷ Ethical conduct in research involves not only protection of the rights of human and animal subjects, but also efforts to maintain high standards of integrity and avoid such forms of **research misconduct** as plagiarism, fabrication of results, or falsification of data.

RESEARCH EXAMPLES | Critical Thinking Activities

 EXAMPLE 1: Quantitative Research

Aspects of a quantitative nursing study, featuring key terms and ethical concepts discussed in this chapter, are presented below, followed by some questions to guide critical thinking. (The full research report is available in *Western Journal of Nursing Research, 25,* 75–92.)

Study

"Resourcefulness and self-care in pregnant women with HIV" (Boonpongmanee, Zauszniewski, & Morris, 2003)

Study Purpose

The purpose of the study was to understand the effects of depression and learned resourcefulness on prenatal self-care among pregnant Thai women who were HIV-positive.

research examples continue on page 104

RESEARCH EXAMPLES *Continued*

Study Methods

A sample of 77 pregnant women who were HIV-positive and 79 pregnant women who were HIV-negative was recruited from antenatal clinics of two Thai hospitals. All women provided information to address the research questions through in-person interviews.

Ethics-Related Procedures

The researchers recruited participants by asking HIV/AIDS counselors to provide information about the study to potential subjects. Women who came forward received "a detailed explanation of the procedures, the potential benefits and risks, and their rights ..." (p. 81). The researchers obtained written informed consent after the women agreed verbally to take part in the study. Each woman was told that "participation was strictly voluntary and had no effect on any services that she was receiving" (p. 82). Participants were also assured that the information they provided would be kept confidential and that results would be reported in aggregate form. To avoid any perception that their participation might be coerced, none of the HIV/AIDS counselors were involved in the data collection process. Trained interviewers collected the data in private rooms, using questionnaires that had been carefully translated into Thai. Interviews lasted about 30 minutes. The researchers obtained approval for the study from their university's IRB and from the research committees of both hospitals where the study took place.

Key Findings

▶ HIV status was not related to the pregnant women's self-care behaviors.
▶ Women who were depressed engaged in fewer prenatal self-care activities than women who were not depressed. Women who scored high on measures of learned resourcefulness tended to score high on the measure of self-care.

Critical Thinking Suggestions*

*See the Student Resource CD-ROM for a discussion of these questions.
1. Answer questions 1–8 from Box 5-3 regarding this study.
2. Also consider the following targeted questions, which may assist you in further assessing the ethical aspects of the study:
   a. Could the data in this study have been collected anonymously? Why do you think anonymity was not used?
   b. What do you think were the benefits of the research (to participants, to others)? What were the risks?
   c. The report did not mention any debriefings or referrals (which does not mean this did not occur). What would you recommend?
   d. If you had an HIV-positive friend or family member who was pregnant, how would you feel about her participating in the study?
3. If the results of this study are valid and reliable, what are some of the uses to which the findings might be put in clinical practice?

RESEARCH EXAMPLES *Continued*

 EXAMPLE 2: Qualitative Research

Aspects of a qualitative nursing study, featuring key terms and ethical concepts discussed in this chapter, are presented below, followed by some questions to guide critical thinking. (The full research report is available in *Journal of Obstetric, Gynecologic, & Neonatal Nursing, 32,* 58–67.)

Study

"Keeping safe: Teenagers' strategies for dealing with perinatal violence" (Renker, 2003)

Study Purpose

Renker explored the actions that teenagers take to keep safe from (or to deal with) violence before, during, and after pregnancy.

Study Methods

Renker recruited 20 teenagers (18- and 19-year-olds) who were no longer pregnant but who had experienced violence during a pregnancy. All women were interviewed in person and asked in-depth questions about their coping strategies relating to violence.

Ethics-Related Procedures

Renker recruited teenagers primarily at two outpatient gynecologic clinics. Teenagers who were deemed eligible for the study were invited to schedule an interview at a location of their choice. All but one of the young women who volunteered chose a public library or a university office rather than their own homes. Teens were offered a $50 stipend to partially compensate them for the time spent in the interview (30–90 minutes). Before beginning the interview, informed consent issues were discussed, including the researcher's responsibility to report child abuse and harm to third parties. Study participants were told that no specific questions would be asked about either of these reportable issues, but that the researcher would assist them in reporting any abuse situations if they so desired. To protect their confidentiality, Renker encouraged each teenager to make up a name for herself, the perpetrator, and other family members. Each interview was assigned an ID number, and the data files contained no information that could identify participants or the locale of their recruitment. Interviews were conducted in a private setting without the presence of the teenagers' partners, parents, or children age 2 or older. At the end of the interview, Renker provided the teenagers with information designed to promote their safety (e.g., danger assessments, review of legal options, information about local community resources). Renker received IRB approval from her university and from the medical systems of the two clinics from which participants were recruited.

Key Findings

▷ The teenagers described experiences of rape, stalking, and physical and sexual violence during their pregnancies.

research examples continue on page 106

▶ Five themes relating to "keeping safe" were identified. One theme, for example, was labeled: "Taking Charge: Being Proactive."

Critical Thinking Suggestions

1. Answer questions 1–8 from Box 5-3 regarding this study.

2. Also consider the following targeted questions, which may assist you in further assessing the ethical aspects of the study:

   a. Renker paid a $50 stipend to participants—do you think this was appropriate?

   b. What dilemma would Renker face if participants told her that during the time they were being abused, they were so stressed that they abused their own children?

   c. What ethical principle(s) did Renker seek to address in providing participants with information to keep them safe?

   d. Did the participants' own use of a pseudonym result in anonymity?

   e. If you had a teenaged friend or family member who had been abused during pregnancy, how would you feel about her participating in the study?

3. If the results of this study are trustworthy, what are some of the uses to which the findings might be put in clinical practice?

 EXAMPLE 3: Quantitative Research

1. Read the method section from Motzer et al.'s study ("Sense of Coherence") in Appendix A of this book, and then answer the relevant questions in Box 5-3.

2. Also consider the following targeted questions, which may further sharpen your critical thinking skills and assist you in assessing ethical aspects of the study:

   a. What was missing in this report with regard to protecting participants' rights? Was the absence of this information critical in your ability to draw conclusions about the ethical aspects of this study?

   b. Where was information about ethical issues located in this report?

   c. Were participants paid a stipend? From an ethical standpoint, do you consider such a payment problematic or beneficial?

   d. If you had a woman friend or family member with irritable bowel syndrome, how would you feel about her participating in the study?

 EXAMPLE 4: Qualitative Research

1. Read the method section from Beck's study ("Birth Trauma") in Appendix B of this book, and then answer the relevant questions in Box 5-3.

2. Also consider the following targeted questions, which may further sharpen your critical thinking skills and assist you in assessing ethical aspects of the study:

   a. Where was information about the ethical aspects of this study located in the report?

   b. What additional information regarding the ethical aspects of Beck's study could the researcher have included in this article?

SUGGESTED READINGS

References on Research Ethics

Holtzclaw, B. J., & Hanneman, S. K. (2002). Use of nonhuman biobehavioral models in critical care nursing research. *Critical Care Nursing Quarterly, 24,* 30–40.

National Commission for the Protection of Human Subjects of Biomedical and Behavioral Research. (1978). *Belmont Report: Ethical principles and guidelines for research involving human subjects.* Washington, DC: U. S. Government Printing Office.

Olsen, D. P. (2003). HIPAA privacy regulations and nursing research. *Nursing Research, 52,* 344–348.

Schrum, L. (1995). Framing the debate: Ethical research in the information age. *Qualitative Inquiry, 1,* 311–326.

Silva, M. C. (1995). *Ethical guidelines in the conduct, dissemination, and implementation of nursing research.* Washington, DC: American Nurses Assocation.

Studies Cited in Chapter 5

Anderson, N. L. R., Nyamathi, A., McAvoy, J. A., Conde, F., & Casey, C. (2001) Perceptions about risk for HIV/AIDS among adolescents in juvenile detention. *Western Journal of Nursing Research, 23,* 336–359.

Bartfay, W. J., & Bartfay, E. (2002). Decreasing effects of iron toxicosis on selenium and glutathione peroxidase activity. *Western Journal of Nursing Research, 24,* 119–131.

Boonpongmanee, C., Zauszniewski, J. A., & Morris, D. L. (2003). Resourcefulness and self-care in pregnant women with HIV. *Western Journal of Nursing Research, 25,* 75–92.

Hentz, P. (2002). The body remembers: Grieving and a circle of time. *Qualitative Health Research, 12,* 161–172.

McKenna, B. G., Smith, N. A., Poole, S. J., & Coverdale, J. H. (2003). Horizontal violence: Experiences of Registered Nurses in their first year of practice. *Journal of Advanced Nursing, 42,* 90–96.

Polit, D. F., London, A. S., & Martinez, J. M. (2001). *The health of poor urban women.* New York: MDRC.

Rankin, M., & Esteves, M. D. (1997). Perceptions of scientific misconduct in nursing. *Nursing Research, 46,* 270–275.

Renker, P. R. (2003). Keeping safe: Teenagers' strategies for dealing with perinatal violence. *Journal of Obstetric, Gynecologic, & Neonatal Nursing, 32,* 58–67.

Spiers, J. A. (2002). The interpersonal contexts of negotiating care in home care nurse-patient interactions. *Qualitative Health Research, 12,* 1033–1057.

Suen, L. W., Morris, D. L., & McDougall, G. J. (2004). Memory functions of Taiwanese American older adults. *Western Journal of Nursing Research, 26,* 222–241.

Wilbur, J., Miller, A. M., Chandler, P., & McDevitt, J. (2003). Determinants of physical activity and adherence to a 24-week home-based walking program in African American and Caucasian women. *Research in Nursing & Health, 26,* 213–224.

Wuest, J., Ford-Gilboe, M., Merritt-Gray, M., & Berman, H. (2003). Intrusion: The central problem for family health promotion among children and single mothers after leaving an abusive partner. *Qualitative Health Research, 13,* 597–622.

Preliminary Steps in the Research Process

Scrutinizing Research Problems, Research Questions, and Hypotheses

STUDENT OBJECTIVES

On completing this chapter, you will be able to:

▶ Evaluate the compatibility of a research problem and a paradigm
▶ Describe the process of developing and refining a research problem
▶ Distinguish statements of purpose and research questions for quantitative and qualitative studies
▶ Describe the function and characteristics of research hypotheses and distinguish different types of hypotheses
▶ Critique statements of purpose, research questions, and hypotheses in research reports with respect to their placement, clarity, wording, and significance
▶ Define new terms in the chapter

RESEARCH PROBLEMS AND RESEARCH QUESTIONS

A study begins as a problem that a researcher would like to solve or as a question that he or she would like to answer. This chapter discusses the formulation and evaluation of research problems, research questions, and hypotheses. We begin by clarifying some related terms.

Basic Terms Relating to Research Problems

At the most general level, researchers select a *topic* or a phenomenon on which to focus. Patient compliance, coping with disability, and pain management are examples of research topics. Within these broad topic areas are many potential research questions or research problems. In this section, we illustrate various terms as we define them using the topic *side effects in chemotherapy patients.*

A **research problem** is an enigmatic, perplexing, or troubling condition. Both qualitative and quantitative researchers identify a research problem within a broad topic area of interest. The purpose of disciplined research is to "solve" the problem—or to contribute to its solution—by accumulating relevant information. A **problem statement** articulates the problem to be addressed. Table 6-1 presents a problem statement related to the topic of side effects in chemotherapy patients.

Research questions are the specific queries researchers want to answer in addressing a research problem. Research questions guide the types of data to be collected in the study. Researchers who make specific predictions regarding the answers to research questions pose **hypotheses** that are tested empirically. Examples of both research questions and hypotheses are presented in Table 6-1.

In a research report, you might also encounter other related terms. For example, many reports include a **statement of purpose** (or purpose statement), which is the researcher's summary of the overall goal. A researcher might also identify several specific *research aims* or *objectives*—the specific accomplishments the researcher hopes to achieve by conducting the study. The objectives include obtaining answers to research questions but may also encompass some broader aims (e.g., developing recommendations for changes to nursing practice based on the study results), as illustrated in Table 6-1.

Research Problems and Paradigms

Some research problems are better suited for studies using qualitative versus quantitative methods. Quantitative studies usually involve concepts that are well developed, about which there is an existing body of literature, and for which reliable methods of measurement have been developed. For example, a quantitative study might be undertaken to determine whether postpartum depression is higher among women who return to work 6 months after delivery than among those who stay home with their babies. There are relatively accurate measures of postpartum depression that would yield quantitative information about the level of depression in a sample of employed and nonemployed postpartum women.

Qualitative studies are often undertaken because some aspect of a concept is poorly understood, and the researcher wants to develop a rich, comprehensive, and context-bound understanding of it. In the example of postpartum depression, qualitative methods would not be

TABLE 6.1	Example of Terms Relating to Research Problems
TERM	**EXAMPLE**
Topic/focus	Side effects of chemotherapy
Research problem	Nausea and vomiting are common side effects among patients on chemotherapy, and interventions to date have been only moderately successful in reducing these effects. New interventions that can reduce or prevent these side effects need to be identified.
Statement of purpose	The purpose of the study is to test an intervention to reduce chemotherapy-induced side effects—specifically, to compare the effectiveness of patient-controlled and nurse-administered antiemetic therapy for controlling nausea and vomiting in patients on chemotherapy.
Research question	What is the relative effectiveness of patient-controlled antiemetic therapy versus nurse-controlled antiemetic therapy with regard to (a) medication consumption and (b) control of nausea and vomiting in patients on chemotherapy?
Hypotheses	(1) Subjects receiving antiemetic therapy by a patient-controlled pump will report less nausea than subjects receiving the therapy by nurse administration; (2) subjects receiving antiemetic therapy by a patient-controlled pump will vomit less than subjects receiving the therapy by nurse administration; (3) subjects receiving antiemetic therapy by a patient-controlled pump will consume less medication than subjects receiving the therapy by nurse administration.
Aims/objectives	This study has as its aim the following objectives: (1) to develop and implement two alternative procedures for administering antiemetic therapy for patients receiving moderate emetogenic chemotherapy (patient controlled versus nurse controlled); (2) to test three hypotheses concerning the relative effectiveness of the alternative procedures on medication consumption and control of side effects; and (3) to use the findings to develop recommendations for possible changes to therapeutic procedures.

well suited to comparing levels of depression among two groups of women, but they would be ideal for exploring, for example, the *meaning* of postpartum depression among new mothers. In evaluating a research report, an important consideration is whether the research problem fits the chosen paradigm (and research tradition) and its associated methods.

Sources of Research Problems

Where do ideas for research problems come from? At the most basic level, research topics originate with researchers' interests. Because research is a time-consuming enterprise, curiosity about and interest in a topic are essential to the success of the project.

Research reports rarely indicate the source of researchers' inspiration for a study, but a variety of explicit sources can fuel their curiosity, including the following:

▶ *Clinical experience.* The nurse's everyday experience is a rich source of ideas for research topics. Problems that need immediate solutions have high potential for clinical significance.

▶ *Nursing literature.* Ideas for studies often come from reading the nursing literature. Research reports may suggest problem areas indirectly by stimulating the reader's imagination and directly by explicitly stating what additional research is needed.

▶ *Social issues.* Topics are sometimes suggested by global social or political issues of relevance to the health care community. For example, the feminist movement has raised questions about such topics as gender equity and domestic violence.

▶ *Theories.* Theories from nursing and other related disciplines are another source of research problems. Researchers ask, If this theory is correct, what would I predict about people's behaviors, states, or feelings? The predictions can then be tested through research.

▶ *Ideas from external sources.* External sources and direct suggestions can sometimes provide the impetus for a research idea. For example, ideas for studies may emerge from reviewing a funding agency's research priorities or from brainstorming with other nurses.

It should be noted that researchers who have developed a program of research on a topic area may get inspiration for "next steps" from their own findings, or from a discussion of those findings with others.

Example of a problem source for a qualitative study

Beck (one of this book's authors) has developed a strong research program on postpartum depression. In 2001, Beck was invited to deliver the keynote address at an international conference in New Zealand. She was asked to speak about perinatal anxiety disorders and, in preparing for her talk, came across a few articles on posttraumatic stress disorder (PTSD) after childbirth. In her keynote address, in which she described the continuum of perinatal anxiety disorders, Beck briefly touched on PTSD due to birth trauma. At the same conference a woman named Sue Watson did a presentation on PTSD after childbirth. She was the chairperson of Trauma and Birth Stress (TABS), a charitable trust in New Zealand dedicated to supporting women who have experienced birth trauma and the resulting PTSD. Watson had herself suffered from PTSD following the birth of her first baby. Her powerful presentation alerted Beck to the devastating effects that birth trauma can have on mothers. Beck then approached Watson to discuss the possibility of conducting a phenomenological study on birth trauma/PTSD with some of the mothers who belonged to TABS. Watson was immediately supportive and helped to recruit mothers into Beck's study. Beck's study is reprinted in Appendix B.

Development and Refinement of Research Problems

The development of a research problem is a creative process. Researchers often begin with interests in a broad topic area, and then develop the topic into a more specific researchable problem. For example, suppose a nurse working on a medical unit begins to wonder why some patients complain about having to wait for pain medication when certain nurses are assigned to them. The general topic is discrepancy in patient complaints about pain medications administered by different nurses. The nurse might ask, What accounts for this discrepancy? This broad question may lead to other questions, such as, How do the two groups of nurses differ? or What characteristics do the complaining patients share? At this point, the nurse may observe that the ethnic background of the patients and nurses could be a relevant factor. This may direct the nurse to a review of the literature for studies concerning ethnic groups and their relationship to nursing behaviors, or it may provoke a discussion of these observations with peers. These efforts may result in several research questions, such as the following:

▶ What is the essence of patient complaints among patients of different ethnic backgrounds?

▶ How do complaints by patients of different ethnic backgrounds get expressed by patients and perceived by nurses?

▶ Is the ethnic background of nurses related to the frequency with which they dispense pain medication?

▶ Is the ethnic background of patients related to the frequency and intensity of their complaints of having to wait for pain medication?

▶ Does the number of patient complaints increase when the patients are of dissimilar ethnic backgrounds as opposed to when they are of the same ethnic background as the nurse?

▶ Do nurses' dispensing behaviors change as a function of the similarity between their own ethnic background and that of patients?

These questions stem from the same general problem, yet each would be studied differently; for example, some suggest a qualitative approach, and others suggest a quantitative one. A quantitative researcher might become curious about nurses' dispensing behaviors, based on some evidence in the literature regarding ethnic differences. Both ethnicity and nurses' dispensing behaviors are variables that can be reliably measured. A qualitative researcher who noticed differences in patient complaints would likely be more interested in understanding the *essence* of the complaints, the patients' *experience* of frustration, the *process* by which the problem got resolved, or the full *nature* of the nurse–patient interactions regarding the dispensing of medications. These are aspects of the research problem that would be difficult to measure quantitatively. Researchers choose a problem to study based on several factors, including its inherent interest to them and its fit with a paradigm of preference.

COMMUNICATING THE RESEARCH PROBLEM, PURPOSE, AND QUESTIONS

Researchers communicate their objectives in various ways in research reports. This section discusses the wording and placement of problem statements, statements of purpose, and research questions; the following major section discusses hypotheses.

Problem Statements

A problem statement is an expression of a dilemma or disturbing situation that needs investigation. A problem statement identifies the nature of the problem that is being addressed in the study and, typically, its context and significance. Generally, the problem statement should be broad enough to include central concerns but narrow enough in scope to serve as a guide to study design.

Example of a problem statement from a quantitative study

Breast cancer is a serious health concern and a major public health challenge in the United States.... Breast cancer is the most common form of cancer, accounting for approximately 30% of new cancer cases, with one in eight women developing breast cancer during their lifetimes.... A significant number of women will experience burdensome side effects associated with their cancer experiences that will have a significant impact on cancer recovery and quality of life.... The most commonly reported psychological side effect of cancer diagnosis and treatment is depression.... Psychosocial interventions are not routinely offered to cancer patients with depression.... To date articles in the literature primarily have been descriptive, with few investigators examining the long-term effectiveness of psychosocial interventions...(Badger, Braden, Mishel, & Longman, 2004).

In this example, the general topic is depression in breast cancer patients. The problem statement asserts the nature of the problem (depression can affect cancer recovery and quality of life) and indicates its breadth (one out of eight women develops breast cancer and a large number experience depression). It also provides a justification for conducting a new study: the dearth of existing studies on the long-term effectiveness of psychosocial interventions for cancer patients.

The problem statement for a qualitative study similarly expresses the nature of the problem, its context, and its significance.

Example of a problem statement from a qualitative study

Hospitalization is a common experience for elderly people in the United States. More than four out of every 10 people 75 years or older are hospitalized each year, with an average stay of almost 7 days.... While hospitalized, elders and hospital staff are concerned about maintaining the elders' dignity.... Gaylin (1984) commented that dignity is often talked about but rarely examined. Almost 20 years later, this statement continues to be true; the few reports on the nature of dignity vary widely in their findings. To support elderly patients' dignity, health care providers must understand the nature of dignity and the strategies employed by patients to maintain it (Jacelon, 2003).

As in the previous example, the researcher articulated the nature of the problem and a justification for conducting a new study. Qualitative studies that are embedded in a particular research tradition generally incorporate terms and concepts in their problem statements that foreshadow their tradition of inquiry. For example, the problem statement in a grounded theory study might refer to the need to develop deeper understandings of social processes. A problem statement for a phenomenological study might note the need to know more about people's experiences or the meanings they attribute to those experiences. And an ethnographer might indicate the desire to describe how cultural forces affect people's behavior.

HOW-TO-TELL TIP

How can you tell a problem statement? Problem statements appear in the introduction to a research report—indeed, the first sentence of a research report is often the starting point of a problem statement. However, problem statements are often interwoven with a review of the literature, which provides context by documenting knowledge gaps. Problem statements are rarely explicitly labeled as such and must therefore be ferreted out.

■

Statements of Purpose

Many researchers first articulate their goals as a broad statement of purpose, worded in the declarative form. The purpose statement captures, in one or two sentences, the essence of the study and establishes the general direction of the inquiry. The words *purpose* or *goal* usually appear in a purpose statement (e.g., "The purpose of this study was. . ." or "The goal of this study was. . ."), but sometimes the words *intent, aim,* or *objective* are used instead.

In a quantitative study, a well-worded statement of purpose identifies the key study variables and their possible interrelationships as well as the population of interest.

Example of a statement of purpose from a quantitative study

The purpose of this descriptive study was to identify urine flow factors contributing to UTI [urinary tract infection] in home care clients who had had an indwelling urinary catheter for at least 3 months (Wilde & Carrigan, 2003).

This statement identifies the population of interest (home care clients with an indwelling urinary catheter), the independent variables (urine flow factors), and the dependent variable (UTI).

In qualitative studies, the statement of purpose indicates the nature of the inquiry, the key concept or phenomenon under investigation, and the group, community, or setting under study.

Example of a statement of purpose from a qualitative study

The purpose of the current study was to describe beliefs and understanding about tobacco use and cessation among current and former users in rural Appalachia (Ahijeyych, Kuun, Christman, Wood, Browning, & Wewers, 2003).

This statement indicates that the central phenomenon of interest is beliefs about tobacco use and that the group under study is former and current users of tobacco in rural Appalachia. In qualitative studies, the statement of purpose may specifically mention the underlying research tradition, if this is relevant.

Example of a statement of purpose from a grounded theory study

The purpose of the study was "to generate a grounded substantive theory of the process of forgiveness in patients with cancer" (Mickley and Cowles, 2001, p. 31).

The statement of purpose communicates more than just the nature of the problem—researchers typically use verbs that suggest how they sought to solve the problem, or what the state of knowledge on the topic is. A study whose purpose is to *explore* or *describe* a phenomenon is likely to focus on a little-researched topic, often involving a qualitative approach. A statement of purpose for a qualitative study may also imply a flexible design through the use of verbs such as *understand, discover,* and *develop.* Creswell (1998) notes that the statement of purpose in qualitative studies often "encode" the tradition of inquiry not only through researchers' choice of verbs but also through the use of certain terms or "buzz words" associated with those traditions, as follows:

▶ *Grounded theory:* Processes; social structures; social interactions
▶ *Phenomenological studies:* Experience; lived experience; meaning; essence
▶ *Ethnographic studies:* Culture; roles; myths; cultural behavior

Quantitative researchers also suggest the nature of the inquiry through their selection of verbs. A purpose statement indicating that the purpose is to *test* the effectiveness of some intervention or to *compare* two alternative nursing strategies suggests a study with a more established knowledge base, using a quantitative approach and a design with tight controls. Note that researchers' choice of verbs in a statement of purpose should connote a certain degree of objectivity. A statement of purpose indicating that the intent of the study was to *prove, demonstrate,* or *show* something suggests a bias.

Research Questions

Research questions are, in some cases, direct rewordings of statements of purpose, phrased interrogatively rather than declaratively. The research questions for the examples cited in the previous section might be as follows:

▶ What are the urine flow factors contributing to urinary tract infection in home care clients with an indwelling urinary catheter?
▶ What are the beliefs and understanding about tobacco use and cessation among current and former users in rural Appalachia?

Questions that are simple and direct invite an answer and help to focus attention on the kinds of data needed to provide that answer. Some research reports thus omit a statement of purpose and state only the research question. Other researchers use a set of research questions to clarify or amplify the purpose statement.

In a quantitative study, research questions identify the key variables (most often, the independent and dependent variable), the relationships among them, and the population under study.

Example of a research question from a quantitative study

Do medical–surgical nurses plan different acute care for a patient because of the presence of a psychiatric diagnosis? (McDonald, Frakes, Apostolidis, Armstrong, Goldblatt, & Bernardo, 2003)

In this example, the independent variable is whether or not a patient has a psychiatric diagnosis; the dependent variable is the medical plan for the patient; and the population under study is medical–surgical nurses.

Researchers in the various qualitative traditions differ in the types of question they believe to be important. Grounded theory researchers are likely to ask *process* questions, phenomenologists tend to ask *meaning* questions, and ethnographers generally ask *descriptive* questions about cultures. The terms associated with the various traditions, discussed earlier in connection with purpose statements, may also be incorporated into the research questions.

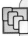

Example of a research question from a phenomenological study

What is the lived experience of individuals when confronted with a life-threatening disease (Albaugh, 2003)?

Not all qualitative studies are rooted in specific research traditions, however. Many researchers use naturalistic methods to describe or explore phenomena without focusing on cultures, meaning, or social processes.

Example of a research question from a descriptive qualitative study

How do bereaving family caregivers of patients who had had advanced cancer perceive the effects of home-based caregiving on their bereavement (Koop & Strang, 2003)?

In qualitative studies, research questions sometimes evolve over the course of the study. Researchers begin with a *focus* that defines the general boundaries of the inquiry, but the boundaries are not cast in stone—they "can be altered and, in the typical naturalistic inquiry, will be" (Lincoln & Guba, 1985, p. 228). Naturalists thus begin with a research question in mind but are sufficiently flexible that the question can be modified as new information makes it relevant to do so.

CONSUMER TIP

Researchers most often state their purpose or research questions at the end of the introduction or immediately after the review of the literature. Sometimes, a separate section of a research report—typically located just before the method section—is devoted to stating the research problem formally and might be labeled "Purpose," "Statement of Purpose," "Research Questions," or, in quantitatve studies, "Hypotheses."

RESEARCH HYPOTHESES IN QUANTITATIVE RESEARCH

In quantitative studies, researchers may present a statement of purpose and then one or more hypotheses. A hypothesis is a tentative prediction about the relationship between two or more variables in the population under study. In a qualitative study, the researcher does not begin with a hypothesis, in part because there is generally too little known about the topic to justify a hypothesis and in part because qualitative researchers want their inquiry to be guided by participants' viewpoints rather than by their own *a priori* hunches (although findings from qualitative studies may *lead to* the formulation of hypotheses). Thus, our discussion here focuses on hypotheses in quantitative research.

Function of Hypotheses in Quantitative Research

A hypothesis translates a research question into a prediction of expected outcomes. For instance, the research question might ask: Does therapeutic touch affect patients' muscle tension levels? The researcher might hypothesize as follows: The muscle tension levels of patients treated with therapeutic touch will be lower than the muscle tension levels of patients treated with physical touch.

Hypotheses sometimes emerge from a theory. Scientists reason from theories to hypotheses and test those hypotheses in the real world. The validity of a theory is never examined directly, but the worth of a theory can be evaluated through hypothesis testing. For example, the theory of reinforcement maintains that behavior or activity that is positively reinforced (rewarded) tends to be learned (repeated). The theory is too abstract to test, but hypotheses based on the theory can be tested. For instance, the following hypotheses are deduced from reinforcement theory:

▹ Elderly patients who are praised (reinforced) for self-feeding require less assistance in feeding than patients who are not praised.
▹ Pediatric patients who are given a reward (e.g., a balloon or permission to watch television) when they cooperate during nursing procedures are more compliant during those procedures than nonrewarded peers.

Both of these propositions can be tested in the real world. The theory gains support if the hypotheses are confirmed.

Even in the absence of a theory, well-conceived hypotheses offer direction and suggest explanations. For example, suppose we hypothesized that widowers experience more psychological distress in the 6 months after the death of their spouse than widows. This prediction could be based on theory (e.g., role expectation theory), earlier studies, or personal observations.

The development of predictions in and of itself forces researchers to think logically, to exercise critical judgment, and to tie together earlier findings.

Now let us suppose the above hypothesis is not confirmed by the evidence collected; that is, we find that men and women experience comparable levels of emotional distress in the 6 months after their spouses' death.

The failure of data to support a prediction forces investigators to analyze theory or previous research critically, to review limitations of the study's methods carefully, and to explore alternative explanations for the findings.

The use of hypotheses in quantitative studies tends to induce critical thinking and, hence, to facilitate interpretation of the data.

To further illustrate the utility of hypotheses, suppose the researcher conducted the study guided only by the research question, Is there a relationship between a person's gender and the degree of distress experienced after losing a spouse? Investigators without a hypothesis are, apparently, prepared to accept any results. The problem is that it is almost always possible to explain something superficially after the fact, no matter what the findings are. Hypotheses guard against superficiality and minimize the possibility that spurious results will be misconstrued.

CONSUMER TIP

Some quantitative research reports explicitly state the hypotheses that guided the study, but most do not. In some cases, the absence of a hypothesis is appropriate, but the absence of a hypothesis often is an indication that the researcher has failed to consider critically the implications of theory or the existing knowledge base, or has failed to disclose the hunches that may have influenced the study design. ■

Characteristics of Testable Hypotheses

Testable research hypotheses state the expected relationship between the independent variable (the presumed cause or antecedent) and the dependent variable (the presumed effect) within a population.

Example of a research hypothesis

Individuals with progressive forms of multiple sclerosis who have higher self-efficacy will be more likely to adhere to glatiramer acetate therapy than those with lower self-efficacy (Fraser, Hadjimichael, & Vollmer, 2003).

In this example, the independent variable is the person's level of self-efficacy, and the dependent variable is adherence to therapy. The hypothesis predicts that these two variables are related—greater adherence is expected among those with higher self-efficacy.

Unfortunately, researchers sometimes state hypotheses that fail to make a relational statement, and such hypotheses are not testable. Consider, for example, the following prediction: "Pregnant women who receive prenatal instruction by a nurse regarding the postpartum experience are not likely to experience postpartum depression." This statement expresses no anticipated relationship; in fact, there is only one variable (postpartum depression), and a relationship by definition requires at least two variables.

When a prediction does not express an anticipated relationship, it cannot be tested. In our example, how would we know whether the hypothesis was supported—what absolute standard could be used to decide whether to accept or reject the hypothesis? To illustrate the problem more concretely, suppose we asked a group of mothers who received prenatal instruction the following question 2 months after delivery: Overall, how depressed have you been since you gave birth? Would you say (1) extremely depressed, (2) moderately depressed, (3) somewhat depressed, or (4) not at all depressed?

Based on responses to this question, how could we compare the actual outcome with the predicted outcome? Would *all* the women in the sample have to say they were "not at all depressed"? Would the prediction be supported if 51% of the women said they were "not at all depressed" *or* "somewhat depressed"? There is no adequate way of testing the accuracy of the prediction.

A test is simple, however, if we modify the prediction to the following: Pregnant women who receive prenatal instruction are less likely to experience postpartum depression than pregnant women with no prenatal instruction. Here, the dependent variable is the women's depression and the independent variable is their receipt or nonreceipt of prenatal instruction. The relational aspect of the prediction is embodied in the phrase *less...than*. If a hypothesis lacks a phrase such as *more than, less than, greater than, different from, related to, associated with*, or something similar, it is not amenable to testing in a quantitative study. To test this revised hypothesis, we could ask two groups of women with different prenatal instruction experiences to respond to the question on depression and then compare the groups' responses. The absolute degree of depression of either group would not be at issue.

Hypotheses should be based on justifiable rationales. The most defensible hypotheses follow from previous research findings or are deduced from a theory. When a relatively new area is being investigated, researchers may have to turn to logical reasoning or personal experience to justify the predictions.

CONSUMER TIP

Hypotheses are typically fairly easy to identify because researchers make statements such as, "The study tested the hypothesis that . . ." or, "It was predicted that . . .".

■

Wording Hypotheses

A hypothesis can predict the relationship between a single independent variable and a single dependent variable (a *simple hypothesis*), or it can predict a relationship between two or more independent variables or two or more dependent variables (a *complex hypothesis*). In the following examples, independent variables are indicated as IVs and dependent variables are identified as DVs:

Example of a simple hypothesis

Central venous catheter–related sepsis (DV) will be lower in patients who do not have a gauze dressing (IV) after the insertion site has healed than in patients who do have a gauze dressing (Olson, Rennie, Hanson, Ryan, Gilpin, Falsetti, et al., 2004).

Example of a complex hypothesis—multiple independent variables

Among men with radical prostatectomy treatment, their quality of life (DV) will be directly affected by their urinary function appraisal, self-esteem, anger suppression, perceived social support, and depression (five IVs) (Rondorff-Klym & Colling, 2003).

Example of a complex hypothesis—multiple dependent variables

Among lactating mothers, those who use hydrogel dressings—versus lanolin ointment—for nipple soreness (IV) will experience (1) greater pain relief and (2) a lower rate of nipple wounds (DVs) (Dodd & Chalmers, 2003).

Hypotheses can be stated in various ways as long as the researcher specifies or implies the relationship that will be tested. Here is an example:

1. Lower levels of exercise postpartum are associated with greater weight retention than higher levels of exercise.
2. There is a relationship between level of exercise postpartum and weight retention.

3. The greater the level of exercise postpartum, the lower the weight retention.
4. Women with different levels of exercise postpartum differ with regard to weight retention.
5. Weight retention postpartum decreases as the woman's level of exercise increases.
6. Women who exercise postpartum have lower weight retention than women who do not.

Other variations are also possible. The important point to remember is that the hypothesis specifies the independent variable (here, level of exercise), the dependent variable (weight retention), and the anticipated relationship between them.

Hypotheses should be worded in the present tense. Researchers make a prediction about a relationship in the population—not just about a relationship that will be revealed in a particular sample of study participants.

Hypotheses can be either directional or nondirectional. A **directional hypothesis** is one that specifies not only the existence but the expected direction of the relationship between variables. In the six versions of the same hypothesis above, versions 1, 3, 5, and 6 are directional because there is an explicit prediction that women who do not exercise postpartum are at greater risk of weight retention than women who do. A **nondirectional hypothesis**, by contrast, does not stipulate the direction of the relationship, as illustrated in versions 2 and 4. These hypotheses predict that a woman's level of exercise and weight retention are related, but they do not stipulate whether the researcher thinks that exercise is related to more weight retention, or less.

Hypotheses based on theory are usually directional because theories provide a rationale for expecting variables to relate in certain ways. Existing studies also offer a basis for specifying directional hypotheses. When there is no theory or related research, when findings from prior studies are contradictory, or when researchers' own experience leads to ambivalent expectations, nondirectional hypotheses may be appropriate. Some people argue, in fact, that nondirectional hypotheses are preferable because they connote a degree of impartiality. Directional hypotheses, it is said, imply that researchers are intellectually committed to certain outcomes, and such commitment might lead to bias. This argument fails to recognize that researchers typically *do* have hunches about the outcomes, whether they state those expectations explicitly or not. We prefer directional hypotheses—when there is a reasonable basis for them—because they clarify the study's framework and demonstrate that researchers have thought critically about the phenomena under study.

Another distinction is the difference between research and null hypotheses. **Research hypotheses** (also referred to as *substantive* or *scientific hypotheses*) are statements of actual expected relationships between variables. All hypotheses presented thus far are research hypotheses that indicate researchers' true expectations.

The logic of statistical inference requires that, for the purposes of statistical analysis, hypotheses be expressed as though no relationship were expected. **Null hypotheses** (or **statistical hypotheses**) state that there is no relationship between the independent variables and dependent variables. The null form of the hypothesis used in our preceding example would be: Weight retention is unrelated to mothers' exercise levels postpartum. A null hypothesis might be compared to the assumption of innocence of an accused criminal in English-based systems of justice; the variables are assumed to be "innocent" of any relationship until they can be shown to be "guilty" through statistical procedures. The null hypothesis is the formal statement of this presumed innocence.

Research reports typically present research rather than null hypotheses. When statistical tests are performed, the underlying null hypotheses are assumed without being explicitly stated. If the researcher's actual research hypothesis is that no relationship among variables exists, the hypothesis cannot be adequately tested using traditional statistical procedures. This issue is explained in Chapter 15.

CONSUMER TIP

If the researcher used any statistical tests (and this is almost always the case in quantitative studies), it means that there were underlying hypotheses—*whether the researcher explicitly stated them or not*—because most statistical tests are designed to test hypotheses.

■

Hypothesis Testing and Proof

Hypotheses are never *proved* (or *disproved*) through hypothesis testing; rather, they are *accepted* or *supported* (or *rejected*). Findings are always tentative. Certainly, if the same results are replicated in numerous investigations, greater confidence can be placed in the conclusions. Hypotheses come to be increasingly supported with mounting evidence.

Let us look more closely at why this is so. Suppose we hypothesized that height and weight are related—which, indeed, they are in a general population. We predict that, on average, tall people weigh more than short people. We would then obtain height and weight measurements from a sample and analyze the data. Now suppose we happened by chance to choose a sample that consisted of short, fat people, and tall, thin people. Our results might indicate that there was no relationship between a person's height and weight. Would we then be justified in stating that this study *proved* or *demonstrated* that height and weight are unrelated?

As another example, suppose we hypothesized that tall people are better nurses than short people. This hypothesis is used here only to illustrate a point because, in reality, we would expect no relationship between height and a nurse's job performance. Now suppose that, by chance again, we draw a sample of nurses in which tall nurses received better job evaluations than short ones. Could we conclude definitively that height is related to a nurse's performance? These two examples demonstrate the difficulty of using observations from a sample to generalize to the population from which the sample has been drawn. Other problems, such as the accuracy of the measures, the validity of underlying assumptions, and the reasonableness of the logical deductions, prohibit researchers from concluding with finality that hypotheses are proved.

CRITIQUING RESEARCH PROBLEMS, RESEARCH QUESTIONS, AND HYPOTHESES

In critiquing research reports, you will need to evaluate the extent to which researchers have adequately communicated their research problem. The researchers' description of the problem, statement of purpose, research questions, and hypotheses set the stage for the description of what was done and what was learned. Ideally, you should not have to dig too deeply to decipher the research problem or to discover the questions.

Critiquing the Substance of a Research Problem

A critique of the research problem involves multiple dimensions, including a substantive dimension. That is, you need to consider whether the problem has significance for nursing. The following issues are relevant in considering the significance of a study problem:

1. *Implications for nursing practice.* A primary consideration in evaluating the significance of a research problem is whether it has the potential to produce evidence for improving nursing practice. The following questions should be posed: Are there practical applications that might stem from research on the problem? Will more knowledge about the problem make a difference that matters to practicing nurses? Will the findings challenge (or lend support to) assumptions about nursing? If the answer to such questions is no, the significance of the problem is bound to be low.

2. *Extension of knowledge base.* A study that extends, refines, or corroborates previous knowledge has a better chance of being significant than a study on an isolated research problem—at least in the short run. Studies that build in a meaningful way on the existing knowledge base are more likely to find immediate applications in nursing practice. For example, Adachi, Shimada, and Usui (2003) tested the effects of different maternal positions on labor pain using a rigorous research design. Their study corroborated earlier findings that had been less conclusive because of their weaker designs (i.e., that the sitting position reduces the intensity of labor pain compared to the supine position). Researchers who develop a systematic *program of research*, building on their own earlier findings, are especially likely to make significant contributions. For example, Beck's series of studies relating to postpartum depression (e.g., Beck, 1993, 1996, 2001; Beck & Gable, 2002, 2003) have influenced women's health care worldwide.

3. *Promotion of theory development.* Studies that either test or develop a theory often have a better chance of making a lasting contribution to knowledge than studies that do not have a conceptual context. For example, Burris and O'Connell (2003) conducted a study that tested a theory (reversal theory) to explain lapses during adolescents' efforts to stop smoking, and the findings have implications for smoking cessation programs aimed at young people.

4. *Correspondence to research priorities.* Research priorities have been established by research scholars, agencies that fund nursing research (such as the National Institute of Nursing Research—NINR), and professional nursing organizations. Clearly, research problems stemming from such priorities have a high likelihood of yielding important new evidence for the nursing profession because they reflect expert opinion about areas of needed research. As an example, in 2001 NINR identified research on behavioral changes and interventions (such as interventions to promote effective sleep) as a high priority. Richardson's (2003) study addressed this priority area with an evaluation of an intervention designed to improve the sleep of critically ill adults.

When critiquing a study, you need to consider whether the research problem was meaningfully based on prior research; has a relationship to a theoretical context; addresses a current research priority; and, most important, can contribute useful evidence for nursing practice.

Critiquing Other Aspects of Research Problems

Another dimension in critiquing the research problem concerns methodologic issues—in particular, whether the research problem is compatible with the chosen research paradigm and its associated methods. You should also evaluate whether the statement of purpose or research questions have been properly worded and lend themselves to empirical inquiry.

BOX 6.1   **Guidelines for Critiquing Reasearch Problems, Research Questions, and Hypotheses**

1. What is the research problem? Is it easy to locate and clearly stated?
2. Does the problem have significance for nursing? How might the research contribute to nursing practice, administration, education, or policy?
3. Is there a good fit between the research problem and the paradigm within which the research was conducted? Is there a good fit with the qualitative research tradition?
4. Does the report formally present a statement of purpose, research question, and/or hypotheses? Is this information communicated clearly and concisely, and is it placed in a logical and useful location?
5. Are purpose statements or questions worded appropriately? (For example, are key concepts/variables identified and the population of interest specified? Are verbs used appropriately to suggest the nature of the inquiry and/or the research tradition?)
6. If there are no formal hypotheses, is their absence justified? Are statistical tests used in analyzing the data despite the absence of stated hypotheses?
7. Do hypotheses (if any) flow from a theory or previous research? Is there a justifiable basis for the predictions?
8. Are hypotheses (if any) properly worded—do they state a predicted relationship between two or more variables? Are they directional or nondirectional, and is there a rationale for how they were stated? Are they presented as research or as null hypotheses?

In a quantitative study, if the research report does not contain explicit hypotheses, you need to consider whether their absence is justified. If there are hypotheses, you should evaluate whether the hypotheses are logically connected to the research problem and whether they are consistent with available knowledge or relevant theory. The wording of the hypothesis should also be assessed. The hypothesis is a valid guidepost to scientific inquiry only if it is testable. To be testable, the hypothesis must contain a prediction about the relationship between two or more variables that can be measured. The hypothesis must imply the criteria by which it could be rejected or accepted through the collection of data.

Specific guidelines for critiquing research problems, research questions, and hypotheses are presented in Box 6-1.

CHAPTER REVIEW

Key new terms introduced in the chapter, together with a summary of major points, are presented in this section. In addition, Chapter 6 of the accompanying *Study Guide to Accompany Essentials of Nursing Research,* 6th edition offers various exercises and study suggestions for reinforcing the concepts presented in this chapter. For additional review, see the Student Self-Study Review Questions section of the Student Resource CD-ROM provided with this book.

KEY NEW TERMS

Directional hypothesis   Research hypothesis
Hypothesis   Research problem
Nondirectional hypothesis   Research questions
Null hypothesis   Statement of purpose
Problem statement   Statistical hypothesis

S U M M A R Y   P O I N T S

▷ A **research problem** is a perplexing or enigmatic situation that a researcher wants to address through disciplined inquiry. The most common sources of ideas for nursing research problems are clinical experience, relevant literature, social issues, theory, and external sources.

▷ Researchers usually identify a broad topic or focus, then narrow the scope of the problem and identify questions consistent with a paradigm of choice.

▷ A **statement of purpose** summarizes the overall goal of the study; in both qualitative and quantitative studies, the purpose statement identifies the key concepts (variables) and the study group or population.

▷ A **research question** states the specific query the researcher wants to answer to address the research problem.

▷ A **hypothesis** is a statement of a predicted relationship between two or more variables. A testable hypothesis states the anticipated association between one or more independent and one or more dependent variables.

▷ A **directional hypothesis** specifies the expected direction or nature of a hypothesized relationship; **nondirectional hypotheses** predict a relationship but do not stipulate the form that the relationship will take.

▷ **Research hypotheses** predict the existence of relationships; **statistical**, or **null**, **hypotheses** express the absence of any relationship.

▷ Hypotheses are never proved or disproved in an ultimate sense—they are accepted or rejected, supported or not supported by the data.

RESEARCH EXAMPLES   Critical Thinking Activities

 EXAMPLE 1: Quantitative Research

Aspects of a quantitative nursing study, featuring terms and concepts discussed in this chapter, are presented below, followed by some questions to guide critical thinking. (The full research report is available in *Western Journal of Nursing Research, 24,* 49–72.)

Study

"Differential predictors of emotional distress in HIV-infected men and women" (van Servellen, Aguirre, Sarna, & Brecht, 2002)

Research Problem

Despite the fact that AIDS rates have been dropping for men but increasing for women, few studies have described the health experiences of HIV-infected women or compared them to those of men. This situation is troubling because of evidence indicating that, once HIV infected, women may be at greater risk than men for illness-related morbidity and adverse outcomes.

research examples continue on page 142

RESEARCH EXAMPLES *Continued*

Statement of Purpose

The purpose of the study was to describe and compare patterns of emotional distress in men and women with symptomatic HIV seeking care in community-based treatment centers.

Framework and Hypotheses

The conceptual framework for the study was attribution theory, which offers explanations of links between life stressors and emotional distress. This framework, together with findings from other studies, guided the development of four hypotheses:

"Hypothesis 1: Sociodemographic vulnerability (less than high school education, etc.) will be associated with emotional distress in both men and women (with symptomatic HIV).
Hypothesis 2: Poor physical and functional health status will be associated with emotional distress in both men and women.
Hypothesis 3: Optimism and social support will be associated with positive mental health outcomes...in both men and women.
Hypothesis 4: Women will have higher levels of emotional distress than men" (pp. 53–54).

Method

Data for the study were collected from 82 low-income men and 44 low-income women with HIV disease in Los Angeles. Respondents were interviewed using formal scales to measure health, emotional status, and demographic characteristics.

Key Findings

▶ Women had greater disruptions in physical and psychosocial well-being than men, consistent with hypothesis 4.
▶ Physical health and optimism were the primary predictors of emotional distress in both men and women, supporting hypotheses 2 and 3.
▶ Contrary to hypothesis 1, there were no significant relationships between any sociodemographic vulnerability indicators and the subjects' level of anxiety or depression.

Critical Thinking Suggestions*

*See the Student Resource CD-Rom for a discussion of these questions.
1. Answer questions 2–5, 7, and 8 from Box 6-1 regarding this study.
2. Also consider the following targeted questions, which may assist you in further assessing aspects of the study:
    a. Where in the research report do you think the researchers would have presented the hypotheses? Where in the research report would the outcomes of the hypothesis tests be placed?
    b. What clues does the summary give you that this study is quantitative?

RESEARCH EXAMPLES *Continued*

    c. Would it have been possible to state the four hypotheses as a single hypothesis? If yes, state what it would be.

    d. Develop a research question for a phenomenological and/or grounded theory study relating to the same general topic area as this study.

3. If the results of this study are valid and reliable, what are some of the uses to which the findings might be put in clinical practice?

 EXAMPLE 2: Qualitative Research

Aspects of a qualitative nursing study, featuring terms and concepts discussed in this chapter, are presented below, followed by some questions to guide critical thinking. (The full research report is available in *Western Journal of Nursing Research, 24,* 7–27.)

Study

"Focused life stories of women with cardiac pacemakers" (Beery, Sommers, & Hall, 2002)

Research Problem

Biotechnical devices such as pacemakers are increasingly being implanted into people to manage an array of disorders, yet relatively little research has examined the emotional impact of such an experience. Women may have distinctive responses to implanted devices due to cultural messages about the masculinity of technology, but little is known about women's unique responses to permanent cardiac pacemakers.

Statement of Purpose

The purpose of the study was to explore women's responses to pacemaker implantation.

Research Questions

The researchers identified two specific research questions: "What is the experience of women living with permanent cardiac pacemakers?" and "How do women incorporate permanent cardiac pacemakers into their lives and bodies?" (p. 8).

Study Methods

A sample of 11 women who were patients at the cardiology service of a large hospital participated in the study. During in-depth interviews, the women were asked a series of questions regarding life events that led up to, and occurred during and after, their pacemaker's implantation. Each woman participated in two interviews.

research examples continue on page 144

RESEARCH EXAMPLES   *Continued*

Key Findings

The researchers' analysis revealed eight themes that emerged from the interview data: relinquishing care, owning the pacemaker, experiencing fears and resistance, imaging their body, normalizing, positioning as caregivers, finding resilience, and sensing omnipotence.

Critical Thinking Suggestions

1. Answer questions 2–6 from Box 6-1 regarding this study.
2. Also consider the following targeted questions, which may assist you in further assessing aspects of the study:
    a. Where in the research report do you think the researchers placed the statement of purpose and research questions?
    b. Does it appear that this study was conducted within one of the three main qualitative traditions? If so, which one?
    c. What clues does the summary give you that this study is qualitative?
    d. Could the findings from this study be used to generate hypotheses?
3. If the results of this study are trustworthy, what are some of the uses to which the findings might be put in clinical practice?

 **EXAMPLE 3: Quantitative Research**

1. Read the abstract and the introduction from Motzer et al.'s study ("Sense of Coherence") in Appendix A of this book, and then answer the relevant questions in Box 6-1.
2. Also consider the following targeted questions, which may further sharpen your critical thinking skills and assist you in assessing aspects of the study:
    a. Are the hypotheses in this study simple or complex?
    b. State the hypotheses from this report as nondirectional hypotheses, then, as null hypotheses.

 EXAMPLE 4: Qualitative Research

1. Read the abstract and the introduction from Beck's study ("Birth Trauma") in Appendix B of this book, and then answer the relevant questions in Box 6-1.
2. Also consider the following targeted questions, which may further sharpen your critical thinking skills and assist you in assessing aspects of the study.
    a. Do you think that Beck provided enough rationale for the significance of her research problem?
    b. Do you think that Beck needed to include research questions in her report, or was the purpose statement clear enough to stand alone?

SUGGESTED READINGS

Methodologic References

Creswell, J. W. (1998). *Qualitative inquiry and research design: Choosing among five traditions*. Thousand Oaks, CA: Sage Publications.

Kerlinger, F. N., & Lee, H. B. (2000). *Foundations of behavioral research* (4th ed.). Orlando, FL: Harcourt College Publishers.

Lincoln, Y. S., & Guba, E. G. (1985). *Naturalistic inquiry*. Newbury Park, CA: Sage Publications.

Polit, D. F., & Hungler, B. P. (2004). *Nursing research: Principles and methods* (7th ed.). Philadelphia: Lippincott Williams & Wilkins.

Studies Cited in Chapter 6

Adachi, K., Shimada, M., & Usui, A. (2003). The relationship beween the parturient's positions and perceptions of labor pain intensity. *Nursing Research, 52,* 47–51.

Ahijeyych, K., Kuun, P., Christman, S., Wood, T., Browning, K., & Wewers, M. E. (2003). Beliefs about tobacco use among Appalachian current and former users. *Applied Nursing Research, 16,* 93–102.

Albaugh, J. A. (2003). Spirituality and life-threatening illness: A phenomenologic study. *Oncology Nursing Forum, 30,* 593–598.

Badger, T. A., Braden, C. J., Mishel, M. H., & Longman, A. (2004). Depression burden, psychological adjustment, and quality of life in women with breast cancer: Patterns over time. *Research in Nursing & Health, 27,* 19–28.

Beck, C. T. (1993). Teetering on the edge: A substantive theory of postpartum depression. *Nursing Research, 42,* 42–48.

Beck, C. T. (1996). Postpartum depressed mothers' experiences interacting with their children. *Nursing Research, 45,* 98–104.

Beck, C. T. (2001). Predictors of postpartum depression: An update. *Nursing Research, 50,* 275–285.

Beck, C. T., & Gable, R. K. (2002). *Postpartum depression screening scale manual*. Los Angeles: Western Psychological Services.

Beck, C. T., & Gable, R. K. (2003). Postpartum Depression Screening Scale-Spanish Version. *Nursing Research, 52,* 296–306.

Beery, T. A., Sommers, M. S., & Hall, J. (2002). Focused life stories of women with cardiac pacemakers. *Western Journal of Nursing Research, 24,* 7–27.

Burris, R. F., & O'Connell, K. A. (2003). Reversal theory states and cigarette availability predict lapses during smoking cessation among adolescents. *Research in Nursing & Health, 26,* 263–272.

Dodd, V., & Chalmers, C. (2003). Comparing the use of hydrogel dressing to lanolin ointment with lactating mothers. *Journal of Obstetric, Gynecologic, & Neonatal Nursing, 32,* 486–494.

Fraser, C., Hadjimichael, O., & Vollmer, T. (2003). Predictors of adherence to glatiramer acetate therapy in individuals with self-reported progressive forms of multiple sclerosis. *Journal of Neuroscience Nursing, 35,* 163–170.

Jacelon, C. S. (2003). The dignity of elders in an acute care hospital. *Qualitative Health Research, 13,* 543–556.

Koop, P. M., & Strang, V. R. (2003). The bereavement experience following home-based family caregiving for persons with advanced cancer. *Clinical Nursing Research, 12,* 127–144.

McDonald, D. D., Frakes, M., Apostolidis, B., Armstrong, B., Goldblatt, S., & Bernardo, D. (2003). Effect of a psychiatric diagnosis on nursing care for nonpsychiatric problems. *Research in Nursing & Health, 26,* 225–232.

Mickley, J. R., & Cowles, K. (2001). Ameliorating the tension: The use of forgiveness for healing. *Oncology Nursing Forum, 28,* 31–37.

Olson, K., Rennie, R., Hanson, J., Ryan, M., Gilpin, J., Falsetti, M., Heffner, T., & Gaudet, S. (2004). Evaluation of a no-dressing intervention for tunneled central venous catheter exit sites. *Infusion Nursing, 27,* 37–44.

Richardson, S. (2003). Effects of relaxation and imagery on the sleep of critically ill adults. *Dimensions of Critical Care Nursing, 22,* 182–190.

Rondorff-Klym, L. M., & Colling, J. (2003). Quality of life after radical prostatectomy. *Oncology Nursing Forum, 30,* E24–32.

van Servellen, G., Aguirre, M., Sarna, L., & Brecht, M (2002). Differential predictors of emotional distress in HIV-infected men and women. *Western Journal of Nursing Research, 24,* 49–72.

Wilde, M. H., & Carrigan, M. J. (2003). A chart audit of factors related to urine flow and urinary tract infection. *Journal of Advanced Nursing, 43,* 254–262.

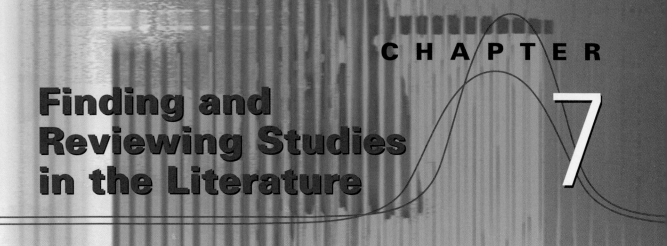

CHAPTER 7

Finding and Reviewing Studies in the Literature

STUDENT OBJECTIVES

On completing this chapter, you will be able to:

◗ Describe several purposes of a research literature review
◗ Identify bibliographic aids for retrieving nursing research reports and locate references for a research topic
◗ Identify appropriate information to include in a research literature review
◗ Understand the steps involved in writing a literature review
◗ Evaluate the style, content, and organization of a traditional literature review
◗ Define new terms in the chapter

PURPOSES AND USES OF LITERATURE REVIEWS

Literature reviews can serve a number of important functions in the research process—and they also play a critical role for nurses seeking to develop an evidence-based practice. This chapter presents information on locating research reports, organizing and preparing a written review, and critiquing reviews prepared by others.

Researchers and Literature Reviews

For researchers, familiarity with relevant research literature can help with the following:

▶ Identifying a research problem and refining research questions or hypotheses
▶ Getting oriented to what is known and not known about a topic, to learn what research can best make a contribution
▶ Determining gaps or inconsistencies in a body of research
▶ Identifying or developing new clinical interventions to test through research
▶ Identifying relevant theoretical or conceptual frameworks for a research problem
▶ Determining suitable designs and data collection methods for a study
▶ Gaining insights for interpreting study findings and developing implications

Literature reviews can inspire new research ideas and help to lay the foundation for studies. A literature review is a crucial early task for most quantitative researchers. As previously noted, however, qualitative researchers have varying opinions about literature reviews, with some deliberately avoiding an in-depth literature search before entering the field. Some of the differences reflect viewpoints associated with various qualitative research traditions. In grounded theory studies, researchers typically begin to collect data before examining the literature. As the data are analyzed and the grounded theory takes shape, researchers then turn to the literature, seeking to relate prior findings to the theory. Phenomenologists, by contrast, often undertake a search for relevant materials at the outset of a study. Ethnographers, although they often do not do a thorough up-front literature review, often review the literature to help shape their choice of a cultural problem before going into the field.

Researchers usually summarize relevant literature in the introduction to research reports, regardless of when they perform the literature search. The literature review provides readers with a background for understanding current knowledge on a topic and illuminates the significance of the new study. Written literature reviews thus serve an integrative function and facilitate the accumulation of evidence on a problem.

Nonresearchers and Literature Reviews

Research reviews are not prepared solely in the context of doing a study. Nursing students, nursing faculty, clinical nurses, nurse administrators, and nurses involved in policy-making organizations also need to review and synthesize evidence on a topic. The specific purpose of the review varies depending on the reviewer's role. Here are a few examples:

▶ Acquiring knowledge on a topic (students, faculty, clinical nurses, administrators)
▶ Evaluating current practices and making recommendations for change (faculty, clinical nurses, administrators, policy-oriented nurses)

▶ Developing evidence-based clinical protocols and interventions to improve clinical practice (clinical nurses, administrators, graduate students)
▶ Developing a theory or conceptual framework (faculty)
▶ Developing or revising nursing curricula (faculty)
▶ Developing policy statements and practice guidelines (policy-oriented nurses)

Thus, both consumers and producers of nursing research need to acquire skills for preparing and critiquing written summaries of knowledge on a problem.

LOCATING RELEVANT LITERATURE FOR A RESEARCH REVIEW

The ability to identify and locate documents on a research topic is an important skill. It is also a skill that requires adaptability—rapid technological changes, such as the expanding use of the Internet, are making manual methods of finding information from print resources obsolete, and more sophisticated methods of searching the literature are being introduced continuously. We urge you to consult with librarians at your institution for updated guidance.

CONSUMER TIP

Locating all relevant information on a research question is a bit like being a detective. The various electronic and print literature retrieval tools are a tremendous aid, but there inevitably needs to be some digging for, and a lot of sifting and sorting of, the clues to knowledge on a topic. Be prepared for sleuthing!

One caveat should be mentioned. You may be tempted to do a literature search through an Internet search engine, such as Yahoo, Google, or Alta Vista. Such a search might yield an array of information, such as advice for lay persons, press releases and notices, connections to advocacy and support groups, and so on. Such Internet searches, however, are unlikely to give you comprehensive bibliographic information on the *research* literature on your topic—and you might become frustrated with searching through the vast number of websites now available.

Electronic Literature Searches

Print-based literature search resources that must be manually searched have become outmoded. Almost all college and university libraries offer students the capability of performing their own searches of **electronic databases**—huge bibliographic files that can be accessed by computer. Most of the electronic databases of interest to nurses can be accessed either through an **online search** (i.e., by directly communicating with a host computer over the Internet) or by CD-ROM (compact discs that store the bibliographic information). Several competing commercial vendors (e.g., Aries Knowledge Finder, Ovid, SilverPlatter) offer information retrieval services for bibliographic databases. Their programs are user friendly—they are menu driven with on-screen support, so that retrieval usually can proceed with minimal instruction. Some of these service providers offer free trial services that allow you to test an online or CD-ROM system before subscribing, and some offer discount rates for students.

Major electronic databases that contain references on nursing studies include the following:

▶ CINAHL (**C**umulative **I**ndex to **N**ursing and **A**llied **H**ealth **L**iterature)
▶ MEDLINE (**Med**ical Literature On**line**)
▶ Cochrane Database
▶ EMBASE (the **E**xcerpta **M**edica data**base**)
▶ PsycINFO (**Psy**chology **Info**rmation)

Most nursing school libraries subscribe to CINAHL, one of the most useful databases for nurses. The CINAHL database (www.cinahl.com) is described more fully in the next section. The MEDLINE database, perhaps the second most important database for nurse researchers, can be accessed free of charge through PubMed (www.ncbi.nlm.nih.gov/PubMed).

Several other types of electronic resources should be mentioned. First, books and other holdings of libraries can almost always be scanned electronically using *online catalog systems*. Moreover, through the Internet, the catalog holdings of libraries across the country can be reviewed. Finally, it may be useful to search through Sigma Theta Tau International's Registry of Nursing Research on the Internet, www.stti.iupui.edu/VirginiaHendersonLibrary/. This registry is an electronic research database with more than 12,000 studies that can be searched by **key words**, variables, and researchers' names. The registry provides access to studies that have not yet been published, which cuts down the publication lag time; however, caution is needed because these studies have not been critiqued by external reviewers. Electronic publishing in general is expanding at a rapid pace; librarians and faculty should be consulted for the most useful websites.

 CONSUMER TIP

It is rarely possible to identify all relevant studies exclusively through literature retrieval mechanisms. An excellent method of identifying additional references is to find recently published studies and examine their bibliographies. Researchers are usually knowledgeable about other relevant works and cite them to provide context for their own studies.

The CINAHL Database

This section illustrates some of the features of an electronic search, through the use of the **CINAHL database**. Our illustrated example relied on the Ovid Search Software for CD-ROM, but similar features are available through other software programs or through direct online access.

The CINAHL database covers references to over 1200 English- and foreign-language nursing journals, as well as to books, book chapters, nursing dissertations, and selected conference proceedings in nursing and allied health fields. The database covers materials dating from 1982 to the present and contains nearly a million records. In addition to providing bibliographic information (i.e., the author, title, journal, year of publication, volume, and page numbers) of a reference), abstracts are available for almost 1000 journals.

Most searches are likely to begin with a **subject search**—a search for references relating to a specific topic. For this type of search, you would type in a word or phrase that captures the essence of the topic, and the computer would then proceed with the search. Fortunately, through *mapping* capabilities, most retrieval software translates (maps) the topic you type in to the most plausible CINAHL subject heading. An important alternative to a subject search is a **textword search** that looks for your specific words in text fields of each record, including the title and the abstract. (If you know the name of a researcher who has worked on a specific research topic, an **author search** might be productive.)

CONSUMER TIP

If you want to identify all major research reports on a topic, you need to be flexible and to think broadly about the key words and subject headings that could be related to your topic. For example, if you are interested in anorexia nervosa, you should search on anorexia, eating disorders, and weight loss, and perhaps under appetite, eating behavior, nutrition, bulimia, body weight changes, and body image.

After you have typed in your topic, the computer will tell you how many "hits" there are in the database (i.e., matches against your topic). In most cases, the number of hits initially will be large, and you will want to constrain the search to ensure that you retrieve only the most relevant references. You can limit your search in a number of ways. For example, you might want only references published in nursing journals; only those that are for research studies; only those published in certain years (e.g., 2000 or later); or only those dealing with participants in certain age groups (e.g., infants).

To illustrate with a concrete example, suppose we were interested in recent research on postoperative pain, which is the term we enter in a subject search. Here is an example of how many hits there were on successive restrictions to the search for studies on therapies for postoperative pain, using the CINAHL database current to September 2003:

Search Topic/Restriction	*Hits*
Postoperative pain	1370
Restrict to therapy subheadings	822
Limit to research reports with abstracts in English-language journals	274
Limit to core nursing journals	86
Limit to 2000–2003 publications	27

This narrowing of the search—from 1370 initial references on postoperative pain to 27 references for recent nursing research reports on postoperative pain therapies—took less than a minute to perform. Next, we would display the 27 references on the monitor, and we could then print full bibliographic information for the ones that appeared especially promising. An example of an abridged CINAHL record entry for a study identified through this search on postoperative pain is presented in Figure 7-1. Each entry shows an accession number, which is the unique identifier for each record in the database; this number can be used to order the full text of the report. Then the authors, their contact information, and the title of the study are displayed, followed by source information. The source indicates the following:

Accession Number
2003092971

Authors
LaMontagne LL, Hepworth JT, Cohen F, Salisbury MH

Institution
School of Nursing, Vanderbilt University, 412 Godchaux Hall, 461 21st Avenue South, Nashville, TN 37240-0008; lynda.lamontagne@vanderbil.edu

Title
Cognitive-behavioral intervention effects on adolescents' anxiety and **pain** following spinal fusion surgery.

Source
Nursing Research, 52 (3): 183–90, 2003 May-Jun, (32 ref)

Cinahl Subject Headings

Adolescence	**Postoperative Pain** / th [Therapy]
Age Factors	**Postoperative** Period
Anxiety/ th [Therapy]	Preoperative Education
Clinical Trials	Psychological Tests
Cognitive Therapy	Repeated Measures
Coping	Spinal Fusion
Descriptive Statistics	State-Trait Anxiety Inventory
Interviews	Surgical patients
Pain Measurement	Videorecording

Instrumentation
State-Trait Anxiety Inventory (STAI) (Spielberger)

Abstract
Background: Cognitive-behavioral interventions, typically effective in reducing anxiety and **pain**, have not been applied to adolescents undergoing major orthopaedic surgery. **Objectives:** To determine the effectiveness of three cognitive-behavioral interventions for reducing adolescents' postoperative anxiety and **pain** following spinal fusion surgery for scoliosis, and whether effectiveness depended on preoperative anxiety and age. **Methods:** A randomized controlled trial with four groups receiving a videotaped intervention (information only, coping only, information plus coping, or control) used a convenience sample of 109 adolescents (88 female, 93 White), 11–18 years of age (M = 14). Speilberger's (1983) State Anxiety scale assessed anxiety preoperative and **postoperatively** on Days 2 and 4. **Results:** Information plus coping was most effective for reducing **postoperative** anxiety and **pain** for adolescents ages 13 and younger. The control group reported the highest level of **pain** on Day 4. **Conclusions:** Cognitive-behavioral interventions designed to prepare adolescents for surgery should be tailored to individual factors and developmental needs, especially the adolescents' preoperative anxiety level and age.

Language
English

Grant Information
NIH-National Institute of Nursing Research, grant # R01NR02673

FIGURE 7.1 Example of a printout from a CINAHL search.

Name of the journal (*Nursing Research*)
Volume (52)
Issue (3)
Page numbers (183–190)
Year and month of publication (2003 May-June)
Number of cited references (32 ref.)

The printout shows all the CINAHL subject headings for this entry, any one of which could have been used to retrieve this reference through a subject search. Note that the subject headings include substantive topics (e.g., coping, postoperative pain), methodologic topics (e.g., descriptive statistics, interviews), and headings relating to the group under study (e.g., adolescence). Note also that the words used in the search (e.g., *pain)* are bolded throughout the printout so they can be easily seen. Next, if formal instruments were used in the study, these are printed under Instrumentation. Then the study abstract is presented. Based on the abstract, you would decide whether this study was pertinent to your literature review; if so, the full research reports could be obtained and read. Reports in the CINAHL database can be ordered by mail or facsimile (fax); therefore, it is not necessary for your library to subscribe to the referenced journal. Moreover, many of the retrieval service providers, such as Ovid, offer *full text* online services, which would enable you to download documents from certain journals. The final entry in Figure 7-1 shows that the study was funded by NINR, and indicates the grant number.

CONSUMER TIP

If your topic includes independent and dependent variables, you may need to do separate searches for each. For example, if you were interested in learning about the effect of stress on the health beliefs of AIDS patients, you might want to read about the effects of stress (in general) and about people's health beliefs (in general). Moreover, you might also want to learn something about AIDS patients and their problems. If you are searching for references electronically, you can also combine searches, so that the references for two independent searches can be linked (e.g., the computer can identify those references that have both stress and health beliefs as subject headings or textwords).

Example of a literature search

Carolan (2003) published a literature review on the relationship between advanced maternal age and pregnancy outcomes. She conducted computerized searches on multiple databases, including CINAHL and MEDLINE, using the following key words: advanced maternal age, pregnancy outcomes for older primiparae and older mothers, and pregnancy risks.

PREPARING WRITTEN REVIEWS OF RESEARCH EVIDENCE

Identifying references, using the guidelines and tools described in the previous section, is an early step in preparing a written review of research literature. Subsequent steps are summarized in Figure 7-2.

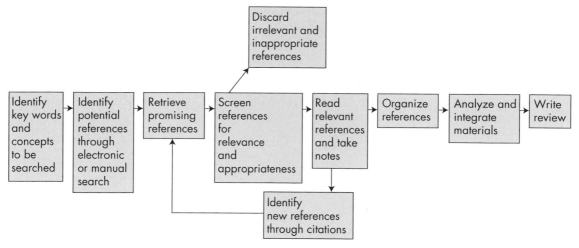

FIGURE 7.2 Flow of tasks in a literature review.

Retrieving and Screening References

As Figure 7-2 shows, after identifying promising references, you need to retrieve the full reports. In addition to obtaining reports through your library or through CINAHL or other electronic databases, many nursing journals (e.g., *Nursing Research* and *Research in Nursing & Health*) are now available online.

The next step is to screen reports for relevance and appropriateness. The report's *relevance*, which concerns whether it really focuses on the topic of interest, usually can be judged quickly by reading the introduction. *Appropriateness* concerns the nature of the information in the report. The most important information for a research review comes from reports that describe study findings. You should rely primarily on **primary source** research reports, which are descriptions of studies written by the researchers who conducted them. **Secondary source** research articles are descriptions of studies prepared by someone other than the original researcher. Literature review articles are secondary sources. Recent review articles are a good place to begin a literature search because they summarize current knowledge, and the reference lists are helpful. However, secondary descriptions of studies should not be considered substitutes for primary sources.

Examples of primary and secondary sources on families and schizophrenia

Primary source—an original qualitative study based on interviews with parents of 22 patients diagnosed with schizophrenia: Experiences of parents with a son or daughter suffering from schizophrenia (Ferriter & Huband, 2003).
Secondary source—a review of the literature on families living with schizophrenia: Families living with severe mental illness: A literature review (Saunders, 2003).

For some literature reviews, it may be important to seek out references from the conceptual literature (i.e., references on a theory or conceptual model). In the conceptual literature, a primary source is a description of a theory written by the developer of the theory, and a secondary source is a discussion or critique of the theory.

In addition to empirical and conceptual references, you may find in your search various nonresearch references, including opinion articles, case reports, anecdotes, and clinical descriptions. Such materials may serve to broaden understanding of a research problem, illustrate a point, demonstrate a need for research, or describe aspects of clinical practice. They may thus play important roles in formulating research ideas, but they generally have limited utility in written research reviews because they do not address the central question of research reviews: What is the current state of *knowledge* on this problem?

Abstracting and Recording Notes

Once you judge a reference to be relevant and appropriate, you should read the entire report carefully and critically, using guidelines that are provided throughout this book. It is useful to work with photocopied articles, so that you can highlight or underline critical information. Even with a copied article, we recommend taking notes or writing a summary of the report's strengths and limitations. A formal protocol is sometimes helpful for recording information in a systematic fashion. An example of such a protocol is presented in Figure 7-3. While many of the terms on this protocol are probably not familiar to you at this point, you will learn their meaning as you progress through this book.

Organizing the Evidence

Organization is crucial in preparing a written review. When literature on a topic is extensive, it is useful to summarize information in a table. The table could include columns with headings such as Author, Type of Study (Qualitative versus Quantitative), Sample, Design, Data Collection Approach, and Key Findings. Such a table provides a quick overview that allows you to make sense of a mass of information.

Most writers find it helpful to work from an outline—a written one if the review is lengthy and complex, a mental one for short reviews. The important point is to work out a structure before starting to write so that the presentation has a meaningful flow. Lack of organization is a common weakness in students' first attempts to write a research review. Although the specifics of the organization differ from topic to topic, the overall goal is to structure the review in such a way that the presentation is logical, demonstrates meaningful integration, and leads to a conclusion of what is known and not known about the topic.

 Example of tabular organization

Glass and her colleagues (2003) reviewed research on adolescent dating violence. Their review included a table summarizing 15 studies that measured the prevalence of dating violence. The column headings were: author and date; number of subjects; ethnicity, gender, and age; design; setting; measure of violence; and prevalence.

After the organization of topics has been determined, you should review your notes or protocols. This not only helps refresh your memory about material read earlier but also lays the groundwork for decisions about where a particular reference fits in the outline. If certain

Citation: Authors: _____
Title: _____
Journal: _____
Year: _____ Volume: _____ Issue: _____ Pages: _____

Type of Study: ☐ Quantitative ☐ Qualitative ☐ Both

Location/setting: _____

Key Concepts/ Concepts: _____
Variables: Intervention/Independent Variable: _____
Dependent Variable: _____
Controlled Variables: _____

Design Type: ☐ Experimental ☐ Quasi-experimental ☐ Pre-experimental ☐ Nonexperimental
Specific Design: _____
Descrip. of Intervention: _____
_____

☐ Longitudinal/prospective ☐ Cross-sectional No. of data collection points: _____
Comparison group(s): _____

Qual. Tradition: ☐ Grounded theory ☐ Phenomenology ☐ Ethnography ☐ Other: _____

Sample: Size: _____ Sampling method: _____
Sample characteristics: _____

Data Sources: Type: ☐ Self-report ☐ Observational ☐ Biophysiologic ☐ Other: _____
Description of measures: _____
_____
Data Quality: _____

Statistical Tests: Bivariate: ☐ t test ☐ ANOVA ☐ Chi-square ☐ Pearson's r ☐ Other: _____
Multivariate: ☐ Multiple regression ☐ MANOVA ☐ ANCOVA ☐ Other: _____

Findings: _____
_____
_____
_____

Recommendations: _____
_____

Strengths: _____
_____
_____

Weaknesses: _____
_____
_____

FIGURE 7.3 Example of a literature review protocol.

references do not seem to fit anywhere, they may need to be put aside; remember that the number of references is less important than their relevance and the overall organization and quality of the review.

CONSUMER TIP

An important principle in organizing a review is to figure out a way to cluster and compare studies. For example, you could contrast studies that have similar findings with studies that have conflicting or inconclusive findings, making sure to analyze why discrepancies may have occurred. Other reviews might have sample characteristics as an organizing scheme if findings vary according to such characteristics (e.g., if results differ for male and female participants). Doing a research review is a bit like doing a qualitative study—you must search for important *themes* in the findings. ■

Writing a Literature Review

Research reviews tend to be written in a particular style and typically include specific types of information.

CONTENT OF A RESEARCH REVIEW

A written research review should provide readers with an objective and thorough summary of the current state of evidence on a topic. A literature review should be neither a series of quotes nor a series of abstracts. The key tasks are to summarize and evaluate the evidence so as to reveal the state-of-the-art knowledge of a topic—not simply to describe what researchers have done. The review should point out both consistencies and contradictions in the literature and offer possible explanations for inconsistencies (e.g., different conceptualizations or data collection methods).

Although important studies should be described in some detail, it is not necessary to provide extensive coverage for every reference. Reports with similar findings sometimes can be summarized together.

Example of grouped studies

In their literature review for a study focusing on family carers of ICU survivors, Foster and Chaboyer (2003, p. 206) summarized several studies as follows: "There is overwhelming evidence that suggests that there is economic, social, and psychological impact for family caregivers as a result of providing care to their relative (Chou et al., 1999; Bell et al., 2001; Johnson et al., 1995; Pearlin et al., 1990)."

The literature should be summarized in your own words. The review should demonstrate that consideration has been given to the cumulative significance of the body of research. Stringing together quotes from various documents fails to show that previous research on the topic has been assimilated and understood.

Another point to bear in mind is that the review should be as objective as possible. Studies that conflict with personal values or hunches should not be omitted. In addition, the review should not deliberately ignore a study because its findings contradict other studies. Inconsistent results should be analyzed and the supporting evidence evaluated objectively.

The literature review should conclude with a critical summary that recaps key study findings and indicates how credible they are; it should also make note of gaps in the research. The summary thus requires critical judgment about the extensiveness and dependability of evidence on a topic.

As you progress through this book, you will become increasingly proficient in critically evaluating research reports. We hope you will understand the mechanics of writing a research review when you have completed this chapter, but we do not expect that you will be in a position to write a state-of-the-art review until you have acquired more skills in research methods.

STYLE OF A RESEARCH REVIEW

Students preparing their first written research review often have trouble adjusting to the standard style of research reviews. One issue is that students sometimes accept research results without criticism or reservation, reflecting a common misunderstanding about the conclusiveness of research. You should keep in mind that no hypothesis or theory can be proved or disproved by empirical testing, and no research question can be definitely answered in a single study. The problem is partly a semantic one: hypotheses are not proved, they are supported by research findings; theories are not verified, but they may be tentatively accepted if a substantial body of evidence demonstrates their legitimacy. When describing study findings, you should generally use phrases indicating tentativeness of the results, such as the following:

▶ Several studies have *found*...
▶ Findings thus far *suggest*...
▶ Results from a landmark study *indicated*...
▶ The data *supported* the hypothesis...
▶ There *appears* to be strong evidence that...

A related stylistic problem among movie reviewers is an inclination to intersperse opinions (their own or someone else's) into the review. The review should include opinions sparingly and should be explicit about their source. Your own opinions do not belong in a review, with the exception of assessments of study quality.

The left-hand column of Table 7-1 presents examples of stylistic flaws. The right-hand column offers recommendations for rewording the sentences to conform to a more acceptable form for a research literature review. Many alternative wordings are possible.

LENGTH OF A RESEARCH REVIEW

There are no easy formulas for how long a review should be. The length depends on several factors, including the complexity of the research question, the extent of prior research, and the purpose for which the review is being prepared. Literature reviews prepared for proposals (e.g., proposals to undertake a study, to test a clinical innovation, or to make a change in practice) tend to be fairly comprehensive. Reviews in theses and dissertations are also lengthy. In these cases, the literature review serves both to summarize knowledge and to document the reviewer's capability.

Because of space limitations in journal articles, literature reviews that appear within research reports are concise. Literature reviews in the introduction to research reports demonstrate the need for the new study and provide a context for the research questions. The literature review sections of qualitative reports tend to be especially brief. However, there are stand-alone research reviews in nursing journals that are more extensive than those appearing in the introductions of research reports. We discuss such reviews next.

| TABLE 7.1 | Examples of Stylistic Difficulties for Research Reviews |

INAPPROPRIATE STYLE OR WORDING	RECOMMENDED CHANGE
1. It is known that unmet expectations engender stress.	Dr. A. Cassard, an expert on stress and anxiety, has found that unmet expectations engender stress (Cassard, 2005).
2. Women who do not participate in childbirth preparation classes tend to manifest a high degree of stress during labor.	Studies have found that women who participate in preparation for childbirth classes manifest less stress during labor than those who do not (Klotz, 2003; Weller, 2004; McTygue, 2005)
3. Studies have proved that doctors and nurses do not fully understand the psychobiologic dynamics of recovery from a myocardial infarction.	Studies by Lowe (2004) and Martin (2003) suggest that doctors and nurses do not fully understand the psychobiologic dynamics of recovery from a myocardial infarction.
4. Attitudes cannot be changed quickly.	Attitudes have been found to be relatively enduring attributes that cannot be changed quickly (Geair, 2003; Casey, 2004).

NOTE: All references are fictitious.

READING AND USING EXISTING RESEARCH REVIEWS

Most of this chapter provides guidance on how to conduct a literature review—how to locate and screen references, what type of information to seek, and how to organize and write a review. However, practicing nurses may not need to perform a full-fledged review if a comprehensive and recent literature review on the topic of interest has been published. Several different types of integrative reviews that can be used to support evidence-based nursing practice are briefly described in this section.

Traditional Narrative Reviews

A traditional narrative literature review synthesizes and summarizes, in a narrative fashion, a body of research literature. The information offered in this chapter has been designed to help you prepare such a review.

Narrative integrated reviews are frequently published in nursing journals, especially in nursing specialty journals. These reviews may have a number of different purposes, including

Example of a narrative research review

Cottrell (2003) did a review of studies on vaginal douching. Studies were identified through searches of the MEDLINE, CINAHL, and Cochrane databases from 1997 through 2001. Her review covered the literature on the prevalence of douching; frequency of douching; characteristics associated with the practice; adverse health effects; and beliefs and misconceptions about douching. Her review concluded with a discussion of practice implications.

providing practitioners with state-of-the-art research-based information; providing a foundation for the development of innovations for clinical practice; and developing an agenda for further research.

Meta-analysis

Meta-analysis is a technique for integrating quantitative research findings statistically. In essence, meta-analysis treats the findings from a study as one piece of data. The findings from multiple studies on the same topic are then combined to create a data set that can be analyzed in a manner similar to that obtained from individuals. Thus, instead of study participants being the **unit of analysis** (the most basic entity on which the analysis focuses), individual studies are the unit of analysis in a meta-analysis. Typically, the meta-analyst takes information about the strength of the relationship between the independent and dependent variables from each study, quantifies that information, and then essentially takes an average across all studies.

Traditional narrative research reviews have some shortcomings that make meta-analysis appealing. For example, if there are many studies and results are inconsistent, it may be difficult in a narrative review to draw conclusions. Furthermore, integration in narrative reviews can be subject to reviewer biases. Another advantage of meta-analysis is that it can take into account the quality of the studies being combined. Meta-analysis provides a convenient and objective method of integrating a large body of findings and of observing patterns and relationships that might otherwise have gone undetected. Meta-analysis can thus serve as an important tool in research utilization. Because of this fact, we discuss meta-analysis at greater length in the final chapter.

Example of a meta-analysis

Taylor-Piliae and Froelicher (2004) conducted a meta-analysis to integrate findings on the effectiveness of Tai Chi exercise in improving aerobic capacity. They integrated results from seven studies. The aggregated evidence suggested that Tai Chi may be effective, especially when the classical Yang style of Tai Chi is performed for 1 year by sedentary adults. (This study appears in its entirety in Appendix F of the accompanying Study Guide.)

Qualitative Metasynthesis

There is an increasing awareness of the need for integrative reviews of qualitative studies so that the understandings gleaned from such studies can be accumulated. Efforts are underway to develop techniques for qualitative metasynthesis, and several strategies have evolved. A qualitative **metasynthesis** involves integrating qualitative research findings on a specific topic that are themselves interpretive syntheses of data, such as from phenomenological, ethnographic, and grounded theory studies (Sandelowski & Barroso, 2003). A metasynthesis of qualitative findings is more than just a summary of findings—it involves interpretation of those findings, and this is where a metasynthesis differs from a meta-analysis. A metasynthesis is less about reducing data and more about amplifying and interpreting data. Sandelowski, Docherty, and Emden (1997) warn researchers that qualitative metasynthesis is a complex process that involves "carefully peeling away the surface layers of studies to find their hearts and souls in a way that does the

Example of a qualitative metasynthesis

Arman and Rehnsfeldt (2003) conducted a metaysnthesis of 14 qualitative studies published between 1990 and 2000 on the experience of suffering and breast cancer. The metasynthesis revealed that after the sudden disruption of their lives in the initial stage of breast cancer, women struggled to restore the balance in their lives. Arman and Rehnsfeldt discovered levels of reported changes or transitions after breast cancer diagnosis. These levels included sudden existential disruption, actions, values and cognitions, and spirituality/existence. The transforming process moved from actions toward healthier lifestyle by renewing values and priorities, to integrating and accepting death—as well as elements of spirituality and finding meaning in the experience.

least damage to them" (p. 370). Various methods have been used to synthesize qualitative findings but to date no firm guidelines exist.

Critiquing Research Reviews

Some nurses never prepare a written research review, and perhaps you will never be required to do one. Most nurses, however, do *read* research reviews (including the literature review sections of research reports) and they should be prepared to evaluate such reviews critically. You may find it difficult to critique a research review, because you are probably a lot less familiar with the topic than the writer. You may thus not be able to judge whether the author has included all relevant literature and has adequately summarized knowledge on that topic. Many aspects of a research review, however, are amenable to evaluation by readers who are not experts on the topic. Some suggestions for critiquing written research reviews are presented in Box 7-1. Additionally, when a literature review—whether it be a traditional review, a meta-analysis, or a metasynthesis—is published as a stand-alone article, it should include information that will help you understand its scope and evaluate its thoroughness. This is discussed in more detail in Chapter 18.

BOX 7.1   **Guidelines for Critiquing Literature Reviews**

1. Does the review seem thorough—does it include all or most of the major studies on the topic? Does it include recent research? Are studies from other related disciplines included, if appropriate?
2. Does the review rely on appropriate materials (e.g., mainly on research reports, using primary sources)?
3. Is the review merely a summary of existing work, or does it critically appraise and compare key studies? Does the review identify important gaps in the literature?
4. Is the review well organized? Is the development of ideas clear?
5. Does the review use appropriate language, suggesting the tentativeness of prior findings? Is the review objective? Does the author paraphrase, or is there an overreliance on quotes from original sources?
6. If the review is part of a research report for a new study, does the review support the need for the study? If it is a critical integrative review designed to summarize evidence for clinical practice, does the review draw appropriate conclusions about practice implications?

In assessing a written literature review, the overarching question is whether the review summarizes the current state of research evidence. If the review is written as part of an original research report, an equally important question is whether the review lays a solid foundation for the new study.

C H A P T E R   R E V I E W

Key new terms introduced in the chapter, together with a summary of major points, are presented in this section. In addition, Chapter 7 of the accompanying *Study Guide to Accompany Essentials of Nursing Research,* 6th edition offers various exercises and study suggestions for reinforcing the concepts presented in this chapter. For additional review, see the Student Self-Study Review Questions section of the Student Resource CD-ROM provided with this book.

K E Y   N E W   T E R M S

Author search
CINAHL database
Electronic database
Key word
Literature review
Meta-analysis
Metasynthesis

Online search
Primary source
Secondary source
Subject search
Textword search
Unit of analysis

S U M M A R Y   P O I N T S

▷ A research **literature review** is a written summary of the state of existing knowledge on a research problem.

▷ Researchers prepare literature reviews to determine knowledge on a topic of interest, to provide a context for a study, and to justify the need for a study; consumers review and synthesize evidence-based information to gain knowledge and improve nursing practice.

▷ An important bibliographic development for locating references is the various **electronic databases**, many of which can be accessed through an **online search** or by way of CD-ROM. For nurses, the **CINAHL database** is especially useful.

▷ Most database searches begin with a **subject search**, but a **textword search** (which looks for specific words) or **author search** are possibilities.

▷ In writing a research review, the reviewer should carefully organize the relevant materials, which should consist primarily of **primary source** research reports.

▷ The role of the reviewer is to point out what has been studied to date, how adequate and dependable those studies are, and what gaps exist in the body of research.

▷ Nurses also need to have skills in using and critiquing integrative research reviews prepared by others, including traditional narrative reviews; **meta-analysis** (the integration of study findings using statistical procedures); and qualitative **metasynthesis** (the integration of qualitative research findings that produce new interpretations that are more substantive than the findings from the individual studies.)

RESEARCH EXAMPLES Critical Thinking Activities

 EXAMPLE 1: Quantitative Research

Aspects of a quantitative nursing study, featuring terms and concepts discussed in this chapter, are presented below, followed by some questions to guide critical thinking. (The full research report is available in *Nursing Research, 52,* 242–248.)

Study

"Backrest angle and cardiac output measurement in critically ill patients" (Giuliano, Scott, Brown, & Olson, 2003)

Statement of Purpose

The purpose of the study was to compare the effect of varying degrees of backrest elevation on cardiac output (CO) in critically ill patients using the continuous cardiac output (CCO) method of measurement.

Method

CCO measurements were taken on 26 critically ill patients at head-of-bed angles of 0°, 30°, and 45°, and at points of time of 0 minutes, 5 minutes, and 10 minutes after each position change.

Literature Review from the Report (Excerpt)

"Studies of the effect of positioning changes on determination of CO in critically ill patients have been very limited. Four studies that specifically measured CO or cardiac index (CI) in response to supine position changes were found...(Driscoll et al., 1995; Grose et al., 1981; Kleven, 1984; Wilson et al., 1996). Grose et al. (1981) reported no clinically significant differences in CO measurements taken at 20° when compared to those at 0° in patients receiving mechanical ventilation with positive-end-expiratory pressure (PEEP), concurrent intravenous infusions, or patients on vasoactive infusions. Kleven (1984) reported a significant decrease in CO measurements taken at 20° when compared to those at 0° in patients receiving mechanical ventilation with PEEP. In Kleven's study, additional measurements were taken 5 minutes after the change in head of bed (HOB) angle. Wilson et al. (1996) also found statistically significant differences in CI between 0°-45°, but these differences were not clinically significant, and the issue of time was not clearly addressed. Driscoll et al. (1995) compared the supine and flat backrest position to a backrest elevation of 45°, and reported 11% decrease in the 40° backrest position. However, the study sample was primarily a cardiac surgery patient population. Literature on measurement intervals of greater than 5 minutes between position changes and measurements of CO were not found.

Optimal care of many critically ill patients depends largely on the accurate measurement of CO....Patient positioning is an aspect of patient care that is left primarily at the disretion of the critical care nurse and it is important that the effect of this intervention on CO measurement be studied. There is some evidence to support that the thermodilution method of CO measurement

RESEARCH EXAMPLES *Continued*

can be accurately reproduced up to a backrest elevation of 20° (Grap et al., 1997; Grose et al., 1981; Kleven, 1984; Wilson et al., 1996). This study was designed to provide further information using CCO as the method of CO measurement" (pp. 243–244).

Key Findings

▶ There were no overall significant differences in CCO values at the various head-of-bed angles and time points in the study sample.

▶ There were also no differences found for stroke volume, heart rate, or mean arterial pressure.

Critical Thinking Suggestions*

*See the Student Resource CD-ROM for a discussion of these questions.
1. Answer the questions from Box 7-1 regarding this study.
2. Also consider the following targeted questions, which may assist you in further assessing aspects of the study:
   a. What were the two independent variables in this study? Did the literature review cover findings from prior studies about both of these variables?
   b. What was the main dependent variable in this study? Did the literature review cover findings from prior studies about this variable and its relationship with the independent variables?
   c. In performing the literature review, what key words might the researchers have used to search for prior studies?
   d. Using the key words, perform a computerized search to see if you can find a recent relevant study to augment the review.
3. If the results of this study are valid and reliable, what are some of the uses to which the findings might be put in clinical practice?

 EXAMPLE 2: Qualitative Research

Aspects of a qualitative nursing study, featuring terms and concepts discussed in this chapter, are presented below, followed by some questions to guide critical thinking. (The full research report is available in *Nursing Research, 51,* 391–397.)

Study

"From 'death sentence' to 'good cancer': Couples' transformation of a prostate cancer diagnosis" (Maliski, Heilemann, & McCorkle, 2002)

Statement of Purpose

The purpose of the study was to describe the experience of men who are diagnosed with prostate cancer and their wives, from the time of diagnosis through staging to the completion of radical prostatectomy.

research examples continue on page 150

RESEARCH EXAMPLES *Continued*

Method

Twenty couples participated in in-depth interviews 3 to 11 months postprostatectomy. Most husbands and wives were interviewed individually with the other spouse present, to facilitate observation of intracouple dynamics.

Literature Review from the Report (Excerpt)

"Although there is some literature on decision-making in prostate cancer treatment, few studies describe the role of wives. Even less is known about the couple's experience at the time of diagnosis while facing treatment decisions, and receiving the treatment itself. As noted by various researchers, few studies have focused on the process of finding meaning within the struggle to deal with cancer and its impact on partners or couples (Germino et al., 1995; Kornblith et al., 1994).

Of the studies that explored the effect of a cancer diagnosis on patients and their spouses, most deal with the impact on husbands of women with breast cancer. Conclusions from these research studies reveal that the spouse sometimes experiences more distress than the patient (Lewis et al., 1993; Northouse et al., 1991, 1997; Northouse & Swain, 1987)....Lewis and Deal (1995) found that couples lived with a breast cancer recurrence by actively balancing their lives, and keeping breast cancer in the background. The investigators concluded that this strategy may have facilitated behavioral functioning, but not mood or marital quality....

Very little research has focused on the couple's experience of the pretreatment phase of prostate cancer. O'Rourke and Germino (1998a) used focus groups to explore prostate cancer treatment decision-making and spousal participation. Twelve patients and six spouses were recruited from a newly formed support group. Few conclusions were drawn by the investigators except that additional studies are needed to explore the pretreatment decision-making process from a family perspective. Citing interview data from a second study, O'Rourke and Germino (1998b) described the wives' roles as that of support person, information-seeker, and advocate for their husbands during the pretreatment phase....Heyman and Rosener (1996) described coping strategies used by husbands and wives in various stages to deal with prostate cancer. They identified the early stage issues including fear of death, dealing with treatment decisions, and coping strategies....Ultimately, the researchers concluded that couples viewed the wife as a partner in managing the disease and expected that she would act on behalf of her husband in all phases of the prostate cancer trajectory. More recently, Harden and colleagues (2002) used focus groups to explore couples' experience of prostate cancer. The themes identified all dealt with post-treatment issues. These findings demonstrate how prostate cancer involves both the patient and his wife" (p. 392).

Key Findings

The researchers' analysis revealed that the diagnosis initially represented a loss of control that led many couples to go through a "crash course" on prostate cancer. The information gathered led them to conclude that prostate cancer was "good cancer," which enabled them to refocus their energies and start their quest for treatment options and surgeons.

RESEARCH EXAMPLES *Continued*

Critical Thinking Suggestions

1. Answer the questions from Box 7-1 regarding this study.
2. Also consider the following targeted questions, which may assist you in further assessing aspects of the study:
   a. What was the central phenomenon that the researchers focused on in this study? Was that phenomenon adequately covered in the literature review?
   b. In performing the literature review, what key words might the researchers have used to search for prior studies?
   c. Using the key words, perform a computerized search to see if you can find a recent relevant study to augment the review.
3. If the results of this study are trustworthy, what are some of the uses to which the findings might be put in clinical practice?

 EXAMPLE 3: Quantitative Research

1. Read the introduction from Motzer et al.'s study ("Sense of Coherence") in Appendix A of this book, and then answer the questions in Box 7-1.
2. Also consider the following targeted questions, which may further sharpen your critical thinking skills and assist you in assessing aspects of the study:
   a. What was the independent variable in this study? Did the literature review cover findings from prior studies about this variable?
   b. What were the dependent variables in this study? Did the literature review cover findings from prior studies about these variables and their relationship with the independent variable?
   c. In performing the literature review, what key words might have been used to search for prior studies?
   d. Using the key words, perform a computerized search to see if you can find a recent relevant study to augment the review.

 EXAMPLE 4: Qualitative Research

1. Read the abstract and the introduction to Beck's study ("Birth Trauma") in Appendix B of this book, and then answer the relevant questions in Box 7-1.
2. Also consider the following targeted questions, which may further sharpen your critical thinking skills and assist you in assessing aspects of the study:
   a. What was the central phenomenon that Beck focused on in this study? Was that phenomenon adequately covered in the literature review?
   b. In what sections of the report did Beck discuss prior research?
   c. In performing her literature review, what key words might Beck have used to search for prior studies?
   d. Using the key words, perform a computerized search to see if you can find a recent relevant study to augment the review.

SUGGESTED READINGS

Methodologic References

Fink, A. (1998). *Conducting research literature reviews: From paper to the Internet.* Thousand Oaks, CA: Sage Publications.

Martin, P. S. (1997). Writing a useful literature review for a quantitative research project. *Applied Nursing Research, 10,* 159–162.

Sandelowksi, M., & Barroso, J. (2003). Creating metasummaries of qualitative findings. *Nursing Research, 52,* 226–233.

Sandelowski, M., Docherty, S., & Emden, C. (1997). Qualitative metasynthesis: Issues and techniques. *Research in Nursing & Health, 20,* 365–371.

Studies Cited in Chapter 7

Arman, M., & Rehnsfeldt, A. (2003). The hidden suffering among breast cancer patients: A qualitative metasynthesis. *Qualitative Health Research, 13,* 510–527.

Carolan, M. (2003). The graying of the obstetric population: Implications for the older mother. *Journal of Obstetric, Gynecologic, & Neonatal Nursing, 32,* 19–27.

Cottrell, B. H. (2003). Vaginal douching. *Journal of Obstetric, Gynecologic, & Neonatal Nursing, 32,* 12–18.

Ferriter, M., & Huband, N. (2003). Experiences of parents with a son or daughter suffering from schizophrenia. *Journal of Psychiatric and Mental Health Nursing, 10,* 552–560.

Foster, M., & Chaboyer, W. (2003). Family carers of ICU survivors: A survey of the burden they experience. *Scandinavian Journal of the Caring Sciences, 17,* 205–214.

Giuliano, K. K., Scott, S. S., Brown, V., & Olson, M. (2003). Backrest angle and cardiac output measurement in critically ill patients. *Nursing Research, 52,* 242–248.

Glass, N., Fredland, N., Campbell, J., Yonas, M., Sharps, P., & Kub, J. (2003). Adolescent dating violence: Prevalance, risk factors, health outcomes, and implications for clinical practice. *Journal of Obstetric, Gynecologic, & Neonatal Nursing, 32,* 227–238.

Maliski, S. L., Heilemann, M. V., & McCorkle, R. (2002). From 'death sentence' to 'good cancer': Couples' transformation of a prostate cancer diagnosis. *Nursing Research, 51,* 391–397.

Saunders, J. C. (2003). Families living with severe mental illness: A literature review. *Issues in Mental Health Nursing, 24,* 175–198.

Taylor-Piliae, R. E., & Froelicher, E. S. (2004). Effectiveness of Tai Chi exercise in improving aerobic capacity: A meta-analysis. *Journal of Cardiovascular Nursing, 19,* 48–57.

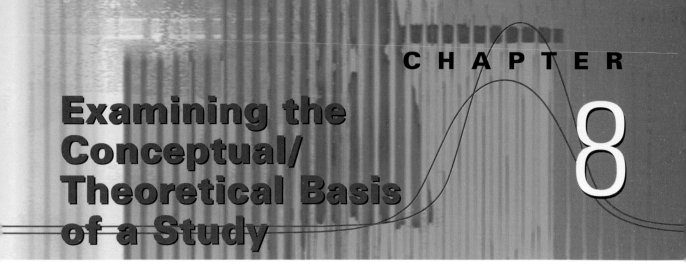

CHAPTER 8

Examining the Conceptual/ Theoretical Basis of a Study

STUDENT OBJECTIVES

On completing this chapter, you will be able to:

▶ Identify the major characteristics of theories, conceptual models, and frameworks
▶ Identify several conceptual models of nursing and other conceptual models frequently
  used by nurse researchers
▶ Describe how theory and research are linked in quantitative and qualitative studies
▶ Critique the appropriateness of a theoretical framework—or its absence—in a study
▶ Define new terms in the chapter

THEORIES, MODELS, AND FRAMEWORKS

Theories and conceptual models are the primary mechanisms by which researchers organize findings into a broader conceptual context. Different terms are used in connection with conceptual contexts for research, including *theories, models, frameworks, schemes,* and *maps*. There is overlap in how these terms are used, partly because they are used differently by different writers. We offer guidance in distinguishing them but note that there is a blurring of these terms in the literature and that our definitions are not universal.

Theories

Nursing instructors and students frequently use the term *theory* to refer to the content covered in classrooms, as opposed to the actual practice of nursing. In both lay and scientific language, *theory* connotes an abstraction.

Classically, theory is defined as an abstract generalization that presents a systematic explanation about how phenomena are interrelated. The traditional definition requires a theory to embody at least two concepts that are related in a manner that the theory purports to explain. As classically defined, theories consist of concepts and a set of propositions that form a logically interrelated system, providing a mechanism for logically deducing new statements from the original propositions. To illustrate, consider the theory of reinforcement, which posits that behavior that is reinforced (i.e., rewarded) tends to be repeated and learned. This theory consists of concepts (reinforcement and learning) and a proposition stating the relationship between them. The proposition readily lends itself to deductive hypothesis generation. For example, if reinforcement theory is valid, we could deduce that hyperactive children who are praised or rewarded when they are engaged in quiet play will exhibit less acting-out behaviors than similar children who are not praised. This prediction, as well as many others based on the theory of reinforcement, could then be tested in a study.

Other researchers use the term *theory* less restrictively to refer to a broad characterization of a phenomenon. Some authors specifically refer to this type of theory as **descriptive theory**—a theory that accounts for (i.e., thoroughly describes) a single phenomenon. Descriptive theories are inductive, empirically driven abstractions that "describe or classify specific dimensions or characteristics of individuals, groups, situations, or events by summarizing commonalities found in discrete observations" (Fawcett, 1999, p. 15). Such theories play an especially important role in qualitative studies.

Both classical and descriptive theory serve to make research findings meaningful and interpretable. Theories allow researchers to knit together observations into an orderly system. Theories also serve to explain research findings: Theory may guide researchers' understanding not only of the "what" of natural phenomena but also of the "why" of their occurrence. Finally, theories help to stimulate research and the extension of knowledge by providing both direction and impetus.

Theories are abstractions that are created and invented by humans. The building of a theory depends not only on observable facts but also on the theorist's ingenuity in pulling those facts together and making sense of them. Because theories are not just "out there" waiting to be discovered, it follows that theories are tentative. A theory can never be proved—a theory simply represents a theorist's best efforts to describe and explain phenomena. Through research, theories evolve and are sometimes discarded.

Theories are sometimes classified in terms of their level of generality. **Grand theories** (also known as **macro-theories**) purport to explain large segments of the human experience. Some learning theorists, such as Clark Hull, or sociologists, such as Talcott Parsons, developed general theoretical systems to account for broad classes of behavior and social functioning. Within nursing, theories are more restricted in scope, focusing on a narrow range of phenomena. Theories that explain a portion of the human experience are sometimes referred to as **middle-range theories**. For example, there are middle-range theories to explain such phenomena as decision-making, infant attachment, and stress.

Models

A **conceptual model** deals with abstractions (concepts) that are assembled because of their relevance to a common theme. Conceptual models provide a conceptual perspective regarding interrelated phenomena, but they are more loosely structured than theories and do not link concepts in a logically derived deductive system. A conceptual model broadly presents an understanding of the phenomenon of interest and reflects the assumptions and philosophical views of the model's designer. There are many conceptual models of nursing that offer broad explanations of the nursing process. Conceptual models are not directly testable by researchers in the same way that theories are, but, like theories, conceptual models can serve as springboards for generating hypotheses.

Some writers use the term **model** to designate a mechanism for representing phenomena with a minimal use of words. Words that define a concept can convey different meanings to different people; thus, a visual or symbolic representation of a phenomenon can sometimes help to express abstract ideas in a more understandable form. Two types of models that are used in research contexts are schematic models and statistical models.

Statistical models, not elaborated on here, are mathematic equations that express the nature and magnitude of relationships among a set of variables. These models are tested using sophisticated statistical methods. A **schematic model** (also called a **conceptual map**) represents a phenomenon of interest in a diagram. Concepts and the linkages between them are represented through boxes, arrows, or other symbols. An example of a schematic model is presented in Figure 8-1. This model, known as Pender's Health Promotion Model (HPM), is described by its designer as "a multivariate paradigm for explaining and predicting the health-promotion component of lifestyle" (Pender, Walker, Sechrist, & Frank-Stromborg, 1990, p. 326). According to this model, a person's decision to engage in health-promoting behaviors is affected by a number of cognitive/perceptual factors (e.g., the person's beliefs about the importance of health) and are modified indirectly by other factors (e.g., gender). Schematic models can be useful in clarifying concepts and their associations.

Frameworks

A **framework** is the conceptual underpinnings of a study. Not every study is based on a theory or conceptual model, but every study has a framework. In a study based on a theory, the framework is referred to as the **theoretical framework**; in a study that has its roots in a specified conceptual model, the framework is often called the **conceptual framework**. (However, the terms *conceptual framework*, *conceptual model*, and *theoretical framework* are often used interchangeably).

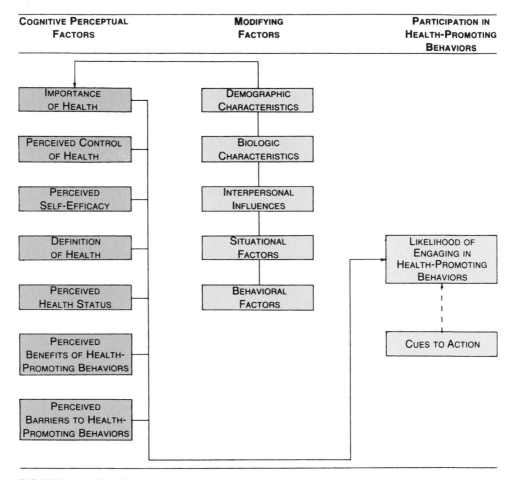

FIGURE 8.1 The Health Promotion Model. (From Pender et al., 1990.)

The framework for a study is often implicit (i.e., not formally acknowledged or described). World views (and views on nursing) shape how concepts are defined and operationalized, but researchers often fail to clarify the conceptual underpinnings of their variables. As noted in Chapter 2, researchers undertaking a study should make clear the conceptual definition of their key variables, thereby providing information about the study's framework.

Example of conceptual and operational definitions

In their study of gender differences in anger among adolescents, Yarcheski, Mahon, and Yarcheski (2002), following the work of psychological theorists, offered the following definitions:

Conceptual definition: The experience of anger includes *state anger,* defined as a condition consisting of subjective feelings of tension, annoyance, irritation, fury, and rage, and *trait anger,* defined as the disposition of individuals to perceive situations as annoying or frustrating (p. 230).

Operational definition: The experience of anger was measured by 20 items on the *State-Trait Anger Expression Inventory (STAXI).* State anger was measured by 10 questions that assess how angry one is feeling right now. Trait anger was measured by 10 questions that assess how angry one generally feels.

Quantitative researchers are generally more guilty of failing to identify their frameworks than qualitative researchers. In most qualitative studies, the frameworks are part of the research tradition within which the study is embedded. For example, ethnographers generally begin their work within a theory of culture. *Grounded theory* researchers incorporate sociological principles into their framework and their approach to looking at phenomena. The questions that most qualitative researchers ask and the methods they use to address those questions inherently reflect certain theoretical formulations.

CONCEPTUAL MODELS AND THEORIES USED BY NURSE RESEARCHERS

Nurse researchers have used both nursing and nonnursing frameworks to provide a conceptual context for their studies. This section briefly discusses some of the more prominent frameworks that have appeared in nursing research studies.

Conceptual Models of Nursing

Nurse theorists have developed a number of conceptual models of nursing that constitute formal explanations of what nursing is. As Fawcett (1995) has noted, four concepts are central to models of nursing: person, environment, health, and nursing. The various nursing models define these concepts differently, link them in diverse ways, and give different emphasis to the relationships among them. Moreover, different models emphasize different processes as being central to nursing. For example, Sister Callista Roy's Adaptation Model identifies adaptation of patients as a critical phenomenon (Roy & Andrews, 1999). Martha Rogers (1986), by contrast, emphasizes the centrality of the individual as a unified whole, and her model views nursing as a process in which individuals are aided in achieving maximum well-being within their potential. The conceptual models were not developed primarily as a base for nursing research. Indeed, these models have had more impact on nursing education and clinical practice than on nursing research. Nevertheless, nurse researchers have turned to these conceptual frameworks for inspiration in formulating research questions and hypotheses. Table 8-1 lists 11 conceptual models of nursing, together with a study for each that claimed the model as its framework.

Let us consider one conceptual model of nursing that has received particular attention among nurse researchers—Roy's Adaptation Model. In this model, human beings are biopsychosocial adaptive systems who cope with environmental change through the process of adaptation. Within the human system, there are four subsystems or response modes: physiologic needs,

 Example of a study using Roy's Adaptation Model

Gagliardi (2003) used Roy's Adaptation Model as the basis for studying the experience of sexuality among people with multiple sclerosis. Themes that emerged from in-depth interviews with eight patients were linked to Roy's model. For example, one theme concerned sexuality as both positive and negative emotionally, which reflected the self-concept and interdependence modes in Roy's model.

TABLE 8.1	Conceptual Models of Nursing Used by Nurse Researchers		
THEORIST EXAMPLE	**NAME OF MODEL/THEORY**	**KEY THESIS OF MODEL**	**RESEARCH**
F. Moyra Allen (In Gottlieb & Rowat, 1987)	McGill Model of Nursing	Nursing is the science of health-promoting interactions. Health promotion is a process of helping individuals cope and develop; the goal of nursing is to work with and actively promote patient and family strengths toward achievement of life goals.	Edgar, et al. (2001) used concepts from the McGill model in the development of a psychoeducational, coping skills training intervention, which they tested in a sample of individuals with newly diagnosed breast or colorectal cancer.
Imogene King, 1981	Open Systems Model	Personal systems, interpersonal systems, and social systems are dynamic and interacting within which transactions occur.	Doornbos (2000) based her framework on King's model; she tested the prediction that family stressors, coping, and other factors affected the health of families with young adults with serious mental illness.
Madeline Leininger, 1991	Theory of Culture Care Diversity and Universality	Caring is a universal phenomenon but varies transculturally.	Van den Brink (2003) incorporated Leininger's theory into a study of diversity and universality of care values relevant to the care of elderly Turkish patients in the Netherlands.
Myra Levine, 1973	Conservation Model	Conservation of integrity contributes to maintenance of a person's wholeness.	Gagner-Tjellesen et al. (2001) used concepts from Levine's model in studying the clinical use of music therapy in acute inpatient settings.
Betty Neuman, 2001	Health Care Systems Model	Each person is a complete system; the goal of nursing is to assist in maintaining client system stability.	Brauer (2001) described common patterns of person–environment interaction in adults with rheumatoid arthritis, based on Neuman's model.
Margaret Newman, 1999	Health as Expanding Consciousness	Health is viewed as an expansion of consciousness with health and disease parts of the same whole; health is seen in an evolving pattern of the whole in time, space, and movement.	Tommet's (2003) study of dialogues between nurses and parents of medically fragile children was guided by Newman's theory.

TABLE 8.1	Conceptual Models of Nursing Used by Nurse Researchers (continued)		
THEORIST EXAMPLE	**NAME OF MODEL/THEORY**	**KEY THESIS OF MODEL**	**RESEARCH**
Dorothea Orem, 2003	Self-Care Model	Self-care activities are what people do on their own behalf to maintain health and well-being; the goal of nursing is to help people meet their own therapeutic self-care demands.	Kreulen and Braden (2004) developed a model of relationships between self-help-promoting nursing interventions and health status outcomes, using concepts from Orem's model.
Rosemarie Rizzo Parse, 1999	Theory of Human Becoming	Health and meaning are co-created by indivisible humans and their environment; nursing involves having clients share views about meanings.	Jonas-Simpson (2003) studied older women's experience of being listened to within the context of Parse's Theory of Human Becoming.
Martha Rogers, 1986	Science of Unitary Human Beings	The individual is a unified whole in constant interaction with the environment; nursing helps individuals achieve maximum well-being within their potential.	Wright (2004) studied the relationship between trust and power in adults (as a way of illuminating nurse–client relationships), using Rogers's theory.
Sr. Callista Roy, 1999	Adaptation Model	Humans are adaptive systems that cope with change through adaptation; nursing helps to promote client adaptation during health and illness.	Shyu, Liang, Lu, and Wu (2004) tested Roy's model in their study of environmental barriers and mobility among elders in Taiwan.
Jean Watson, 1999	Theory of Caring	Caring is the moral ideal, and entails mind–body–soul engagement with one another.	Erci et al. (2003) studied the effectiveness of nurses who had been trained according to Watson's model on the quality on life of patients with hypertension.

self-concept, role function, and interdependence. These subsystems constitute adaptive modes that provide mechanisms for coping with environmental stimuli and change. The goal of nursing, according to this model, is to promote patient adaptation during health and illness.

Other Models Developed by Nurses

In addition to conceptual models that describe and characterize the entire nursing process, nurses have developed other models and theories that focus on specific phenomena of interest to nurses. An important example is Nola Pender's Health Promotion Model (2001), a conceptual map for which was presented in Figure 8-1. Another example is Mishel's Uncertainty in Illness Theory (1988), which focuses on the concept of uncertainty—the inability of a person to determine the meaning of illness-related events. According to this theory, a situation appraised as uncertain will mobilize individuals to use their resources to adapt to the situation. Mishel's conceptualization of uncertainty has been used as a framework for both qualitative and quantitative studies.

Examples of studies based on uncertainty theory

Santacroce (2002) used Uncertainty in Illness Theory to test hypothesized relationships between uncertainty, anxiety, and symptoms of posttraumatic stress in parents of children diagnosed with cancer. Brashers and colleagues (2003) conducted a qualitative study of the medical, personal, and social factors contributing to uncertainty in HIV illness.

Other Models Used by Nurse Researchers

Many concepts of interest to nurse researchers are not unique to nurses, and therefore nursing studies are sometimes linked to frameworks that are not models from the nursing profession. Four conceptual models that have been used frequently in nursing studies are as follows:

▶ *Becker's Health Belief Model* (HBM). The HBM is a framework for explaining people's health-related behavior, such as health care use and compliance with a medical regimen. According to the model, health-related behavior is influenced by a person's perception of a threat posed by a health problem as well as by the value associated with actions aimed at reducing the threat (Becker, 1976). Nurse researchers have used the HBM extensively—for example, Jirojwong and MacLennan (2003) used the HBM in their study of factors associated with breast self-examination among Thai immigrants in Australia.

▶ *Lazarus and Folkman's Theory of Stress and Coping.* This model, which explains people's methods of dealing with stress, posits that coping strategies are learned, deliberate responses to stressors, used to adapt to or change the stressors. According to this model, people's perception of mental and physical health is related to the ways they evaluate and cope with the stresses of living (Lazarus & Folkman, 1984). An example of a nursing study based on this theory is Carter's (2003) study of sleep loss and depression over time among adult family caregivers of patients with cancer.

▶ *Ajzen's Theory of Planned Behavior* (TPB). The TPB, an extension of a theory called the Theory of Reasoned Action (Ajzen & Fishbein, 1980), provides a framework for understanding the relationships among a person's attitudes, intentions, and behaviors. According to the TPB, behavioral intentions are the best predictor of a person's actual behavior, and behavioral intentions are a function of attitude toward performing the behavior, perceived control over the behavior, and subjective norms—the person's belief in whether others think the behavior should be performed (Azjen, 1988). The TPB has been used in many nursing studies, including a study of exercise intentions and behavior among survivors of breast and prostate cancer (Blanchard et al., 2002). A research example using the TPB is described in greater detail at the end of this chapter.

▶ *Bandura's Social Cognitive Theory.* Social Cognitive Theory (Bandura, 1997) offers an explanation of human behavior using the concepts of self-efficacy, outcome expectations, and incentives. Self-efficacy expectations are focused on people's belief in their own capacity to carry out particular behaviors (e.g., smoking cessation). Self-efficacy expectations determine the behaviors a person chooses to perform, their degree of perseverance, and the quality of the performance. Many nurses have applied this theory to their research, such as Conn and colleagues (2003), who sought to identify social cognitive theory–based predictors of exercise in community-dwelling elders.

The use of theories and conceptual models from other disciplines such as psychology (**borrowed theories**) has not been without controversy—some commentators advocate the development of unique nursing theories. However, nursing research is likely to continue on its current path of conducting studies within a multidisciplinary and multitheoretical perspective. Moreover, when a borrowed theory is tested and found to be empirically adequate in health-relevant situations of interest to nurses, it becomes **shared theory**.

CONSUMER TIP

Among nursing studies that are linked to a conceptual model or theory, about half are based on borrowed or shared theories. Among the models of nursing, those of Roy, Orem, and Rogers are especially likely to be used as the basis for research. ▬

TESTING, USING, AND DEVELOPING THEORY THROUGH RESEARCH

The relationship between theory and research is a reciprocal one. Theories and conceptual models are built inductively from observations, and research findings provide an important source of observations. Concepts and relations that are validated in studies can be the foundation for theory development. The theory, in turn, must be tested by subjecting deductions from it (hypotheses) to further empirical inquiry. Thus, research plays a dual and continuing role in theory building and testing. Theory can guide and generate ideas for research; research can assess the worth of the theory and provide a foundation for new ones.

Theories and Qualitative Research

Qualitative research traditions provide researchers with an overarching framework and theoretical grounding, although different traditions involve theory in different ways.

Sandelowski (1993) makes a useful distinction between **substantive theory** (inductively derived conceptualizations of the target phenomenon under study) and theory that reflects a conceptualization of human inquiry. Some qualitative researchers insist on an atheoretical stance vis-a-vis the phenomenon of interest, with the goal of suspending *a priori* conceptualizations (substantive theories) that might bias their collection and analysis of data. For example, phenomenologists are generally committed to theoretical naiveté and explicitly try to hold preconceived views of the phenomenon in check. Nevertheless, phenomenologists are guided in their inquiries by a framework or philosophy that focuses their analysis on certain aspects of a person's lifeworld. That framework is based on the premise that human experience is an inherent property of the experience itself, not constructed by an outside observer.

Ethnographers typically bring a strong cultural perspective to their studies, and this perspective shapes their initial fieldwork. Fetterman (1998) has observed that most ethnographers adopt one of two cultural theories: *ideational theories*, which suggest that cultural conditions and adaptation stem from mental activity and ideas, or *materialistic theories*, which view material conditions (e.g., resources, money, production) as the source of cultural developments.

The theoretical underpinning of grounded theory studies is *symbolic interactionism*, which stresses that behavior is developed through ongoing processes of negotiation and renegotiation within human interactions. Similar to phenomenologists, however, grounded theory researchers attempt to hold prior substantive theory (existing conceptualizations about the phenomenon) in abeyance until their own substantive theory begins to emerge. Once the theory takes shape, grounded theorists use previous literature for comparison with the emerging and developing categories of the theory. The goal of grounded theory is to use the data, grounded in reality, to provide a description or an explanation of events as they occur in reality—not as they have been conceptualized in preexisting theories. Grounded theory methods are designed to facilitate the generation of theory that is *conceptually dense*, i.e., with many conceptual patterns and relationships.

Example of theory in a grounded theory study

Rose, Mallinson, and Walton-Moss (2002) conducted a grounded theory study of families responding to mental illness of a relative. Living with the ambiguity of mental illness was the central concern of these families. The underlying process that was revealed was *pursuing normalcy*, and this process included *confronting the ambiguity, seeking to control the impact of the illness*, and *seeing possibilities for the future*.

In grounded theory studies, substantive theory is produced "from the inside," but theory can also enter a qualitative study "from the outside." Some qualitative researchers use existing theory or models as an interpretive framework. For example, a number of qualitative nurse researchers acknowledge that the philosophical roots of their studies lie in conceptual models of nursing such as those developed by Neuman, Parse, and Rogers.

Example of existing theory as an interpretive framework in a qualitative study

Bournes (2002) studied the structure of the experience of *having courage* as an aspect of human becoming (Parse's theory) among persons with spinal cord injuries.

Other qualitative researchers use substantive theories about the target phenomenon as a comparative context for interpreting data *after* the researcher has undertaken a preliminary analysis. Sandelowski (1993) notes that previous substantive theories or conceptualizations, when used in this manner, are essentially data themselves, and can be taken into consideration, along with study data, as part of inductively driven new conceptualization.

Another strategy that can lead to theory development involves an integrative review of qualitative studies on a specific topic, as in a metasynthesis. In such integrative reviews, qualitative studies are combined to identify their essential elements. These findings from different sources are then used for theory building. Paterson (2001), for example, used the results of 292 qualitative studies that described the experiences of adults with chronic illness to develop the shifting perspectives model of chronic illness. This model depicts living with chronic illness as an ongoing, constantly shifting process in which individuals' perspectives change in the degree to which illness is in the foreground or background in their lives.

Theories and Quantitative Research

Quantitative researchers, like qualitative researchers, link research to theory or models in several ways. The classic approach is to test hypotheses deduced from an existing theory. The process of theory testing begins when a researcher extrapolates the implications of the theory or conceptual model for a problem of interest. The researcher asks: If this theory or model is correct, what kinds of behavior or outcomes would I expect to find in specified situations? or What evidence would support this theory? Through such questioning, the researcher deduces implications of the theory in the form of research hypotheses. These hypotheses are predictions about how variables would be related, if the theory were correct. For example, a researcher might conjecture that, if Orem's Self-Care Model is valid, nursing effectiveness could be enhanced in environments more conducive to self-care (e.g., a birthing room versus a delivery room). Comparisons between the observed outcomes of research and the relationship predicted by the hypotheses are the major focus of the testing process.

Researchers sometimes base a new study on a theory or model in an effort to explain findings from previous research. For example, suppose that several researchers discovered that nursing home patients demonstrate greater levels of depression, anxiety, and noncompliance with nursing staff around bedtime than at other times. These descriptive findings are provocative, but they shed no light on the underlying cause of the problem and consequently suggest no way to ameliorate it. Several explanations, rooted in models such as the Lazarus and Folkman's Stress and Coping Model or Neuman's Health Care Systems Model may be relevant in explaining the behavior and moods of the nursing home patients. By directly testing the theory in a new study (i.e., deducing hypotheses derived from the theory), a researcher could gain some understanding of why bedtime is a vulnerable period for the elderly in nursing homes.

CONSUMER TIP

When a quantitative study is based on a theory or conceptual model, the research report generally states this fact fairly early—often in the first paragraph, or even in the title. Many studies also have a subsection of the introduction called "Conceptual Framework" or "Theoretical Framework." The report usually includes a brief overview of the theory so that even readers with no background in the theory can understand, in a general way, the conceptual context of the study.

Tests of a theory sometimes take the form of testing a theory-based intervention. If a theory is correct, it has implications for strategies to influence people's attitudes or behaviors, including health-related ones. The impetus for an intervention may be a theory developed within the context of qualitative research. The actual tests of the effectiveness of the intervention—which are also indirect tests of the theory—are generally done in structured quantitative research.

Example of theory testing in an intervention study

Mishel and colleagues (2003) developed an Uncertainty Management Intervention to assist patients with prostate cancer to manage uncertainty. The Uncertainty in Illness theory predicted that the intervention would have positive effects on such outcomes as problem solving, cognitive reframing, and management of treatment side effects. The theory was also used as a basis for predicting that the intervention would have differential effects depending on such patient characteristics as education, ethnicity, and religiosity. The findings indicated that men's levels of education and extrinsic religiosity influenced the efficacy of the intervention on important outcomes.

A few nurse researchers have begun to adopt a useful strategy for furthering knowledge through the direct testing of two competing theories in a single study. Almost all phenomena can be explained in alternative ways. Researchers who directly test alternative explanations, using a single sample of subjects, are in a position to make powerful comparisons about the utility of the competing theories.

Example of testing competing theories

Mahon and Yarcheski (2002) tested two alternative models of happiness in early adolescents: a theory relating happiness to enabling mechanisms and a theory of happiness based on adolescents' personality traits. The findings suggested that enabling mechanisms had more explanatory power than personality characteristics in predicting happiness.

It should also be noted that many researchers who cite a theory or model as their framework are not directly *testing* the theory. Silva (1986), in her analysis of 62 studies that used five nursing models, found that only nine were direct and explicit tests of the models cited by the researchers. She found that the most common use of nursing models in empirical studies was to provide an organizing structure. In such an approach, a researcher begins with a broad conceptualization of nursing (or stress, health beliefs, and so on) that is consistent with that of the model. These researchers *assume* that the models they espouse are valid, and then use the model's constructs or proposed schemas to provide a broad organizational or interpretive context. Silva noted that using models in this fashion can serve a valuable organizing purpose, but such studies offer little evidence about the validity of the theory itself. To our knowledge, Silva's study has not been replicated with a more recent sample of studies. However, we suspect that, even today, many quantitative studies that offer models and theories as their conceptual frameworks are using them primarily as organizational or interpretive tools.

Example of using a model as an organizing structure

Kirchhoff, Conradt, and Anumandia (2003) studied ICU nurses' preparation of families for death of patients following withdrawal of ventilator support. Their descriptive study used Self-Regulation Theory (SRT) as a framework. SRT was used as the basis for asking nurses about types of activities in which they engaged, but the validity of the SRT was not tested.

CRITIQUING CONCEPTUAL AND THEORETICAL FRAMEWORKS

You will find references to theories and conceptual frameworks in some (but not all) of the studies you read. It is often challenging to critique the theoretical context of a published research report—or its absence—but we offer a few suggestions.

In a qualitative study in which a grounded theory is presented, you will not be given enough information to refute the proposed descriptive theory; only evidence supporting the theory is presented. However, you can determine whether the theory seems logical, whether the conceptualization is truly insightful, and whether the evidence is solid and convincing. In a phenomenological study you should look to see if the researcher addresses the philosophical underpinnings of the study. The researcher should briefly discuss the philosophy of phenomenology upon which the study was based.

Critiquing a theoretical framework in a quantitative report is also difficult, especially because most of you are not likely to be familiar with the range of relevant models in nursing and related disciplines. Some suggestions for evaluating the conceptual basis of a quantitative study are offered in the following discussion and in Box 8-1.

The first task is to determine whether the study does, in fact, have a theoretical or conceptual framework. If there is no mention of a theory or conceptual model, you should consider whether the study's contribution to knowledge is likely to be diminished by the absence of such a framework. Nursing has been criticized for producing many pieces of isolated research that are difficult to integrate because of the absence of a theoretical foundation, but in many cases, the research may be so pragmatic that it does not really need a theory to enhance its usefulness. For example, research designed to determine the optimal frequency of turning patients has a utilitarian goal; it is difficult to see how a theory would enhance the value of the findings.

CONSUMER TIP

In most quantitative nursing studies, the research problem is *not* linked to a specific theory or conceptual model. Thus, students may read many studies before finding a study with an explicit theoretical underpinning. ■

If the study does involve an explicit framework, you must then ask whether this particular framework is appropriate. You may not be able to challenge the researcher's use of a particular theory or model or to recommend an alternative because that would require a solid theoretical grounding. However, you can evaluate the logic of using a particular framework and assess whether the link

---

BOX 8.1   Guidelines for Critiquing Theoretical and Conceptual Frameworks

1. Does the report describe an explicit theoretical or conceptual framework for the study? If not, does the absence of a framework detract from the usefulness or significance of the research?
2. Does the report adequately describe the major features of the theory or model so that readers can understand the conceptual basis of the study?
3. Is the theory or model appropriate for the research problem? Would a different framework have been more fitting?
4. Is the theory or model used as the basis for generating hypotheses that were tested, or is it used as an organizational or interpretive framework? Was this appropriate?
5. Do the research problem and hypotheses (if any) naturally flow from the framework, or does the purported link between the problem and the framework seem contrived? Are deductions from the theory logical?
6. Are the concepts adequately defined in a way that is consistent with the theory?
7. Is the framework based on a conceptual model of nursing or on a model developed by nurses? If it is borrowed from another discipline, is there adequate justification for its use?
8. Did the framework guide the study methods? For example, was the appropriate research tradition used if the study was qualitative? If quantitative, do the operational definitions correspond to the conceptual definitions? Were hypotheses tested statistically?
9. Does the researcher tie the findings of the study back to the framework at the end of the report? How do the findings support or undermine the framework? Are the findings interpreted within the context of the framework?

---

between the problem and the theory is genuine. Does the researcher present a convincing rationale for the framework used? Do the hypotheses flow from the theory? Will the findings contribute to the validation of the theory? Does the researcher interpret the findings within the context of the framework? If the answer to such questions is no, students may have grounds for criticizing the study's framework, even though they may not be in a position to articulate how the conceptual basis of the study could be improved.

 CONSUMER TIP

Some studies (in nursing as in any other discipline) claim theoretical linkages that are not justified. This is most likely to occur when researchers first formulate the research problem and then find a theoretical context to fit it. An after-the-fact linkage of theory to a research question may prove useful, but it is usually problematic because the researcher will not have taken the nuances of the theory into consideration in designing the study. If a research problem is truly linked to a conceptual framework, then the design of the study, the measurement of key constructs, and the analysis and interpretation of data will flow from that conceptualization. ■

C H A P T E R   R E V I E W

Key new terms introduced in the chapter, together with a summary of major points, are presented in this section. In addition, Chapter 8 of the *Study Guide to Accompany Essentials of Nursing Research*, 6th edition offers various exercises and study suggestions for reinforcing the concepts presented in this chapter. For additional review, see the Student Self-Study Review Questions section of the Student Resource CD-ROM provided with this book.

KEY NEW TERMS

Borrowed theory
Conceptual framework
Conceptual model
Descriptive theory
Framework
Grand theory
Macro-theory
Middle-range theory

Model
Schematic model
Shared theory
Substantive theory
Statistical model
Theoretical framework
Theory

SUMMARY POINTS

▷ A **theory** is a broad and abstract characterization of phenomena. As classically defined, a theory is an abstract generalization that systematically explains the relationships among phenomena. **Descriptive theory** thoroughly describes a phenomenon.

▷ The overall objective of theory is to make research findings meaningful, summarize existing knowledge into coherent systems, stimulate new research by providing direction and impetus, and explain the nature of relationships among variables.

▷ The basic components of a theory are concepts; classically defined theories consist of a set of propositions about the interrelationships among concepts, arranged in a logically interrelated system that permits new statements to be derived from them.

▷ Concepts are also the basic elements of **conceptual models**, but the concepts are not linked to one another in a logically ordered, deductive system.

▷ **Schematic models** (sometimes called **conceptual maps**) are symbolic representations of phenomena that depict a conceptual model through the use of symbols or diagrams.

▷ A **framework** is the conceptual underpinnings of a study. In many studies, the framework is implicit and not fully explicated.

▷ Several conceptual models of nursing have been developed and have been used in nursing research (e.g., Orem's Self-Care Model). The concepts that are central to models of nursing are person, environment, health, and nursing.

▷ Nonnursing models used by nurse researchers (e.g., Lazarus and Folkman's Theory of Stress and Coping) are referred to as **borrowed theories**; when the appropriateness of borrowed theories for nursing inquiry is confirmed, the theories become **shared theories**.

▷ In some qualitative research traditions (e.g., phenomenology), the researcher strives to suspend previously held substantive conceptualizations of the phenomena under study, but nevertheless there is a rich theoretical underpinning associated with the tradition itself.

▷ Some qualitative researchers specifically seek to develop *grounded theories*, data-driven explanations to account for phenomena under study (**substantive theories**) through inductive processes.

▷ In the classical use of theory, quantitative researchers test hypotheses deduced from an existing theory. A particularly fruitful approach involves testing two competing theories in one study.

▷ In both qualitative and quantitative studies, researchers sometimes use a theory or model as an organizing framework, or as an interpretive tool.

▷ Researchers sometimes develop a problem, design a study, and *then* look for a conceptual framework; such an after-the-fact selection of a framework is less compelling than the systematic testing of a particular theory.

RESEARCH EXAMPLES **Critical Thinking Activities**

 **EXAMPLE 1: Quantitative Research**

Aspects of a quantitative nursing study, featuring terms and concepts discussed in this chapter, are presented below, followed by some questions to guide critical thinking. (The full research report is available in *Nursing Research*, *52,* 148–158.)

Study

"Theory of planned behavior-based models for breastfeeding duration among Hong Kong mothers" (Dodgson, Henly, Duckett, & Tarrant, 2003)

Statement of Purpose

The purpose of the study was to evaluate the cross-cultural application of models based on the Theory of Planned Behavior (TPB) to explain the duration of breastfeeding among new mothers in Hong Kong. The TPB had previously been used to explain breastfeeding behaviors in Western cultures.

Method

A sample of 209 first-time breastfeeding mothers completed questionnaires during postpartum hospitalization and provided information about breastfeeding at 1, 3, 6, 9, and 12 months postdelivery or until they weaned.

Theoretical Framework

The TPB, as described earlier, predicts people's behaviors based on a constellation of factors that include their intentions, attitudes, perceived control, and subjective norms. In the present study, the researchers used the TPB to predict new mothers' duration of breastfeeding over a 1-year period based on their intention to breastfeed, which was operationalized as the mothers' judgment about the number of weeks they would breastfeed immediately postpartum. Intention to breastfeed, according to the TPB model, is in turn shaped by three types of factors: the mothers' attitudes toward breastfeeding (which are influenced by their beliefs about breastfeeding outcomes); perceived social pressure to breastfeed (which is influenced by the mothers' beliefs about social expectations—subjective norms); and perceptions that they can control breastfeeding duration (which are influenced by factors that can help or hinder breastfeeding). All of these predictor variables were measured during postpartum hospitalization, and then the dependent variable, duration of breastfeeding, was measured in follow-up contact in the year that followed.

Dodgson and her colleagues tested the utility of three predictive models. The first was a strict interpretation of the TPB, with two added predictors of breastfeeding duration (breastfeeding problems and daily proximity of mother and baby to each other). The second was a TPB-based model with modifications derived from a previous study of one of the investigators. The third was another TPB-based model that ordered the chain of influence among predictor variables somewhat differently than in the original model. In this model (shown in Figure 8-2), perceived control over breastfeeding is viewed as mediating the relationship between attitudes and subjective norms on the one hand and breastfeeding intention on the other.

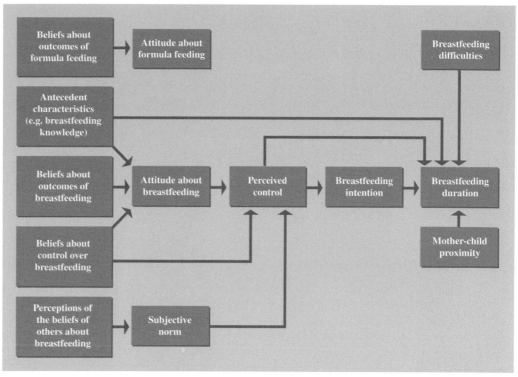

FIGURE 8.2 TPB Perceived Control Mediated Model. (Adapted from Dodgson et al., 2003.)

RESEARCH EXAMPLES *Continued*

Key Findings

▶ All of the models had fairly good ability to predict breastfeeding duration in this sample of Chinese women.

▶ The model that worked least well in predicting breastfeeding behavior was the original TPB model. The other two models were equally good.

▶ All hypothesized paths of influence in the third model—the TPB Perceived Control Mediated Model shown in Figure 8-2—were statistically significant (i.e., they had a high probability of being reliable).

Critical Thinking Suggestions*

* See the Student Resource CD-ROM for a discussion of the questions.

1. Answer questions 1 and 3–9 from Box 8-1 regarding this study.

research examples continue on page 170

RESEARCH EXAMPLES *Continued*

2. Also consider the following targeted questions, which may assist you in further assessing aspects of the study:
   a. What was the value of testing three competing models in a single study?
   b. Is there another model or theory that was described in this chapter that could have been used to study breastfeeding duration? If yes, would this model have been a better choice for a framework than the TPB?
   c. Based on the description of the TPB, where would the "box" for *perceived control* be placed in a schematic model of the original TPB—that is, how would Figure 8.2 need to be changed?
   d. What do the findings suggest about the cross-cultural utility of the TPB?
3. If the results of this study are valid and reliable, what are some of the uses to which the findings might be put in clinical practice?

 EXAMPLE 2: Qualitative Research

Aspects of a qualitative nursing study, featuring terms and concepts discussed in this chapter, are presented below, followed by some questions to guide critical thinking. (The full research report is available in *Nursing Research, 52,* 234–241, and in Appendix B of the associated *Study Guide to Accompany Essentials of Nursing Research*, 6th edition.)

Study

"A theory of taking care of oneself grounded in experiences of homeless youth" (Rew, 2003)

Statement of Purpose

The purpose of the study was to explore self-care attitudes and behaviors of homeless adolescents and to develop a descriptive substantive theory.

Method

Grounded theory methods were used. Data were collected through individual interviews with 15 youths. The two main questions posed in the interviews were: What helps you to remain healthy, living as you do? and What would you like to tell me about how you take care of yourself?

Theoretical Framework

A grounded theory method was adopted "because of its potential to address the patterns of behavior within and between members of a particular social group" (p. 235). Although Rew's grounded theory approach ensured that the end product of her study would be a descriptive theory of homeless youth's health-related behaviors, she consciously focused on an aspect of their behaviors that is linked to a conceptual model of nursing, Orem's Self-Care Model. The report pointed out features of Orem's model and noted that the concept of self-care had not previously been explored with high-risk youth.

RESEARCH EXAMPLES ❘ *Continued*

Key Findings

▸ Based on in-depth interviews, Rew identified an underlying social process that she labeled "Taking Care of Oneself in a High-Risk Environment." This basic social process linked together three categories to form a descriptive theory of self-care for homeless youth.

▸ The three categories linked together in Rew's theory were: Becoming Aware of Oneself; Staying Alive with Limited Resources; and Handling One's Own Health. As shown in the schematic model in Figure 8-3, each category contains two processes.

▸ Taking care of oneself for homeless youth was found to be "a process of deciding and acting in ways that enhance basic self-respect (caring about yourself) and that promote health" (p. 237).

Critical Thinking Suggestions

1. Answer questions 1 and 3–9 from Box 8-1 regarding this study.

2. Also consider the following targeted questions, which may assist you in further assessing aspects of the study:

   a. Was Rew testing Orem's theory in this study?

   b. In what way was the use of theory different in Rew's study than in the previous study by Dodgson et al.?

   c. Comment on the utility of the schematic model shown in Figure 8-3.

3. If the results of this study are trustworthy, what are some of the uses to which the findings might be put in clinical practice?

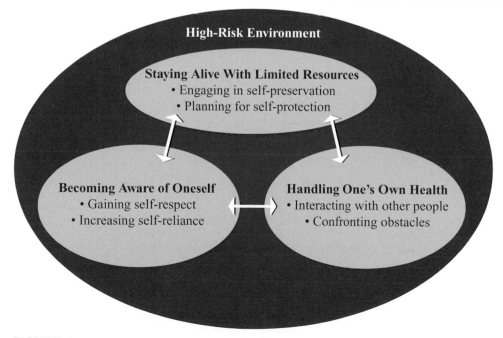

FIGURE 8.3 Taking care of oneself in a high-risk environment. (Adapted from Rew, 2003.)

research examples continue on page 172

RESEARCH EXAMPLES *Continued*

 EXAMPLE 3: Quantitative Research

1. Read the introduction and results section from the Motzer et al. study ("Sense of Coherence") in Appendix A of this book, and then answer the questions in Box 8-1.
2. Also consider the following targeted questions, which may further sharpen your critical thinking skills and assist you in assessing aspects of the study's merit:
   a. The study articulated two hypotheses. Were both based directly on salutogenic theory?
   b. Would a schematic model have helped readers to better understand the framework? Attempt to draw one that captures major variables in this study.
   c. Develop a research question for a new study in which salutogenic theory might be appropriate.

 EXAMPLE 4: Qualitative Research

1. Read the introduction and results section of Beck's study ("Birth Trauma") in Appendix B of this book, and then answer the relevant questions in Box 8-1.
2. Also consider the following targeted questions, which may further sharpen your critical thinking skills and assist you in assessing aspects of the study.
   a. Do you think that a schematic model would have helped to present the findings in this report?
   b. Does Beck present convincing evidence to support her use of the philosophy of phenomenology?

SUGGESTED READINGS

Theoretical References

Azjen, I. (1988). *Attitudes, personality, and behavior.* Chicago: Dorsey Press.

Azjen, I., & Fishbein, M. (1980). *Understanding attitudes and predicting social behavior.* Englewood Cliffs, NJ: Prentice Hall.

Bandura, A. (1997). *Self-efficacy: The exercise of control.* New York: W. H. Freeman.

Becker, M. (1976). *Health belief model and personal health behavior.* Thorofare, NJ: Slack, Inc.

Fawcett, J. (1995). *Analysis and evaluation of conceptual models of nursing* (3rd ed.). Philadelphia: F. A. Davis.

Fawcett, J. (1999). *The relationship between theory and research* (3rd ed.). Philadelphia: F. A. Davis.

Fetterman, D. M. (1998). *Ethnography: Step by step* (2nd ed.). Newbury Park, CA: Sage Publications.

Gottlieb, L. N., & Rowat, K. (1987). The McGill Model of Nursing: A practice-derived model. *Advances in Nursing Science, 9,* 51–61.

Greenwood, J. (2000). *Nursing theory in Australia: Development and application.* (2nd ed.). Sydney: Prentice Hall Health.

King, I. M. (1981). *A theory for nursing: Systems, concept, and process.* New York: John Wiley & Sons.

Lazarus, R. S., & Folkman, S. (1984). *Stress, appraisal, and coping.* New York: Springer Publishing Co.

Leininger, M. (1991). *Culture care diversity and universality: A theory of nursing.* New York: National League for Nursing.

Levine, M. E. (1973). *Introduction to clinical nursing* (2nd ed.). Philadelphia: F. A. Davis.

Mishel, M. H. (1988). Uncertainty in illness. *Image—The Journal of Nursing Scholarship, 20,* 225–232.

Neuman, B., & Fawcett, J. (2001). *The Neuman systems model* (4th ed.). Englewood, NJ: Prentice Hall.

Newman, M. (1999). *Health as expanding consciousness.* New York: National League for Nursing.

Orem, D. E., Taylor, S. G., Renpenning, K. M., & Eisenhandler, S. A. (2003). *Self-care theory in nursing: Selected papers of Dorothea Orem.* New York: Springer Publishing Co.

Parse, R. R. (1999). *Illuminations: The human becoming theory in practice and research.* Sudbury, MA: Jones & Bartlett.

Pender, N., & Pender, A. R. (2001). *Health promotion in nursing practice* (4th ed.). Englewood Cliffs, NJ: Prentice Hall.

Reed, P. G., Shearer, N., & Nicoll, L. H. (2003). *Perspectives on nursing theory* (4th ed.). Philadelphia: Lippincott Williams & Wilkins.

Designs
for
Nursing
Research

CHAPTER 9

Scrutinizing Quantitative Research Design

STUDENT OBJECTIVES

On completing this chapter, you will be able to:

▷ Discuss decisions that are embodied in a research design for a quantitative study
▷ Describe and evaluate experimental, quasi-experimental, preexperimental, and
  nonexperimental designs
▷ Distinguish between and evaluate cross-sectional and longitudinal designs
▷ Identify and evaluate alternative methods of controlling extraneous variables
▷ Understand various threats to the validity of quantitative studies
▷ Evaluate a quantitative study in terms of its overall research design and methods of
  controlling extraneous variables
▷ Define new terms in the chapter

DIMENSIONS OF RESEARCH DESIGN IN QUANTITATIVE STUDIES

The research design of a quantitative study incorporates key methodologic decisions about the fundamental form of a study and spells out the strategies researchers plan to adopt to develop information that is accurate and interpretable. Thus, it is crucial for you to understand the implications of researchers' design decisions. Typically, developing a quantitative research design involves decisions with regard to the following aspects of the study:

▶ *Will there be an intervention?* In some studies, nurse researchers examine the effects of a new intervention (e.g., an innovative program to promote smoking cessation); in others, researchers gather information about phenomena as they exist. As noted in Chapter 2, this is a distinction between experimental and nonexperimental research. When there is an intervention, the research design specifies its features.

▶ *What types of comparisons will be made?* Researchers usually design their studies to involve comparisons that enhance the interpretability of the results. Consider the example presented in Chapter 4 (Box 4-2), in which women who had an abortion were compared with women who delivered a baby in terms of their emotional well-being. Without a comparison group, the researchers would not have known whether the abortion group members' emotional status was anomalous. Sometimes, researchers use a before–after comparison (e.g., preoperative versus postoperative), and sometimes different groups are compared.

▶ *How will extraneous variables be controlled?* The complexity of relationships among variables makes it difficult to test hypotheses unambiguously unless efforts are made to control factors extraneous to the research question (i.e., to control *extraneous variables*). This chapter discusses techniques for achieving such control.

▶ *When and how many times will data be collected?* In many studies, data are collected from participants at a single point in time, but some studies include multiple contacts with participants, for example, to determine how things have changed over time. The research design designates the frequency and timing of data collection.

▶ *In what setting will the study take place?* Data for quantitative studies sometimes are collected in real-world settings, such as in clinics or people's homes. Other studies are conducted in highly controlled environments established for research purposes (e.g., laboratories).

There is no single typology of research designs, because they vary along a number of dimensions. As shown in Table 9-1, the dimensions involve whether researchers have control over the independent variable, what type of comparison is made, how many times data are collected, and whether researchers look forward or backward in time for the occurrence of the independent and dependent variables. Each dimension is, with a few exceptions, independent of the others. For example, an experimental design can be a between-subjects or within-subjects

CONSUMER TIP

Research reports typically present information about the research design early in the method section. Complete information about the design is not always provided, however, and some researchers use terminology that is different from that used in this book. (Occasionally, researchers even misidentify the study design.)

▬

Table 9.1	Dimensions of Quantitative Research Design	
DIMENSION	**DESIGN**	**MAJOR FEATURES**
Control over independent variable	Experimental	Manipulation of independent variable; control group; randomization
	Quasi-experimental	Manipulation of independent variable; no randomization and/or no comparison group; but efforts to compensate for this lack
	Preexperimental	Manipulation of independent variable; no randomization or no comparison group; limited control over extraneous variables
	Nonexperimental	No manipulation of independent variable
Type of group comparison	Between-subjects	Subjects in groups being compared are different people
	Within-subjects	Subjects in groups being compared are the same people at different times or in different conditions
Timeframes	Cross-sectional	Data are collected at a single point in time
	Longitudinal	Data are collected at two or more points in time over an extended period
Observance of independent and dependent variables	Retrospective	Study begins with dependent variable and looks backward for cause or influence
	Prospective	Study begins with independent variable and looks forward for the effect
Setting	Naturalistic setting	Data collected in real-world setting
	Laboratory	Data collected in contrived laboratory setting

design; experiments can also be cross-sectional or longitudinal, and so on (these terms are discussed later). The sections that follow elaborate on different designs for quantitative nursing research. Qualitative research design is discussed in Chapter 10.

EXPERIMENTAL, QUASI-EXPERIMENTAL, AND NONEXPERIMENTAL DESIGNS

This section describes designs that differ with regard to the amount of control the researcher has over the independent variable. We begin with research designs that offer the greatest amount of control: experimental designs.

Experiments

Experiments differ from nonexperimental studies in one important respect: Researchers using an experimental design are active agents rather than passive observers. Early physical scientists found that, although observation of natural phenomena is valuable, the complexity of naturally occurring events often obscures relationships. This problem was addressed by isolating phenomena in laboratories and controlling the conditions under which they occurred. Procedures developed by physical scientists were adopted by biologists during the 19th century, resulting in many achievements in physiology and medicine. Researchers interested in human behavior began using experimental methods in the 20th century.

CHARACTERISTICS OF EXPERIMENTS

Experiments can be conducted in any setting, not just in laboratories. To qualify as an experiment, a research design must have three properties:

1. *Manipulation.* Experimenters do something to participants in the study.
2. *Control.* Experimenters introduce controls over the experimental situation, including the use of a control group.
3. *Randomization.* Experimenters assign participants to control or experimental groups randomly.

Using **manipulation**, experimenters consciously vary the independent variable and then observe its effect on the dependent variable. Researchers manipulate the independent variable by administering an experimental *treatment* (or *intervention*) to some subjects while withholding it from others. To illustrate, suppose we were investigating the effect of physical exertion on mood in healthy young adults. One experimental design for this research problem is a **pretest–posttest design** (or *before–after design*). This design involves the observation of the dependent variable (mood) at two points in time: before and after the treatment. Participants in the experimental group are subjected to a physically demanding exercise routine, whereas those in the control group undertake a sedentary activity. This design permits us to examine what changes in mood were *caused* by the exertion because only some people were subjected to it, providing an important comparison. In this example, we met the first criterion of a true experiment by manipulating physical exertion, the independent variable.

This example also meets the second requirement for experiments, the use of a control group. Campbell and Stanley (1963), in a classic monograph on research design, noted that scientific evidence requires at least one comparison. But not all comparisons provide equally persuasive evidence. Let us look at an example. If we were to supplement the diet of a sample of premature neonates with special nutrients for 2 weeks, the infants' weight at the end of the 2-week period would give us no information about the treatment's effectiveness. At a minimum, we would need to compare their posttreatment weight with their pretreatment weight to determine whether, at least, their weights had increased. But suppose we find an average weight gain of half a pound. Does this finding indicate that there is a causal relationship between the nutritional supplements (the independent variable) and weight gain (the dependent variable)? No, it does not. Infants normally gain weight as they mature. Without a control group—a group that does not receive the supplements—it is impossible to separate the effects of maturation from those of the treatment. The term **control group** refers to a group of participants whose performance on a dependent variable is used to evaluate the performance of the **experimental group** (the group receiving the treatment of interest) on the same dependent variable.

Experimental designs also involve placing subjects in groups at random. Through **randomization** (or *random assignment*), every participant has an equal chance of being included in any group. If people are randomly assigned, there is no systematic bias in the groups with respect to attributes that may affect the dependent variable. *Randomly assigned groups are expected to be comparable, on average, with respect to an infinite number of biologic, psychological, and social* *traits at the outset of the study.* Group differences observed after random assignment can therefore be inferred as resulting from the treatment.

Random assignment can be accomplished by flipping a coin or pulling names from a hat. Researchers typically either use computers to perform the randomization or rely on a *table of random numbers*, a table displaying hundreds of digits arranged in a random order.

HOW-TO-TELL TIP

How can you tell if a study is experimental? Researchers usually indicate in their reports (in the method section) when they have used an experimental design, but they may also refer to the design as a *randomized design* or *clinical trial* (see Chapter 11). If such terms are missing, you can conclude that a study is experimental if the report says that a goal of the study was to "test," "evaluate," "assess," or "examine the effectiveness of" an "intervention," "treatment," or "innovation," AND if individual participants were put into groups (or exposed to different conditions) in a *random* fashion.

EXPERIMENTAL DESIGNS
Basic Designs

The most basic experimental design involves randomizing subjects to different groups and subsequently measuring the dependent variable. This design is called a **posttest-only** (or *after-only*) **design**. A more widely used design, discussed previously, is the pretest–posttest design, which involves the collection of **pretest data** (also known as **baseline data**) on the dependent variable before the intervention and **posttest data** (or *outcome data*) after it.

Example of a before–after design

Schachman, Lee, and Lederman (2004) used a before–after design to test the effects of a nursing intervention on maternal role adaptation among military wives. One group of primigravid women received the special "Baby Boot Camp" intervention and the other group received a traditional childbirth education program. Maternal role adaptation was assessed before the intervention (32–37 weeks' gestation), immediately after the intervention, and 6 weeks postpartum.

Factorial Design

Researchers sometimes manipulate two or more variables simultaneously. Suppose we were interested in comparing two therapeutic strategies for premature infants: tactile stimulation versus auditory stimulation. We are also interested in learning whether the daily amount of stimulation affects infants' progress. Figure 9-1 illustrates the structure of this experiment. This factorial design allows us to address three questions: (1) Does auditory stimulation have a different effect on infant development than tactile stimulation? (2) Is the amount of stimulation (independent of modality) related to infant development? (3) Is auditory stimulation most effective when linked to a certain dose and tactile stimulation most effective when coupled with a different dose?

The third question demonstrates a strength of factorial designs: They permit us to evaluate not only **main effects** (effects resulting from the manipulated variables, as exemplified in questions 1 and 2) but also **interaction effects** (effects resulting from combining the treatments). Our results may indicate, for example, that 15 minutes of tactile stimulation and 45 minutes

TYPE OF STIMULATION

	Auditory A1	*Tactile* A2
15 min. B1	A1 B1	A2 B1
DAILY EXPOSURE 30 min. B2	A1 B2	A2 B2
45 min. B3	A1 B3	A2 B3

FIGURE 9.1 Schematic diagram of a factorial experiment.

of auditory stimulation are the most beneficial treatments. We could not have learned this by conducting two separate experiments that manipulated one independent variable at a time.

In factorial experiments, subjects are assigned at random to a combination of treatments. In our example, premature infants would be assigned randomly to one of the six cells. The term *cell* is used in experimental research to refer to a treatment condition and is represented in a schematic diagram as a box. In a factorial design, the independent variables are referred to as *factors*. Type of stimulation is factor A and amount of exposure is factor B. Each factor must have two or more *levels*. Level one of factor A is *auditory*, and level two of factor A is *tactile*. The research design in Figure 9-1 would be described as a 2×3 factorial design: two levels of factor A times three levels of factor B.

Example of a factorial design

McDonald, Wiczorek, and Walker (2004) used a 2×2 factorial design to study the effect of background noise (noice versus no noise) and interruption (interruption versus no interruption) on learning health information in a sample of college students.

Crossover Design

Thus far, we have described experiments in which subjects who are randomly assigned to treatments are different people. For instance, the infants given 15 minutes of auditory stimulation in the factorial experiment are not the same infants as those exposed to other treatment conditions.

This broad class of designs is called **between-subjects designs** because the comparisons are *between* different people. When the same subjects are compared, the designs are **within-subjects designs**.

A **crossover design** (sometimes called a *repeated measures design*) involves exposing participants to more than one treatment. Such studies are true experiments only if participants are randomly assigned to different orderings of treatment. For example, if a crossover design were used to compare the effects of auditory and tactile stimulation on infants, some subjects would be randomly assigned to receive auditory stimulation first followed by tactile stimulation, and others would receive tactile stimulation first. In such a study, the three conditions for an experiment have been met: There is manipulation, randomization, and control—with *subjects serving as their own control group.*

A crossover design has the advantage of ensuring the highest possible equivalence among subjects exposed to different conditions. Such designs are inappropriate for certain research questions, however, because of possible *carryover effects.* When subjects are exposed to two different treatments, they may be influenced in the second condition by their experience in the first. Drug studies rarely use a crossover design because drug B administered after drug A is not necessarily the same treatment as drug B before drug A.

CONSUMER TIP

Research reports do not always identify the specific experimental design that was used; this may have to be inferred from information about the data collection plan (in the case of after-only and before–after designs) or from such statements as: The subjects were used as their own controls (in the case of a crossover design). Before–after and crossover designs are the most commonly used experimental designs in nursing research.

Example of a crossover design

Schenider, Prince-Paul, Allen, Silverman, and Talaba (2004) compared the symptom distress levels of women receiving chemotherapy with and without virtual reality as a distraction intervention. A sample of 20 women were randomly assigned to an ordering of chemotherapy with distraction versus without it.

EXPERIMENTAL AND CONTROL CONDITIONS

In designing experiments, researchers make many decisions about what the experimental and control conditions entail, and these decisions can affect the results.

To give an experimental intervention a fair test, researchers need to carefully design one that is appropriate to the problem and of sufficient intensity and duration that effects on the dependent variable might reasonably be expected. Researchers delineate the full nature of the intervention in formal *protocols* that stipulate exactly what the treatment is for those in the experimental group; research protocols usually are summarized in research reports.

The control group condition used as a basis of comparison is sometimes called the *counterfactual.* Researchers have choices about what to use as the counterfactual, and the decision has implications for the interpretation of the findings. Among the possibilities for the counterfactual are the following:

- No intervention—the control group gets no treatment at all;
- An alternative treatment (e.g., auditory versus tactile stimulation);
- A **placebo** or pseudo-intervention presumed to have no therapeutic value;
- Standard methods of care—normal procedures used to treat patients;
- A lower dose or intensity of treatment, or only parts of the treatment; and
- Delayed treatment, i.e., exposure to the experimental treatment at a later point

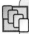

Example of a delayed treatment

Goodfellow (2003) tested the effect of a therapeutic back massage on psychophysiologic variables and immune function in spouses of patients with cancer. Experimental group subjects got the massage and control group subjects did not get the massage—until after all outcome variables were measured.

Methodologically, the best possible test is between two conditions that are as different as possible, as when the experimental group gets a strong treatment and the control group gets no treatment. Ethically, however, the most appealing counterfactual is probably the "delay of treatment" approach, which may be difficult to do pragmatically. Testing two alternative interventions is also appealing ethically, but the risk is that the results will be inconclusive because it may be difficult to detect differential effects on the outcomes. Ideally, subjects should be *blinded* to which treatment group they are in.

ADVANTAGES AND DISADVANTAGES OF EXPERIMENTS

Experiments are the most powerful designs for testing hypotheses of cause-and-effect relationships. Because of its special controlling properties, an experiment offers greater corroboration than any other research design that the independent variable (e.g., diet, drug dosage, teaching approach) affects the dependent variable (e.g., weight loss, blood pressure, learning).

Lazarsfeld (1955) identified three criteria for causality. First, a cause must precede an effect in time. To test the hypothesis that saccharin causes bladder cancer, we would need to ensure that subjects had not developed cancer before exposure to saccharin. Second, there must be an empirical relationship between the presumed cause and the presumed effect. Thus, we would need to demonstrate an association between the ingestion of saccharin and the presence of cancer (i.e., that people who used saccharin experienced a higher incidence of cancer than those who did not). The final criterion for causality is that the relationship cannot be due to the influence of a third variable. Suppose, for instance, that people who use saccharin tend also to drink more coffee than nonusers. Thus, a relationship between saccharin use and bladder cancer may reflect an underlying causal relationship between a substance in coffee and bladder cancer. It is particularly because of this third criterion that experimental designs are so strong. Through the controlling properties of manipulation, control groups, and randomization, alternative explanations to a causal interpretation can often be ruled out.

Despite the advantages of experiments, they have some limitations. First, a number of interesting variables simply are not amenable to manipulation. A large number of human characteristics, such as disease or health habits, cannot be randomly conferred on people.

Second, there are many variables that could technically—but not ethically—be manipulated. For example, to date there have been no experiments to study the effect of cigarette smoking on lung cancer. Such an experiment would require us to assign people randomly to a smoking group (people forced to smoke) or a nonsmoking group (people prohibited from smoking). Experimentation with humans is subject to ethical constraints.

In many health care settings, experimentation may not be feasible because it is impractical. It may, for instance, be impossible to secure the necessary cooperation from administrators or other key people to conduct an experiment.

Another potential problem is the **Hawthorne effect**, a term derived from a series of experiments conducted at the Hawthorne plant of the Western Electric Corporation in which various environmental conditions (e.g., light, working hours) were varied to determine their effect on worker productivity. Regardless of what change was introduced (i.e., whether the light was made better or worse), productivity increased. Thus, knowledge of being in a study may cause people to change their behavior, thereby obscuring the effect of the research variables.

In health care settings, researchers sometimes contend with a double Hawthorne effect. For example, if an experiment investigating the effect of a new postoperative procedure were conducted, nurses as well as patients might be aware of participating in a study, and both groups could alter their actions accordingly. It is for this reason that **double-blind experiments**, in which neither the subjects nor those administering the treatment know who is in the experimental or control group, are so powerful. Unfortunately, the double-blind approach is not feasible in most nursing research because nursing interventions are often difficult to disguise.

Example of a double-blind study

Niesen, Harris, Parkin, and Henn (2003) compared the effects of heparin versus normal saline for maintaining patency in intravenous locks during pregnancy. Women were randomly assigned to the two treatment groups. The hospital pharmacy prepared batches of the two treatment solutions, and only pharmacy staff (not the patients nor any nurses) had access to the list of group assignments.

In summary, experimental designs have some limitations that make them difficult to apply to real-world problems; nevertheless, experiments have a clear-cut superiority to other designs for testing causal hypotheses.

Quasi-Experiments

Quasi-experimental research looks much like experiments because **quasi-experiments** also involve the manipulation of an independent variable (i.e., the institution of a treatment). Quasi-experiments, however, lack either the randomization or control-group features of true experiments—features whose absence weakens the ability to make causal inferences.

QUASI-EXPERIMENTAL DESIGNS
There are several quasi-experimental designs, but only the two most commonly used by nurse researchers are discussed here.

Nonequivalent Control Group Design
The most frequently used quasi-experimental design is the **nonequivalent control-group before–after design**, which involves two or more groups of subjects observed before and after

the implementation of an intervention. As an example, suppose we wanted to study the effect of primary nursing on nursing staff morale in an urban hospital. The new system of nursing care is being implemented throughout the hospital, and so randomization of nurses is not possible. Therefore, we decide to collect comparison data from nurses in a similar hospital that is not instituting primary nursing. We gather data on staff morale in both hospitals before implementing the primary nursing system (the pretest) and again after its implementation (the posttest).

This quasi-experimental research design is identical to the before–after experimental design discussed in the previous section, *except* subjects were not randomly assigned to the groups. The quasi-experimental design is weaker because, without randomization, *it cannot be assumed that the experimental and comparison groups are equivalent at the outset.* The design is, nevertheless, a strong one because the collection of pretest data allows us to determine whether the groups had similar morale initially. If the comparison and experimental groups were similar, on average, at the pretest, we could be relatively confident that posttest differences in self-reported morale resulted from the intervention. (Note that in quasi-experiments, the term **comparison group** is generally used in lieu of *control group* to refer to the group against which experimental group outcomes are evaluated.)

Now suppose we had been unable to collect pretest data before primary nursing care was introduced (i.e., only posttest data were collected). This design has a serious flaw because we have no basis for judging the initial equivalence of the two nursing staffs. If we found higher morale in the experimental group, could we conclude that primary nursing caused an improvement in staff morale? There could be several alternative explanations for such differences. Campbell and Stanley (1963), in fact, called this *nonequivalent control group after-only design* a **preexperimental design** rather than a quasi-experimental design because we would be constrained from making the desired inferences. Thus, even though quasi-experiments lack some of the controlling properties of experiments, the hallmark of quasi-experiments is the effort to introduce some controls.

Example of a nonequivalent control group before–after design

Maas and her colleagues (2004) used a strong quasi-experimental design to assess the effects of the Family Involvement in Care partnership intervention for caregivers of individuals with dementia. Seven matched pairs of nursing home dementia care units (i.e., 14 units) were randomly assigned to experimental and control conditions; family members could not be randomized. Outcomes of interest, including family members' perceptions of the caregiving role and satisfaction with the care of their relatives, were measured prior to the intervention and at several points after it.

Time-Series Design

In the designs just described, a control group was used, but randomization was not. The next design has neither a control group nor randomization. Suppose that a hospital was adopting a requirement that all its nurses accrue a certain number of continuing education credits before being eligible for a promotion. The nurse administrators want to assess the consequences of this mandate on turnover rate, absentee rate, and number of promotions awarded. Let us assume there is no other hospital that can serve as a reasonable comparison for this study, and so the only kind of comparison that can be made is a before–after contrast. If the requirement were inaugurated in January, one could compare the turnover rate, for example, for the 3-month period before the new rule with the turnover rate for the subsequent 3-month period.

This **one-group before–after design** seems logical, but it has a number of problems. What if one of the 3-month periods is atypical, apart from the mandate? What about the effect of any other rules instituted during the same period? What about the effects of external factors, such as changes in the local economy? The design in question, which is also preexperimental, offers no way of controlling any of these factors.

The inability to obtain a meaningful control group, however, does not eliminate the possibility of conducting research with integrity. The previous design could be modified so that at least some of the alternative explanations for change in nurses' turnover rate could be ruled out. One such design is the **time-series design**, which involves collecting data over an extended time period and introducing the treatment during that period. The present study could be designed with four observations before the new continuing education rule and four observations after it. For example, the first observation might be the number of resignations between January and March in the year before the new rule, the second observation might be the number of resignations between April and June, and so forth. After the rule is implemented, data on turnover similarly would be collected for four consecutive 3-month periods, giving us observations 5 through 8.

Although the time-series design does not eliminate all the problems of interpreting changes in turnover rate, the extended time perspective strengthens our ability to attribute change to the intervention. This is because the time-series design rules out the possibility that changes in resignations represent a random fluctuation of turnover measured at only two points.

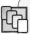

Example of a time-series design

Edwards and Beck (2002) used a powerful time series design to assess the effect of animal-assisted therapy (aquariums) on the nutritional intake of individuals with Alzheimer's disease. Weight (one of the outcomes) was measured on the first of each month for 3 months prior to the intervention, and for 4 months after it in a sample of residents in specialized units in three facilities. The researchers found that, over this 7-month period, weight declined in the 3 months prior to the intervention and then increased significantly in the month the aquariums were introduced, and continued to increase in the following months.

ADVANTAGES AND DISADVANTAGES OF QUASI-EXPERIMENTS

A strength of quasi-experiments is that they may be practical—it is sometimes not feasible to conduct true experiments. Nursing research often occurs in natural settings, where it is difficult to deliver an innovative treatment randomly to some people but not to others. Quasi-experimental designs introduce some research control when full experimental rigor is not possible.

The major disadvantage of quasi-experiments is that cause-and-effect inferences cannot be made as easily as with experiments. With quasi-experiments, there are alternative explanations for observed results. Suppose we wanted to evaluate the effect of a nursing intervention for infants of heroin-addicted mothers on infants' weight gain. If we use no comparison group or if we use a nonequivalent control group and then observe a weight gain, we must ask the following questions: Is it plausible that some external factor influenced the gain? Is it plausible that pretreatment group differences resulted in differential weight gains? Is it plausible that the changes would have occurred without an intervention? If the answer to any of these *rival hypotheses* is yes, inferences about treatment effectiveness are weakened. With quasi-experiments, there is almost always at least one plausible rival explanation.

HOW-TO-TELL TIP

How can you tell if a study is quasi-experimental? Researchers do not always identify their studies as quasi-experimental (or preexperimental). If a study involves an intervention (*i.e.*, if the researcher has control over the independent variable) and if the report does not explicitly mention random assignment, it is probably safe to conclude that the design is quasi-experimental or preexperimental. Oddly, quite a few researchers *misidentify* true experimental designs as quasi-experimental. If individual subjects are randomized to groups or conditions, the design is *not* quasi-experimental.

Nonexperimental Studies

Many research problems cannot be addressed with an experimental or quasi-experimental design. For example, suppose we were interested in studying the effect of widowhood on physical and psychological functioning. Our independent variable here is widowhood versus nonwidowhood. Clearly, we cannot manipulate widowhood; people lose their spouses by a process that is neither random nor subject to control. Thus, we would have to proceed by taking the two groups (widows and nonwidows) as they naturally occur and comparing their psychological and physical well-being. There are various reasons for doing a **nonexperimental study**—sometimes referred to as an *observational study* by medical researchers because the study involves making observations rather than intervening. For example, there are situations in which the independent variable inherently cannot be manipulated or in which it would be unethical to manipulate the independent variable. There are also research questions for which an experimental design is not appropriate, such as studies whose purpose is description.

TYPES OF NONEXPERIMENTAL STUDIES

One class of nonexperimental research is known as **correlational** (or *ex post facto*) **research**. The literal translation of the Latin term *ex post facto* is "from after the fact," indicating that the research has been conducted after variation in the independent variable has occurred.

The basic purpose of correlational research is the same as that of experimental research: to study relationships among variables. However, it is difficult to infer causal relationships in correlational studies. In experiments, investigators make a prediction that a deliberate variation in *X*, the independent variable, will result in changes to *Y*, the dependent variable. In correlational research, on the other hand, investigators do not control the independent variable—the presumed causative factor—because it has already occurred. It is risky to draw cause-and-effect conclusions in such a situation. A famous research dictum is relevant: *Correlation does not prove causation.* That is, the mere existence of a relationship between variables is not enough to warrant the conclusion that one variable caused the other, even if the relationship is strong.

Correlational research that is designed to explore causal relationships sometimes is described as either retrospective or prospective. Correlational studies with a **retrospective design** are ones in which a phenomenon observed in the present is linked to phenomena occurring in the past. In a retrospective study, the investigator focuses on a presently occurring outcome and then tries to ascertain the antecedent factors that have caused it. For example, in retrospective lung cancer research, the investigator begins with a sample of those who have lung cancer and a sample of those who do not. The researcher then looks for differences between the groups in antecedent behaviors or conditions, such as smoking habits.

Correlational studies with a **prospective design**, by contrast, start with a presumed cause and then go forward to the presumed effect. For example, in prospective lung cancer studies, researchers start with samples of smokers and nonsmokers and later compare the two groups in terms of lung cancer incidence. Prospective studies are more costly than retrospective studies but are considerably stronger. For one thing, any ambiguity concerning the temporal sequence of phenomena is resolved in prospective research (i.e., the smoking is known to precede the lung cancer). In addition, samples are more likely to be representative of smokers and nonsmokers, and investigators may be in a position to impose controls to rule out competing explanations for observed effects.

Example of a prospective nonexperimental study

Schuurmans and colleagues (2003) conducted a prospective study of risk factors for delirium among elderly patients with a hip fracture. Data were collected on predisposing and precipitating factors for delirium from 92 patients undergoing surgery. Within the first 6 days of admission, 18 patients developed delirium. Patients' prefracture cognitive and functional capacities were predictive of postsurgical delirium.

Researchers can sometimes strengthen a retrospective study, using a **case-control design**. This design involves comparing "cases" with a certain condition (e.g., breast cancer) with controls (women without breast cancer) who are selected to be similar to the cases with regard to key background factors (e.g., age, family history of breast cancer) that could be linked to the condition. If the researcher can demonstrate similarity between cases and controls with regard to such extraneous traits, the inferences regarding the contribution of the independent variable (e.g., dietary factors) to the disease are enhanced.

Example of a retrospective case-control study

Hendrich, Bender, and Nyhuis (2003) conducted a large case-control study of hospitalized patients to determine risk factors for falls. A sample of 355 fall cases and 780 nonfall controls (patients who had been admitted on the same day as a fall case) were assessed retrospectively for more than 600 risk factors.

A second broad class of nonexperimental studies is **descriptive research**. The purpose of descriptive studies is to observe, describe, and document aspects of a situation. For example, an investigator may wish to determine the percentage of teenaged mothers who receive adequate prenatal care. Sometimes, a report refers to the study design as **descriptive correlational**, meaning that researchers were interested in describing relationships among variables, without seeking to establish causal connections. For example, researchers might be interested in describing the relationship between fatigue and psychological distress in HIV patients. Because the intent in these situations is not to explain or to understand the underlying causes of the variables of interest, a nonexperimental design is appropriate.

Example of a descriptive correlational study

Tanyi and Werner (2003) conducted a study to describe relationships between adjustment, spiritual well-being, and self-perceived health in women with end-stage renal disease.

ADVANTAGES AND DISADVANTAGES OF NONEXPERIMENTAL RESEARCH

The major disadvantage of nonexperimental research is its inability to reveal causal relationships with assurance. Although this is not a problem when the aim is purely descriptive, correlational studies are often undertaken with an underlying desire to discover causes. Yet, correlational studies are susceptible to faulty interpretation because researchers work with preexisting groups that have formed through **self-selection**. Kerlinger and Lee (2000) indicate that "self-selection occurs when the members of the groups being studied are in the groups, in part, because they differentially possess traits or characteristics extraneous to the research problem, characteristics that possibly influence or are otherwise related to the variables of the research problem" (p. 560). In other words, preexisting differences may be a plausible alternative explanation for any observed group differences on the dependent variable.

As an example of such interpretive problems, suppose we studied differences in depression levels of cancer patients who do or do not have adequate social support (i.e., emotional sustenance through a social network). The independent variable is social support, and the dependent variable is depression. Suppose we found that patients without social support were more depressed than patients with adequate social support. We could interpret this to mean that people's emotional state is influenced by the adequacy of their social support, as diagrammed in Figure 9-2A. There are, however, alternative explanations for the findings. Perhaps a third variable influences *both* social support and depression, such as patients' family structure (e.g., whether they are married). It may be that the availability of a significant other affects how depressed cancer patients feel *and* the quality of their social support. These relationships are diagrammed in Figure 9-2B. A third possibility may be reversed causality, as shown in Figure 9-2C. Depressed cancer patients may find it more difficult to elicit social support than patients who are more cheerful. In this interpretation, it is the person's emotional state that causes the amount of received social support, and not the other way around. The point here is that correlational results should be interpreted cautiously, especially if the research has no theoretical basis.

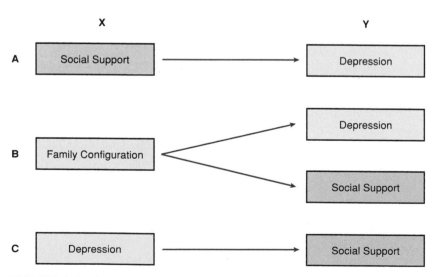

FIGURE 9.2 Alternative explanations for relationship between depression and social support in cancer patients.

CONSUMER TIP

Be prepared to think critically when a researcher claims to be studying the "effects" of an independent variable on a dependent variable in a nonexperimental study. For example, if a report title were "The Effects of Dieting on Depression," the study would likely be nonexperimental (i.e., subjects were not randomly assigned to dieting or not dieting). In such a situation, you might ask, did dieting have an effect on depression—or did depression have an effect on dieting? Or, did a third variable (e.g., being overweight) have an effect on both?

Despite interpretive problems, correlational studies play a crucial role in nursing because many interesting problems are not amenable to experimentation. Correlational research is often an efficient and effective means of collecting a large amount of data about a problem area. For example, it would be possible to collect extensive information about people's health problems and eating habits. Researchers could then examine which health problems correlate with which nutritional patterns. By doing this, many relationships could be discovered in a short time. By contrast, an experimenter looks at only a few variables at a time. For example, one experiment might manipulate foods with different cholesterol levels to observe the effects on physical symptoms, whereas another experiment might manipulate protein consumption, and so forth.

Quantitative Designs and Research Evidence

Evidence for nursing practice depends upon descriptive, correlational, and experimental research. There is often a logical progression to knowledge expansion that begins with rich description, including description from qualitative research. Descriptive studies can be invaluable in documenting the prevalence, nature, and intensity of health-related conditions and behaviors, and are critical in the conceptualization of effective interventions.

Correlational studies are often undertaken in the next phase of developing a knowledge base. Exploratory retrospective studies may pave the way for more rigorous case-control studies and for prospective studies. As the evidence builds, conceptual models may be developed and tested using nonexperimental theory-testing strategies. These studies can provide hints about how to structure an intervention, who can most profit from it, and when it can best be instituted. Thus, the next important phase is to design interventions to improve health outcomes. Evidence regarding the effectiveness of interventions and health strategies is strongest when it comes from experiments. For this reason, experimental designs have earned the reputation among many of being the "gold standard" in an evidence-based practice (EBP) environment.

RESEARCH DESIGN AND THE TIME DIMENSION

The research design incorporates decisions about when and how often data will be collected in a study. In many nursing studies, data are collected in a single time period; other studies involve data collection on multiple occasions. Indeed, several designs involving multiple measurements have already been discussed, such as the pretest–posttest experimental design, the time-series design, and the prospective design.

There are four situations in which it is appropriate to design a study with multiple points of data collection:

1. *Time-related processes.* Certain research problems involve phenomena that evolve over time. Examples include healing, growth, recidivism, and learning.
2. *Time-sequenced phenomena.* It is sometimes important to ascertain the sequencing of phenomena. For example, if it is hypothesized that infertility contributes to depression, it would be important to determine that depression did not precede fertility problems.
3. *Comparative purposes.* Sometimes, multiple data points are used to compare phenomena over time. For example, a study might document trends in the incidence of child abuse over a 10-year period. Another example is a time-series study, in which the intent is to determine whether changes over time can be attributed to an intervention.
4. *Enhancement of research control.* Some research designs collect data at multiple points to enhance the interpretability of the results. For example, in nonequivalent control-group designs, the collection of preintervention data allows the researcher to detect and control for initial group differences.

Because of the importance of the time dimension in designing research, studies are sometimes categorized in terms of how they deal with time. The major distinction is between cross-sectional and longitudinal designs—terms that are most often (although not always) used to describe nonexperimental studies.

Cross-Sectional Designs

Cross-sectional designs involve the collection of data at one point in time (or multiple times in a short time period, such as 2 hours and 4 hours postoperatively). All phenomena under study are captured during one data collection period. Cross-sectional designs are especially appropriate for describing the status of phenomena or relationships among phenomena at a fixed point. For example, a researcher might study whether psychological symptoms in menopausal women are correlated contemporaneously with physiologic symptoms. Retrospective studies are almost always cross-sectional. Data with regard to the independent and dependent variables are collected concurrently (e.g., the lung cancer status of respondents and their smoking habits), but the independent variable usually captures events or behaviors occurring in the past.

When cross-sectional designs are used to study time-related phenomena, the designs are weaker than longitudinal ones. Suppose, for example, we were studying changes in children's health promotion activities between ages 7 and 10. One way to investigate this would be to interview the children at age 7 and then 3 years later at age 10—a longitudinal design. On the other hand, we could use a cross-sectional design by interviewing children ages 7 and 10 at one point in time and then comparing their responses. If 10-year-olds engaged in more health-promoting activities than the 7-year-olds, it might be inferred that children became more conscious of making good health choices as they age. To make this kind of inference, we would have to assume that the older children would have responded as the younger ones did had they been questioned 3 years earlier, or, conversely, that 7-year-olds would report more health-promoting activities if they were questioned again 3 years later.

The main advantage of cross-sectional designs is that they are economical and easy to manage. There are, however, problems in inferring changes and trends over time using a cross-sectional design. The amount of social and technological change that characterizes our society makes it questionable to assume that differences in the behaviors, attitudes, or characteristics of different age groups are the result of the passage through time rather than cohort or generational differences. In the previous example, 7- and 10-year-old children may have different attitudes toward health and health promotion independent of maturational factors. In such cross-sectional studies, there are often alternative explanations for observed differences.

Example of a cross-sectional study

Using a cross-sectional design, Ferrario (2003) studied the relationship between nursing experience and the use of mental representations in diagnostic reasoning. Expert nurses (those with 5 or more years of experience) were compared with novice nurses (less than 5 years of experience).

Longitudinal Designs

Studies designed to collect data at more than one point in time over an extended period use a **longitudinal design**. Longitudinal designs are useful for examining changes over time and for ascertaining the temporal sequencing of phenomena, which is an essential criterion for establishing causality.

Three types of longitudinal studies deserve special mention: trend, panel, and follow-up studies. **Trend studies** are investigations in which samples from a population are studied over time with respect to some phenomenon. Different samples are selected from the same population at repeated intervals. In trend studies, researchers can examine patterns of change and make predictions about future directions. For example, trend studies have been conducted to analyze the number of students entering nursing programs and to forecast future supplies of nurses.

In **panel studies**, the same people provide data at two or more points in time. The term *panel* refers to the sample of people in the study. Panel studies typically yield more information than trend studies because researchers can examine patterns of change and reasons for the changes. Researchers can identify individuals who did and did not change and then explore characteristics that differentiate the two groups. Panel studies are appealing as a method of studying change but are difficult and expensive to manage. The most serious challenge is the loss of participants over time—a problem known as **attrition**. Subject attrition is problematic because those who drop out of the study may differ in important respects from those who continue to participate, resulting in potential biases and concerns about the generalizability of the findings.

Example of a panel study

Miller, Ratner, and Johnson (2003) used data from the Survey on Smoking in Canada, a national panel study with four rounds of data collection. In this study, all those who reported that they were former smokers in round 1 were divided into two groups: those who had a smoking relapse at some point during the next three rounds, and those who were continuously abstinent. The study focused on identifying predictors of smoking relapse prospectively.

Follow-up studies are undertaken to determine the subsequent status of subjects with a specified condition or those who received a specified intervention. For example, patients who have received a particular nursing intervention or clinical treatment may be followed up to ascertain the long-term effects of the treatment. To take a nonexperimental example, samples of premature infants may be followed up to assess their later perceptual and motor development.

Example of follow-up study

Chang and Hancock (2003) followed up a group of new nurses in Australia 2–3 months after initial employment and then 11–12 months later. The researchers investigated sources of, and changes to, role stress in the new nurses and examined the relationship between their role stress and job satisfaction over time.

In longitudinal studies, the number of data collection points and the time intervals between them depend on the nature of the study. When change or development is rapid, numerous data collection points at relatively short intervals may be required to document the pattern and to make accurate forecasts. By convention, however, the term *longitudinal* implies multiple data collection points over an extended period of time.

CONSUMER TIP

Not all longitudinal studies are prospective, because sometimes the independent variable occurred well before the initial wave of data collection. And not all prospective studies are longitudinal in the classic sense. For example, an experimental study that collects data at 2, 4, and 6 hours after an intervention would be considered prospective but not longitudinal (i.e., data are not collected over a long time period). ■

TECHNIQUES OF RESEARCH CONTROL

A major purpose of research design in quantitative studies is to maximize researchers' control over extraneous variables. There are two basic types of extraneous variables that need to be controlled—those that are intrinsic to study participants and those that are external, stemming from the research situation.

Controlling External Factors

Various external factors, such as the research environment, can affect study outcomes. In carefully controlled quantitative research, steps are taken to minimize situational contaminants (i.e., to achieve **constancy of conditions** for the collection of data) so that researchers can be confident that the conditions are not affecting the data.

The environment has been found to influence people's emotions and behavior, and so, in designing quantitative studies, researchers strive to control the environmental context. Control over the environment is most easily achieved in laboratory experiments, in which all subjects are brought into an environment structured by the experimenter. Researchers have less control over the environment in studies that occur in natural settings, but some opportunities exist. For example, in interview studies, researchers can restrict data collection to one type of setting (e.g., respondents' homes).

A second external factor that may need to be controlled is time. Depending on the research topic, the dependent variable may be influenced by the time of day or the time of year in which data are collected. In these cases, researchers should ensure that constancy of time is maintained. If an investigator were studying fatigue, for example, it would matter whether the data were gathered in the morning, afternoon, or evening, and so data from all subjects should be collected at the same time of day.

Another issue concerns constancy of communications to subjects. Formal scripts are often prepared to inform subjects about the study purpose, the use that will be made of the data, and so forth. In research involving an intervention, formal research protocols, or specifications for the interventions, are developed. For example, in an experiment to test the effectiveness of a new medication, care would be needed to ensure that the subjects in the experimental group received the same chemical substance and the same dosage, that the substance was administered in the same way, and so forth.

Example of controlling external factors

Wipke-Tevis, Stotts, Williams, Froelicher, and Hunt (2001) took great care to ensure constancy of conditions in their quasi-experimental study, which compared tissue oxygenation in four body positions among people with venous ulcers. As examples of how the researchers controlled environmental factors, all measurements were made in the early morning; subjects had been instructed to fast so that a fasting blood sample could be drawn; subjects were then provided the same breakfast; and after breakfast all subjects rested in bed supine for 30 minutes before testing began.

Controlling Intrinsic Factors

Control of study participants' extraneous characteristics is especially important. For example, suppose we were investigating the effects of an innovative physical training program on the cardiovascular functioning of nursing home residents. In this study, variables such as the subjects' age, gender, and smoking history would be extraneous variables; each is likely to be related to the outcome variable (cardiovascular functioning), independent of the physical training program. In other words, the effects that these variables have on the dependent variable are extraneous to the study. In this section, we review methods of controlling extraneous subject characteristics.

METHODS OF CONTROLLING SUBJECT CHARACTERISTICS
Randomization
We have already discussed the most effective method of controlling subject characteristics: randomization. The primary function of randomization is to secure comparable groups, that is, to equalize groups with respect to the extraneous variables. A distinct advantage of randomization, compared with other methods of controlling extraneous variables, is that it controls all possible sources of extraneous variation, without any conscious decision by researchers about which variables need to be controlled. In our example of the physical training intervention, random assignment of subjects to an experimental (intervention) group and control (no intervention) group would be an excellent control mechanism. Presumably, the two groups would be comparable in terms of age, gender, smoking history, and thousands of other preintervention characteristics. Randomization within a crossover design is especially powerful: Participants serve as their own controls, thereby totally controlling all extraneous variables.

Example of randomization

Gallagher, McKinley, & Dracup (2003) tested the effect of a postdischarge telephone counseling intervention on women's psychosocial adjustment after a cardiac event. A sample of 196 women, recruited from four hospitals in Sydney, Australia, were randomized to usual care or telephone counseling.

Homogeneity

When randomization is not feasible, other methods of controlling extraneous subject characteristics can be used. One alternative is **homogeneity,** in which only subjects who are homogeneous with respect to extraneous variables are included in the study. Extraneous variables, in this case, are not allowed to vary. In the physical training example, if gender were considered a confounding variable, we could recruit only men (or women) as participants. If we were concerned about the confounding effect of participants' age on physical fitness, participation could be limited to those within a specified age range. This strategy of using a homogeneous sample is easy, but its limitation is that the findings can be generalized only to the type of subjects who participated. If the physical training program were found to have beneficial effects on the cardiovascular functioning of men aged 65 to 75 years, its usefulness for improving the cardiovascular status of women in their 80s would need to be tested in a separate study.

Example of control through homogeneity

Kozuki and Froelicher (2003) studied the relationship between schizophrenic patients' lack of awareness of symptoms and their nonadherence to psychotropic medications. Because mental retardation and substance abuse could affect symptom awareness and nonadherence, patients who had comorbidity with substance abuse and mental retardation were not included in the sample.

Matching

A third method of dealing with extraneous variables is matching. **Matching** involves using information about subject characteristics to form comparison groups. For example, suppose we began with a sample of nursing home residents already set to participate in the physical training program. A comparison group of nonparticipating residents could be created by matching subjects, one by one, on the basis of important extraneous variables (e.g., age and gender). This procedure results in groups known to be comparable in terms of the extraneous variables of concern. Matching is the technique used to form comparable groups in case-control designs.

Matching has some drawbacks as a control method. To match effectively, researchers must know in advance what the relevant extraneous variables are. Second, after two or three variables, it becomes difficult to match. Suppose we wanted to control the age, gender, race, and length of nursing home stays of the participants. In this situation if participant 1 in the physical training program were an African-American woman, aged 80 years, whose length of stay was 5 years, we would have to seek another woman with these same or similar characteristics as a comparison group counterpart. With more than three variables, matching becomes cumbersome. Thus, matching as a control method is usually used only when more powerful procedures are not feasible.

Example of matching

Mahon, Yarcheski, and Yarcheski (2003) compared early adolescents from divorced families with those from intact families in terms of anger, anxiety, and depression. To control extraneous variables, adolescents from divorced families were matched to those from intact families in terms of gender, age, race, and grade in school.

Statistical Control

Yet another method of controlling extraneous variables is through statistical analysis. You may be unfamiliar at this point with basic statistical procedures, let alone sophisticated techniques such as those referred to here. Therefore, a detailed description of powerful statistical control mechanisms, such as **analysis of covariance**, will not be attempted. You should recognize, however, that nurse researchers are increasingly using powerful statistical techniques to control extraneous variables. A brief description of methods of statistical control is presented in Chapter 15.

Example of statistical control

Li and Holm (2003) used a 2 × 2 nonexperimental design to compare the vasomotor symptoms (e.g., hot flashes) of postmenopausal women who were high or low on physical activity (factor A) and who used or did not use hormone replacement therapy (factor B). To make the four groups of women more comparable, the researchers statistically controlled the women's level of education and their body mass index.

EVALUATION OF CONTROL METHODS

Overall, random assignment is the most effective approach to controlling extraneous variables because randomization tends to cancel out individual variation on all possible extraneous variables. Crossover designs are especially powerful, but they cannot be applied to all nursing research problems because of the possibility of carryover effects. The three remaining alternatives described here have two disadvantages in common. First, researchers must know which variables to control in advance. To select homogeneous samples, match, or perform an analysis of covariance, researchers must decide which variables to control. Second, these three methods control only for identified characteristics, possibly leaving others uncontrolled.

Although randomization is the best mechanism for controlling extraneous subject characteristics, randomization is not always possible. If the independent variable cannot be manipulated, other techniques should be used. It is far better to use matching or analysis of covariance than simply to ignore the problem of extraneous variables.

CONSUMER TIP

In nursing studies that are not experimental, statistical procedures such as analysis of covariance are the most frequently used methods of controlling extraneous variables. Matching, which was a commonly used control technique a few decades ago, has become much less prevalent since computers have become widely available for statistical analysis.

■

CHARACTERISTICS OF GOOD DESIGN

In evaluating the merits of a quantitative study, one overarching question is whether the research design did the best possible job of providing valid and reliable evidence. Cook and Campbell (1979), in their classic book on research design, describe four important considerations for evaluating research design in studies that focus on relationships among variables. The questions that must be addressed by researchers (and evaluated by consumers) regarding research design are as follows:

1. What is the strength of the evidence that a relationship exists between two variables?
2. If a relationship exists, what is the strength of the evidence that the independent variable of interest (e.g., an intervention), rather than extraneous factors, caused the outcome?
3. What is the strength of evidence that observed relationships are generalizable across people, settings, and time?
4. What are the theoretical constructs underlying the related variables, and are those constructs adequately captured?

These questions, respectively, correspond to four aspects of a study's validity: (1) statistical conclusion validity; (2) internal validity; (3) external validity; and (4) construct validity. In this section we discuss certain aspects of the first three types of validity; construct validity, which concerns the measurement of variables, is discussed in Chapter 14.

Statistical Conclusion Validity

As noted earlier in this chapter, the first criterion for establishing causality is demonstrating that there is, in fact, an empirical relationship between the independent and dependent variable. Statistical methods are used to determine if such a relationship exists. Design decisions can influence whether statistical tests will actually detect true relationships, and so researchers need to make decisions that protect against reaching false statistical conclusions. Although we cannot at this point in the text discuss all aspects of **statistical conclusion validity**, we can describe a few design issues that can be threats to making valid statistical inferences.

One issue concerns **statistical power**, which is the ability of the design to detect true relationships among variables. Adequate statistical power can be achieved in various ways, the most straightforward of which is to use a sufficiently large sample. When small samples are used, statistical power tends to be low, and the analyses may fail to show that the independent and dependent variables are related—*even when they are*. Power and sample size are discussed in Chapter 12.

Another aspect of a powerful design concerns the construction or definition of the independent variable and the counterfactual. Both statistically and substantively, results are clearer when differences between the groups (or treatment conditions) being compared are large. To enhance statistical conclusion validity, researchers should aim to maximize group differences on the independent variables so as to maximize differences on the dependent variables. If the groups or treatments are not very different, the statistical analysis might not be sufficiently sensitive to detect true differences that actually exist. A related issue is that the strength of an intervention (and hence statistical power) can be undermined if the intervention is not as powerful in reality as it is "on paper." An intervention can be weakened by a number of factors, such as lack of standardization, inadequate training, or premature withdrawal of subjects from the intervention. It is the researchers' responsibility to monitor the integrity of treatments in studies and to report deficiencies in achieving it.

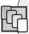

Example of monitoring treatment integrity

Cowan, Pike, and Budzynski (2001) conducted a rigorous experimental study of the effectiveness of a psychosocial nursing therapy for reducing mortality in patients who experienced sudden cardiac arrest. Subjects were randomized to the intervention (individual therapeutic sessions) or to a control group. Those administering the intervention protocol were trained extensively; subject adherence to the intervention was carefully monitored and deemed to be excellent.

Thus, if you are evaluating a study that indicates that groups being compared were not statistically different with respect to outcomes (e.g., an experimental and control group), one possibility is that the study had low statistical conclusion validity. The report might give clues about this possibility (e.g., too small a sample or substantial subject attrition) that should be taken into consideration in drawing conclusions about the study's evidence.

Internal Validity

Internal validity refers to the extent to which it is possible to make an inference that the independent variable is truly causing or influencing the dependent variable. Experiments possess a high degree of internal validity because randomization to different groups enables researchers to rule out competing explanations. With quasi-experiments and correlational studies, investigators must contend with rival hypotheses. Competing explanations, or *threats to internal validity*, have been grouped into several classes.

THREATS TO INTERNAL VALIDITY
History
The **history threat** is the occurrence of events concurrent with the independent variable that can affect the dependent variable. For example, suppose we were studying the effectiveness of an outreach program to encourage flu shots among community-dwelling elders using a time-series design. Now let us further suppose that, at about the same time the outreach program was initiated, there was a national public media campaign focusing on the flu. Our dependent variable in this case, number of flu shots administered, is subject to the influence of at least two forces, and it would be difficult for us to disentangle the two effects. In experiments, history is not typically an issue because external events are as likely to affect one group as another. The designs most likely to be affected by the history threat are one-group before–after designs and time-series designs.

Selection
The **selection threat** encompasses biases resulting from preexisting differences between groups. When people are not assigned randomly to groups, the possibility always exists that groups being compared are not equivalent. In such a situation, researchers contend with the possibility that any difference in the dependent variable is due to extraneous factors rather than to the independent variable. Selection biases are the most problematic threats to the internal validity of

studies not using an experimental design (e.g., nonequivalent control group designs, case-control designs) but can be partially addressed using the control mechanisms described in the previous section.

Maturation

In a research context, the **maturation threat** arises from processes occurring as a result of time (e.g., growth, fatigue) rather than the independent variable. For example, if we wanted to evaluate the effect of a special sensorimotor-development program for developmentally retarded children, we would have to contend with the fact that progress would occur even without the intervention. Maturation is a relevant consideration in many areas of nursing research. Remember that the term here does not refer to developmental changes exclusively but rather to any kind of change that occurs as a function of time. Phenomena such as wound healing, postoperative recovery, and other bodily changes can occur with little nursing intervention, and thus maturation may be a rival explanation for any positive posttreatment outcomes. One-group before–after designs are especially vulnerable to the maturation threat.

Mortality

The **mortality threat** stems from differential attrition from groups. The loss of subjects during the study may differ among groups because of initial differences in interest, motivation, and the like. For example, suppose we used a nonequivalent control-group design to assess nurses' morale in two different hospitals, one of which initiated primary nursing. The dependent variable, nursing staff satisfaction, is measured before and after the intervention. The comparison group, which may have no particular commitment to the study, may be reluctant to complete a posttest questionnaire. Those who do fill it out may be unrepresentative of the group as a whole; they may be highly critical of their work environment, for example. Thus, on the average, it may appear that the morale of nurses in the comparison hospital declined, but this might only be an artifact of the mortality of a select segment of this group.

INTERNAL VALIDITY AND RESEARCH DESIGN

Quasi-experimental, preexperimental, and correlational studies are especially susceptible to threats to internal validity. These threats represent alternative explanations (rival hypotheses) that compete with the independent variable as a cause of the dependent variable. *The aim of a good quantitative research design is to rule out these competing explanations.* The control mechanisms previously reviewed are strategies for improving the internal validity of studies—and thus for strengthening the quality of evidence they yield.

An experimental design normally eliminates competing explanations, but this is not always the case. For example, if constancy of conditions is not maintained for experimental and control groups, history might be a rival explanation for obtained results. Experimental mortality is, in particular, a salient threat in experiments. Because the experimenter does different things with the experimental and control groups, members of the two groups may drop out of the study differentially. This is particularly likely to happen if the experimental treatment is stressful, inconvenient, or time-consuming, or if the control condition is boring or aggravating. When this happens, participants remaining in the study may differ from those who left, thereby nullifying the initial equivalence of the groups.

You should pay careful attention to the possibility of competing explanations for reported results, especially in studies that do not use an experimental design. When the investigator does not have control over critical extraneous variables, caution in interpreting results and drawing conclusions about using the evidence in practice is appropriate.

CONSUMER TIP

As classically defined, internal validity concerns the strength of the evidence that the independent variable (rather than other factors) caused or influenced the dependent variable. Such a concern typically arises when significant group differences are found and there is an interest in ruling out rival hypotheses. However, internal validity is also of concern when group differences are *not* statistically significant. In such situations, the question is, Is it plausible that extraneous or competing factors *masked* the relationship between the independent and dependent variables?

External Validity

External validity is the generalizability of research findings to other settings or samples, an issue of great importance for those interested in an evidence-based practice. Quantitative studies are rarely conducted with the intention of discovering relationships among variables for a single group of people. If a nursing intervention is found to be effective—and if the study results are internally valid—then others will want to adopt it. Therefore, an important question is whether an intervention will work in another setting or with different patients.

One aspect of a study's external validity concerns the adequacy of the sampling design. If the characteristics of the sample are representative of those of the population, the generalizability of the results to the population is enhanced. Sampling designs are described in Chapter 12.

Various aspects of a research situation also affect the study's external validity. For example, when a treatment is new (e.g., a new protocol for pain management), subjects and researchers alike might alter their behavior. People may be either enthusiastic or skeptical about new methods of doing things. Thus, the results may reflect reactions to the novelty rather than to the intrinsic qualities of the treatment. Results may also reflect study participants' awareness of being in a study (the Hawthorne effect) or their expectations about benefits of an intervention, independent of the actual intervention (a **placebo effect**).

Example of a possible Hawthorne effect

Hundley and a team of Scottish nurse researchers (2000) designed an intervention aimed at raising research awareness among midwives and nurses. The treatment group got an educational program, while the control group did not. Both groups showed a knowledge gain from pretest to posttest, which the researchers interpreted as a Hawthorne effect.

Sometimes, the demands for internal and external validity conflict. If a researcher exercises tight control in a study to maximize internal validity, the setting may become too artificial to generalize to a more naturalistic environment. Therefore, a compromise must sometimes be reached. The importance of replicating studies in different settings with new subjects cannot be overemphasized.

CRITIQUING QUANTITATIVE RESEARCH DESIGNS

The overriding consideration in evaluating a research design is whether the design enables the researcher to answer the research question conclusively. This must be determined in terms of both substantive and methodologic considerations.

Box 9.1   Guidelines for Critiquing Research Designs in Quantitative Studies

1. Does the study involve an intervention? If yes, was an experimental, quasi-experimental, or preexperimental design used—and was this the most appropriate design?
2. If the study was experimental or quasi-experimental, was "blinding" used? Who was blinded?
3. If the study was nonexperimental, why didn't the researcher manipulate the independent variable? Was the decision regarding manipulation appropriate?
4. Was the study longitudinal or cross-sectional? Was the number of data collection points appropriate, given the research question?
5. What type of comparisons were called for in the research design (e.g., was the study design within-subjects or between-subjects)? Are the comparisons the most appropriate for illuminating the relationship between the independent and dependent variables?
6. What did the researcher do to control extraneous external factors and intrinsic subject characteristics? Were the procedures appropriate and adequate?
7. What steps did the researcher take in designing the study to enhance statistical conclusion validity? Were these steps adequate?
8. What steps did the researcher take to enhance the internal validity of the study? To what extent were those steps successful? What types of alternative explanations must be considered—what are the threats to internal validity? Does the design enable the researcher to draw causal inferences about the relationship between the independent and dependent variables?
9. To what extent is the study externally valid?
10. What are the major limitations of the design used? Are these limitations acknowledged by the researcher and taken into account in interpreting results?

Substantively, the issue is whether the researcher selected a design that matches the aims of the research. If the research purpose is descriptive or exploratory, an experimental design is not appropriate. If the researcher is searching to understand the full nature of a phenomenon about which little is known, a highly structured design that allows little flexibility might block insights (flexible designs are discussed in Chapter 10). We have discussed research control as a mechanism for reducing bias, but in certain situations, too much control can introduce bias, for example, when the researcher tightly controls the ways in which the phenomena under study can be manifested and thereby obscures their true nature.

Methodologically, the main design issue in quantitative studies is whether the research design provides the most accurate, unbiased, interpretable, and replicable evidence possible. Indeed, there usually is no other aspect of a quantitative study that affects the quality of evidence as much as the research design. Box 9-1 provides questions to assist you in evaluating the methodologic aspects of quantitative research designs; these questions are key to a meaningful critique of a quantitative study.

C H A P T E R   R E V I E W

Key new terms introduced in the chapter, together with a summary of major points, are presented in this section. In addition, Chapter 9 of the *Study Guide to Accompany Essentials of Nursing Research*, 6th edition offers various exercises and study suggestions for reinforcing the concepts presented in this chapter. For additional review, see the Student Self-Study Review Questions section of the Student Resource CD-ROM provided with this book.

KEY NEW TERMS

Analysis of covariance	Main effects
Attrition	Manipulation
Baseline data	Matching
Between-subjects design	Maturation threat
Case-control design	Mortality threat
Comparison group	Nonequivalent control group before–after design
Constancy of conditions	Nonexperimental study
Control group	One group before-after design
Correlational research	Panel study
Crossover design	Placebo
Cross-sectional design	Placebo effect
Descriptive correlational	Posttest-only design
Descriptive research	Preexperimental design
Double-blind experiment	Pretest–posttest design
Experiments	Prospective design
Experimental group	Quasi–experiment
External validity	Random assignment (randomization)
Factorial design	Retrospective design
Follow-up study	Selection threat
Hawthorne effect	Statistical conclusion validity
History threat	Statistical power
Homogeneity	Time-series design
Interaction effects	Trend study
Internal validity	Within-subjects design
Longitudinal design	

SUMMARY POINTS

◊ The **research design** is the researcher's overall plan for answering research questions. In quantitative studies, the design indicates whether there is an intervention, the nature of any comparisons, the methods used to control extraneous variables, and the timing and location of data collection.

◊ **Experiments** involve **manipulation** (the researcher manipulates the independent variable by introducing a *treatment* or *intervention*), control (including the use of a **control group** that is compared to the **experimental group**), and **randomization** (wherein subjects are allocated to groups at random to make them comparable at the outset).

◊ **Posttest only** (or *after-only*) **designs** involve collecting data only once—after random assignment and the introduction of the treatment; in **pretest–posttest** (*before–after*) **designs**, data are collected both before and after the experimental manipulation.

◊ **Factorial designs**, in which two or more variables are manipulated simultaneously, allow researchers to test both **main effects** (effects from the experimentally manipulated variables) and **interaction effects** (effects resulting from combining the treatments).

◊ **Between-subjects designs**, in which different sets of people are compared, contrast with **within-subjects designs**, which involve comparisons of the same subjects.

▷ In a **crossover** (or *repeated-measures*) **design**, subjects are exposed to more than one experimental condition in random order and serve as their own controls.

▷ **Quasi-experiments** involve manipulation but lack a comparison group or randomization. Quasi-experimental designs introduce controls to compensate for these missing components. By contrast, **preexperimental designs** have no such safeguards.

▷ The **nonequivalent control-group before–after design** involves the use of a **comparison group** that was not created through random assignment, and the collection of pretreatment data that permits an assessment of initial group equivalence.

▷ In a **time-series design**, there is no comparison group; information on the dependent variable is collected over a period of time before and after the treatment.

▷ **Nonexperimental research** includes **descriptive research**—studies that summarize the status of phenomena—and **correlational** (or *ex post facto*) **studies** that examine relationships among variables but involve no manipulation of the independent variable.

▷ Researchers use **retrospective** and **prospective** correlational designs to infer causality, but the findings from such studies are generally open to several interpretations.

▷ **Cross-sectional designs** involve the collection of data at one time period, whereas **longitudinal designs** involve data collection at two or more times over an extended period. Three types of longitudinal studies, which are used to study changes or development over time, are **trend studies, panel studies,** and **follow-up studies.**

▷ Quantitative researchers strive to control external factors that could affect the study outcomes (e.g., the environment) and subject characteristics that are extraneous to the research question.

▷ Techniques for controlling subject characteristics include **homogeneity** (restricting the selection of subjects to eliminate variability on the extraneous variable); **matching** (matching subjects on a one-to-one basis to make groups comparable on the extraneous variables); statistical procedures, such as **analysis of covariance**; and randomization—the most effective control procedure because it controls all possible extraneous variables without researchers having to identify or measure them.

▷ A well-designed study attends to statistical conclusion validity, internal validity, external validity, and construct validity.

▷ **Statistical conclusion validity** concerns the strength of evidence that a relationship exists between two variables. Threats to statistical conclusion validity include low **statistical power** (the ability to detect true relationships among variables) and a weak treatment.

▷ **Internal validity** concerns the degree to which outcomes can be attributed to the independent variable. *Threats to internal validity* include **history, selection, maturation,** and **mortality** (caused by subject **attrition**).

▷ **External validity** refers to the generalizability of study findings to other samples and situations.

RESEARCH EXAMPLES | **Critical Thinking Activities**

 EXAMPLE 1: Experimental Design

Aspects of an experimental nursing study, featuring terms and concepts discussed in this chapter, are presented below, followed by some questions to guide critical thinking. (The full research report is available in *Nursing Research, 52,* 183–190.)

RESEARCH EXAMPLES *Continued*

Study

"Cognitive-behavioral intervention effects on adolescents' anxiety and pain following spinal fusion surgery" (LaMontagne, Hepworth, Cohen, & Salisbury, 2003)

Statement of Purpose

The purpose of the study was to determine the effectiveness of three cognitive-behavioral interventions for reducing adolescents' postoperative pain and anxiety following spinal fusion surgery.

Treatment Conditions

The three interventions consisted of (1) concrete-objective information (procedural and sensory information about the surgery) plus instruction in specific coping behaviors that adolescents could perform during recovery; (2) concrete-objective information only; and (3) coping instruction only. Subjects in a control condition (group 4) were given standard information about the surgery experience. All interventions were delivered by videotape.

Method

A sample of 109 adolescents aged 11 to 18 and their parents was recruited in a medical center on the day before surgery and provided informed consent. Study participants, who included only English-speaking children with no learning or developmental problems, were randomly assigned to one of the four groups using a computer-generated list of numbers. After completing a pretest measure of anxiety, the adolescents and their parents viewed the assigned videotaped intervention with a researcher. Those who received coping instruction (groups 1 and 3) practiced the coping skills taught on the videotape with the researcher. On the second postoperative day (between noon and 3:00 PM), participants were verbally administered scales to measure both pain and anxiety. Pain was measured a second time on the fourth postoperative day.

Key Findings

▶ The four groups of adolescents were comparable (not statistically different) in terms of age, ethnicity, gender, socioeconomic status, and anxiety level prior to surgery.
▶ Overall, there were no significant group differences with respect to postoperative anxiety. Pain decreased significantly from day 2 to day 4 in all groups except those in the coping only group.
▶ Although the interventions did not affect anxiety and pain for experimental group subjects as a whole, the information-plus-coping intervention was effective for reducing postoperative anxiety among adolescents who had high anxiety scores preoperatively.
▶ Among adolescents aged 13 and younger, the coping instruction (alone or with concrete-objective information) was significantly more effective for reducing postoperative pain than conditions without coping instruction.

research examples continue on page 206

RESEARCH EXAMPLES *Continued*

*Critical Thinking Suggestions**

* See the Student Resource CD-ROM for a discussion of these questions.
1. Answer questions 1, 2 and 3–10 from Box 9-1 regarding this study.
2. Also consider the following targeted questions, which may assist you in further assessing aspects of the study:
   a. What specific experimental design was used in this study? Was this appropriate?
   b. Could a crossover design have been used?
   c. Would you describe this study as a 4 × 1 design or a 2 × 2 design?
   d. Was randomization successful?
3. If the results of this study are valid and reliable, what are some of the uses to which the findings might be put in clinical practice?

 EXAMPLE 2: Quasi-Experimental Design

Aspects of a quasi-experimental nursing study, featuring terms and concepts discussed in this chapter, are presented below, followed by some questions to guide critical thinking. (The full research report is available in *Clinical Nursing Research, 12,* 210–225.)

Study

"Reducing hydration-linked events in nursing home residents" (Mentes & Culp, 2003).

Statement of Purpose

The purpose of the study was to test the effectiveness of an 8-week hydration intervention in reducing hydration-linked events (HLEs) in nursing home residents.

Treatment Conditions

The hydration intervention used with experimental group subjects involved the use of a hydration management guideline. The guideline called for the calculation of a daily individual fluid goal for each participant adjusted for his or her weight. Various strategies for providing adequate fluids were included in the guidelines. Those in the comparison group received usual care, with no special attention paid to fluid intake.

Method

Four nursing homes in eastern Iowa (two Veteran's Affairs facilities and two comparable community nursing homes) were randomly assigned by a coin toss to be a treatment or comparison facility. Randomization of individual study participants was not possible because of the nature and visibility of the hydration intervention. Participants (25 in the treatment group and 24 in the comparison group) were recruited from the nursing homes if they were capable of participating in data collection activities, were aged 65 or older, and met other health criteria. Participants were chosen in a manner that ensured gender balance in the two groups. At baseline, the researchers collected extensive information about the demographic and clinical characteristics of participants, including a dehydration risk assessment. Outcome data (weekly urinalysis, fluid records, infection information) were collected by RN research assistants over an 8-week period. The RN research assistant in the comparison group sites were blinded with regard to the participants' fluid goals. The main dependent variable was incidence of an HLE, defined as any episode of acute confusion or urinary or respiratory tract infection preceded by a urine specific gravity (SG) of ≥1.020.

Key Findings

▶ At baseline, the two groups were comparable demographically, but experimental group partici-pants were found to be more at risk for acute confusion, more likely to have a diagnosis of dementia, and physically more frail than comparison group members; they also had lower urine SGs than comparison group members.

▶ The incidence of HLE was three events per 63 days of follow-up in the treatment group versus six events per 60 days of follow-up in the comparison group, but this difference was not statis-tically significant (i.e., could have occurred by chance).

▶ Comparison group members were more likely than treatment group members to exceed their fluid goals at baseline, but by the end of the intervention, the reverse was true; however, group differences at the end of the study narrowly missed being statistically significant at conven-tional levels.

Critical Thinking Suggestions

1. Answer questions 1, 2, and 4–9 from Box 9-1 regarding this study.
2. Also consider the following targeted questions, which may assist you in further assessing aspects of the study:
    a. What specific quasi-experimental design was used in this study? Was this appropriate?
    b. Comment on the researchers' decision to randomize nursing homes to conditions.
    c. Comment on the researchers' decision to balance the groups in terms of gender.
3. If the results of this study are valid and reliable, what are some of the uses to which the find-ings might be put in clinical practice?

 EXAMPLE 3: Nonexperimental Design

1. Read the method section from the Motzer et al. study ("Sense of Coherence") in Appendix A of this book, and then answer the relevant questions in Box 9-1.
2. Also consider the following targeted questions, which may further sharpen your critical think-ing skills and assist you in assessing aspects of the study's merit:
    a. Was this study retrospective or prospective?
    b. In this study, the researchers conceptualized irritable bowel syndrome as the independent variable and sense of coherence as one of the dependent variables, and a relationship between these two variables was observed. Provide 3 interpretations of this relationship.
    c. Suggest a design that might help to rule out one of these three explanations.

SUGGESTED READINGS

Methodologic References

Campbell, D. T., & Stanley, J. C. (1963). *Experimental and quasi-experimental designs for research.* Chicago: Rand McNally.

Cook, T. D., & Campbell, D. T. (1979). *Quasi-experimental design and analysis issues for field settings.* Chicago: Rand McNally.

Kerlinger, F. N., & Lee, H. B. (2000). *Foundations of behavioral research* (4th ed.). Orlando, FL: Harcourt College Publishers.

Lazarsfeld, P. (1955). Foreword. In H. Hyman (Ed.), *Survey design and analysis.* New York: The Free Press.

Polit, D. F., & Beck, C. T. (2003). *Nursing research: Principles and methods* (7th ed.). Philadelphia: Lippincott Williams & Wilkins.

Studies Cited in Chapter 9

Chang, E., & Hancock, K. (2003). Role stress and role ambiguity in new nursing graduates in Australia. *Nursing Health Science, 5,* 155–163.

Cowan, M. J., Pike, K. C., Budzynski, H. K. (2001). Psychosocial nursing therapy following sudden cardiac arrest: Impact on two-year survival. *Nursing Research, 50,* 68–76.

Edwards, N. E., & Beck, A. M. (2002). Animal-assisted therapy and nutrition in Alzheimer's disease. *Western Journal of Nursing Research, 24,* 697–712.

Ferrario, C. G. (2003). Experienced and less-experienced nurses' diagnostic reasoning: Implications for fostering students' critical thinking. *International Journal of Nursing Terminologies and Classifications, 14,* 41–52.

Gallagher, R., McKinley, S., & Dracup, K. (2003). Effects of a telephone counseling intervention on psychosocial adjustment in women following a cardiac event. *Heart & Lung, 32,* 79–87.

Goodfellow, L. M. (2003). The effects of therapeutic back massage on psychophysiologic variables and immune function in spouses of patients with cancer. *Nursing Research, 52,* 318–328.

Hendrich, A. L., Bender, P. S., & Nyhuis, A. (2003). Validation of the Hendrich II Fall Risk Model. *Applied Nursing Research, 16,* 9–21.

Hundley, V., Milne, J., Leighton-Beck, L., Graham, W., & Fitmaurice, A. (2000). Raising research awareness among midwives and nurses. *Journal of Advanced Nursing, 31,* 78–88.

Kozuki, Y., & Froelicher, E. S. (2003). Lack of awareness and nonadherence in schizophrenia. *Western Journal of Nursing Research, 25,* 57–74.

LaMontagne, L. L., Hepworth, J. T., Cohen, F., & Salisbury, M. H. (2003). Cognitive-behavioral intervention effects on adolescents' anxiety and pain following spinal fusion surgery. *Nursing Research, 52,* 183–190.

Li, S., & Holm, K. (2003). Physical activity alone and in combination with hormone replacement therapy on vasomotor symptoms in postmenopausal women. *Western Journal of Nursing Research, 25,* 274–288.

Maas, M., Reed, D., Park, M., Specht, J., Schutte, D., Kelley, L., Swanson, E., Tripp Reimer, T., & Buckwalter, K. (2004). Outcomes of family involvement in care intervention for caregivers of individuals with dementia. *Nursing Research, 53,* 76–86.

Mahon, N. E., Yarcheski, A., & Yarcheski, T. J. (2003). Anger, anxiety, and depression in early adolescents from intact and divorced families. *Journal of Pediatric Nursing, 18,* 267–273.

McDonald, D. D., Wiczorek, M., & Walker, C. (2004). Factors affecting learning during health education sessions. *Clinical Nursing Research, 13,* 156–167.

Mentes, J. C., & Culp, K. (2003). Reducing hydration-linked events in nursing home residents. *Clinical Nursing Research, 12,* 210–225.

Miller, C. E., Ratner, P. A., & Johnson, J. L. (2003). Reducing cardiovascular risk: Identifying predictors of smoking relapse. *Canadian Journal of Cardiovascular Nursing, 13,* 7–12.

Niesen, K. M., Harris, D. Y., Parkin, L. S., & Henn, L. T. (2003). The effects of heparin versus normal saline for maintenance of peripheral intravenous locks in pregnant women. *Journal of Obstetric, Gynecologic & Neonatal Nursing, 32,* 503–508.

Schachman, K. A., Lee, R. K., & Lederman, R. P. (2004). Baby Boot Camp: Facilitating maternal role adaptation among military wives. *Nursing Research, 53,* 107–115.

Schneider, S. M., Prince-Paul, M., Allen, M. J., Silverman, P., & Talaba, D. (2004). Virtual reality as a distraction intervention for women receiving chemotherapy. *Oncology Nursing Forum, 31,* 81–88.

Schuurmans, M. J., Duursma, S. A., Shortridge-Baggett, L. M., Clevers, G., & Pel-Little, R. (2003). Elderly patients with a hip fracture: The risk for delirium. *Applied Nursing Research, 16,* 75–84.

Tanyi, R. A., & Werner, J. S. (2003). Adjustment, spirituality, and health in women on hemodialysis. *Clinical Nursing Research, 12,* 229–245.

Wipke-Tevis, D. D., Stotts, N. A., Williams, D. A., Froelicher, E. S., & Hunt, T. K. (2001). Tissue oxygenation, perfusion, and position in patients with venous leg ulcers. *Nursing Research, 50,* 24–32.

Understanding Qualitative Research Design

STUDENT OBJECTIVES

On completing this chapter, you will be able to:

▶ Discuss the rationale for an emergent design in qualitative research and describe qualitative design features
▶ Identify the major research traditions for qualitative research and describe the domain of inquiry of each
▶ Describe the main features of ethnographic, phenomenological, and grounded theory studies
▶ Discuss the goals and methods of various types of research with an ideological perspective
▶ Define new terms in the chapter

THE DESIGN OF QUALITATIVE STUDIES

Quantitative researchers specify a research design before collecting their data and adhere to that design after the study is underway; they *design* and then they *do*. In qualitative research, by contrast, the study design typically evolves over the course of the project; qualitative researchers *design* as they *do*. Decisions about how best to obtain data, from whom to obtain data, how to schedule data collection, and how long each data collection session should last are made in the field, as the study unfolds. The design for qualitative studies is an **emergent design**—a design that emerges as researchers make ongoing decisions reflecting what has already been learned. As noted by Lincoln and Guba (1985), an emergent design in qualitative studies is not the result of researchers' sloppiness or laziness, but rather of their desire to base the inquiry on the realities and viewpoints of those under study—realities and viewpoints that are not known at the outset.

CONSUMER TIP

Design decisions for a qualitative study are usually summarized in the method section of a report (e.g., a decision to interview a subset of study participants a second time), but the decision-making process for design decisions is rarely described. ■

Characteristics of Qualitative Research Design

Qualitative inquiry has been guided by a number of different disciplines, and each has developed methods best suited to address questions of particular interest. However, some general characteristics of qualitative research design tend to apply across disciplines. Qualitative design:

- is flexible and elastic, capable of adjusting to what is being learned during the course of data collection;
- requires researchers to become intensely involved, often remaining in the field for lengthy periods of time;
- requires researchers to become the research instruments;
- requires ongoing analysis of the data to formulate subsequent strategies and to determine when fieldwork is done;
- tends to be holistic, striving for an understanding of the whole; and
- typically involves a merging together of various data collection strategies.

With regard to the last characteristic, qualitative researchers tend to put together a complex array of data, derived from various sources. This tendency has been described as **bricolage**, and qualitative researchers have been referred to as *bricoleurs,* people who are "adept at performing a large number of diverse tasks, ranging from interviewing to observing, to interpreting personal and historical documents, to intensive reflection and introspection" (Denzin & Lincoln, 1994, p. 2).

Qualitative Design and Planning

Although design decisions are not specified in advance, qualitative researchers typically do advance planning that supports their flexibility in developing an emergent design. In the absence of planning, design choices might actually be constrained. For example, a researcher initially might anticipate a 6-month data collection period, but may need to be prepared (financially and emotionally) to spend even longer in the field to pursue emerging data collection opportunities. In other words, qualitative researchers plan for broad contingencies that may be expected to pose decision opportunities after the study has begun. Advance planning is usually important with regard to the following:

▸ Selection of the research tradition (described in the next section) that will guide certain design and analytic decisions

▸ Selection of a study site and identification of settings within the site that are likely to be especially fruitful for data collection

▸ Identification of the key "gatekeepers" who can provide (or deny) access to important sources of data and can make arrangements for gaining entrée

▸ Determination of the maximal time available for the study, given costs and other constraints

▸ Identification of all needed equipment for the collection and analysis of data in the field (e.g., audio and video recording equipment, laptop computers, and so forth)

Thus, qualitative researchers plan for a variety of circumstances, but decisions about how they will deal with them must be resolved when the social context of time, place, and human interactions is better understood.

One further task that qualitative researchers typically undertake before (as well as during) collecting data is an analysis of their own biases and ideology. Qualitative researchers tend to accept that research is subjective and may be ideologically driven. Decisions about research design and research approaches are not value-free. Qualitative researchers, then, are more inclined to take on as an early research challenge the identification of their own biases and presuppositions. Such an identification is particularly important in qualitative inquiry because of the intensely personal nature of the data collection and data analysis experience.

Example illustrating disclosure of possible bias

Rashid (2001) studied women's views about the use of the Norplant contraceptive implant in rural Bangladesh. She wrote: "My writing on this subject is influenced by my position as a native (born in Bangladesh) and as an outsider (I grew up overseas from 1979 to 1993). The kind of fieldwork I carried out was influenced by my cultural background, Muslim identity, status as an unmarried Bengali woman, and mixed cultural upbringing..." (p. 89).

Phases in a Qualitative Study

Although the exact form of a qualitative study is not specified in advance, Lincoln and Guba (1985) noted that a naturalistic inquiry typically progresses through three broad phases while in the field:

1. *Orientation and overview.* Quantitative researchers generally believe they know what they do not know (i.e., they know the type of knowledge they expect to obtain by doing a study and then strive to obtain it). A qualitative researcher, by contrast, enters the study "not knowing what is not known" (i.e., not knowing what it is about the phenomenon that will drive the inquiry forward). Therefore, the first phase of many qualitative studies is to get a handle on what is salient about the phenomenon or culture of interest.

2. *Focused exploration.* The second phase is a more focused scrutiny and in-depth exploration of aspects of the phenomenon judged to be salient. The questions asked and the types of people invited to participate in the study are shaped by the understandings developed in the first phase.

3. *Confirmation and closure.* In the final phase, qualitative researchers undertake efforts to establish that their findings are trustworthy, often by going back and discussing their understanding with study participants. Phase 3 activities, which are crucial in the critique of a qualitative study, are described in Chapter 14.

The three phases are not discrete but rather overlap to a greater or lesser degree in different projects. For example, even the first few interviews or observations are typically used as a basis for selecting subsequent informants, even though the researcher is still striving to understand the scope of the phenomenon and to identify its major dimensions. The various phases might take only a few weeks to complete—or they may take many months.

Janesick (2004), who also conceptualized qualitative design as having three phases, has likened it to choreography. The first phase is the warm-up and preparation or prechoreograhic stage of design decisions early in a study. The second phase is the exploration or tryout and total work phase. Just as in choreography, qualitative design is viewed as a work in progress. The final stage is the cooling down period, which Janesick calls illumination and formulation. The design decisions made toward the end of the study include deciding when to actually leave the field setting. Just as choreographers depend on the spine of the dancer for power and cohesion, qualitative researchers depend on the design of the study. Both the spine of the dancer and the design of a qualitative study should be elastic and flexible.

Qualitative Design Features

Some of the design features of quantitative studies also apply to qualitative studies. However, qualitative design features are often *post hoc* characterizations of what happened in the field rather than features specifically planned in advance. To further contrast qualitative and quantitative research design, we refer to the design elements identified in Table 9-1 in Chapter 9.

Experimental versus Nonexperimental. Qualitative research is almost always nonexperimental—although, as discussed in the next chapter, a qualitative study sometimes is embedded within an experimental project. Qualitative researchers do not conceptualize their studies as having independent and dependent variables and do not control or manipulate any aspect of the people or environment under study. The goal of most qualitative studies is to develop a rich understanding of a phenomenon as it exists in the real world and as it is constructed by individuals within the context of that world.

Comparisons. Qualitative researchers typically do not plan in advance to make group comparisons because the intent of most qualitative studies is to thoroughly describe and explain a phenomenon. Nevertheless, patterns emerging in the data sometimes suggest that certain comparisons are relevant and illuminating.

Example of qualitative comparisons

Rossen and Knafl (2003) studied older women's responses to a residential move to congregate living facilities. As they analyzed their data, they realized that there were three separate relocation styles, each of which was associated with a distinct configuration of conditions, characteristics, and outcome themes.

Data Collection Points. Qualitative research, like quantitative research, can be either cross-sectional, with one data collection point, or longitudinal, with multiple data collection points over an extended time period, to observe the evolution of some phenomenon. Sometimes, a qualitative researcher plans in advance for multiple sessions, but in other cases, the decision to study a phenomenon longitudinally may be made in the field after preliminary data have been collected and analyzed.

Examples of the time dimension in qualitative studies

Cross-sectional: McCurry and Thomas (2002) studied spouses' experience in heart transplantation through interviews at a single point in time. The time since the transplant ranged from 2 to almost 9 years, which the researchers regarded as desirable as a means of understanding variation in the experience over time.

Longitudinal: Schneider (2002) conducted a grounded theory study of Australian women's experiences of their first pregnancy. She interviewed 13 women three times during their pregnancies—near the end of each trimester.

Retrospective versus Prospective. Qualitative researchers do not typically apply the terms *retrospective* or *prospective* to their studies. Nevertheless, in trying to elucidate the full nature of a phenomenon, they may look back retrospectively (with the assistance of study participants) for antecedent events leading to the occurrence of some phenomenon. Qualitative researchers may also study the evolution of a phenomenon prospectively.

Examples of exploring influences and causes in qualitative designs

Retrospective exploration: Beery, Sommers, and Hall (2002) studied the emotional impact of living with permanent cardiac pacemakers. The 11 women in their sample were asked questions about life events that led up to, and occurred during and after, their pacemaker's implantation.

Prospective exploration: Olson and her coresearchers (2002) conducted a prospective qualitative study to explore the evolution of routines among Canadian cancer patients who were able to prevent fatigue; participants were interviewed before, during, and after treatment.

Research Setting. Qualitative researchers collect their data in real-world, naturalistic settings. And, whereas quantitative researchers usually strive to collect data in one type of setting to maintain constancy of conditions (e.g., conducting all interviews in study participants' homes), qualitative researchers may deliberately strive to study their phenomena in a variety of natural contexts.

Example of variation in settings

Long, Kneafsey, Ryan, and Berry (2002) conducted a 2-year qualitative study to examine nurses' role within multiprofessional rehabilitation teams in the United Kingdom. Forty-nine clients were recruited. Their pathways through rehabilitation services were observed for 6 months in a variety of settings, including homes, outpatient clinics, hospital wards, and nursing homes.

QUALITATIVE RESEARCH TRADITIONS

Although qualitative research designs share some common features, there is a wide variety of over-all approaches. There is no readily agreed-upon taxonomy, but one useful system is to describe qualitative research according to disciplinary traditions. As we have already noted in previous chapters, these traditions vary in their conceptualization of what questions are important to ask in understanding human experiences. This section provides an overview of qualitative research traditions (some of which we have previously introduced), and subsequent sections describe ethnographies, phenomenological studies, and grounded theory studies in greater detail. In the discussion that follows, we describe "traditional" qualitative inquiry, but a later section examines qualitative studies that adopt a "critical" perspective.

Overview of Qualitative Research Traditions

The research traditions that have provided an underpinning for qualitative studies come primarily from anthropology, psychology, and sociology. As shown in Table 10-1, each discipline has tended to focus on one or two broad domains of inquiry.

TABLE 10.1	Overview of Qualitative Research Traditions		
DISCIPLINE	**DOMAIN**	**RESEARCH TRADITION**	**AREA OF INQUIRY**
Anthropology	Culture	Ethnography Ethnoscience (cognitive anthropology)	Holistic view of a culture Mapping of the cognitive world of a culture; a culture's shared meanings, semantic rules
Psychology/ philosophy	Lived experience	Phenomenology Hermeneutics	Experiences of individuals within their lifeworld Interpretations and meanings of individuals' experiences
Psychology	Behavior and events	Ethology Ecologic psychology	Behavior observed over time in natural context Behavior as influenced by the environment
Sociology	Social settings	Grounded theory Ethnomethodology	Social structural processes within a social setting Manner by which shared agreement is achieved in social settings
Sociolinguistics	Human communication	Discourse analysis	Forms and rules of conversation
History	Past behavior, events, and conditions	Historical analysis	Description and interpretation of historical events

The discipline of anthropology is concerned with human cultures. **Ethnography** is the primary research tradition within anthropology and provides a framework for studying the meanings, patterns, and experiences of a defined cultural group in a holistic fashion. **Ethnoscience** (or *cognitive anthropology*) focuses on the cognitive world of a culture, with particular emphasis on the semantic rules and the shared meanings that shape behavior. Ethnoscientific studies may rely on quantitative as well as qualitative data.

Example of an ethnoscientific study

Hirst (2002) used methods of ethnoscience to articulate a definition of resident abuse as perceived by nurses working in long-term care settings. She focused on the linguistic symbols and "folk terms" of the culture in long-term care institutions.

Phenomenology has its disciplinary roots in both philosophy and psychology. As noted in Chapter 3, phenomenology is concerned with the lived experiences of humans. A closely related research tradition is **hermeneutics**, which uses the lived experiences of people as a tool for better understanding the social, cultural, political, and historical context in which those experiences occur. Hermeneutic inquiry almost always focuses on meaning and interpretation—how socially and historically conditioned individuals interpret the world within their given context.

The discipline of psychology has several qualitative research traditions that focus on behavior. Human **ethology**, which is sometimes described as the biology of human behavior, studies behavior as it evolves in its natural context. Human ethologists use observational methods to explore universal behavioral structures.

Example of an ethological study

Morse and Pooler (2002) used ethological methods to study the interactions of patients' family members with the patients and with nurses in the trauma-resuscitation room of an emergency department. The analysis was based on 193 videotapes of trauma room care.

Ecological psychology focuses on the environment's influence on human behavior and attempts to identify principles that explain the interdependence of humans and their environmental context. Viewed from an ecological context, people are affected by (and affect) a multilayered set of systems, including family, peer group, and neighborhood; the more indirect effects of health care and social services systems; and the larger cultural belief and value systems of the society in which individuals live.

Example of an ecological study

Rose and Garwick (2003) conducted a community-based study of urban American Indian family caregivers of children with asthma to determine their perceptions of the multifaceted barriers they faced in managing the illness.

Sociologists study the social world and have developed several research traditions of importance to qualitative researchers. The grounded theory tradition (described earlier and elaborated on in a later section of this chapter) seeks to understand the key social psychological and structural processes that occur in a social setting.

Ethnomethodology seeks to discover how people make sense of everyday activities and interpret their social world in order to behave in socially acceptable ways. Within this tradition, researchers attempt to understand a social group's norms and assumptions that are so deeply ingrained that members no longer think about the underlying reasons for their behaviors.

Example of an ethnomethodologic study

Montbriand (2004) explored the meaning that seniors from a Canadian prairie city ascribe to illness and healing. Seniors' analyses of their own lives revealed that their perceptions of surviving war and the Great Depression were related to their perceptions about current illnesses.

The domain of inquiry for sociolinguists is human communication. The tradition often referred to as **discourse analysis** seeks to understand the rules, mechanisms, and structure of conversations. The data for discourse analysis typically are transcripts from naturally occurring conversations, such as those between nurses and their patients.

Example of a discourse analysis

Mitchell, Gale, Garand, and Wesner (2003) applied discourse analysis to the dialogue of members of a support group that had been organized to help suicide survivors cope with their grief.

Finally, **historical research**—the systematic collection and critical evaluation of data relating to past occurrences—is also a tradition that relies primarily on qualitative data. Generally, historical research is undertaken to answer questions concerning causes, effects, or trends relating to past events that may shed light on present behaviors or practices. It is important not to confuse historical research with a review of the literature about historical events. Like other types of research, historical inquiry has as its goal the discovery of *new* knowledge. Nurses have used historical research methods to examine a wide range of phenomena in both the recent and more distant past.

Example of historical research

Meehan (2003) undertook an analysis of historical documentation of *careful nursing*, a system of nursing that was developed in Ireland by Catherine McAuley in the early 19th century, used by Irish nurses in the Crimean War, and considered Ireland's legacy to nursing.

It should be noted that some qualitative research reports do not identify a research tradition but simply refer to the study as qualitative. In some cases a research tradition can be inferred from information about the types of questions that were asked and the methods used to collect and analyze data. However, not all qualitative research *has* a link to one of the qualitative traditions we have discussed. Some *descriptive qualitative studies* simply focus on describing a phenomenon in a holistic fashion.

Example of a descriptive qualitative study

Marshall, Olsen, Mandleco, Dyches, Allred, and Sansom (2003) described the role of religion on the ability of families of the Church of Jesus Christ of Latter-Day Saints to deal with the stresses of having a child with disabilities.

CONSUMER TIP

A research report will sometimes identify more than one tradition as having provided the framework for a qualitative inquiry (e.g., a phenomenological study using the grounded theory method). However, such "method slurring" (Baker, Wuest, & Stern, 1992) has been criticized because each research tradition has different intellectual assumptions and methodologic prescriptions. ■

Ethnography

Ethnographies are qualitative inquiries that involve the description and interpretation of cultural behavior. Ethnographies are a blend of a process and a product: fieldwork and a written text. *Fieldwork* is the process by which ethnographers inevitably come to understand a culture; ethnographic texts are how that culture is communicated and portrayed. Because culture is, in itself, not visible or tangible, it must be constructed through ethnographic writing. Culture is inferred from the words, actions, and products of members of a group.

Ethnographic research is in some cases concerned with broadly defined cultures (e.g., a Ghanaian village culture), in what is sometimes referred to as a *macroethnography*. However, ethnographies sometimes focus on more narrowly defined cultures in a *microethnography*. Microethnographies are exhaustive, fine-grained studies of either small units within a group or culture (e.g., the culture of homeless shelters), or of specific activities within an organizational unit (e.g., how nurses communicate with children in an emergency room). An underlying assumption of ethnographers is that every human group eventually evolves a culture that guides the members' view of the world and the way they structure their experiences.

Example of a microethnography

Mohr (2003) conducted a microethnographic study of the culture of a family-run advocacy organization for families of children and youth with mental health needs. The data were collected during 2½ years of fieldwork.

Ethnographers seek to learn from (rather than to study) members of a cultural group. Ethnographers sometimes refer to emic and etic perspectives. An **emic perspective** is the way the members of the culture envision their world—it is the insiders' view. The emic is the local language, concepts, or means of expression that are used by the members of the group under study to name and characterize their experiences. The **etic perspective**, by contrast, is the outsiders' interpretation of the experiences of that culture; it is the language used by those doing the research to refer to the same phenomena. Ethnographers strive to acquire an emic perspective of a culture being studied. Moreover, they strive to reveal **tacit knowledge**, information about the culture that is so deeply embedded in cultural experiences that members do not talk about it or may not even be consciously aware of it.

Ethnographic research typically is a labor-intensive and time-consuming endeavor—months and even years of fieldwork may be required to learn about the cultural group of interest. The study of a culture requires a certain level of intimacy with members of the cultural group, and such intimacy can only be developed over time and by working directly with those members as active participants. The concept of *researcher as instrument* is frequently used by anthropologists to describe the significant role ethnographers play in analyzing and interpreting a culture.

Three broad types of information are usually sought by ethnographers: cultural behavior (what members of the culture do); cultural artifacts (what members of the culture make and use); and cultural speech (what members of the culture say). This implies that ethnographers rely on various data sources, including observations, in-depth interviews, records, and other types of physical evidence (photographs, diaries, letters, and so forth). Ethnographers typically conduct in-depth interviews with about 25 to 50 informants. They also typically use a strategy known as **participant observation** in which they make observations of a community or group while participating in its activities (see Chapter 13).

The products of ethnographic research are rich and holistic descriptions of the culture under study. Ethnographers also make interpretations of the culture, describing normative behavioral and social patterns. Among health care researchers, ethnography provides information about the health beliefs and health-related practices of a culture or subculture. Ethnographic inquiry can thus facilitate understanding of behaviors affecting health and illness. Many nurse researchers have undertaken ethnographic studies. Indeed, Madeleine Leininger has coined the phrase **ethnonursing research**, which she defines as "the study and analysis of the local or indigenous people's viewpoints, beliefs, and practices about nursing care behavior and processes of designated cultures" (1985, p. 38).

 Example of an ethnonursing study

Ohm (2003) used ethnonursing methods to explore the African-American experience in the Islam faith, from the Nation of Islam to universal Islam.

Ethnographers are often, but not, for example, always, "outsiders" to the culture under study. However, if nurse researchers studied the culture of an intensive care unit, this would be called **insider research** or *peer research* or an *auto-ethnography*. There are numerous practical and substantive advantages to such a study, including ease of entry into the culture, access to information and informants that might not otherwise be available, avoidance of disruption to the culture, and an abundance of prior knowledge. The drawback is that an "insider" may have developed biases about certain issues or may be so entrenched in the culture that valuable pieces of data get overlooked. Insider research demands that researchers maintain a high level of consciousness about their role and monitor their internal state and interactions with others.

Example of insider research

Lipson (2001) conducted an ethnographic study about the experiences of people with multiple chemical sensitivity (MCS). She gathered her data over a 2-year period through in-depth interviews and observations in two U.S. and two Canadian settings, and through participation in a weekly MCS chat room. Lipson, who herself suffers from MCS, included a valuable discussion of issues relating to the conduct of insider research.

Phenomenology

Phenomenology, rooted in a philosophical tradition developed by Husserl and Heidegger, is an approach to thinking about people's life experiences.

Phenomenological researchers ask: What is the *essence* of this phenomenon as experienced by these people and what does it *mean?* Phenomenologists assume there is an essence—an essential invariant structure—that can be understood, in much the same way that ethnographers assume that cultures exist. Phenomenologists investigate subjective phenomena in the belief that critical truths about reality are grounded in people's lived experiences. The phenomenological approach is especially useful when a phenomenon has been poorly defined or conceptualized. The topics appropriate to phenomenology are ones that are fundamental to the life experiences of humans; for health researchers, these include such topics as the meaning of stress, the experience of bereavement, and the quality of life with chronic pain.

Phenomenologists believe that lived experience gives meaning to each person's perception of a particular phenomenon. The goal of phenomenological inquiry is to understand fully lived experience and the perceptions to which it gives rise. Four aspects of lived experience that are of interest to phenomenologists are *lived space*, or spatiality; *lived body*, or corporeality; *lived time*, or temporality; and *lived human relation*, or relationality.

Phenomenologists view human existence as meaningful and interesting because of people's consciousness of that existence. The phrase **being-in-the-world** (or *embodiment*) is a concept that acknowledges people's physical ties to their world—they think, see, hear, feel, and are conscious through their bodies' interaction with the world.

In phenomenological studies, the main data source typically is in-depth conversations, with researchers and informants as co-participants. Researchers help informants to describe lived experiences without leading the discussion. Through in-depth conversations, researchers strive to gain entrance into the informants' world, to have full access to their experiences as lived. Two or more separate interviews or conversations are sometimes needed. Typically, phenomenological studies involve a small number of study participants—often 10 or fewer. For some phenomenological researchers, the inquiry includes not only gathering information from informants but also efforts to experience the phenomenon in the same way, typically through participation, observation, and introspective reflection.

Example of a phenomenological study

Wilkin and Slevin (2004) conducted a phenomenological study of the meaning of caring to nurses working in an intensive care unit in Ireland. The descriptive accounts of the nurses' experiences of caring were used to illuminate the nature of intensive care nursing.

There are a number of variants and methodologic interpretations of phenomenology. The two main schools of thought are descriptive phenomenology and interpretive phenomenology (hermeneutics).

DESCRIPTIVE PHENOMENOLOGY

Descriptive phenomenology was developed first by Husserl (1962), who was primarily interested in the question: What do we know as persons? His philosophy emphasized descriptions of human experience. Descriptive phenomenologists insist on the careful description of ordinary conscious experience of everyday life—a description of "things" as people experience them. These "things" include hearing, seeing, believing, feeling, remembering, deciding, evaluating, acting, and so forth.

Descriptive phenomenological studies often involve the following four steps: bracketing, intuiting, analyzing, and describing. **Bracketing** refers to the process of identifying and holding in abeyance preconceived beliefs and opinions about the phenomenon under study. Although bracketing can never be achieved totally, researchers strive to bracket out the world and any presuppositions in an effort to confront the data in pure form. Bracketing is an iterative process that involves preparing, evaluating, and providing systematic ongoing feedback about the effectiveness of the bracketing. Phenomenological researchers (as well as other qualitative researchers) often maintain a **reflexive journal** in their efforts to bracket.

Intuiting, the second step in descriptive phenomenology, occurs when researchers remain open to the meanings attributed to the phenomenon by those who have experienced it. Phenomenological researchers then proceed to the analysis phase (i.e., extracting significant statements, categorizing, and making sense of the essential meanings of the phenomenon). Chapter 16 provides further information regarding the analysis of data collected in phenomenological studies. Finally, the descriptive phase occurs when researchers come to understand and define the phenomenon.

Example of a descriptive phenomenological study

Beitz and Zuzelo (2003) did a phenomenological study designed to describe the experience of living with a neobladder and to explore the essence of this experience. They elicited richly detailed narrative descriptions of the experience in 1 to 2 hour interviews with 14 men and women who had a neobladder.

INTERPRETIVE PHENOMENOLOGY

Heidegger, a student of Husserl, moved away from his professor's philosophy into **interpretive phenomenology** or hermeneutics. To Heidegger (1962), the critical question is: What is being? He stressed interpreting and understanding—not just describing—human experience.

Heidegger argued that hermeneutics ("understanding") is a basic characteristic of human existence. Indeed, the term hermeneutics generally refers to the art and philosophy of interpreting the meaning of an object (such as a *text*, work of art, human utterances, and so on). Hermeneutics is viewed as a primary and universal way of our being in the world. The goals of interpretive phenomenological research are to enter another's world and to discover the practical wisdom, possibilities, and understandings found there.

It should be noted that an important distinction between descriptive and interpretive phenomenology is that in an interpretive phenomenological study, bracketing does not occur. For Heidegger, it was not possible to bracket one's being-in-the-world. Hermeneutics presupposes prior understanding on the part of the researcher.

Example of an interpretive phenomenological study

Öhman, Söderberg, and Lundman (2003) used a hermeneutic approach to elucidate the meaning of the experience of living with serious chronic illness, which they interpreted as hovering between suffering and enduring. The researchers interviewed 10 men and women in Sweden who had different chronic illnesses and used a three-phase hermeneutic process to interpret the texts.

Interpretive phenomenologists, like descriptive phenomenologists, rely primarily on in-depth interviews with individuals who have experienced the phenomenon of interest, but they sometimes augment their understandings of the phenomenon through an analysis of supplementary texts, such as novels, poetry, or other artistic expressions—or they use such materials in their conversations with study participants.

Example of a hermeneutic study using artistic expression

Lauterbach (2001) studied the phenomenon of maternal mourning over the death of a wished-for baby. She increased her "attentive listening" to this phenomenon by turning to examples of infant death experiences as illustrated in the arts, literature, and poetry. For example, she included a poem written by Shakespeare as he mourned his son's death. She also described the painting "Rachel Weeping" by Charles Wilson Peale. This painting depicted the artist's daughter, who had died of smallpox in 1772, laid out in her burial dress. Lauterbach also visited cemeteries to discover memorial art on babies' grave stones, such as a section of a cemetery near Philadelphia called "Babyland." She used the examples of memorial art and of literature to validate the themes of mothers' experiences in her research.

HOW-TO-TELL TIP

How can you tell if a phenomenological study is descriptive or interpretive? Phenomenologists often use key terms in their report that can help you determine whether the study is descriptive or interpretive. In a descriptive phenomenological study, such terms may be bracketing, description, essence, Husserl, and phenomenological reduction. The names of Colaizzi, Van Kaam, and Giorgi may be found in the method section. In an interpretive phenomenological study, key terms can include being-in-the-world, shared interpretations, hermeneutics, understanding, and Heidegger. The names van Manen, Benner, and Diekelmann may appear in the method section. These names will be discussed in the chapter on qualitative data analysis.

▬

Grounded Theory

Grounded theory has become an important research method for the study of nursing phenomena and has contributed to the development of many middle-range theories of phenomena of relevance to nurses. Grounded theory began more as a systematic method of qualitative research than as a philosophy. It was developed in the 1960s by two sociologists, Glaser and Strauss (1967), whose theoretical roots were in *symbolic interactionism*, which focuses on the manner in which people make sense of social interactions and the interpretations they attach to social symbols (e.g., language).

As noted in Chapter 3, grounded theory comprises methods for studying social processes and social structures. The focus of most grounded theory studies is on the discovery of a basic social psychological problem that a defined group of people experience, and on the social psychological stages or phases that characterize the process used to cope with or resolve this basic problem. The primary purpose is to generate a theory that explains a pattern of behavior that is problematic and relevant to the participants involved in the study.

Grounded theory methods constitute an entire approach to the conduct of field research. For example, a study that truly follows Glaser and Strauss's precepts does not begin with the identification of a specific research problem. In grounded theory both the research problem and the process used to resolve it are discovered during the study. A fundamental feature of grounded theory research is that data collection, data analysis, and sampling of participants occur simultaneously. The grounded theory process is recursive: Researchers collect data, categorize them, describe the emerging central phenomenon, and then recycle earlier steps.

A procedure referred to as **constant comparison** is used to identify the basic problem and to develop and refine theoretically relevant categories. The categories elicited from the data are constantly compared with data obtained earlier so that commonalities and variations can be determined and categories can be condensed and collapsed. As data collection proceeds, the inquiry becomes increasingly focused on emerging theoretical concerns and on core processes. Data analysis within a grounded theory framework is described more fully in Chapter 16.

In-depth interviews are the most common data source in grounded theory studies, but observation (including participant observation) and existing documents may also be used. Typically, a grounded theory study involves interviews with a sample of about 25 to 50 informants.

Example of a grounded theory study

Mok, Martinson, and Wong (2004) conducted a grounded theory study that focused on how Chinese cancer patients in Hong Kong were able to overcome powerlessness and attain individual empowerment.

HOW-TO-TELL TIP

Grounded theory studies often use gerunds in their titles, which suggest action and change. A gerund is a part of speech ending in "ing." It is part verb (signifying action) and part noun. An example is the title of one of Beck's studies, "Teetering on the edge: A substantive theory of postpartum depression." ■

ALTERNATIVE VIEWS OF GROUNDED THEORY

In 1990 Strauss and Corbin published what was to become a controversial book, *Basics of Qualitative Research: Grounded Theory and Procedures*. Strauss and Corbin stated that the purpose of the book was to provide beginning grounded theory students with a more concrete description of the procedures involved in building theory at the substantive level.

Glaser, however, disagreed with some of the procedures advocated by Strauss (his original co-author) and Corbin (a nurse researcher). Glaser published a rebuttal in 1992, *Emergence Versus Forcing: Basics of Grounded Theory Analysis.* Glaser believed that Strauss and Corbin developed a method that is not grounded theory but rather what he calls "full conceptual description." According to Glaser, the purpose of grounded theory is to generate concepts and theories about their relationships that explain, account for, and interpret variation in behavior in the substantive area under study. *Conceptual description*, in contrast, is aimed at describing the full range of behavior of what is occurring in the substantive area, "irrespective of relevance and accounting for variation in behavior" (Glaser, 1992, p. 19).

Nurse researchers have conducted grounded theory studies using both the original Glaser and Strauss and the Strauss and Corbin approaches. We discuss aspects of the two approaches in more detail in the chapter on data analysis (Chapter 16).

Example of grounded theory alternatives

Kendall (1999) provided a comparison of the two approaches to grounded theory from her research on families with a child with attention deficit hyperactivity disorder. She described study results two ways: (1) results using Strauss and Corbin's approach and (2) findings using Glaser and Strauss's original grounded theory approach. Kendall felt that Strauss and Corbin's coding procedure was a distraction that hindered her ability to reach a higher level of abstract thinking needed in grounded theory analysis.

FORMAL GROUNDED THEORY

Glaser and Strauss (1967) distinguished two types of grounded theory: substantive and formal. **Substantive theory** is grounded in data on a specific substantive area, such as postpartum depression. It can serve as a springboard for **formal grounded theory**, which involves developing a higher, more abstract level of theory from a compilation of substantive grounded theory studies regarding a particular phenomenon. Glaser and Strauss' (1971) theory of status passage is an example of a formal grounded theory.

Kearney (1998) used an interesting analogy to differentiate substantive theories (custom-tailored clothing) and formal theory (ready-to-wear clothing). Formal grounded theories were likened to clothing sold in department stores that can fit a wider variety of users. Formal grounded theory is not personally tailored like substantive theory, but rather provides a conceptualization that applies to a broader population experiencing a common phenomenon. Formal grounded theories are not situation specific. The best data for constructing grounded formal theories are substantive grounded theories.

Example of a formal grounded theory

Kearney and O'Sullivan (2003) used a formal grounded theory approach to synthesize the findings of 14 studies, with the goal of identifying common elements of individuals' efforts to change a variety of unhealthy behaviors. The concept of *identity shift* was discovered as a core process.

CONSUMER TIP

Avoid jumping to conclusions about the qualitative research tradition of a study based on the content in a report's title. For example, the study "Hardships and personal strategies of Vietnam War nurses" (Scannell-Desch, 2000) is not a historical study, but rather a phenomenological study. As another example, despite the title's reference to a culture, "Older South Asian patient and carer perceptions of culturally sensitive care in a community hospital setting" (Clegg, 2003) is a study involving the application of grounded theory to service delivery issues in the United Kingdom.

■

RESEARCH WITH IDEOLOGICAL PERSPECTIVES

An emerging trend in nursing research—especially outside of the United States—is to conduct inquiries within ideological frameworks, typically to draw attention to certain social problems or the needs of certain groups. These approaches, which represent important investigative avenues, usually rely primarily on qualitative data and interpretive methods of analysis.

Critical Theory

Critical theory originated within a group of Marxist-oriented German scholars in the 1920s, collectively referred to as the Frankfurt School. Variants of critical theory abound in the social sciences. Essentially, critical researchers are concerned with a critique of society and with envisioning new possibilities.

Critical research is typically action-oriented. Its broad aim is to integrate theory and practice such that people become aware of contradictions and disparities in their beliefs and social practices and become inspired to change them. Critical researchers reject the idea of an objective and disinterested inquirer and are oriented toward a transformation process. An important feature of critical theory is that it calls for inquiries that foster enlightened self-knowledge and sociopolitical action. Moreover, critical theory involves a self-reflexive aspect. To prevent a critical theory of society from becoming yet another self-serving ideology, critical theorists must account for their own transformative effects.

The design of research within critical theory often begins with a thorough analysis of certain aspects of a problem. For example, critical researchers might analyze and critique taken-for-granted assumptions that underlie a problem, the language used to depict the situation, and the biases of prior researchers investigating the problem. Critical researchers often triangulate multiple methodologies and emphasize multiple perspectives (e.g., alternative racial or social class perspectives) on problems. Critical researchers typically interact with study participants in ways that emphasize participants' expertise. Some of the features that distinguish more traditional qualitative research and critical research are summarized in Table 10-2.

Critical theory has been applied in a number of disciplines and has played an especially important role in ethnography. **Critical ethnography** focuses on raising consciousness and aiding emancipatory goals in the hope of effecting social change. Critical ethnographers address the historical, social, political, and economic dimensions of cultures and their value-laden agendas. An assumption in critical ethnographic research is that actions and thoughts are mediated by power relationships. Critical ethnographers attempt to increase the political dimensions of cultural research and undermine oppressive systems.

Example of a critical ethnography

Elliott, Berman, and Kim (2002) undertook a critical ethnographic study to examine how menopause is experienced by Korean women living in Canada. Through dialogic interviews, the researchers explored how the lack of understanding of cultural health practices can result in misunderstanding and the provision of care that is culturally inappropriate.

Feminist Research

Feminist research uses approaches that are similar to those of critical theory research, but the focus is sharply on gender domination and discrimination within patriarchal societies. Similar to critical researchers, feminist researchers seek to establish collaborative and nonexploitive relationships with their informants, to place themselves within the study to avoid objectification, and to conduct research that is transformative. Feminist researchers stress *intersubjectivity* between researchers and participants and the mutual creation of knowledge.

Gender is the organizing principle in feminist research, and investigators seek to understand how gender and a gendered social order have shaped women's lives and their consciousness. The aim is to ameliorate the "invisibility and distortion of female experience in ways relevant to ending women's unequal social position" (Lather, 1991, p. 71). The purpose of feminist research is to provide information *for* women, rather than merely *about* women.

Although feminist researchers generally agree that it is important to focus on women's diverse situations and the institutions and relationships that frame those situations, there are many variants of feminist inquiry. Three broad models (within each of which there is diversity) have been identified: (1) *feminist empiricism*, whose adherents generally work within fairly standard norms of qualitative inquiry but who seek to portray more accurate pictures of the social realities of women's lives; (2) *feminist standpoint research*, which holds that inquiry ought to begin in and

TABLE 10.2	Comparison of Traditional Qualitative Research and Critical Research	
ISSUE	**TRADITIONAL QUALITATIVE RESEARCH**	**CRITICAL RESEARCH**
Research aims	Understanding; reconstruction of multiple constructions	Critique; transformation; consciousness-raising; advocacy
View of knowledge	Transactional/subjective; knowledge is created in interaction between investigator and participants	Transactional/subjective; value-mediated and value-dependent; importance of historical insights
Methods	Dialectic: truth arrived at logically through conversations	Dialectic and didactic: dialogue designed to transform naivety and misinformation
Evaluative criteria for inquiry quality	Authenticity; trustworthiness	Historical situatedness of the inquiry; erosion of ignorance; stimulus for change
Researcher's role	Facilitator of multivoice reconstruction	Transformative agent; advocate; activist

be tested against the lived everyday sociopolitical experiences of women, and that women's views are particular and privileged; and (3) *feminist postmodernism*, which stresses that "truth" is a destructive illusion and views the world as endless stories, texts, and narratives. In nursing and health care, feminist empiricism and feminist standpoint research have been most prevalent.

The scope of feminist research ranges from studies of the particular and subjective views of individual women to studies of social movements, structures, and broad policies that affect (and often exclude) women. Olesen (1994), a sociologist who studied nurses' career patterns and definitions of success, has noted that some of the best feminist research on women's subjective experiences has been done in the area of women's health.

Feminist research methods generally include in-depth, interactive, and collaborative individual interviews or group interviews that offer the possibility of reciprocally educational encounters. Feminists generally seek to negotiate the meanings of the results with those participating in the study, and to be self-reflexive about what they themselves are experiencing and learning. In feminist research, the researcher's history, assumptions, interests, motives, and interpretations are explicitly scrutinized in the process of the study.

Feminist research, like other research that has an ideological perspective, has raised the bar for the conduct of ethical research. With the emphasis on trust, empathy, and nonexploitive relationships, proponents of these newer modes of inquiry view any type of deception or manipulation as abhorrent. As Punch (1994) has noted in speaking about ethics and feminist research, "You do not rip off your sisters" (p. 89).

Example of a feminist research

Kushner and Harrison (2002) conducted a feminist grounded theory study to examine how employed mothers in Canada managed multiple responsibilities in family, work, and health. Twenty employed mothers participated in repeated interviews over a 2-year period. The women experienced stress from continuous and sometimes conflicting demands, compromised personal resources, and inadequate support. The researchers indicated that the findings underscore the need to explicate social–ecological influences such as relational power.

Participatory Action Research

A type of research known as **participatory action research** is closely allied to both critical research and feminist research. Participatory action research, one of several types of *action research* that originated in the 1940s with social psychologist Kurt Lewin, is based on a recognition that the use and production of knowledge can be political and can be used to exert power. Researchers in this approach typically work with groups or communities that are vulnerable to the control or oppression of a dominant group or culture.

Participatory action research (PAR) is, as the name implies, participatory. There is collaboration between researchers and study participants in the definition of the problem, the selection of an approach and research methods, the analysis of the data, and the use to which findings are put. The aim of PAR is to produce not only knowledge, but action and consciousness-raising as well. Researchers specifically seek to empower people through the process of constructing and using knowledge. The PAR tradition has as its starting point a concern for the powerlessness of the group under study. Thus, a key objective is to produce action that is directly used to make improvements through education and sociopolitical action.

In participatory action research, the research methods take second place to emergent processes of collaboration and dialogue that can motivate, increase self-esteem, and generate community solidarity. Thus, the "data-gathering" strategies used are not only the traditional methods of interview and observation (including both qualitative and quantitative approaches), but may include storytelling, sociodrama, drawing and painting, plays and skits, and other activities designed to encourage people to find creative ways to explore their lives, tell their stories, and recognize their own strengths.

Example of participatory action research

Brackley and colleagues (2003) described a participatory action project involving a community readiness model for preventing intimate partner violence in Bexar County, Texas. The project involved determining the county's state of readiness to prevent partner violence, engaging the community in determining the usefulness and accuracy of the assessment, developing targeted strategies to enhance readiness, and evaluating the results.

CRITIQUING QUALITATIVE DESIGNS

Evaluating a qualitative design is often difficult. Qualitative researchers do not always document design decisions and are even less likely to describe the process by which such decisions were made. Researchers often do, however, indicate whether the study was conducted within a specific qualitative tradition. This information can be used to come to some conclusions about the study design. For example, if a report indicated that the researcher conducted 1 month of fieldwork for an ethnographic study, there would be reason to suspect that insufficient time had been spent in the field to obtain a true emic perspective of the culture under study. Ethnographic studies may also be critiqued if their only source of information was from interviews, rather than from a broader range of data sources including observations.

In a grounded theory study, you might also be concerned if the researcher relied exclusively on data from interviews; a stronger design might have been obtained by including participant observations. Also, look for evidence about when the data were collected and analyzed. If the researcher collected all the data before analyzing any of it, you might question whether the constant comparative method was used correctly.

In critiquing a phenomenological study, you should first determine if the study is descriptive or interpretive. This will help you to assess how closely the researcher kept to the basic tenets of that qualitative research tradition. For example, in a descriptive phenomenological study, did the researcher bracket?

No matter what qualitative design is identified in a study, look to see if the researchers stayed true to a single qualitative tradition throughout the study or if they mixed qualitative

CONSUMER TIP

In this age of the Internet, students and researchers have access to information on qualitative design at their fingertips. Two important websites are:
 www.phenomenologyonline.com
 www.groundedtheory.com

BOX 10.1   Guidelines for Critiquing Qualitative Designs

1. Is the research tradition for the qualitative study identified? If none was identified, can one be inferred? If more than one was identified, is this justifiable or does it suggest "method slurring"?
2. Is the research question congruent with a qualitative approach and with the specific research tradition (i.e., is the domain of inquiry for the study congruent with the domain encompassed by the tradition)? Are the data sources, research methods, and analytic approach congruent with the research tradition?
3. How well is the research design described? Are design decisions explained and justified? Does it appear that the researcher made all design decisions up-front, or did the design emerge during data collection, allowing researchers to capitalize on early information?
4. Is the design appropriate, given the research question? Does the design lend itself to a thorough, in-depth, intensive examination of the phenomenon of interest? What design elements might have strengthened the study (e.g., a longitudinal perspective rather than a cross-sectional one)?
5. Was there appropriate evidence of reflexivity in the design?
6. Was the study undertaken with an ideological perspective? If so, is there evidence that ideological methods and goals were achieved? (e.g., Was there evidence of full collaboration between researchers and participants? Did the research have the power to be transformative, or is there evidence that a transformative process occurred?)

---

traditions and weakened the rigor of the study. For example, did the researcher state that a grounded theory design was used, but then present results that described *themes* instead of generating a substantive theory?

The guidelines in Box 10-1 are intended to assist you in critiquing the designs of qualitative studies.

CHAPTER REVIEW

Key new terms introduced in the chapter, together with a summary of major points, are presented in this section. In addition, Chapter 10 of the *Study Guide to Accompany Essentials of Nursing Research,* 6th edition offers various exercises and study suggestions for reinforcing the concepts presented in this chapter. For additional review, see the Student Self-Study Review Questions section of the Student Resource CD-ROM provided with this book.

KEY NEW TERMS

Being-in-the-world	Ecological psychology
Bracketing	Emergent design
Bricolage	Emic perspective
Constant comparison	Ethnomethodology
Critical ethnography	Ethnonursing research
Critical theory	Ethnoscience
Descriptive phenomenology	Ethology
Discourse analysis	Etic perspective

Feminist research Intuiting
Formal grounded theory Participant observation
Hermeneutics Participatory action research (PAR)
Historical research Reflexive journal
Insider research Substantive theory
Interpretive phenomenology Tacit knowledge

S U M M A R Y   P O I N T S

▷ Qualitative research typically involves an **emergent design**—a design that emerges as the study unfolds.

▷ As **bricoleurs**, qualitative researchers tend to be creative and intuitive, putting together an array of data drawn from many sources in an effort to arrive at a holistic understanding of a phenomenon or culture.

▷ Although qualitative design is elastic and flexible, qualitative researchers nevertheless can plan for broad contingencies that are expected to pose decision opportunities for the design of the study in the field.

▷ A naturalistic inquiry typically progresses through three broad phases in the field: an orientation and overview phase to determine what it is about the phenomenon under investigation that is salient; a focused exploration phase that closely examines important aspects of the phenomenon; and a confirmation and closure phase to confirm findings.

▷ Qualitative research traditions have their roots in anthropology (e.g., *ethnography* and **ethnoscience**); philosophy (*phenomenology* and **hermeneutics**); psychology (**ethology, ecological psychology**); sociology (**grounded theory, ethnomethodology**); sociolinguistics (**discourse analysis**); and history (**historical research**).

▷ Some *descriptive qualitative* studies are not linked to any research tradition and are designed to describe some phenomenon in an in-depth and holistic fashion.

▷ Ethnography focuses on the culture of a group of people and relies on extensive fieldwork. The ethnographer strives to acquire an **emic** (or insider's) **perspective** of the culture under study and strives to discover deeply embedded **tacit knowledge**; the outsider's perspective is known as the **etic perspective**.

▷ Phenomenology seeks to discover the essence and meaning of a phenomenon as it is experienced by people.

▷ In **descriptive phenomenology**, researchers strive to describe lived experiences by **bracketing** out any preconceived views and **intuiting** the essence of the phenomenon by remaining open to the meanings attributed to it by those who have experienced it.

▷ Bracketing is not a feature of **interpretive phenomenology (hermeneutics)**, which focuses on interpreting the meaning of experiences.

▷ *Grounded theory* is an approach to generating a theory to explain a pattern of behavior that is problematic and relevant to study participants. This approach uses **constant comparison**: Categories elicited from the data are constantly compared with data obtained earlier so that shared patterns and variations can be determined.

▷ There are two types of grounded theory: **substantive theory**, which is grounded in data on a specific substantive area, and **formal grounded theory** (often using data from substantive theory studies), which is at a higher level of abstraction.

▷ Research is sometimes conducted within an ideological perspective, and such research tends to rely primarily on qualitative research.

▷ **Critical theory** is concerned with a critique of existing social structures; critical researchers strive to conduct inquiries that involve collaboration with participants and foster enlightened self-knowledge and transformation. Critical ethnography uses the principles of critical theory in the study of cultures.

▷ **Feminist research**, like critical research, is designed to be transformative, but the focus is sharply on how gender domination and discrimination shape women's lives and their consciousness.

▷ **Participatory action research (PAR)** produces knowledge through close collaboration with groups or communities that are vulnerable to control or oppression by a dominant culture; in PAR, research methods take second place to emergent processes that can motivate people and generate community solidarity.

RESEARCH EXAMPLES Critical Thinking Activities

 EXAMPLE 1: Critical/Feminist Ethnography

Aspects of an ethnographic nursing study, featuring terms and concepts discussed in this chapter, are presented below, followed by some questions to guide critical thinking. (The full research report is available in *Western Journal of Nursing Research, 23,* 126–147.)

Study

"First Nations women's encounters with mainstream health services," (Browne & Fiske, 2001)

Statement of Purpose

The purpose of the study was to address two central questions: How do First Nations women describe their encounters with local mainstream health care services? and How are these encounters shaped by social, political, and economic factors?

Community Setting and Sociopolitical Context

The research was conducted in partnership with a First Nations reserve community with a population of 600 in rural northwest Canada. The community believed it would benefit from a thorough description of women's encounters as it developed plans to improve health and health care for its members. Women from the community (including one of the researchers) were renowned locally as leaders in health, and yet First Nations people were rarely invited to join nearby mainstream health boards or decision-making bodies.

Theoretical Perspectives

The construct of *cultural safety,* originally developed by indigenous nurses in postcolonial New Zealand to address the health concerns of the Maori, informed this research. The emphasis of cultural safety is on transforming attitudes and practices in health care by gaining an awareness of the forces shaping the health and status of indigenous people.

RESEARCH EXAMPLES *Continued*

Method

The study was a critical ethnography drawing on feminist perspectives. The researchers made efforts to "equalize power within the research team and between the participants and researchers" (p. 132). This was accomplished in a variety of ways, including the adoption of a "critically reflective research process." Using input from community leaders and elders, the researchers selected 10 women to participate in two rounds of interviews. Each woman was interviewed separately for 1 to 2 hours. The second interviews were used to clarify and verify information from the first interviews. Participants were asked to describe both positive encounters (model cases) and negative encounters (contrary cases) with the health care establishment. An interpretive thematic analysis was conducted with transcripts from these interviews. The initial analysis was subjected to critical questioning, reflection, and discussions with participants.

Key Findings

▶ The narratives revealed that the "women's encounters were shaped by racism, discrimination, and structural inequalities that continue to marginalize and disadvantage First Nations women" (p. 126).

▶ Participants described situations in which their health concerns or reported symptoms were not taken seriously or were trivialized. Encounters that revealed health care workers' discriminatory attitudes and behaviors were found to be pervasive.

Critical Thinking Suggestions*

*See the Student Resource CD-ROM for a discussion of these questions.

1. Answer questions 1–6 from Box 10-1 regarding this study.

2. Also consider the following targeted questions, which may assist you in further assessing aspects of the study:

    a. Would you consider this an example of insider research? If yes, explain some of the issues the researchers faced—and how they appeared to handle those issues.

    b. The report did not indicate over how long a period the researchers conducted their fieldwork. Comment on their fieldwork for this ethnographic study.

    c. Could this study have been conducted as a phenomenological study? As a grounded theory study? Why or why not?

3. If the results of this study are trustworthy, what are some of the uses to which the findings might be put in clinical practice?

 EXAMPLE 2: Grounded Theory Study

Aspects of a grounded theory study, featuring terms and concepts discussed in this chapter, are presented below, followed by some questions to guide critical thinking. (The full research report is available in *Qualitative Health Research, 13,* 675–688.)

research examples continue on page 232

RESEARCH EXAMPLES *Continued*

Study

"Reconstructing a meaning of pain: Older Korean American women's experiences with the pain of osteoarthritis" (Dickson & Kim, 2003)

Statement of Purpose

The purpose of this cross-cultural grounded theory study was to develop a substantive theory about the reconstruction of the meaning of chronic osteoarthritic pain for older Korean American women.

Context

The researchers noted that culture is a major factor affecting the way people perceive and respond to chronic pain. Moreover, Koreans traditionally have had two treatment modes: Western medicine or ethnic medicine. Even in the United States, Koreans are less likely than other patients to choose Western medicine exclusively. The study explored the cultural context of the study participants.

Method

A sample of seven Korean women (aged 63–80) living in a Northeastern U.S. community provided data through two individual interviews and a follow-up telephone interview (21 interviews in all). Participants were recruited through an advertisement in a Korean American physician's office. Each participant was interviewed in her own home on two occasions, with each interview lasting about 1 hour. Tape-recorded interviews were transcribed in both Korean and English, and the transcription of the first interview was completed before the second interview was scheduled. The researchers also observed the women, their interactions, and their environments during each interview and made notes of their observations. Follow-up telephone interviews lasting about 15 to 30 minutes were conducted to confirm emerging concepts with participants and to address questions to clarify the data. One of the two researchers maintained a reflexive log that recorded conjectures and personal information about the data collection experience. The researchers used constant comparative analysis in an ongoing fashion to analyze and reanalyze the data within and among interviews, until no new knowledge was gleaned. The principles of grounded theory as articulated by Strauss and Corbin were followed. The researchers achieved triangulation by having both of them review the data and arrive at consensus about the analysis.

Key Findings

▶ The core variable was *Reconstructing a Meaning of Pain,* which revealed a process through which the women learned to manage and tolerate the pain. The process involved giving meaning to their pain as a sign of aging rather than as a symptom of a disease, and integrating aging and culture to manage and tolerate pain.
▶ The women moved through a five-stage basic social process: suffering with pain; struggling to remove pain; stumbling along with pain; striving to reduce pain; and managing and tolerating pain.

RESEARCH EXAMPLES *Continued*

Critical Thinking Suggestions

1. Answer questions 1–6 from Box 10-1 regarding this study.
2. Also consider the following targeted questions, which may assist you in further assessing aspects of the study:
   a. Was the theory the researchers developed a substantive theory or a formal theory?
   b. Would you describe this study as longitudinal?
   c. Could this study have been conducted as a phenomenological study? As an ethnographic study? Why or why not?
   d. Could this study have been conducted as a feminist inquiry? If yes, what might the researchers have done differently?
3. If the results of this study are valid and reliable, what are some of the uses to which the findings might be put in clinical practice?

 EXAMPLE 3: Phenomenological Study

1. Read the method section from Beck's phenomenological study ("Birth Trauma") in Appendix B of this book, and then answer the relevant questions in Box 10-1.
2. Also consider the following targeted questions, which may further sharpen your critical thinking skills and assist you in assessing aspects of the study's merit:
   a. Was this study a descriptive or interpretive phenomenology?
   b. Could this study have been conducted as a grounded theory study? As an ethnographic study? Why or why not?
   c. Could this study have been conducted as a feminist inquiry? If yes, what might Beck have done differently?

SUGGESTED READINGS

Methodologic References

Baker, C., Wuest, J., & Stern, P. N. (1992). Method slurring: The grounded theory/phenomenology example. *Journal of Advanced Nursing, 17,* 1355–1360.

Creswell, J. W. (1998). Qualitative inquiry and research design: Choosing among five traditions. Thousand Oaks, CA: Sage Publications.

Denzin, N. K., & Lincoln, Y. S. (Eds.). (2000). *Handbook of qualitative research* (2nd ed.). Thousand Oaks, CA: Sage Publications.

Glaser, B. G., & Strauss, A. L. (1967). The discovery of grounded theory: Strategies for qualitative research. Chicago: Aldine.

Glaser, B., & Strauss, S. (1971). *Status passage: A formal theory.* Mill Valley, CA: Sociology Press.

Heidegger, M. (1962). *Being and time.* New York: Harper & Row.

Husserl, E. (1962). Ideas: General introduction to pure phenomenology. New York: MacMillan.

Janesick, V. J. (2004). *Stretching exercises for qualitative researchers.* Thousand Oaks, CA: Sage Publications.

Kearney, M. H. (1998). Ready-to-wear: Discovering grounded formal theory. *Research in Nursing & Health, 21,* 179–186.

Lather, P. (1991). *Getting smart: Feminist research and pedagogy within the postmodern.* New York: Routledge.

Leininger, M. M. (Ed.). (1985). *Qualitative research methods in nursing.* New York: Grune & Stratton.

Lincoln, Y. S., & Guba, E. G. (1985). *Naturalistic inquiry.* Newbury Park, CA: Sage Publications.

Morse, J. M. (1991). *Qualitative nursing research: A contemporary dialogue.* Newbury Park, CA: Sage Publications.

Morse, J. M. (1999). Qualitative methods: The state of the art. *Qualitative Health Research, 9,* 393–406.

Morse, J. M., & Field, P. A. (1995). *Qualitative research methods for health professionals* (2nd ed.). Thousand Oaks, CA: Sage Publications.

Olesen, V. (1994). Feminism and models of qualitative research. In N. K. Denzin & Y. S. Lincoln (Eds.), *Handbook of qualitative research.* Thousand Oaks, CA: Sage Publications.

Punch, M. (1994). Politics and ethics in qualitative research. In N. K. Denzin & Y .S. Lincoln (Eds.), *Handbook of qualitative research.* Thousand Oaks, CA: Sage.

Streubert, H. J., & Carpenter, D. R. (1995). *Qualitative research in nursing: Advancing the humanistic imperative.* Philadelphia: J. B. Lippincott.

Studies Cited in Chapter 10

Beery, T. A., Sommers, M. S., & Hall, J. (2002). Focused life stories of women with cardiac pacemakers. *Western Journal of Nursing Research, 24,* 7–23.

Beitz, J. M., & Zuzelo, P. R. (2003). The lived experience of having a neobladder. *Western Journal of Nursing Research, 25,* 294–316.

Brackley, M., Davila, Y., Thornton, J., Leal, C., Mudd, G., Shafer, J., et al. (2003). Community readiness to prevent intimate partner violence in Bexar County, Texas. *Journal of Transcultural Nursing, 14,* 227–236.

Browne, A. J., & Fiske, J. (2001). First Nations women's encounters with mainstream health services. *Western Journal of Nursing Research, 23,* 126–147.

Clegg, A. (2003). Older South Asian patient and carer perceptions of culturally sensitive care in a community hospital setting. *Journal of Clinical Nursing, 12,* 283–290.

Dickson, G. L., & Kim, J. I. (2003). Reconstructing a meaning of pain: Older Korean American women's experiences with the pain of osteoarthritis. *Qualitative Health Research, 13,* 675–688.

Elliott, J., Berman, H., & Kim, S. (2002). A critical ethnography of Korean Canadian women's menopause experience. *Health Care Women International, 23,* 377–388.

Hirst, S. P. (2002). Defining resident abuse within the culture of long-term care institutions. *Clinical Nursing Research, 11,* 267–284.

Kearney, M. H., & O'Sullivan, J., (2003). Identity shifts as turning points in health behavior change. *Western Journal of Nursing Research, 25,* 134–152.

Kendall, J. (1999). Axial coding and the grounded theory controversy. *Western Journal of* Nursing Research, 21, 743–757.

Kushner, K. E., & Harrison, M. J. (2002). Employed mothers: Stress and balance-focused coping. *Canadian Journal of Nursing Research, 34,* 47–65.

Lauterbach, S. S. (2001). Longitudinal phenomenology: An example of "doing" phenomenology over time. Phenomenology of maternal mourning: Being-a-mother in another world (1992) and five years later (1997). In P. L. Munhall (Ed.), *Nursing research: A qualitative perspective.* Sudbury MA: Jones and Bartlett Publishers.

Lipson, J. G. (2001). We are the canaries: Multiple chemical sensitivity sufferers. *Qualitative Health Research, 11,* 103–116.

Long, A. F., Kneafsey, R., Ryan, J., and Berry, J. (2002). The role of the nurse within the multi-professional rehabilitation team. *Journal of Advanced Nursing, 37,* 70–78.

Marshall, E. S., Olsen, S. F., Mandleco, B. L., Dyches, T. T., Allred, K. W., & Sansom, N. (2003). "This is a spiritual experience": Perspectives of Latter-Day Saint families living with a child with disabilities. *Qualitative Health Research, 13,* 57–76.

McCurry, A. H., & Thomas, S. P. (2002). Spouses' experience in heart transplantation. *Western Journal of Nursing Research, 24,* 180–194.

Meehan, T. C. (2003). Careful nursing: A model for contemporary nursing practice. *Journal of Advanced Nursing, 44,* 99–107.

Mitchell, A. M., Gale, D. D., Garand, L., & Wesner, S. (2003). *Issues in Mental Health Nursing, 24,* 91–106.

Mohr, W. K. (2003). The substance of a support group. *Western Journal of Nursing Research, 25,* 676–692.

Mok, E., Martinson, I., & Wong, T. K. S. (2004). Individual empowerment among Chinese cancer patients in Hong Kong. *Western Journal of Nursing Research, 26,* 59–75.

Montbriand, M. J. (2004). Seniors' survival trajectories and the illness connection. *Qualitative Health Research, 14,* 449–461.

Morse, J. M., & Pooler, C. (2002). Patient-family-nurse interactions in the trauma-resuscitation room. *American Journal of Critical Care, 11,* 240–249,

Öhman, M., Söderberg, S., & Lundman, B. (2003), Hovering between suffering and enduring: The meaning of living with serious chronic illness. *Qualitative Health Research, 13,* 528–542.

Ohm, R. (2003). The African American experience in the Islamic faith. *Public Health Nursing, 20,* 478–486.

Olson, K., Tom, B., Hewitt, J., Whittingham, J., Buchanan, L., & Ganton, G. (2002). Evolving routines: Preventing fatigue associated with lung and colorectal cancer. *Qualitative Health Research, 12,* 655–670.

Rashid, S. F. (2001). Indigenous notions of the workings of the inner body: Conflicts and dilemmas with Norplant use in rural Bengladesh. *Qualitative Health Research, 11,* 85–102.

Rose, D., & Garwick, A. (2003). Urban American Indian family caregivers' perceptions of barriers to management of childhood asthma. *Journal of Pediatric Nursing, 18,* 2–11.

Rossen, E. K., & Knafl, K. A. (2003). Older women's response to residential relocation: Description of transition styles. *Qualitative Health Research, 13,* 20–36.

Scannell-Desch, E. A. (2000). Hardships and personal strategies of Vietnam war nurses. *Western Journal of Nursing Research, 22,* 526–550.

Schneider, Z. (2002). An Australian study of women's experiences of their first pregnancy. *Midwifery, 18,* 238–249.

Wilkin, K., & Slevin, E. (2004). The meaning of caring to nurses: An investigation into the nature of caring work in an intensive care unit. *Journal of Clinical Nursing, 13,* 50–59.

Examining Specific Types of Research

STUDENT OBJECTIVES

On completing this chapter, you will be able to:

▶ Identify the purposes and some of the distinguishing features of specific types of research (e.g., clinical trials, surveys)
▶ Determine whether researchers' primary approach (qualitative versus quantitative) and their design were appropriate for the type of research
▶ Identify several advantages of mixed-method research and describe specific applications
▶ Define new terms in the chapter

All quantitative studies can be categorized as either experimental, quasi-experimental/ pre-experimental, or nonexperimental in design as discussed in Chapter 9. And, most qualitative studies lie within one of the research traditions described in Chapter 10. This chapter describes types of qualitative and quantitative research that vary according to the study purpose rather than according to research design or tradition. The chapter also describes mixed method research that combines qualitative and quantitative approaches in a single project.

STUDIES THAT ARE TYPICALLY QUANTITATIVE

The research described in this section usually uses quantitative approaches, but it is important to note that for certain types of research (e.g., evaluation research), qualitative methods may also be added as a component used in a mixed-method strategy.

Clinical Trials

Clinical trials are studies designed to assess the effectiveness of clinical interventions. Methods associated with clinical trials have been developed for medical and epidemiologic research, but nurse researchers are increasingly adopting these methods to test nursing interventions.

Clinical trials undertaken to test innovative therapies or drugs often are designed in a series of phases.

▶ *Phase I* of the trial occurs after the initial development of the drug or therapy, and is designed primarily to determine things like drug dose (or strength of the therapy), safety, and patient tolerance. This phase typically uses pre-experimental designs (e.g., before– after without a control group). The focus is not on efficacy, but on developing the best possible (and safest) treatment.

▶ *Phase II* of the trial involves seeking preliminary evidence of the effectiveness of the treatment as it has been designed in phase I, typically using a pre- or quasi-experimental design, but sometimes a true experimental design with a small sample. During this phase, researchers ascertain the feasibility of launching a larger and more rigorous test, seek evidence that the treatment holds promise, and look for signs of possible side effects. This phase is sometimes considered a *pilot test* of the treatment. There have been clinical trials of drug therapies that have shown such powerful effects during this phase that further phases were considered unnecessary (and even unethical), but this would rarely be the case in nursing studies.

Example of a Phase II clinical trial

Olson, Hanson, and Michaud (2003) conducted a Phase II trial that compared pain levels, quality of life, and analgesic use with a sample of 24 Canadian cancer patients who received either standard opioid pain management plus Reiki or standard pain opioid management plus rest.

▶ *Phase III* is a full experimental test of the treatment, involving random assignment to an experimental or control group (or to orderings of treatment conditions). The objective of this phase is to determine the efficacy of the innovation compared to the standard treatment or an alternative counterfactual. When the term *clinical trial* is used in the nursing literature, it most often is referring to a Phase III trial, which may also be referred to as a **randomized clinical trial (RCT)**. Phase III clinical trials usually involve the use of a large and heterogeneous sample of subjects, frequently selected from multiple, geographically dispersed sites to ensure that findings are not unique to a single setting, and to enhance the power of the statistical tests through larger samples.

▶ *Phase IV* of the trial occurs after the decision to adopt an innovative treatment has been made. In this phase, researchers focus primarily on monitoring the long-term consequences of the intervention as it is used in actual practice, including both benefits and side effects. This phase might use a nonexperimental, pre-experimental, or quasi-experimental design.

Example of a multisite randomized clinical trial

A nurse-managed intervention called the Women's Initiative for Nonsmoking (WINS), developed on the basis of a well-tested smoking-cessation intervention, was tailored specifically to meet the needs of women (Martin, Froelicher, & Miller, 2000). Ten hospitals in the San Francisco area participated in the clinical trial. In each hospital, half of the subjects were assigned to either the 3-month experimental condition or to a "usual care" group. Follow-up data were collected at 6, 12, 24, and 30 months after baseline (Froelicher & Christopherson, 2000). Findings from this large clinical trial are beginning to emerge (e.g., Mahrer-Imhof, Froelicher, Li, Parker, & Benowitz, 2002; Froelicher et al., 2004).

Whittemore and Grey (2002) have proposed guidelines for the systematic and progressive testing of nursing innovations within a clinical trial framework. They suggest a fifth phase: wide-scale implementation of an intervention and an assessment of its effects on public health.

Evaluations

Evaluations are used to find out how well a program, treatment, practice, or policy works. Clinical nurses, nurse administrators, and nursing educators often need to pose such questions as the following: How are current practices working? Is there a better way to do things? Should a new practice be adopted? and Which approach is most effective? In this era of accountability, evaluations of the effectiveness of nursing actions are common. Evaluations can employ experimental, quasi-experimental, or nonexperimental designs and can be either cross-sectional or longitudinal. Although most evaluations are quantitative, certain aspects of programs can be evaluated using qualitative methods.

Clinical trials are sometimes evaluations. The multisite clinical trial of the WINS program described earlier is an evaluation of that program. A clinical trial is being undertaken to determine if the WINS program is meeting the objective of reducing smoking. Generally, the term *evaluation research* is used when researchers are testing to determine the effectiveness of a rather complex program, rather than when they are testing a specific entity (e.g., alternative drugs or sterilizing solutions). Thus, not all clinical trials would be called evaluations, and not all evaluations use methods associated with clinical trials. Moreover, evaluations often try to answer broader questions than simply whether an intervention is more effective clinically than care as usual. Evaluations may involve determining how the intervention was actually put into place, for example.

There are various types of evaluations. A **process analysis** (or an **implementation analysis**) is undertaken to obtain descriptive information about the process of implementing a

new program or procedure and about its functioning in actual operation. Process evaluations, which often rely on both qualitative and quantitative data, are designed to address such questions as the following: What are the strongest and weakest aspects of the program? What exactly *is* the treatment, and how does it differ (if at all) from traditional practices? What were the barriers to implementing the program successfully?

Example of a process analysis

A team of nurse researchers in Canada (Chalmers et al., 2004) used a participatory process to develop a community-based smoking cessation intervention for perinatal women. Their report summarized descriptive information about the development and implementation of the intervention and participants' reactions to its various components.

An **outcome analysis** documents the extent to which the goals of a program are attained, as a means of obtaining preliminary evidence about program success (e.g., the extent to which positive outcomes are in line with the original intent). Outcome analyses tend to be descriptive and do not use rigorous experimental designs; before–after designs without a comparison group are especially common.

Example of an outcome analysis

Lyder, Shannon, Empleo-Frazier, McGeHee, and White (2002) studied the outcomes of a comprehensive program to prevent pressure ulcers in long-term care. Pressure ulcer incidence in two long-term care facilities was studied before and after implementing the program.

An **impact analysis** attempts to identify the *impacts* or *net effects* of an intervention (i.e., the effects over and above what would have occurred in its absence). Impact analyses use an experimental or quasi-experimental design because their goal is to attribute a causal connection between outcomes and the intervention. Many nursing evaluations are impact analyses, although they are not necessarily labeled as such.

Example of an impact analysis

Keele-Smith and Leon (2003) evaluated the effectiveness of a theory-driven individualized exercise prescription on exercise consistency, body fat, and exercise motivation for faculty, staff, and students at a U.S. university. An experimental pretest-posttest design was used.

Finally, evaluations sometimes include a **cost–benefit analysis** to determine whether the monetary benefits of a program outweigh the costs. Administrators and public policy officials make decisions about resource allocations for health services not only on the basis of whether something "works," but also on the basis of whether it is economically viable. Cost–benefit analyses are typically done in connection with impact analyses and phase III clinical trials, that is, when researchers establish solid evidence regarding program effectiveness.

Example of a cost–benefit analysis

Capasso and Munro (2003) undertook a study to compare the costs and efficacy of two alternative wound treatments (set-to-dry normal saline gauze dressings and amorphous hydrogel dressings) for patients with infrainguinal arterial disease and diabetes. The analysis revealed a similar rate of healing, but the overall costs were significantly higher for patients in the normal saline group.

Outcomes Research

Outcomes research, designed to document the effectiveness of health care services, is gaining momentum in nursing and health care fields. Outcomes research overlaps with evaluation research, but evaluations typically appraise a specific new intervention, whereas outcomes research is a more global assessment of health care services. The impetus for outcomes research comes from the quality assessment and quality assurance functions that grew out of the professional standards review organizations (PSROs) in the 1970s. Outcomes research represents a response to the increasing demand from policy makers, insurers, and the public to justify care practices and systems in terms of both improved patient outcomes and costs. The focus of outcomes research in the 1980s was predominantly on patient health status and costs associated with medical care, but there is a growing interest in studying broader patient outcomes in relation to nursing care.

Although many nursing studies are concerned with examining patient outcomes and patient satisfaction, specific efforts to appraise and document the quality of nursing care—as distinct from the care provided by the overall health care system—are not numerous. A major obstacle is attribution—that is, linking patient outcomes to specific nursing actions or interventions, distinct from the actions of other members of the health care team. It is also difficult in some cases to determine a causal connection between outcomes and health care interventions because factors outside the health care system (e.g., patient characteristics) affect outcomes in complex ways.

Nevertheless, outcomes research has been gaining momentum. There is increasing interest, for example, in describing the work that nurses do in terms of established classification systems and taxonomies, and there is also interest in maintaining complete, accurate, and systematic records of nursing actions in computerized data sets (often referred to as *nursing minimal data sets* or *NMDS*). A number of research-based classification systems of nursing interventions are being developed, refined, and tested, including the Nursing Diagnoses Taxonomy of the North American Nursing Diagnosis Association, or NANDA, and the Nursing Intervention Classification (NIC), developed at the University of Iowa. Studies with these classification systems have thus far focused on descriptions of patient problems and nursing interventions, and assessments of the utility of these systems.

Just as there have been efforts to develop classifications of nursing interventions, work has been undertaken to develop outcome classification systems. Of particular note is the Nursing Outcomes Classification (NOC), which has been developed by nurses at the University of Iowa College of Nursing to complement the Nursing Intervention Classification (Johnson & Maas, 1998). The NOC system was developed as a way to measure patient outcomes that are sensitive to nursing care and to help standardize these outcomes. The NOC includes 260 patient outcomes categorized into seven domains: functional health, physiological health, psychosocial health, health knowledge and behavior, perceived health, family health and community health. Measuring outcomes and linking them to nursing actions is critical in developing an evidence-based practice and in launching quality-improvement efforts.

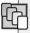

Example of outcomes research

Aiken, Clarke, Cheung, Sloane, and Silber (2003) studied patient outcomes (risk-adjusted mortality and failure to rescue) in relation to the education composition of nurses in hospitals, using data from over 200,000 surgical patients discharged from hospitals in Pennsylvania. They found that in hospitals with higher proportions of nurses educated at the baccalaureate level or higher, surgical patients experienced lower mortality and failure-to-rescue rates.

Surveys

A **survey** obtains information regarding the prevalence, distribution, and interrelationships of variables within a population. Political opinion polls, such as those conducted by Gallup, are examples of surveys. Surveys collect information on people's actions, knowledge, intentions, opinions, and attitudes.

Survey data are based on **self-reports**; that is, respondents answer questions posed by researchers. Survey data can be collected in a number of ways, but the most respected method is through **personal interviews** (or *face-to-face interviews*), in which interviewers meet in person with respondents to ask them questions. Generally, personal interviews are rather costly because they tend to involve a lot of personnel time. Nevertheless, personal interviews are regarded as the best method of collecting survey data because the quality of information they yield is higher than other methods and because relatively few people refuse to be interviewed in person. **Telephone interviews** are a less costly, but often less effective, method of gathering survey information. When the interviewer is unknown, respondents may be uncooperative on the telephone. Telephoning can, however, be a convenient method of collecting information if the interview is short, specific, and not too personal. Telephone interviews may be difficult for certain groups of respondents, including low-income people (who do not always have a telephone) or the elderly (who may have hearing problems).

Another mode of conducting a survey is by distributing **questionnaires**, which are self-administered. Because respondents differ in their reading levels and in their ability to communicate in writing, questionnaires are *not* merely a printed form of an interview. Self-administered questionnaires are economical but are not appropriate for surveying certain populations (e.g., the elderly, children). Survey questionnaires are generally distributed through the mail, but may also be distributed in other ways (e.g., through the Internet).

Survey research is highly flexible: It can be applied to many populations, it can focus on a wide range of topics, and its information can be used for many purposes. Survey information tends, however, to be relatively superficial. Survey research is better suited to extensive rather than intensive analysis. Although surveys can be performed within the context of large-scale experiments, surveys are usually done as part of a nonexperimental study.

Example of a survey

Robinson, Clements, and Land (2003) studied the prevalence, distribution, correlates, and predictors of vicarious trauma and burnout among registered psychiatric nurses in Canada. Questionnaires were distributed to over 1000 nurses in Manitoba.

STUDIES THAT CAN BE QUALITATIVE OR QUANTITATIVE

The studies described in the previous section are typically conducted with formal instruments designed to yield quantitative data, although qualitative methods can sometimes be used in these studies as well. The types of studies described in this section can be either qualitative or quantitative.

Case Studies

Case studies are in-depth investigations of a single entity or a small number of entities. The entity may be an individual, family, group, institution, community, or other social unit. In a case study, researchers obtain a wealth of descriptive information and may examine relationships among different phenomena or examine trends over time. Case study researchers attempt to analyze and understand issues that are important to the history, development, or circumstances of the person or entity under study.

One way to think of a case study is to consider what is center stage. In most studies, whether qualitative or quantitative, a certain phenomenon or variable (or set of variables) is the core of the inquiry. In a case study, the *case* itself is central. As befits an intensive analysis, the focus of case studies is typically on determining the dynamics of *why* an individual thinks, behaves, or develops in a particular manner rather than on *what* his or her status, progress, or actions are. It is not unusual for probing research of this type to require detailed study over a considerable period. Data are often collected that relate not only to the person's present state but also to past experiences and situational factors relevant to the problem being examined.

The greatest strength of case studies is the depth that is possible when a limited number of individuals or groups is being investigated. On the other hand, this same strength is a potential weakness because researchers' familiarity with the person or group may make objectivity more difficult. Perhaps the biggest criticism of case studies concerns generalizability: If researchers discover important relationships, it is difficult to know whether the same relationships would occur with others. However, case studies can often play a critical role in challenging generalizations based on other types of research. It is important to recognize that case study research is not simply anecdotal descriptions of a particular incident or patient. Case study research is a disciplined process and typically requires an extended period of systematic data collection.

Example of a quantitative case study

Kolanowski, Litaker, and Catalano (2002) studied the self-reported mood and affective pattern of an older man with severe cognitive impairments. Data were collected through observation of the man and through his self-reports of mood collected three times a day over a 35-day period.

Example of a qualitative case study

Fleming (2003) explored the meaning of the experience of abdominal hysterectomy for one woman in Scotland using in-depth case study methods.

Secondary Analysis

Secondary analysis involves the use of data gathered in a previous study to test new hypotheses or explore new phenomena or relationships. In a typical study, researchers collect far more data than are actually analyzed. Secondary analysis of existing data is efficient and economical because data collection is typically the most time-consuming and expensive part of a research project. Nurse researchers have done secondary analyses with both large national data sets and smaller, localized sets, and with both qualitative and quantitative data.

A number of avenues are available for making use of an existing set of quantitative data. For example, variables and relationships among variables that were previously unanalyzed can be examined (e.g., a dependent variable in the original study could become the independent variable in the secondary analysis). Or, the secondary analysis can focus on a particular subgroup rather than on the full original sample (e.g., survey data about health habits from a national sample could be analyzed to study smoking among urban teenagers). As another example, the unit of analysis can be changed. A **unit of analysis** is the basic unit that yields data for an analysis; in nursing studies, each individual subject is typically the unit of analysis. However, data are sometimes aggregated to yield information about larger units (e.g., a study of individual nurses from 25 hospitals could be converted to aggregated data about the hospitals). In qualitative studies, wider theories can be generated by using data from several different data sets. Or, a qualitative researcher could scrutinize an existing data set for particular themes or content coverage that was previously unexplored.

The use of available data makes it possible to bypass time-consuming and costly steps in the research process, but there are some noteworthy disadvantages in working with existing data. In particular, if researchers do not play a role in collecting the data, the chances are pretty high that the data set will be deficient in one or more ways, such as in the sample used, the variables measured, and so forth. Researchers may continuously face "if only" problems: if only they had asked questions on a certain topic or had measured a particular variable differently. Nevertheless, existing data sets present exciting opportunities for exploring phenomena of importance to nurses.

Example of a secondary analysis of quantitative data

Young, Nikolette, McCaul, Twigg, and Morey (2002) used existing data from three annual cross-sectional pressure ulcer prevalence studies in a western Australia hospital. The combined sample of 1394 patients was used to explore risk factors associated with pressure ulcer development.

Example of a secondary analysis of qualitative data

Thorne, Con, McGuinness, McPerson, and Harris (2004) analyzed previously collected qualitative data from a larger study that explored patterns in health care communication across several different chronic diseases. Their study involved an analysis of how persons with multiple sclerosis described helpful and unhelpful communication in their health care.

Methodologic Research

Methodologic research examines methods of obtaining and analyzing data and addresses the development, validation, and evaluation of research tools or methods. Nurse researchers have become increasingly interested in methodologic research; this is not surprising in light of growing demands for sound and reliable outcome measures and for sophisticated procedures for obtaining and analyzing qualitative and quantitative data.

Quantitative methodologic studies often focus on instrument development and testing. For example, suppose we developed and evaluated an instrument to accurately measure patients' satisfaction with nursing care. In such a study, we would not examine levels of patient satisfaction, nor how satisfaction relates to characteristics of nurses, hospitals, or patients. Our goal would be to develop an effective and trustworthy instrument that could be used by others and to determine our success.

Most methodologic studies are descriptive and nonexperimental, but occasionally quantitative researchers use an experimental or quasi-experimental design to test competing methodologic strategies. For example, a researcher might test whether a financial incentive increases the number of volunteers willing to participate in a study. Potential subjects could be randomly assigned to an incentive or no-incentive condition. The dependent variable in this case is whether people agree to participate.

In qualitative research, methodologic issues often arise within the context of a substantive study, rather than having a study originate as a purely methodologic endeavor. In such instances, however, the researcher typically performs separate analyses designed to highlight a methodologic issue and to generate strategies for solving a methodologic problem.

Methodologic research may appear less provocative than substantive research, but it is virtually impossible to produce high-quality research evidence on a substantive topic with inadequate research methods.

Example of a quantitative methodologic study

Beck and Gable (2003) undertook a rigorous methodologic study to develop and test the Spanish version of their widely used Postpartum Depression Screening Scale. Their analysis suggested that the translated Spanish version would yield good-quality data for screening mothers postpartum.

Example of a qualitative methodologic study

Janet Mentes undertook a quasi-experimental multisite study to test the effectiveness of a hydration management intervention in nursing homes (see the research example at the end of Chapter 9). Mentes and Tripp-Reimer (2002) analyzed qualitative data that were collected during the course of that study to gain an understanding of factors that were barriers and facilitators to such research, to better prepare future researchers for the challenges of clinical research in nursing home settings.

MIXED METHOD STUDIES

An emerging trend, and one that we believe will gain momentum, is the planned integration of qualitative and quantitative data within single studies or coordinated clusters of studies. This section discusses the rationale for such **mixed method** (or **multimethod**) **studies** and presents a few applications.

Rationale for Mixed Method Studies

The dichotomy between quantitative and qualitative data represents a key methodologic distinction in the social, behavioral, and health sciences. Some argue that the paradigms that underpin qualitative and quantitative research are fundamentally incompatible. Others, however, believe that many areas of inquiry can be enriched and the evidence base enhanced through the judicious blending of qualitative and quantitative data. The advantages of an integrated design include the following:

▶ *Complementarity.* Qualitative and quantitative data represent words and numbers, the two fundamental languages of human communication. The strengths and weaknesses of these two types of data and associated methods are complementary. By using multiple methods, researchers can allow each method to do what it does best, possibly avoiding the limitations of a single approach.

▶ *Incrementality.* Progress on a topic tends to be incremental, relying on multiple feedback loops. Qualitative findings can generate hypotheses to be tested quantitatively, and quantitative findings sometimes need clarification through in-depth probing. It can be productive to build such a loop into the design of a single study.

▶ *Enhanced validity.* When a hypothesis or model is supported by multiple and complementary types of data, researchers can be more confident about the validity of their results.

▶ *Creating new frontiers.* Sometimes qualitative and quantitative findings are inconsistent with each other. This lack of congruity—when it happens in a single investigation—can lead to insights that can push a line of inquiry further. Inconsistencies in separate studies may reflect differences in study participants and circumstances rather than theoretically meaningful distinctions. In a single study, discrepancies can be used as a springboard for further exploration.

CONSUMER TIP

Mixed method studies rarely combine qualitative and quantitative findings in a single report. Typically, the quantitative findings are reported in one journal article, and the qualitative findings appear in a separate article in a different journal. This sometimes makes it difficult for readers to grasp the contributions of all the components.

Applications of Mixed Method Research

Researchers make decisions about study design and procedures based on the specific objectives of their investigations. The integration of qualitative and quantitative data can be used to address various research goals.

1. *Instrumentation.* Researchers sometimes collect qualitative data for the development and validation of formal, quantitative instruments used in research or clinical applications. The questions for a formal instrument are sometimes derived from clinical experience, theory, or prior research. When a construct is new, however, these mechanisms may be inadequate to capture its full complexity and dimensionality. A researcher's knowledge base, no matter how rich, is subjective and limited, and thus nurse researchers sometimes gather qualitative data as the

basis for generating questions for quantitative instruments that are subsequently subjected to rigorous testing in methodologic studies.

Example of instrumentation

Beck and Gable (2000) developed the Postpartum Depression Screening Scale (PDSS), an instrument that screens new mothers for the mood disorder that can develop after delivering a baby. Scale items were based on in-depth interviews of mothers suffering from postpartum depression in a grounded theory study and two phenomenological studies. Here is an example of how items on the PDSS were developed from mothers' quotes. The quote "I was extremely obsessive with my thoughts. They would never stop. I could not control them" was developed into the item: I could not control the thoughts that kept coming into my mind (Beck and Gable, 2001).

2. *Hypothesis generation and testing.* In-depth qualitative studies are often fertile with insights about constructs or relationships among them. These insights then can be tested and confirmed in quantitative studies, and the generalizability of the insights can be assessed. This most often happens in the context of discrete investigations. One problem, however, is that it usually takes years to do a study and publish the results, which means that considerable time may elapse between the qualitative insights and the formal quantitative testing of hypotheses based on those insights. A research team interested in a phenomenon might wish to collaborate in a research program that has hypothesis generation and testing as an explicit goal.

Example of hypothesis generation

Wendler (2001) described how a *meta-matrix* can be used to facilitate pattern recognition across data from different sources—including qualitative and quantitative sources—and to generate hypotheses. In Wendler's example of a mixed-method study of Tellington touch (Ttouch), use of a meta-matrix led to a discovery of the relationship between the administration of Ttouch and the practitioner's physical state (e.g., caffeine intake).

3. *Illustration.* Qualitative data are sometimes used to illustrate the meaning of quantitative descriptions or relationships. Such illustrations help to clarify important concepts and further serve to corroborate the findings from the statistical analysis. The illustrations help to illuminate the analysis and give guidance to the interpretation of results. Qualitative materials can be used to illustrate specific statistical findings and to provide more global and dynamic views of the phenomena under study, often in the form of illustrative case studies.

Example of illustrating with qualitative data

Polit, London, and Martinez (2000, 2001) used data from the ethnographic component of a study of poor urban families to illustrate how food insecurity and hunger—reported by more than half of the sample from the survey component—were actually experienced and managed. The following excerpt illustrates the sustenance problems some women had: "*It was hard, especially when you got kids at home saying, 'I'm hungry.'... I started working at the church as a babysitter. I was getting paid $20 a week and a bag of food every Thursday.... Then I was doing very odd jobs that most people would not dare to do. I was making deliveries on pizza in bad neighborhoods where most people wouldn't go. I mean, I literally took my life in my own hands*" (2001, p. 58).

4. *Understanding relationships and causal processes.* Quantitative methods can demonstrate that variables are systematically related but may fail to provide insights about *why* they are related. Interpretations are often speculative, representing hypotheses that could be tested in another study. When a study integrates qualitative and quantitative data, however, the researcher may be in a stronger position to derive meaning immediately from the statistical findings.

Example of illuminating with qualitative data

Tilden, Tolle, Nelson, and Fields (2001) collected both qualitative and quantitative data about family members' decision to withdraw life-sustaining treatments from hospitalized patients. The quantitative data indicated that family members' stress scores were lower if the patient had left advance directives. The rich qualitative data shed light on how people with low stress scores were more convinced that they made the right decision, because they knew what the patient wanted.

5. *Theory building, testing, and refinement.* The most ambitious application of mixed method research is in the area of theory development. A theory gains acceptance as it escapes disconfirmation, and the use of multiple methods provides great opportunity for potential disconfirmation of a theory. If the theory can survive these assaults, it can provide a stronger context for the organization of clinical and intellectual work.

Example of theory building

Morgan and Stewart (2002) conducted a mixed-method evaluation of a dementia special care unit in a midwestern Canadian city that involved a quasi-experimental component and a grounded theory component. The study led to a better understanding of how the nursing home environment affects residents with dementia, which in turn helped to advance theory development in person–environment interaction.

Mixed Method Strategies

The ways in which researchers can design studies to integrate qualitative and quantitative methods are almost limitless. The three following scenarios are especially common:

1. *Adding qualitative methods to a survey.* Once researchers have gained the cooperation of survey respondents, they may be in a good position to collect more in-depth data with a subset of them. If the collection of in-depth data can be postponed until after the analysis of quantitative data, researchers can probe into the reasons for any obtained results. The second-stage respondents, in other words, can be used as informants to help researchers interpret outcomes.

Example of a qualitative component following a survey

Wilson and Williams (2000) were involved in a three-phase study on telephone consultation among community nurses in England. The first phase involved a national survey of community nurses, via mailed questionnaire. In the second phase, which involved in-depth interviews with a subset of 14 survey respondents, nurses were probed about their experiences with telephone consultations. The third phase involved a survey of clients from the interviewees' caseload who had used telephone services.

2. *Embedding quantitative measures into an ethnography.* Although qualitative data prevail in ethnographic field studies, ethnographers can often profit from the collection of more structured information, either from the study participants or from a larger or more representative sample. Having already gained entrée into the community and the trust and cooperation of its members, ethnographers may be in an ideal position to pursue a survey or a record-extraction activity. For example, if a researcher's in-depth field work focused on family violence, community-wide police and hospital records could be used to gather systematic data amenable to statistical analysis.

Example of a multimethod ethnography

Clark (2002) conducted a focused ethnography of Mexican-origin mothers' experiences of obtaining and using health services for their children in an urban Latino community in the United States. In addition to gathering in-depth ethnographic data through multiple interviews and detailed observations, Clark gathered and analyzed quantitative information from the children's medical records (e.g., number of emergency department visits, number of well-child visits).

3. *Embedding qualitative approaches into experimental research.* Qualitative data can often enrich clinical trials and evaluations that rely on experimental (or quasi-experimental) designs. Through in-depth, unstructured approaches, researchers can, for example, better understand qualitative differences between groups, including differences in the experiences and processes underlying experimental effects. Qualitative data may be especially useful when researchers are evaluating complex interventions. When an experimental treatment is straightforward (e.g., a new drug), it might be easy to interpret the results. However, many nursing interventions are more complicated; they may involve new ways of interacting with patients or new approaches to organizing the delivery of care. At the end of the experiment, even when hypothesized results are obtained, people may ask, What was it that really caused the group differences? In-depth qualitative data may help researchers to address the **black box** question—understanding what it is about the intervention that is driving any observed effects. The use of qualitative methods in nursing intervention studies can play a role in making nursing work more visible and accessible to other nurses, policy makers, and the public (Sandelowski, 1996).

Example of qualitative data collection in the development of a clinical trial

Maliski, Heilemann, and McCorkle (2001, 2002) embedded a grounded theory study in a large clinical trial of a Standardized Nursing Intervention Protocol postprostatectomy. A subsample of 20 participants in the trial (10 experimental and 10 control group members) were interviewed in depth to gain an understanding of postprostatectomy incontinence and impotence, and to describe their evolving experiences from diagnosis through treatment.

Sometimes mixed method approaches are useful in the early stages of an experiment or clinical trial. For example, through in-depth questioning, researchers can gather information about the feasibility and acceptability of an intervention, or about how best to "package" or promote it.

Example of qualitative data early in a clinical trial

Ross and Johansen (2002) conducted in-depth interviews as an initial part of a large randomized intervention study of the effect of home visits to Danish patients with colorectal cancer. The qualitative component was designed to provide information about how the home visits should be carried out and what the content of the intervention should be.

CRITIQUING STUDIES DESCRIBED IN THIS CHAPTER

It is somewhat difficult to provide guidance on critiquing the types of studies described in this chapter because they are so varied and because many of the fundamental methodologic issues that would be critiqued concern the overall design. Table 11-1 provides a very crude guide to the types of quantitative research designs that are usually considered appropriate for the various types of studies described in this chapter. Note that qualitative approaches could be integrated as an adjunct in *any* of these types in a mixed method study, and in some cases (e.g., a process analysis) qualitative data could be collected exclusively in lieu of quantitative data. Despite the limitations of the table, you can see, for example, that an impact analysis or Phase III clinical trial that used a pre-experimental design would be problematic.

TABLE 11.1	**Guide to Study Types and Quantitative Research Designs**
TYPE OF STUDY	**USUAL TYPE OF QUANTITATIVE DESIGN**
Clinical trial	
Phase I	Pre-experimental, nonexperimental*
Phase II	Small-scale experimental, quasi-experimental
Phase III	Experimental
Phase IV	Nonexperimental, pre-experimental, quasi-experimental
Evaluation	
Process analysis	Nonexperimental*
Outcome analysis	Pre-experimental
Impact analysis	Experimental, quasi-experimental
Cost–benefit analysis	Experimental, quasi-experimental
Outcomes research	Nonexperimental,* pre-experimental, quasi-experimental, experimental
Survey	Nonexperimental
Case study	Nonexperimental*
Secondary analysis	Nonexperimental*
Methodologic	Nonexperimental, pre-experimental, quasi-experimental, experimental*

* Information collected could be qualitative data rather than quantitative data. In deliberately mixed-method studies, both qualitative and quantitative data could be gathered for *any* of these types of study.

BOX 11.1   Guidelines for Critiquing Studies Described in This Chapter

1. Does the study purpose match the study design? Was the best possible design (or research tradition) used to address the study purpose?
2. Is the study exclusively qualitative or exclusively quantitative? If so, could the study have been strengthened by including both types of data?
3. If both qualitative and quantitative data were collected, was the use of both types justified? How (if at all) did the inclusion of both types of data strengthen the study and further the aims of the research?

You should also consider whether researchers took appropriate advantage of the possibilities of a mixed method design. Collecting both qualitative and quantitative data is not always necessary or practical, but in critiquing studies you can consider whether the study would have been strengthened by triangulating different types of data. In studies in which mixed methods were used, you should carefully consider whether the inclusion of both types of data were justified and whether the researcher really made use of both types of data to enhance knowledge on the research topic.

Box 11-1 offers a few specific questions for critiquing the types of studies included in this chapter.

CHAPTER REVIEW

Key new terms introduced in the chapter, together with a summary of major points, are presented in this section. In addition, Chapter 11 of the *Study Guide to Accompany Essentials of Nursing Research,* 6th edition offers various exercises and study suggestions for reinforcing the concepts presented in this chapter. For additional review, see the Student Self-Study Review Questions section of the Student Resource CD-ROM provided with this book.

KEY NEW TERMS

Black box question
Case study
Clinical trial
Cost–benefit analysis
Evaluation
Impact analysis
Implementation analysis
Methodologic research
Mixed method (multimethod)
   study

Outcome analysis
Outcomes research
Personal interview
Process analysis
Questionnaire
Randomized clinical trial (RCT)
Secondary analysis
Self reports
Survey
Telephone interview

SUMMARY POINTS

▷ Quantitative and qualitative studies vary according to purpose as well as design and tradition. Several specific types of study are described in this chapter.

▷ **Clinical trials**—studies designed to assess the effectiveness of clinical interventions—are often designed in a series of phases. *Phase I* is designed to finalize the features of the intervention; *Phase II* involves seeking preliminary evidence of treatment effectiveness; *Phase III* is a full experimental test of the treatment, often called a **randomized clinical trial (RCT)**; and *Phase IV* monitors generalizability and long-term consequences, including both benefits and side effects.

▷ **Evaluations**, which assess the effectiveness of a program, policy, or procedure, can answer a variety of questions. **Process** or **implementation analyses** describe the process by which a program gets implemented and how it functions in practice. **Outcome analyses** describe the status of some condition after the introduction of an intervention. **Impact analyses** test whether an intervention caused any *net effects* relative to a counterfactual. **Cost–benefit analyses** seek to determine whether the monetary costs of a program are outweighed by benefits.

▷ **Outcomes research** is undertaken to document the quality and effectiveness of health care and nursing services. Classification systems that help to standardize descriptions of nursing actions and outcomes sensitive to nursing care can contribute to outcomes research.

▷ **Surveys** examine people's characteristics, behaviors, attitudes, and intentions by asking them questions. The preferred survey method is through **personal interviews**, in which interviewers meet respondents face-to-face and question them. **Telephone interviews** are more economical, but are not suitable for lengthy surveys or for ones with sensitive or personal questions. **Questionnaires** are self-administered; i.e., questions are read by respondents, who then give written responses.

▷ **Case studies** are intensive investigations of a single entity or small number of entities (e.g., people, organizations). Such studies, which can be qualitative or quantitative, typically involve data collection over an extended period.

▷ **Secondary analysis** refers to studies in which researchers analyze previously collected data—either qualitative or quantitative. The secondary analyst may examine unanalyzed concepts, focus on a particular subsample, or change the *unit of analysis*.

▷ In **methodologic research**, investigators are concerned with the development and assessment of methodologic tools or strategies.

▷ **Mixed method** (or **multimethod**) **studies** blend qualitative and quantitative data in a single project and can be advantageous in developing an evidence base for nursing practice. Qualitative and quantitative methods have complementary strengths and weaknesses, and an integrated approach can lead to theoretical and substantive insights into the multidimensional nature of reality.

▷ In nursing, one of the most frequent uses of multimethod research has been in the area of instrument development and refinement. Qualitative data are also used to illustrate, clarify, or amplify the meaning of quantified descriptions or relationships. Multimethod studies can help to interpret and give shape to relationships and causal processes and can also be used to generate and test hypotheses.

▷ Researchers can implement a multimethod study in a variety of ways, including the use of qualitative data as an adjunct in clinical trials, experimental evaluations, and surveys. The collection of quantitative data within the context of a primarily qualitative study is somewhat less common, but is most likely to happen in ethnographies.

RESEARCH EXAMPLES | Critical Thinking Activities

EXAMPLE 1: Mixed Method Research—Qualitative Inquiry Following a Survey

Aspects of a mixed method nursing study, featuring terms and concepts discussed in this chapter, are presented below, followed by some questions to guide critical thinking. (The research reports are available in (1) *Nursing Research, 51,* pp. 168–174 and (2) *Journal of Nursing Scholarship, 34,* 139–145.

Study

(1) "Planning a sexual health promotion intervention with homeless adolescents" (Rew, Chambers, & Kulkarni, 2002) and (2) "Sexual health practices of homeless youth" (Rew, Fouladi, & Yockey, 2002)

Statement of Purpose

The overall project involved gathering information about the sexual health practices of homeless adolescents with the aim of developing an appropriate intervention for these high-risk youths.

Method

The project included a survey component, followed by in-depth group interviews with some of the survey respondents. A sample of 425 homeless young men and women aged 16–20 years were recruited to complete the survey through a street outreach program. The youths completed the questionnaires at the program site. Respondents were asked specific questions on a range of topics, including their sexual orientation, safe sex behaviors, social support, perceived health status, time away from home, and future time perspective. From the survey sample, 32 youths were selected at random and invited to participate in an in-depth group interview; 22 youths actually participated in one of four group interview sessions. These interviews, which were conducted at the church drop-in center where the outreach program offered services, focused on the youths' knowledge about sexually transmitted diseases (STDs) and their prevention, and on suggestions for an intervention that might best serve their needs for preventing and treating STDs.

Key Findings

▶ In the survey, sexual orientation was reported as a reason for leaving home; 35% reported homosexual or bisexual orientation. Over half the youths had a history of sexual abuse.
▶ The youths' safe sex behaviors were found to be related to cognitive–perceptual variables (e.g., future time perspective), which are potentially amenable to a culturally relevant intervention.
▶ In the in-depth group interviews, the youths identified a variety of barriers to seeking diagnosis and treatment for symptoms of STDs. They thought that any intervention should be brief, gender-specific, easily accessible, and focused on the unique circumstances of homeless youths.

Critical Thinking Suggestions*

*See the Student Resource CD-ROM for a discussion of these questions.
1. Answer the questions from Box 11-1 regarding this study.

RESEARCH EXAMPLES *Continued*

2. Also consider the following targeted questions, which may assist you in further assessing aspects of the study:

    a. Comment on the researchers' decision to collect survey data via a self-administered questionnaire.

    b. Comment on the sequencing of the survey and group interviews.

3. If the results of this study are valid and trustworthy, what are some of the uses to which the findings might be put in clinical practice?

EXAMPLE 2: Mixed Method Research—Secondary Analysis, Ethnography, and Medical Records Analysis

Aspects of a mixed method nursing study, featuring terms and concepts discussed in this chapter, are presented below, followed by some questions to guide critical thinking. (The research reports are available in (1) *Western Journal of Nursing Research*, *25*, pp. 854–871 and (2) *Journal of Refugee Studies, 13,* 303–327.)

Study

(1) "Bosnian and Soviet refugees' experiences with health care" (Lipson, Weinstein, Gladstone, & Sarnoff, 2003) and (2) "Physical and psychological health issues of resettled refugees in the United States" (Weinstein, Sarnoff, Gladstone, & Lipson, 2000)

Statement of Purpose

The overall project was designed to provide a comprehensive understanding of the health status and health care needs of refugees in Santa Clara County, California, in the first few years after resettlement in the United States.

Method

The study had three parts. The first involved a secondary analysis of an administrative data set containing health records from 2361 refugees who sought services from all county health facilities between 1995 and 1998. The second part involved an analysis of 187 randomly selected medical records from the County Refugee Clinic with regard to diagnosis, use of services, and quality of care. The third component involved ethnographic studies of the Bosnian and former Soviet Union refugee communities. In the ethnography, the researchers made observations of community events, interviewed refugees in their homes, and interviewed health care providers. Data from the ethnographic component, which indicated that certain health problems were especially common in the refugee population, helped to focus certain aspects of the medical records component.

Key Findings

▶ The quantitative portions of the study revealed a high prevalence of ill-defined symptoms (malaise, headache, fatigue, pain) among the refugees; there was, however, a low rate of

research examples continue on page 254

RESEARCH EXAMPLES *Continued*

diagnosis of mental disorder. Elevated rates of TB, parasites, and liver disease were
observed.

▷ Most refugee women were not receiving gynecologic care. The refugees were infrequent users
of county emergency services and saw few specialists.

▷ The ethnographic data revealed that the U.S. health care system was confusing and the lack of
interpreters at most facilities made it difficult for refugees to secure satisfactory health care.

▷ The refugees worried about adequate health insurance coverage and choice, and disliked the
red tape of managed care; they also were troubled by the long waits for appointments.

▷ Several participants said they avoided seeing physicians for fear of finding a severe problem or
because a diagnosed illness could lead to job loss.

Critical Thinking Suggestions

1. Answer the questions from Box 11-1 regarding this study.
2. Also consider the following targeted questions, which may assist you in further assessing
aspects of the study:
   a. Comment on the researchers' decision to conduct a secondary analysis of an existing data
   set.
   b. Do you think that information about the incidence and prevalence of refugees' health problems and use of services could have been collected in the ethnography? Why or why not?
   c. What other types of data could have been gathered in this study to supplement the
   researchers' understanding of refugee health care issues?
3. If the results of this study are valid and trustworthy, what are some of the uses to which the
findings might be put in clinical practice?

 EXAMPLE 3: Mixed Method Study: Randomized Clinical Trial and In-Depth Interviews

Aspects of a mixed method nursing study, featuring terms and concepts discussed in this
chapter, are presented below, followed by some questions to guide critical thinking. (The
research report is available in *Lippincott's Case Management*, *7*, 170–179, and in Appendix
E of the associated *Study Guide to Accompany Essentials of Nursing Research*, 6th edition.)

Study

"A randomized control trial of nursing-based case management for patients with chronic obstructive pulmonary disease" (Egan, Clavarino, Burridge, Teuwen, & White, 2002)

Statement of Purpose

The main purpose of the study was to test the effectiveness of nursing-based case management for
patients with chronic obstructive pulmonary disease (COPD). The study also investigated issues
relating to the implementation of the intervention and satisfaction with it among patients, caregivers, and health care staff.

RESEARCH EXAMPLES | *Continued*

Method

A sample of 66 hospitalized patients with COPD in Brisbane, Australia, were randomly assigned either to an intervention group (which received individualized nursing-based case management during and after hospitalization over a 6-week period) or to a control group (which received normal care). The following outcomes were measured upon admission and then 1 month and 3 months post-discharge: health-related quality of life, including frequency and severity of respiratory symptoms; social support availability; anxiety; depression; and subjective well-being. Nurses in the hospital were surveyed to determine their perceptions about the case management intervention. Additionally, two physicians, 10 patients, and eight caregivers of the patients were interviewed in-depth regarding their experiences during the study period.

Key Findings

▶ The experimental and control groups did not differ significantly in terms of unplanned re-admissions, depression, symptoms, support, and subjective well-being.

▶ The in-depth interviews indicated that intervention group patients placed a high value on case management, noting that they had access to resources they otherwise would not have had.

▶ Most nursing and medical staff found case management beneficial to patients.

Critical Thinking Suggestions:

1. Answer the questions from Box 11-1 regarding this study.

2. Also consider the following targeted questions, which may assist you in further assessing aspects of the study:

   a. What phase of a clinical trial would you consider this research?

   b. Would you consider this study an evaluation? Why or why not? If yes, what type of evaluation would this be?

   c. The results of the qualitative and quantitative portions of the study are not totally congruent. Why do you think that might be the case?

3. If the results of this study are valid and trustworthy, what are some of the uses to which the findings might be put in clinical practice?

SUGGESTED READINGS

Methodologic References

Johnson, M., & Maas, M. (1998). The nursing outcomes classification. *Journal of Nursing Care Quality, 12*, 9–20.

Kerlinger, F. N., & Lee, H. B. (2000). *Foundations of behavioral research* (4th ed.). Orlando, FL: Harcourt College Publishers.

Morse, J. M. (1991). Approaches to qualitative-quantitative methodological triangulation. *Nursing Research, 40*, 120–122.

Polit, D. F., & Beck, C. T. (2004). *Nursing Research: Principles and Methods.* (7th ed.) Philadelphia: Lippincott Williams & Wilkins.

Sandelowski, M. (1996). Using qualitative methods in intervention studies. *Research in Nursing & Health, 19*, 359–364.

Sandelowski, M. (2000). Combining qualitative and quantitative sampling, data collection, and analysis techniques in mixed-method studies. *Research in Nursing & Health, 23*, 246–255.

Whittemore, R., & Grey, M. (2002). The systematic development of nursing interventions. *Journal of Nursing Scholarship, 34,* 115–120.

Studies Cited in Chapter 11

Aiken, L. H., Clarke, S. P., Cheung, R. B., Sloane, D. M., & Silber, J. H. (2003). Educational levels of hospital nurses and surgical patient mortality. *Journal of the American Medical Association, 290,* 1617–1623.

Beck, C. T., & Gable, R. K. (2000). Postpartum Depression Screening Scale: Development and psychometric testing. *Nursing Research, 49,* 272–282.

Beck, C. T., & Gable, R. K. (2001). Ensuring content validity: An illustration of the process. *Journal of Nursing Measurement, 9,* 201–215.

Beck, C. T., & Gable, R. K. (2003). Postpartum Depression Screening Scale: Spanish version. *Nursing Research, 52,* 296–306.

Capasso, V. A., & Munro, B. H. (2003). The cost and efficacy of two wound treatments. *AORN Journal, 77,* 984–992.

Chalmers, K., Gupton, A., Katz, A., Hack, T., Hildes-Ripstein, E., Brown, J., McMillan, D., Labossiere, D., Mackay, M., Pickerl, C., Savard-Preston, Y., Vincent, J. A., Morris, H. M., & Cann, B. (2004). The description and evaluation of a longitudinal pilot study of a smoking relapse/reduction intervention for perinatal women. *Journal of Advanced Nursing, 45,* 162–171.

Clark, L. (2002). Mexican-origin mothers' experiences using children's health care services. *Western Journal of Nursing Research, 24,* 159–179.

Dickerson, S. S. (2002). Redefining life while forestalling death: Living with an implantable cardioverter defibrillator after a sudden cardiac death experience. *Qualitative Health Research, 12,* 360–372.

Doran, D. I., Sidani, S., Keatings, M., & Dodge, D. (2002). An empirical test of the Nursing Role Effectiveness Model. *Journal of Advanced Nursing, 38,* 29–39.

Egan, E., Clavarino, A., Burridge, L., Teuwen, M., & White, E. (2002). A randomized control trial of nursing-based case management for patients with chronic obstructive pulmonary disease. *Lippincott's Case Management, 7,* 170–179.

Fleming, V. (2003). Hysterectomy: A case study of one woman's experience. *Journal of Advanced Nursing, 44,* 575–582.

Froelicher, E. S., & Christopherson, D. J. (2000). Women's Initiative for Nonsmoking (WINS) I: Design and methods. *Heart & Lung, 29,* 429–437.

Froelicher, E. S., Miller, N. H., Christopherson, D. J., Martin, K., Parker, K., Amonetti, M., Lin, Z., Sohn, M., Benowitz, N., Taylor, C. B., & Bacchetti, P. (2004). High rates of sustained smoking cessation in women hospitalized with cardiovascular disease: The women's initiative for nonsmoking (WINS). *Circulation, 109,* 587–593.

Keele-Smith, R., & Leon, T. (2003). Evaluation of individually tailored interventions on exercise adherence. *Western Journal of Nursing Research, 25,* 623–640.

Kolanowski, A. M., Litaker, M. S., & Catalano, P. A. (2002). Emotional well-being in a person with dementia. *Western Journal of Nursing Research, 24,* 28–48.

Lipson, J. G., Weinstein, H. M., Glastone, E. A., & Sarnoff, R. H. (2003). Bosnian and Soviet refugees' experiences with health care. *Western Journal of Nursing Research, 25,* 854–871.

Lyder, C. H., Shannon, R., Empleo-Frazier, O., McGeHee, D., & White, C. (2002). A comprehensive program to prevent pressure ulcers in long-term care: Exploring costs and outcomes. *Ostomy & Wound Management, 48,* 52–62.

Mahrer-Imhof, R., Froelicher, E. S., Li, W. W., Parker, K. M., & Benowitz, N. (2002). Women's Initiative for Nonsmoking (WINS) V: Under-use of nicotine replacement therapy. *Heart & Lung, 31,* 368–373.

Maliski, S. L., Heilemann, M. V., & McCorkle, R. (2001). Mastery of postprostatectomy incontinence and impotence: His work, her work, our work. *Oncology Nursing Forum, 28,* 985–992.

Maliski, S. L., Heilemann, M. V., & McCorkle, R. (2002). From 'death sentence' to 'good cancer': Couples' transformation of a prostate cancer diagnosis. *Nursing Research, 51,* 391–397.

Martin, K., Froelicher, E. S., & Miller, N. H. (2000). Women's Initiative for Nonsmoking (WINS) I: The intervention. *Heart & Lung, 29,* 438–445.

Mentes, J., & Tripp-Reimer, T. (2002). Barriers and facilitators in nursing home intervention research. *Western Journal of Nursing Research, 24,* 918–936.

Morgan, D. G., & Stewart, N. J. (2002). Theory building through mixed-method evaluation of a dementia special care unit. *Research in Nursing & Health, 25,* 479–488.

Olson, K., Hanson, J., Michaud, M. (2003). A phase II trial of Reiki for the management of pain in advanced cancer patients. *Journal of Pain & Symptom Management, 26,* 990–997.

Polit, D. F., London, A. S., & Martinez, J. M. (2000). *Food security and hunger in poor, mother-headed families in four U. S. cities.* New York: MDRC. Available at http://www.mdrc.org

Polit, D. F., London, A. S., & Martinez, J. M. (2001). *The health of poor urban women.* New York: MDRC (available at www.mdrc.org).

Rew, L., Chambers, K. B., & Kulkarni, S. (2002). Planning a sexual health promotion intervention with homeless adolescents. *Nursing Research, 51,* 168–174.

Rew, L., Fouladi, R. T., & Yockey, R. D. (2002). Sexual health practices of homeless youth. *Journal of Nursing Scholarship, 34,* 139–145.

Robinson, J. R., Clements, K., & Land, C. (2003). Workplace stress among psychiatric nurses. Prevalence, distribution, correlates, & predictors. *Journal of Psychosocial Nursing and Mental Health Services, 41*, 32–41.

Root, S. D. (2000). Implementing a shared governance model in the perioperative setting. *AORN Journal, 72*, 95–102.

Ross, L., & Johansen, C. (2002). Psychosocial home visits in cancer treatment: A qualitative study on the content of home visits. *Cancer Nursing, 25*, 350–357.

Thorne, S., Con, A., McGuinness, L., McPerson, G., & Harris, S. R. (2004). Health care communication issues in multiple sclerosis: An interpretive description. *Qualitative Health Research, 14*, 5–22.

Tilden, V. P., Tolle, S. W., Nelson, C. A., & Fields, J. (2001). Family decision-making to withdraw life-sustaining treatments from hospitalized patients. *Nursing Research, 50*, 105–115.

Weinstein, H. M., Sarnoff, R., Gladstone, E., & Lipson, J. (2000). Physical and psychological health issues of resettled refugees in the United States. *Journal of Refugee Studies, 13*, 303–327.

Wendler, M. C. (2001). Triangulation using a meta-matrix. *Journal of Advanced Nursing, 35*, 521–525.

Wilson, K., & Williams, A. (2000). Visualism in community nursing: Implications for telephone work with service users. *Qualitative Health Research, 10*, 507–520.

Young, J., Nikolette, S., McCaul, K., Twigg, D., & Morey, P. (2002). Risk factors associated with pressure ulcer development at a major western Australian teaching hospital from 1998 to 2000: Secondary data analysis. *Journal of Wound Ostomy & Continence Nursing, 29*, 234–241.

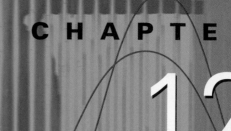

Examining Sampling Plans

12

BASIC SAMPLING CONCEPTS
Populations
Samples and Sampling
Strata
**SAMPLING DESIGNS IN QUANTITATIVE
   RESEARCH**
Nonprobability Sampling
Probability Sampling
Sample Size in Quantitative Studies
SAMPLING IN QUALITATIVE RESEARCH
The Logic of Qualitative Sampling
Types of Qualitative Sampling
Sample Size in Qualitative Studies

Sampling in the Three Main Qualitative
   Traditions
CRITIQUING THE SAMPLING PLAN
Critiquing Quantitative Sampling Plans
Critiquing Qualitative Sampling Plans
CHAPTER REVIEW
Key New Terms
Summary Points
**RESEARCH EXAMPLES: CRITICAL THINKING
   ACTIVITIES**
SUGGESTED READINGS
Methodologic References
Studies Cited in Chapter 12

STUDENT OBJECTIVES

On completing this chapter, you will be able to:

▶ Describe the rationale for sampling in research
▶ Identify differences in the logic and evaluation criteria used in sampling for quantitative versus qualitative studies
▶ Distinguish between nonprobability and probability samples and compare their advantages and disadvantages in both qualitative and quantitative studies
▶ Identify several types of sampling in qualitative and quantitative studies and describe their main characteristics
▶ Evaluate the appropriateness of the sampling method and sample size used in a study
▶ Define new terms in the chapter

S ampling is a process familiar to all of us—we gather information, make decisions, and formulate predictions about phenomena based on contact with a limited portion of them. Researchers, too, derive knowledge and draw conclusions from samples. In testing the efficacy of a nursing intervention for cancer patients, nurse researchers reach conclusions without testing the intervention with every victim of the disease. However, researchers cannot afford to draw conclusions about nursing interventions and other health-related phenomena based on faulty samples. The consequences of erroneous inferences are more momentous in drawing research conclusions than in private decision making.

BASIC SAMPLING CONCEPTS

Sampling is an important step in the research process. In quantitative studies in particular, the findings can be seriously compromised by sampling inadequacies. Let us first consider some terms associated with sampling—terms that are used primarily (but not exclusively) in connection with quantitative studies.

Populations

A **population** is the entire aggregation of cases that meet specified criteria. For instance, if a researcher were studying American nurses with doctoral degrees, the population could be defined as all U.S. citizens who are RNs and who have acquired a DNSc, PhD, or other doctoral-level degree. Other possible populations might be: all the cardiac patients hospitalized in Suffolk Hospital in 2004; all women in treatment for breast cancer who live in San Francisco; or all the children in New Zealand with cystic fibrosis. Thus, a population may be broadly defined, involving millions of people, or narrowly specified to include only several hundred people.

Populations are not restricted to human subjects. A population might consist of all the shift reports from the Gold Coast Hospital from 2001 to 2004, or all the U.S. high schools with a school-based clinic that dispenses contraceptives. Whatever the basic unit, the population comprises the aggregate of entities in which a researcher is interested.

Quantitative researchers (and sometimes qualitative researchers) specify the characteristics that delimit the study population through the **eligibility criteria** (or *inclusion criteria*). For example, consider the population of American nursing students. Would this population include part-time students? Would RNs returning to school for a bachelor's degree be included? Researchers establish these criteria to determine whether a person qualifies as a member of the population. Readers of a research report (especially in quantitative studies) need to know the eligibility criteria to understand the population to which the findings apply. Sometimes, a population

Example of eligibility criteria in a quantitative study

Allison and Keller (2004) studied the effectiveness of an intervention for older postcardiac patients in Texas. To be included, patients had to be (a) aged 65 to 80 years old; (b) diagnosed with coronary heart disease; and (c) referred to Phase I cardiac rehabilitation. Patients were excluded if they (a) terminated Phase I cardiac rehabilitation; (b) had complex dysrhythmias; (c) had disorders that affected mobility; and (d) could not understand either English or Spanish.

is defined in terms of characteristics that people must *not* possess through *exclusion criteria* (e.g., the population may be defined to exclude people who do not speak English).

Example of eligibility criteria in a qualitative study

Kvigne and Kirkevold (2003) conducted a phenomenological study of Norwegian women's experiences with their changing body following stroke. The eligibility criteria for the study included the following: (1) female; (2) hospitalized for a first-time stroke; (3) no serious mental or linguistic disorder; and (4) not suffering from other serious disorders that might overshadow the experience of stroke.

Quantitative researchers sample from an accessible population in the hope of generalizing to a target population. The **target population** is the entire population in which a researcher is interested. The **accessible population** comprises cases from the target population that are accessible to the researcher as a pool of subjects. For example, the researcher's target population might consist of all diabetic patients in the United States, but, in reality, the population that is accessible to him or her might consist of diabetic patients who are members of a particular health plan.

CONSUMER TIP

The development of an evidence-based practice is dependent upon good information about the population about whom research has been conducted. Many quantitative researchers fail to identify their target populations or discuss the issue of the generalizability of their findings. Researchers should carefully communicate their populations so that users will know whether the findings have external validity and are relevant to groups with whom they work.

■

Samples and Sampling

Sampling is the process of selecting a portion of the population to represent the entire population. A **sample**, then, is a subset of the population. The entities that make up the samples and populations are *elements*. In nursing research, the elements are usually humans.

Researchers work with samples rather than with populations because it is more economical and practical to do so. Researchers have neither the time nor the resources to study all members of a population. Furthermore, it is unnecessary to study everyone because it is usually possible to obtain reasonably good information from a sample.

Still, information from samples can lead to erroneous conclusions, and this is especially a concern in quantitative studies.

In quantitative studies, *the overriding criterion of adequacy is a sample's representativeness*—the extent to which the sample is similar to the population. Unfortunately, there is no method for ensuring that a sample is representative. Certain sampling plans are less likely to result in biased samples than others, but there is never a guarantee of a representative sample. Researchers operate under conditions in which error is possible, but quantitative researchers strive to minimize or control those errors. Consumers must assess their success in having done so—their success in minimizing sampling bias.

Sampling bias is the systematic overrepresentation or underrepresentation of some segment of the population in terms of a characteristic relevant to the research question. Sampling bias is affected by many things, including the homogeneity of the population. If the elements in a population were all identical on the critical attribute, any sample would be as good as any other. Indeed, if the population were completely homogeneous (i.e., exhibited no variability at all), a single element would be a sufficient sample for drawing conclusions about the population. For many physical or physiologic attributes, it may be safe to assume a reasonable degree of homogeneity. For example, the blood in a person's veins is relatively homogeneous; hence, a single blood sample chosen haphazardly from a patient is adequate for clinical purposes. Most human attributes, however, are not homogeneous. Variables, after all, derive their name from the fact that traits vary from one person to the next. Age, blood pressure, and stress level, for example, are all attributes that reflect the heterogeneity of humans.

Strata

Populations consist of subpopulations, or **strata**. Strata are mutually exclusive segments of a population based on a specific characteristic. For instance, a population consisting of all RNs in the United States could be divided into two strata based on gender. Alternatively, we could specify three strata consisting of nurses younger than 30 years, nurses aged 30 to 45 years, and nurses aged 46 years or older. Strata are used in the sample selection process in quantitative studies to enhance the sample's representativeness.

CONSUMER TIP

The sampling plan is usually discussed in a report's method section, sometimes in a subsection called "Sample," "Subjects," or "Participants." A description of sample characteristics, however, may be reported in the results section. If researchers have undertaken analyses to detect sample biases, these may be described in either the method or results section (e.g., researchers might compare the characteristics of patients who were invited to participate in the study but who declined to do so with those of patients who actually became subjects).

SAMPLING DESIGNS IN QUANTITATIVE STUDIES

Quantitative and qualitative researchers have different approaches to sampling. Quantitative researchers select samples that allow them to generalize their results by developing an appropriate plan before data collection begins. Qualitative researchers are not as concerned with generalizability but rather want to achieve an in-depth, holistic understanding of the phenomenon of interest. They allow sampling decisions to emerge during the course of data collection based on informational and theoretical needs. This section discusses sampling strategies used by quantitative researchers and the next section focuses on sampling in qualitative investigations.

The two main sampling design issues in quantitative studies are how the sample is selected and how many elements are included. There are two broad types of sampling designs in quantitative research: probability sampling and nonprobability sampling.

Nonprobability Sampling

In **nonprobability sampling**, researchers select elements by nonrandom methods. There is no way to estimate the probability of including each element in a nonprobability sample, and every element usually does not have a chance for inclusion. Three primary methods of nonprobability sampling are used in quantitative studies: convenience, quota, and purposive sampling.

CONVENIENCE AND SNOWBALL SAMPLING

Convenience sampling (or *accidental sampling*) entails using the most conveniently available people as participants. A nurse who distributes questionnaires about vitamin use to the first 100 available community-dwelling elders is using a convenience sample. The problem with convenience sampling is that available subjects might be atypical of the population; therefore, the price of convenience is the risk of bias.

Another type of convenience sampling is **snowball sampling** (or *network sampling* or *chain sampling*). With this approach, early sample members are asked to refer others who meet the eligibility criteria. This method of sampling is most often used when the population consists of people with specific traits who might be difficult to identify by ordinary means (e.g., people who are afraid of hospitals).

Convenience sampling is the weakest (but most widely used) form of sampling for quantitative studies. In heterogeneous populations, there is no other sampling method in which the risk of bias is greater—and there is no way to evaluate the biases. Caution is needed in interpreting findings and generalizing results from quantitative studies based on convenience samples.

Example of a convenience sample

Shaker, Scott, and Reid (2004) studied the infant feeding attitudes (breastfeeding versus formula feeding) of expectant parents. Their sample was a convenience sample of 108 expectant mothers and their partners attending three maternity clinics in Scotland.

QUOTA SAMPLING

In **quota sampling**, researchers identify strata of the population and then determine how many participants are needed from each stratum to meet a quota. By using information about population characteristics, researchers can ensure that diverse segments are adequately represented.

As an example, suppose we were interested in studying the attitudes of undergraduate nursing students toward working on an AIDS unit. The accessible population is a nursing school with an enrollment of 500 undergraduates; a sample size of 100 students is desired. With a convenience sample, we could distribute questionnaires to 100 students as they entered the nursing school library. Suppose, however, that we suspect that male and female students have different attitudes toward working with AIDS victims. A convenience sample might result in too many men, or too few. Table 12-1 presents some fictitious data showing the gender distribution for the population and for a convenience sample (second and third columns). In this example, the convenience sample seriously overrepresents women and underrepresents men. In a quota sample, researchers can guide the selection of subjects so that the sample includes an appropriate number of cases from both strata. The far-right panel of Table 12-1 shows the number of men and women required for a quota sample for this example.

If we pursue this example a bit further, you may better appreciate the dangers of a biased sample. Suppose the key question in this study was: Would you be willing to work on a unit that cared exclusively for AIDS patients? The percentage of students in the population who would respond "yes" to this question is shown in the first column of Table 12-2. Of course, these values

TABLE 12.1 **Numbers and Percentages of Students in Strata of a Population, Convenience Sample, and Quota Sample**

STRATA	POPULATION	CONVENIENCE SAMPLE	QUOTA SAMPLE
Male	100 (20%)	5 (5%)	20 (20%)
Female	400 (80%)	95 (95%)	80 (80%)
Total	500 (100%)	100 (100%)	100 (100%)

would not be known; they are displayed to illustrate a point. Within the population, male students are more likely than female students to express willingness to work on an AIDS unit, yet men were underrepresented in the convenience sample. As a result, there is a notable discrepancy between the population and sample values: Nearly twice as many students in the population are favorable toward working with AIDS victims (20%) than in the convenience sample (11%). The quota sample, on the other hand, does a reasonably good job of reflecting the population's views.

Except for identifying key strata, quota sampling is procedurally similar to convenience sampling: Subjects are a convenience sample from each population stratum. Because of this fact, quota sampling shares many of the weaknesses of convenience sampling. For instance, if we were required by the quota sampling plan to interview 20 male nursing students, a trip to the dormitories might be a convenient method of recruiting those subjects. Yet this approach would fail to give any representation to male students living off campus, who may have distinctive views about working with AIDS patients. Despite its problems, however, quota sampling is an important improvement over convenience sampling for quantitative studies. Quota sampling is a relatively easy way to enhance the representativeness of a nonprobability sample and does not require sophisticated skills or a lot of effort. Surprisingly, few researchers use this strategy.

Example of a quota sample

Reyes, Meininger, Liehr, Chan, and Mueller (2003) examined differences in adolescents' anger by gender, age, and ethnicity. They used quota sampling to ensure adequate representation of diverse subgroups of adolescents.

TABLE 12.2 **Students Willing to Work on AIDS Unit: Population, Convenience Sample, and Quota Sample**

	NUMBER IN POPULATION	NUMBER IN CONVENIENCE SAMPLE	NUMBER IN QUOTA SAMPLE
Willing males	28 (out of 100)	2 (out of 5)	6 (out of 20)
Willing females	72 (out of 400)	9 (out of 95)	13 (out of 80)
Total number of willing students	100 (out of 500)	11 (out of 100)	19 (out of 100)
Percentage willing	20%	11%	19%

PURPOSIVE SAMPLING

Purposive sampling (or *judgmental sampling*), is based on the belief that researchers' knowledge about the population can be used to hand pick the cases (or types of cases) to be included in the sample. Researchers might decide purposely to select the widest possible variety of respondents or might choose subjects who are judged to be typical of the population in question or particularly knowledgeable about the issues under study. Sampling in this subjective manner, however, provides no external, objective method for assessing the typicalness of the selected subjects. Nevertheless, this method can be used to advantage in certain instances. For example, sometimes researchers want to ask questions of a group of experts. Also, as discussed in a later section, purposive sampling is often used productively by qualitative researchers.

Example of a purposive sample

Staggers, Gassert, and Curran (2002) conducted a study to identify informatics competencies needed for nurses at various levels of practice. They conducted a 3-round survey with a purposive sample of expert nurses who had at least 5 years of experience in nursing informatics and had high visibility within the specialty.

EVALUATION OF NONPROBABILITY SAMPLING

Nonprobability samples are rarely representative of the target population—some segment of the population is likely to be systematically underrepresented. And, when there is sampling bias, there is a good chance that the results will be misleading or erroneous. Why, then, are nonprobability samples used at all in quantitative research? Clearly, the advantage of these sampling designs lies in their convenience and economy. Probability sampling requires resources and time. There may be no option but to use a nonprobability sampling plan. Researchers using a nonprobability sample out of necessity should be cautious about their conclusions, and you as reader should be alert to the possibility of sampling bias.

HOW-TO-TELL TIP

How can you tell what type of sampling design was used in a quantitative study? Researchers who have made explicit efforts to achieve a representative sample usually indicate the type of sampling design in the method section. If the sampling design is not specified, it is probably safe to assume that a sample of convenience was used. ■

Probability Sampling

Probability sampling involves the random selection of elements from the population. *Random selection* should not be confused with *random assignment*, which was described in Chapter 9. Random assignment is the process of allocating subjects to different treatments on a random basis in experimental designs. Random assignment has no bearing on how subjects in the experiment were selected in the first place. A **random selection** process is one in which each element in the population has an equal, independent chance of being selected. Because probability samples involve selecting units at random, some confidence can be placed in their representativeness.

The four most commonly used probability sampling designs are simple random, stratified random, cluster, and systematic sampling.

SIMPLE RANDOM SAMPLING

Simple random sampling is the most basic probability sampling design. Because more complex probability sampling designs incorporate features of simple random sampling, the procedures are briefly described so that you can understand what is involved.

After defining the population, researchers establish a *sampling frame*, the technical name for the actual list of the population elements. If nursing students at the University of Connecticut were the accessible population, then a student roster would be the sampling frame. If the population were 300-bed or larger general hospitals in the United Kingdom, then a list of all those hospitals would be the sampling frame. Populations are sometimes defined in terms of an existing sampling frame. For example, a researcher might use a telephone directory as a sampling frame. In such a case, the population would be defined as the residents of a certain community who have telephones and who have a listed number. After a list of population elements has been developed, the elements are numbered consecutively. A table of random numbers or a computer program is then used to draw, at random, a sample of the desired size.

Samples selected randomly in such a fashion are not subject to researcher biases. There is no *guarantee* that the sample will be representative of the population, but random selection does guarantee that differences between the sample and the population are purely a function of chance. The probability of selecting a markedly deviant sample through random sampling is low, and this probability decreases as the sample size increases.

Simple random sampling is a laborious process. The development of the sampling frame, enumeration of all the elements, and selection of the sample elements are time-consuming chores, particularly with a large population. Moreover, it is rarely possible to get a complete listing of population elements; hence, other methods are often used.

Example of a random sample

Criste (2003) examined whether nurse anesthetists demonstrate gender bias in treating pain. Questionnaires were mailed to a national random sample of 450 currently practicing Certified Registered Nurse Anesthetists in the United States.

STRATIFIED RANDOM SAMPLING

In **stratified random sampling**, the population is divided into homogeneous subsets from which elements are selected at random. As in quota sampling, the aim of stratified sampling is to enhance the sample's representativeness. The most common procedure for drawing a stratified random sample is to group together those elements that belong to a stratum and to randomly select the desired number of elements.

Researchers may sample either proportionately (in relation to the size of the stratum) or disproportionately. If a population of students in a nursing school in the United States consisted of 10% African Americans, 5% Hispanics, and 85% Whites, a **proportionate sample** of 100 students, stratified on race/ethnicity, would consist of 10, 5, and 85 students from the respective strata. Researchers often use a **disproportionate sample** whenever comparisons between strata of unequal size are desired. In our example, the researcher might select 20 African Americans,

20 Hispanics, and 60 Whites to ensure a more adequate representation of the viewpoints of the two racial minorities. (When disproportionate sampling is used, however, it is necessary to make a mathematical adjustment—known as **weighting**—to the data to arrive at the best estimate of overall population values.)

By using stratified random sampling, researchers can sharpen the precision and representativeness of their samples. Stratified sampling may, however, be impossible if information on the stratifying variables is unavailable (e.g., a student roster might not include information on race and ethnicity). Furthermore, a stratified sample requires even more labor than simple random sampling because the sample must be drawn from multiple enumerated listings.

Example of a stratified random sample

Ulrich, Soeken, and Miller (2003) studied the views of nurse practitioners (NPs) regarding ethical conflicts associated with managed care. The researchers mailed questionnaires to a stratified random sample of 700 NPs licensed to practice in the state of Maryland. The stratifying variable was primary care specialty (Family Health, Pediatrics, Obstetrics/Gynecology, and Adult Health) as listed with the Maryland State Board of Nursing.

CLUSTER SAMPLING

For many populations, it is impossible to obtain a listing of all elements. For example, there is no listing of all full-time nursing students in the United States. Large-scale quantitative studies rarely use simple or stratified random sampling. The most common procedure for national surveys is cluster sampling.

In **cluster sampling**, there is a successive random sampling of units. The first unit to be sampled is large groupings, or clusters. For example, in drawing a sample of nursing students, researchers might first draw a random sample of nursing schools and then sample students from the selected schools. The usual procedure for selecting samples from a general population is to sample such administrative units as states, cities, census tracts, and then households, successively. Because of the successive stages of sampling, this approach is sometimes referred to as *multistage sampling*.

For a specified number of cases, cluster sampling tends to contain more sampling error than simple or stratified random sampling. Nevertheless, cluster sampling is more economical and practical when the population is large and widely dispersed.

Example of a cluster/multistage sample

Thato, Charron-Prochownik, Dorn, Albrecht, and Stone (2003) studied predictors of condom use among adolescent Thai vocational students. In the first stage, the researchers randomly selected eight private vocational schools in Bangkok, and then randomly selected students from the school. A total of 425 students aged 18 to 22 were sampled.

SYSTEMATIC SAMPLING

Systematic sampling involves the selection of every *k*th case from some list or group, such as every 10th person on a patient list. Systematic sampling designs can be applied in such a way that an essentially random sample is drawn. First, the size of the population is divided by the size of the desired sample to obtain the sampling interval width. The *sampling interval* is the standard distance between the selected elements. For instance, if we wanted a sample of 50 from a population of 5000, our sampling interval would be 100 (5000/50 = 100). In other words, every 100th case on the sampling frame would be sampled. Next, the first case would be selected randomly (e.g., by using a table of random numbers). If the random number chosen were 73, the people corresponding to numbers 73, 173, 273, and so forth would be included in the sample. Systematic sampling conducted in this manner is essentially identical to simple random sampling and often is preferable because the same results are obtained in a more convenient manner.

Example of a systematic random sample

Ruchala, Metheny, Essenpreis, and Borcherding (2003) surveyed a national sample of obstetric units in the United States to determine the types of intravenous fluids used to dilute oxytocin for labor induction. They mailed questionnaires to a systematic random sample of nurse managers in 700 obstetric units with 50 or more births per year as listed by the American Hospital Association.

EVALUATION OF PROBABILITY SAMPLING

Probability sampling is the only reliable method of obtaining representative samples in quantitative studies. Probability sampling avoids the risk of conscious or unconscious biases. If all the elements in the population have an equal probability of being selected, there is a high likelihood that the sample will represent the population adequately. A further advantage is that probability sampling allows researchers to estimate the magnitude of sampling error. **Sampling error** is the difference between population values (e.g., the average heart rate of the population) and sample values (e.g., the average heart rate of the sample). It is rare that a sample is perfectly representative of a population and contains no sampling error; however, probability sampling permits estimates of the degree of expected error. On the other hand, probability sampling is expensive and demanding. Unless the population is narrowly defined, it is beyond the scope of most researchers to draw a probability sample.

CONSUMER TIP

The quality of the sampling plan is of particular importance in survey research, because the purpose of surveys is to obtain descriptive information about the prevalence or average values for a population. All national surveys, such as the National Health Interview Survey in the United States use probability samples (usually cluster samples). Probability samples are rarely used in experimental and quasi-experimental studies, in part because the main focus of such inquiries is on between-group differences rather than absolute values for a population.
▬

Sample Size in Quantitative Studies

Sample size—the number of subjects in a sample—is a major issue in conducting and evaluating quantitative research. There is no simple equation to determine how large a sample is needed, but quantitative researchers are generally advised to use the largest sample possible. The larger the sample, the more representative it is likely to be. Every time researchers calculate a percentage or an average based on sample data, the purpose is to estimate a population value. The larger the sample, the smaller the sampling error.

Let us illustrate this with an example of estimating monthly aspirin consumption in a nursing home (Table 12-3). The population is 15 nursing home residents whose aspirin consumption averages 16 per month. Two simple random samples with sample sizes of 2, 3, 5, and 10 were drawn from the population of 15 residents. Each sample average on the right represents an estimate of the population average, which we know is 16. (Under ordinary circumstances, the population value would be unknown, and we would draw only one sample.) With a sample size of 2, our estimate might have been wrong by as many as eight aspirins (sample 1B). As the sample size increases, the average gets closer to the population value, and differences in the estimates between samples A and B get smaller. As the sample size increases, the probability of getting a deviant sample diminishes because large samples provide the opportunity to counterbalance atypical values.

Sophisticated researchers estimate how large their samples should be to adequately test their research hypotheses through **power analysis** (Cohen, 1988). A simple example can illustrate basic principles of power analysis. Suppose a researcher were testing a new intervention to help people quit smoking; smokers would be randomly assigned to either an experimental or a control group. The question is, how many subjects should be used in this study? When using power analysis, researchers estimate how large the group difference will be (e.g., the difference in the average number of cigarettes smoked in the week after the intervention). This estimate might be based on previous research, on the researchers' personal experience, or on other factors. When expected differences are large, it does not take a large sample to ensure that the differences will be revealed in a statistical analysis; but when small differences are predicted, large samples are needed. Cohen (1988) claimed that, for new areas of research, group differences are likely to be small. In our example, if a small group difference in postintervention smoking were

TABLE 12.3	Comparison of Population and Sample Values and Averages in Nursing Home Aspirin Consumption Example		
NUMBER IN GROUP	**GROUP**	**VALUES (MONTHLY NUMBER OF ASPIRINS CONSUMED)**	**AVERAGE**
15	Population	2, 4, 6, 8, 10, 12, 14, 16, 18, 20, 22, 24, 26, 28, 30	16.0
2	Sample 1A	6, 14	10.0
2	Sample 1B	20, 28	24.0
3	Sample 2A	16, 18, 8	14.0
3	Sample 2B	20, 14, 26	20.0
5	Sample 3A	26, 14, 18, 2, 28	17.6
5	Sample 3B	30, 2, 26, 10, 4	14.4
10	Sample 4A	18, 16, 24, 22, 8, 14, 28, 20, 2, 6	15.8
10	Sample 4B	14, 18, 12, 20, 6, 14, 28, 12, 24, 16	16.4

expected, the sample size needed to test the effectiveness of the new program, assuming standard statistical criteria, would be about 800 smokers (400 per group). If a medium-sized difference were expected, the total sample size would still need to be several hundred smokers.

When samples are too small, quantitative researchers run the risk of gathering data that will not support their hypotheses—even when those hypotheses are correct. As we discussed in Chapter 9, this would undermine the study's statistical conclusion validity. Large samples are no assurance of accuracy, however. With nonprobability sampling, even a large sample can harbor extensive bias. The famous example illustrating this point is the 1936 U. S. presidential poll conducted by the magazine *Literary Digest,* which predicted that Alfred M. Landon would defeat Franklin D. Roosevelt by a landslide. A large sample of about 2.5 million people participated in this poll, but biases arose because the sample was drawn from telephone directories and automobile registrations during a Depression year when only the well-to-do (who favored Landon) had a car or telephone.

A large sample cannot correct for a faulty sampling design; nevertheless, a large non-probability sample is preferable to a small one. When critiquing quantitative studies, you must assess both the sample size and the sample selection method to judge how representative the sample likely was.

CONSUMER TIP

The sampling plan is often one of the weakest aspects of quantitative nursing studies (this is also true of quantitative research in other disciplines). Most nursing studies use samples of convenience, and many are based on samples that are too small to provide an adequate test of the research hypotheses. Most quantitative studies are based on samples of fewer than 200 subjects, and a great many studies have fewer than 100 subjects. Power analysis is not used by many nurse researchers, and research reports typically offer no justification for the size of the study sample. Small samples run a high risk of leading researchers to erroneously reject their research hypotheses. Therefore, you should be especially prepared to critique the sampling plan of studies that fail to support research hypotheses.

SAMPLING IN QUALITATIVE RESEARCH

Qualitative studies typically use small, nonrandom samples. This does not mean that qualitative researchers are unconcerned with the quality of their samples, but rather that they use different criteria for selecting participants. This section examines sampling considerations in qualitative studies.

The Logic of Qualitative Sampling

Quantitative research is concerned with measuring attributes and relationships in a population, and therefore a representative sample is needed to ensure that the measurements accurately reflect and can be generalized to the population. The aim of most qualitative studies is to discover meaning and to uncover multiple realities; therefore, generalizability, as quantitative researchers use this term, is not a guiding criterion.

Qualitative researchers ask such sampling questions as: Who would be an information-rich data source for my study? and Whom should I talk to, or what should I observe, to maximize my understanding of the phenomenon? A critical first step in qualitative sampling is selecting settings with high potential for "information richness."

As the study progresses, new sampling questions emerge, such as the following: Whom can I talk to or observe to confirm my understandings? Challenge or modify my understandings? Enrich my understandings? Thus, as with the overall design in qualitative studies, sampling design is an emergent one that capitalizes on early learning to guide subsequent direction.

Another point worth mentioning is that individuals are not always considered the *unit of analysis* in qualitative studies. For example, Glaser and Strauss (1967) have noted that "incidents" or experiences are the basis for analysis. An information-rich informant can therefore contribute dozens of incidents, and so even a small number of informants can generate a large sample for analysis.

Example of a large sample of incidents in a qualitative study

Thulesius, Håkansson, and Petersson (2003) conducted a grounded theory study of basic processes in end-of-life cancer care in Sweden. They interviewed 64 participants (nurses, physicians, patients, and relatives) over an 8-year period. Their interviews generated over 1000 incidents, which were used to identify *balancing* as the main social process.

Types of Qualitative Sampling

Qualitative researchers usually eschew probability samples. A random sample is not the best method of selecting people who will make good informants—people who are knowledgeable, articulate, reflective, and willing to talk at length with a researcher.

CONVENIENCE AND SNOWBALL SAMPLING

Qualitative researchers sometimes use or begin with a convenience sample, which is sometimes referred to as a **volunteer sample**. Volunteer samples are especially likely to be used when researchers need participants to come forward to identify themselves (*e.g.*, by placing notices in newspapers for people with certain experiences) or when they need to rely on referrals from others.

Sampling by convenience is often efficient, but it is not usually a preferred sampling approach, even in qualitative studies. The key aim in qualitative studies is to extract the greatest possible information from the small number of informants in the sample, and a convenience sample may not provide the most information-rich sources. However, a convenience sample may be an economical way to begin the sampling process.

Example of a convenience sample

Porter (2003) conducted a phenomenological study to describe older frail widows' experience of having a personal emergency response system. She recruited a convenience sample of eight frail widows aged 80 years or older through representatives of social service agencies in six counties in central Missouri.

Qualitative researchers also use snowball sampling, asking early informants to make referrals for other study participants. This method is sometimes referred to as *nominated sampling* because it relies on the nominations of others already in the sample. Researchers may use this method to gain access to people who are difficult to identify. A weakness of this approach is that the eventual sample might be restricted to a rather small network of acquaintances.

Moreover, the quality of the referrals may be affected by whether the referring sample member trusted the researcher and truly wanted to cooperate.

Example of a snowball sample

Dickinson and Digman (2002) used snowball sampling to identify mothers in New Zealand for their descriptive study of how mothers manage a preschool child's acute asthma episode.

PURPOSIVE SAMPLING

Qualitative sampling may begin with volunteer informants and may be supplemented with new participants through snowballing, but many qualitative studies eventually evolve to a purposive (or *purposeful*) sampling strategy—to a strategy in which researchers hand pick the cases or types of cases that will best contribute to the information needs of the study. That is, regardless of how initial participants are selected, qualitative researchers often strive to select sample members purposefully based on the information needs emerging from the early findings. Whom to sample next depends on who has been sampled already.

Example of a purposive sample

Woodgate and Degner (2003) undertook a descriptive qualitative study to describe the cancer symptom course experienced by children with cancer and their families in Manitoba, Canada. Their sample included a purposive sample of 39 children chosen to represent a variety of cancer diagnoses.

Within purposive sampling, several strategies have been identified (Patton, 2002), only some of which are mentioned here. Note that researchers themselves do not necessarily refer to their sampling plans with Patton's labels; his classification shows the kind of diverse strategies qualitative researchers have adopted to meet the theoretical needs of their research:

▶ *Maximum variation sampling* involves purposefully selecting cases with a range of variation on dimensions of interest
▶ *Homogeneous sampling* involves a deliberate reduction of variation to permit a more focused inquiry
▶ *Extreme/deviant case sampling* provides opportunities for learning from the most unusual and extreme informants (e.g., outstanding successes and notable failures)
▶ *Typical case sampling* involves selecting participants who will illustrate or highlight what is typical or average
▶ *Criterion sampling* involves studying cases that meet a predetermined criterion of importance

Example of maximum variation sampling

McCarthy (2003) used maximum variation sampling to explore nurses' clinical reasoning in their differentiation of acute confusion and dementia in elderly patients. Nurses were purposely selected to represent a range of acute-care settings, nursing specialty areas, and types of training.

Maximum variation sampling is often the sampling mode of choice in qualitative research because it is useful in documenting the scope of a phenomenon and in identifying important patterns that cut across variations. Other strategies can also be used advantageously, however, depending on the nature of the research question.

CONSUMER TIP

A qualitative research report will not necessary use such terms as "maximum variation sampling," but may describe the researcher's intent in selecting a diverse sample of participants. ■

A strategy of sampling confirming and disconfirming cases is another purposive strategy that is often used toward the end of data collection in qualitative studies. As researchers note trends and patterns in the data, emerging conceptualizations may need to be checked. **Confirming cases** are additional cases that fit researchers' conceptualizations and offer enhanced credibility. **Disconfirming cases** are new cases that do not fit and serve to challenge researchers' interpretations. These "negative" cases may offer new insights about how the original conceptualization needs to be revised or expanded.

CONSUMER TIP

Some qualitative researchers appear to call their sample purposive simply because they "purposely" selected people who were exposed to the phenomenon of interest. However, exposure to the phenomenon is actually an eligibility criterion—the population of interest comprises people with that exposure. If the researcher then recruits *any* person with that exposure, the sample is selected by convenience, not purposively. Purposive sampling implies an intent to carefully choose *particular* exemplars or *types* of people who can best enhance the researcher's understanding of the phenomenon. ■

THEORETICAL SAMPLING

Theoretical sampling is a method of sampling that is most often used in grounded theory studies. Glaser (1978) defined this sampling approach as "the process of data collection for

Example of a theoretical sample

Beck (2002) used theoretical sampling in her grounded theory study of mothering twins during the first year of life, in which 16 mothers of twins were interviewed. An example of theoretical sampling concerned what the mothers kept referring to as the "blur period"—the first few months of caring for the twins. Initially, Beck interviewed mothers whose twins were around 1 year old. Her rationale was that these mothers would be able to reflect back over the entire first year of mothering the multiples. When these mothers referred to the "blur period," Beck asked them to describe this period more fully, but they could not provide many details because the period was "such a blur!" Beck then chose to interview mothers whose twins were 3 months old or younger, to ensure that mothers still immersed in the "blur period" would be able to provide rich detail about what this phase of mothering twins was like.

generating theory whereby the analyst jointly collects, codes, and analyzes his data and decides what data to collect next and where to find them, in order to develop his theory as it emerges" (p. 36). This complex sampling technique requires researchers to be involved with multiple lines and directions as they go back and forth between data and categories as the theory emerges.

Glaser stressed that theoretical sampling is not the same as purposeful sampling. The purpose of theoretical sampling is to discover categories and their properties and to offer interrelationships that occur in the substantive theory. Glaser noted that the basic question in theoretical sampling is: What groups or subgroups should the researcher turn to next? The groups are chosen as they are needed for their theoretical relevance in furthering the emerging conceptualization.

Sample Size in Qualitative Studies

There are no established rules for sample size in qualitative research. Sample size is largely a function of the purpose of the inquiry, the quality of the informants, and the type of sampling strategy used. For example, a larger sample is likely to be needed with maximum variation sampling than with typical case sampling. Patton argues that purposive sample sizes should "be judged on the basis of the purpose and rationale of each study.... The sample, like all other aspects of qualitative inquiry, must be judged in context..." (2002, p. 245).

In qualitative research, sample size is usually determined based on informational needs. Hence, a guiding principle in sampling is **data saturation** (i.e., sampling to the point at which no new information is obtained and redundancy is achieved). Redundancy can typically be achieved with a fairly small number of cases, if the information from each is of sufficient depth. Morse (2000) noted that the number of participants needed to reach saturation depends on a number of factors. For example, the broader the scope of the research question, the more participants will likely be needed. Data quality can also affect sample size. If participants are good informants who are able to reflect on their experiences and communicate effectively, saturation can be achieved with relatively few informants. Also, if longitudinal data are collected, fewer participants may be needed, because each will provide a greater amount of information. As discussed in the next section, sample size is also partly a function of the type of qualitative inquiry that is undertaken.

CONSUMER TIP

The sample size adequacy of quantitative studies can be estimated by consumers after the fact through power analysis. However, sample size adequacy in a qualitative study is more difficult to critique on the basis of reading a research report because the main criterion is redundancy of information, which is difficult for consumers to judge. Some qualitative reports explicitly state that data saturation was achieved.

Sampling in the Three Main Qualitative Traditions

There are similarities among the various qualitative traditions with regard to sampling: Samples are generally small, probability sampling is almost never used, and final sampling decisions generally take place during data collection. However, there are some differences as well.

SAMPLING IN ETHNOGRAPHIC STUDIES

Ethnographers often begin by adopting a "big net" approach—that is, mingling with and having conversations with as many members of the culture under study as possible. Starting with this wide angle lens of the culture provides ethnographers with the "lay of the land."

While they may converse with many people (usually 25 to 50), ethnographers often rely heavily on a smaller number of **key informants**, who are highly knowledgeable about the culture and who develop special, ongoing relationships with them. These key informants are often ethnographers' main link to the "inside." Different informants belong to different groups of constituents; they allow ethnographers access to some people, but may prevent access to others, and ethnographers must be sensitive to possible informant biases.

Key informants usually are chosen purposively, guided by ethnographers' informed judgments (although sampling may become more theoretical as the study progresses). Developing a pool of potential key informants often depends on ethnographers' prior knowledge to construct a relevant framework. For example, an ethnographer might make decisions about different types of key informants to seek out based on roles (e.g., physicians, nurse practitioners) or on some other theoretically meaningful distinction. Once a pool of potential key informants is developed, the main considerations for final selection are their level of knowledge about the culture and how willing they are to collaborate with the ethnographer in revealing and interpreting the culture. Ethnographers typically attempt to develop relationships with as diverse a group of informants as possible.

Sampling in ethnography typically involves more than selecting informants, because observation and other means of data collection play a big role in helping researchers understand a culture. Ethnographers have to decide not only *whom* to sample, but *what* to sample as well. For example, ethnographers have to make decisions about observing *events* and *activities*, about examining *records* and *artifacts*, and about exploring *places* that provide clues about the culture. Key informants can play an important role in helping ethnographers decide what to sample.

Example of an ethnographic sample

Kirkham (2003) conducted an institutional ethnography, informed by feminist and cultural theories, to examine the theme of "belonging" within the social context of intercultural health care in Canada. Fieldwork was undertaken in three medical–surgical units in two hospitals. Kirkham began with a core of 11 nurses in one of the units. She then "buddied" with 20 nurses during the course of several shifts and had formal and informal interviews with them. Sampling was purposive: She sought to represent a range of nursing experiences and ethnocultural backgrounds. In addition to nurses, she interviewed administrators and patients, as well as policy makers and educators from outside the settings.

SAMPLING IN PHENOMENOLOGICAL STUDIES

Phenomenologists tend to rely on very small samples of participants—typically 10 or fewer. There is one guiding principle in selecting the sample for a phenomenological study: All participants must have experienced the phenomenon under study and must be able to articulate what it is like to have lived that experience. Although phenomenological researchers seek participants who have had the targeted experiences, they also want to explore diversity of individual experiences. Thus, as described by Porter (1999), they may specifically look for people with demographic or other differences who have shared a common experience. To study a phenomenon of interest in depth, phenomenologists may also sample experiences of place and of events in time because a person's experience of the phenomenon under study is situated in a specific place and time.

Example of a sample in a phenomenological study

McCabe (2004) conducted a hermeneutic inquiry to study patients' experiences of how nurses communicate. McCabe purposively sampled and conducted in-depth interviews with eight patients in a general hospital in Ireland.

Interpretive phenomenologists may, in addition to sampling people, sample artistic or literary sources. Experiential descriptions of the phenomenon may be selected from a wide array of literature, such as poetry, novels, biographies, autobiographies, diaries, and journals. These sources can help increase phenomenologists' insights into the phenomena under study. Art—including paintings, sculpture, film, photographs, and music—is viewed as another source of lived experience by interpretive phenomenologists. Each artistic medium is viewed as having its own specific language or way of expressing the experience of the phenomenon.

SAMPLING IN GROUNDED THEORY STUDIES

Grounded theory research is typically done with samples of about 20 to 30 people, using theoretical sampling. The goal in a grounded theory study is to select informants who can best contribute to the evolving theory. Sampling, data collection, data analysis, and theory construction occur concurrently, and so study participants are selected serially and contingently—i.e., contingent on the emerging conceptualization. Theoretical sampling is used to develop and refine categories. As grounded theorists identify gaps or holes in their emerging theory, they go back to the field and sample data to fill in these thin areas. At this point in their research grounded theorists become very selective in their sampling: Participants are sampled only in regard to specific issues. Theoretical sampling is used not to increase the sample size but to refine the developing theory and to gain more insight into the properties of the categories. Sampling might evolve as follows:

1. The researcher begins with a general notion of where and with whom to start. The first few cases may be solicited purposively, by convenience, or through snowballing.

Example of a sample in a grounded theory study

Meeker (2004) investigated end-of-life decision making among family surrogates using grounded theory methods. The sample consisted of 20 persons who had functioned as family surrogate decision-maker during the terminal phase of a family member's cancer illness. She used theoretical sampling "to provide data needed to describe the categories thoroughly" (p. 208). For example, early participants reported that other family members had been supportive, and so she sought participants who had experienced conflict.

2. In the early part of the study, a strategy such as maximum variation sampling might be used to gain insights into the range and complexity of the phenomenon under study.
3. The sample is adjusted in an ongoing fashion. Emerging conceptualizations help to focus the sampling process to maximize understanding of the categories.
4. Sampling continues until saturation is achieved.
5. Final sampling often includes a search for confirming and disconfirming cases to test, refine, and strengthen the theory.

CRITIQUING THE SAMPLING PLAN

The sampling plan of a research study—particularly a quantitative study—merits particular scrutiny because, if the sample is seriously biased or too small, the findings may be misleading or just plain wrong. In critiquing a description of a sampling plan, you should consider two issues. The first is whether the researcher has adequately described the sampling strategy. Ideally, research reports should include a description of the following aspects of the sample:

▶ The type of sampling approach used (e.g., convenience, snowball, purposive, simple random)
▶ The population under study and the eligibility criteria for sample selection in quantitative studies; the nature of the setting and study group in qualitative ones (qualitative studies may also articulate eligibility criteria)
▶ The number of participants in the study and a rationale for the sample size
▶ A description of the main characteristics of participants (e.g., age, gender, medical condition, race/ethnicity, and so forth) and, in a quantitative study, of the population
▶ In quantitative studies, the number and characteristics of potential subjects who declined to participate in the study

If the description of the sample is inadequate, you may not be in a position to deal with the second and principal issue, which is whether the researcher made good sampling decisions.

Critiquing Quantitative Sampling Plans

We have stressed that the main criterion for assessing the adequacy of a sampling plan in quantitative research is whether the sample is representative of the population. You will never be able to know for sure, of course, but if the sampling strategy is weak or if the sample size is small, there is reason to suspect some bias. When researchers have adopted a sampling plan in which the risk for bias is high, they should take steps to estimate the direction and degree of this bias so that readers can draw some informed conclusions.

Even with a rigorous sampling plan, the sample may contain some bias if not all people invited to participate in a study agree to do so. If certain segments of the population refuse to participate, then a biased sample can result, even when probability sampling is used. The research report ideally should provide information about **response rates** (i.e., the number of people participating in a study relative to the number of people sampled), and about possible **nonresponse bias**—differences between participants and those who declined to participate (also sometimes referred to as *response bias*).

In developing the sampling plan, quantitative researchers make decisions about the specification of the population as well as the selection of the sample. If the target population is

BOX 12.1   Guidelines for Critiquing Quantitative Sampling Designs

1. Is the population under study identified and described? Are eligibility criteria specified? Are the sample selection procedures clearly delineated?
2. What type of sampling plan was used? Would an alternative sampling plan have been preferable? Was the sampling plan one that could be expected to yield a representative sample?
3. How were subjects recruited into the sample? Does the method suggest potential biases?
4. Did some factor other than the sampling plan (e.g., a low response rate) affect the representativeness of the sample?
5. Are possible sample biases or weaknesses identified?
6. Are key characteristics of the sample described (e.g., mean age, percent female)?
7. Is the sample size sufficiently large? Was the sample size justified on the basis of a power analysis or other rationale?
8. To whom can the study results reasonably be generalized?

defined broadly, researchers may have missed opportunities to control extraneous variables, and the gap between the accessible and the target population may be too great. Your job as reviewer is to come to conclusions about the reasonableness of generalizing the findings from the researcher's sample to the accessible population and from the accessible population to a broader target population. If the sampling plan is seriously flawed, it may be risky to generalize the findings at all without replicating the study with another sample.

Box 12-1 presents some guiding questions for critiquing the sampling plan of a quantitative research report.

Critiquing Qualitative Sampling Plans

In a qualitative study, the sampling plan can be evaluated in terms of its adequacy and appropriateness (Morse, 1991). *Adequacy* refers to the sufficiency and quality of the data the sample yielded. An adequate sample provides data without any "thin" spots. When the researcher has truly obtained saturation with a sample, informational adequacy has been achieved, and the resulting description or theory is richly textured and complete.

Appropriateness concerns the methods used to select a sample. An appropriate sample is one resulting from the identification and use of study participants who can best supply information according to the conceptual requirements of the study. Researchers must use a strategy that will yield the fullest possible understanding of the phenomenon of interest. A sampling approach that excludes negative cases or that fails to include participants with unusual experiences may not meet the information needs of the study.

Another important issue to consider concerns the potential for transferability of the findings. The degree of transferability of study findings is a direct function of the similarity between the sample of the original study and the people at another site to which the findings might be applied. **Fittingness** is the degree of congruence between these two groups. Thus, in critiquing a report you should see whether the researcher provided an adequately thick description of the sample, setting, and context in which the study was carried out so that someone interested in transferring the findings could make an informed decision.

Further guidance to critiquing sampling in a qualitative study is presented in Box 12-2.

BOX 12.2   Guidelines for Critiquing Qualitative Sampling Designs

1. Is the setting or context adequately described? Is the setting appropriate for the research question?
2. Are the sample selection procedures clearly delineated? What type of sampling strategy was used?
3. Were the eligibility criteria for the study specified? How were participants recruited into the study? Did the recruitment strategy yield information-rich participants?
4. Given the information needs of the study—and, if applicable, its qualitative tradition— was the sampling approach appropriate? Are dimensions of the phenomenon under study adequately represented?
5. Is the sample size adequate and appropriate for the qualitative tradition of the study? Did the researcher indicate that information redundancy had been achieved? Do the findings suggest a richly textured and comprehensive set of data without any apparent "holes" or thin areas?
6. Are key characteristics of the sample described (e.g., age, gender)? Is a rich description of participants provided, allowing for an assessment of the transferability of the findings?

CHAPTER REVIEW

Key new terms introduced in the chapter, together with a summary of major points, are presented in this section. In addition, Chapter 12 of the *Study Guide to Accompany Essentials of Nursing Research,* 6th edition offers various exercises and study suggestions for reinforcing the concepts presented in this chapter. For additional review, see the Student Self-Study Review Questions section of the Student Resource CD-ROM provided with this book.

KEY NEW TERMS

Accessible population	Proportionate sample
Cluster sampling	Purposive sampling
Confirming case	Quota sampling
Convenience sampling	Random selection
Criterion sampling	Response rate
Data saturation	Sample
Disconfirming case	Sample size
Disproportionate sample	Sampling
Eligibility criteria	Sampling bias
Extreme/deviant case sampling	Sampling error
Fittingness	Simple random sampling
Key informant	Snowball sampling
Homogenous sampling	Strata
Maximum variation sampling	Stratified random sampling
Nonprobability sampling	Systematic sampling
Nonresponse bias	Target population
Population	Theoretical sampling
Power analysis	Typical case sampling
Probability sampling	Weighting

SUMMARY POINTS

▷ **Sampling** is the process of selecting a portion of the **population**, which is an entire aggregate of cases.

▷ An *element* (the basic unit about which information is collected) can be included in a sample if it meets the **eligibility criteria**.

▷ The main consideration in assessing a sample in a quantitative study is its *representativeness*—the extent to which the sample is similar to the population and avoids bias. **Sampling bias** refers to the systematic overrepresentation or underrepresentation of some segment of the population.

▷ Quantitative researchers usually sample from an **accessible population** but typically want to generalize to a larger **target population**.

▷ **Nonprobability sampling** (wherein elements are selected by nonrandom methods) includes convenience, quota, and purposive sampling. Nonprobability sampling designs are convenient and economical; a major disadvantage is their potential for bias.

▷ **Convenience sampling** (or *accidental sampling*) uses the most readily available or most convenient group of people for the sample. **Snowball sampling** is a type of convenience sampling in which referrals for potential participants are made by those already in the sample.

▷ **Quota sampling** divides the population into homogeneous **strata** (subgroups) to ensure representation of those subgroups in the sample; within each stratum, researchers select participants by convenience sampling.

▷ In **purposive** (or *judgmental*) **sampling**, participants (or types of participants) are hand picked based on the researcher's knowledge about the population.

▷ **Probability sampling** designs, which involve the **random selection** of elements from the population, yield more representative samples than nonprobability designs and permit estimates of the magnitude of **sampling error**. Probability samples, however, are expensive and inconvenient.

▷ **Simple random sampling** involves the selection of elements on a random basis from a *sampling frame* that enumerates all the elements.

▷ **Stratified random sampling** divides the population into homogeneous subgroups from which elements are selected at random.

▷ **Cluster sampling** (or *multistage sampling*) involves the successive selection of random samples from larger to smaller units by either simple random or stratified random methods.

▷ **Systematic sampling** is the selection of every *k*th case from a list. By dividing the population size by the desired sample size, the researcher establishes the *sampling interval*, which is the standard distance between the selected elements.

▷ In addition to representativeness, **sample size** is another important concern in quantitative studies, especially with regard to a study's statistical conclusion validity.

▷ Advanced researchers use **power analysis** to estimate sample size needs. Large samples are preferable to small ones in quantitative studies because larger samples tend to be more representative. However, even a large sample does not guarantee representativeness.

▷ Qualitative researchers use the theoretical demands of the study to select articulate and reflective informants with certain types of experience in an emergent way, capitalizing on early learning to guide subsequent sampling decisions.

▷ Qualitative researchers most often use purposive or, in grounded theory studies, **theoretical sampling** to guide them in selecting data sources that maximize information richness.

▷ Various purposive sampling strategies have been used by qualitative researchers. One strategy is **maximum variation sampling**, which entails purposely selecting cases with a wide range of variation. Other strategies include **homogeneous sampling** (deliberately reducing variation); **extreme case sampling** (selecting the most unusual or extreme cases); and **criterion sampling** (studying cases that meet a predetermined criterion of importance).

▷ Another important strategy in qualitative research is sampling **confirming** and **disconfirming cases**, that is, selecting cases that enrich and challenge the researchers' conceptualizations.

▷ Samples in qualitative studies are typically small and based on information needs. A guiding principle is **data saturation**, which involves sampling to the point at which no new information is obtained and redundancy is achieved.

▷ Ethnographers make numerous sampling decisions, including not only *whom* to sample but *what* to sample (e.g., activities, events, documents, artifacts); these decisions are often aided by their **key informants** who serve as guides and interpreters of the culture.

▷ Phenomenologists typically work with a small sample of people (10 or fewer) who meet the criterion of having lived the experience under study.

▷ Grounded theory researchers typically use theoretical sampling and work with samples of about 20 to 30 people.

▷ Criteria for evaluating qualitative sampling are informational adequacy and appropriateness; potential for transferability is another issue of concern.

RESEARCH EXAMPLES | Critical Thinking Activities

 EXAMPLE 1: Quantitative Research

Aspects of a quantitative nursing study, featuring terms and concepts discussed in this chapter, are presented below, followed by some questions to guide critical thinking. (The full research report is available in *AAOHN, 49,* 130–136.)

Study

"Exposure risks and tetanus immunization in women of family owned farms" (Holland & Carruth, 2001)

Purpose

The purposes of the study were to examine the risk factors of farm women who engage in activities that could have exposed them to tetanus and to study circumstances related to tetanus immunization.

Design

The researchers conducted a cross-sectional telephone survey. The interviews lasted approximately 30 minutes, on average.

Sampling Plan

The researchers first used a purposive sampling method to select 10 parishes (counties) in southeast Louisiana. The counties were hand picked to reflect agricultural and geographic diversity.

RESEARCH EXAMPLES *Continued*

The researchers had access to a sampling frame of 4808 farm owners in these 10 parishes (a list maintained by Louisiana State University Agricultural Centers and Farm Service Agency). A stratified random sample of farm owners was drawn, with parish as the stratifying variable. That is, in each parish, a random sample of farm owners was selected. Sampled farm owners were screened to determine whether an eligible woman lived in the household. Women were deemed eligible if they were 18 years or older and were members of a family participating in a farming operation. A total of 1141 farms were determined to have an eligible sample member. Interviews were completed with 657 women, for a response rate of 57.6% among known eligible farms.

Key Findings

▸ Only 54% of the women had had a tetanus booster within the prior 10 years.
▸ Just as many women received a tetanus vaccination for an injury or accident as for prevention.
▸ Older women were much less likely than younger women to be up-to-date on their immunizations.

Critical Thinking Suggestions*

*See the Student Resource CD-ROM for a discussion of these questions.
1. Answer questions 1–5, 7, and 8 from Box 12-1 regarding this study.
2. Also consider the following targeted questions, which may assist you in further assessing aspects of the study:
    a. Comment on the researchers' decision to purposefully sample parishes in the first stage.
    b. The report did not mention whether the sampling in the second stage was proportionate or disproportionate. What would you recommend?
    c. Identify some of the major potential sources of bias in the final sample of 657 participants.
3. If the results of this study are valid and reliable, what are some of the uses to which the findings might be put in clinical practice?

 EXAMPLE 2: Qualitative Research

Aspects of a qualitative nursing study, featuring terms and concepts discussed in this chapter, are presented below, followed by some questions to guide critical thinking. (The full research report is available in *Qualitative Health Research, 13,* 1252–1271.)

Study

"Deciding whether to continue, share, or relinquish caregiving: Caregiver views" (Caron & Bowers, 2003)

Research Purpose

The researchers conducted a study of informal caregiving in an effort to develop a substantive caregiving theory to explain the complex decision making involved in providing care to older family members.

research examples continue on page 282

RESEARCH EXAMPLES *Continued*

Method

Caron and Bowers used Glaser and Strauss's grounded theory method with the goal of generating a substantive theory of caregiving decisions from their data. They conceptualized caregiving as a complex social process that lent itself well to a grounded theory approach. Each study participant was interviewed once.

Sampling Plan

The researchers generated a sample of 16 family caregivers. They first recruited five caregivers from a social service program, the Wisconsin Partnership Program (WPP). As the analysis progressed, sample selection was guided by factors emerging in the theory. These factors included presence or absence of cognitive impairment (Alzheimer's disease or early dementia) in the care recipient, living arrangement (same or separate households), and use or nonuse of external social services in support of the caregiving. Their sample of 6 male and 10 female caregivers included 10 who were caring for relatives with cognitive impairment and 7 who were living with the family member. Four of the 16 caregivers did not have supplemental assistance from outside service providers. Although initial sample members were recruited with the WPP, the researchers recruited the remainder of their sample outside the WPP to ensure that they would be able to learn about caregiving in the absence of outside help. The remaining participants were recruited through an Alzheimer's disease association and by word of mouth.

Key Findings

▶ The analysis revealed various *purposes* of caregiving for an older adult. These purposes were found to influence whether—and how—caregivers continued to provide care or decided to share or relinquish caregiving to health care professionals.

▶ The two main purposes of caregiving were an interrelational purpose (in which caregivers protected and maintained the caregiver–care recipient relationship) and a pragmatic purpose (providing physical comfort and appropriate care).

▶ The purposes were often linked to phases of caregiving (i.e., an interrelational phase and a pragmatic phase), with a nonlinear progression between the phases.

Critical Thinking Suggestions

1. Answer questions 1–6 from Box 12-2 regarding this study.
2. Also consider the following targeted questions, which may assist you in further assessing aspects of the study:
   a. Comment on the characteristics of the participants, given the researchers' aims.
   b. What do you think the eligibility criteria for the study were?
   c. Do you think it was a strength or a weakness of the sampling plan for the researchers to use three different approaches to recruit participants (i.e., WPP, Alzheimer's disease association, and word of mouth)?

RESEARCH EXAMPLES *Continued*

3. If the results of this study are trustworthy, what are some of the uses to which the findings might be put in clinical practice?

 ### EXAMPLE 3: Quantitative Research

1. Read the abstract and the introduction from Motzer et al.'s study ("Sense of Coherence") in Appendix A of this book, and then answer the relevant questions in Box 12-1.
2. Also consider the following targeted questions, which may further sharpen your critical thinking skills and assist you in assessing aspects of the study:
  a. What type of sampling plan might have improved the representativeness of the sample?
  b. Why do you think the researchers used sample members from four other studies?

 ### EXAMPLE 4: Qualitative Research

1. Read the abstract and the introduction from Beck's study ("Birth Trauma") in Appendix B of this book, and then answer the relevant questions in Box 12-2.
2. Also consider the following targeted questions, which may further sharpen your critical thinking skills and assist you in assessing aspects of the study:
  a. Comment on the characteristics of the participants, given the purpose of this study.
  b. Do you think that Beck should have limited her sample to women from one country only? Provide a rationale for your answer.

SUGGESTED READINGS

Methodologic References
Cohen, J. (1988). *Statistical power analysis for the behavioral sciences* (2nd ed.). Mahwah, NJ: Erlbaum.

Glaser, B. (1978). *Theoretical sensitivity*. Mill Valley, CA: Sociology Press.

Glaser, B., & Strauss, A. (1967). *The discovery of grounded theory: Strategies for qualitative research*. Mill Valley, CA: Sociology Press.

Morse, J. M. (1991). Strategies for sampling. In J. M. Morse (Ed.), *Qualitative nursing research: A contemporary dialogue*. Newbury Park, CA: Sage Publications.

Morse, J. M. (2000). Determining sample size. *Qualitative Health Research, 10*, 3–5.

Patton, M. Q. (2002). *Qualitative evaluation and research methods* (3rd ed.). Newbury Park, CA: Sage Publications.

Polit, D. F. & Beck, C. T. (2004). *Nursing research: principles and methods* (7th ed.). Philadelphia: Lippincott Williams & Wilkins.

Porter, E. J. (1999). Defining the eligible, accessible population for a phenomenological study. *Western Journal of Nursing Research, 21*, 796–804.

Studies Cited in Chapter 12
Allison, M. J., & Keller, C. (2004). Self-efficacy intervention effect on physical activity in older adults. *Western Journal of Nursing Research, 26,* 31–46.

Beck, C. T. (2002). Releasing the pause button: Mothering twins during the first year of life. *Qualitative Health Research. 12,* 593–608.

Caron, C. D., & Bowers, B. J. (2003). Deciding whether to continue, share, or relinquish caregiving: Caregiver views. *Qualitative Health Research, 13,* 1252–1271.

Criste, A. (2003). Do nurse anesthetists demonstrate gender bias in treating pain? A national survey using a standardized pain model. *AANA Journal, 71,* 206–209.

Dickinson, A. R., & Digman, D. (2002). Managing it: A mother's perspective of managing a pre-school child's acute asthma episode. *Journal of Child Health Care, 6,* 7–18.

Holland, C., & Carruth, A. K. (2001). Exposure risks and tetanus immunization in women of family owned farms. *AAOHN, 49,* 130–136.

Kirkham, S. R. (2003). The politics of belonging and intercultural health care. *Western Journal of Nursing Research, 25,* 762–780.

Kvigne, K., & Kirkevold, M. (2003). Living with bodily strangeness: Women's experiences of their changing and unpredictable body following a stroke. *Qualitative Health Research, 13,* 1291–1310.

McCabe, C. (2004). Nurse-patient communication: An exploration of patients' experiences. *Journal of Clinical Nursing, 13,* 41–49.

McCarthy, M. (2003). Situated clinical reasoning: Distinguishing acute confusion from dementia in hospitalized older adults. *Research in Nursing & Health, 26,* 90–101.

Meeker, M. A. (2004). Family surrogate decision making at the end of life: Seeing them through with care and respect. *Qualitative Health Research, 14,* 204–225.

Porter, E. J. (2003). Moments of apprehension in the midst of a certainty: Some frail older widows' lives with a personal emergency response system. *Qualitative Health Research, 13,* 1311–1323.

Reyes, L. R., Meininger, J. C., Liehr, P., Chan, W., & Mueller, W. H. (2003). Anger in adolescents: Sex, ethnicity, age differences, and psychometric properties. *Nursing Research, 52,* 2–11.

Ruchala, P. L., Metheny, N., Essenpreis, H., & Borcherding, K. (2003). Current practice in oxytocin dilution and fluid administration for induction of labor. *Journal of Obstetric, Gynecologic, & Neonatal Nursing, 31,* 545–550.

Shaker, I., Scott, J. A., & Reid, M. (2004). Infant feeding attitudes of expectant parents: Breastfeeding versus formula feeding. *Journal of Advanced Nursing, 45,* 260–268.

Staggers, N., Gassert, C. A., & Curran, C. (2002). A Delphi study to determine informatics competencies for nurses at four levels of practice. *Nursing Research, 51,* 383–390.

Thato, S., Charron-Prochownik, D., Dorn, L. D., Albrecht, S. A., & Stone, C. A. (2003). Predictors of condom use among adolescent Thai vocational students. *Journal of Nursing Scholarship, 35,* 157–163.

Thulesius, H., Håkansson, A., & Petersson, K. (2003). Balancing: A basic process in end-of-life care. *Qualitative Health Research, 13,* 1353–1377.

Ulrich, C. M., Soeken, K. L., & Miller, N. (2003). Ethical conflict associated with managed care: Views of nurse practitioners. *Nursing Research, 52,* 168–175.

Woodgate, R. L., & Degner, L. F. (2003). Expectations and beliefs about children's cancer symptoms: Perspectives of children with cancer and their families. *Oncology Nursing Forum, 30,* 479–491.

Data
Collection

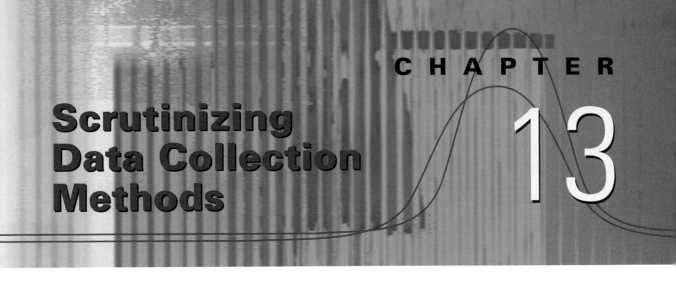

CHAPTER 13

Scrutinizing Data Collection Methods

STUDENT OBJECTIVES

On completing this chapter, you will be able to:

▪ Evaluate a researcher's decision to use existing data versus collecting new data
▪ Discuss the four dimensions along which data collection approaches vary
▪ Identify phenomena that lend themselves to self-reports, observation, and physiologic measurement
▪ Distinguish between and evaluate structured and unstructured self-reports; open-ended and closed-ended questions; and interviews and questionnaires
▪ Distinguish between and evaluate structured and unstructured observations and describe various methods of collecting, sampling, and recording such observational data
▪ Describe the major features, advantages, and disadvantages of biophysiologic measures
▪ Critique a researcher's decisions regarding the data collection plan (degree of structure, general method, mode of administration) and its implementation
▪ Define new terms in the chapter

T he phenomena in which researchers are interested must be translated into concepts that can be measured, observed, or recorded. The task of selecting or developing methods for gathering data is among the most challenging in the research process. Without appropriate data collection methods, the validity of research conclusions is easily challenged.

OVERVIEW OF DATA COLLECTION AND DATA SOURCES

There are many alternative approaches to data collection, and these approaches vary along several dimensions. This introductory section provides an overview of some of the important dimensions.

Existing Data Versus New Data

One of the first data decisions an investigator makes concerns the use of existing data versus new data gathered specifically for the study. Most of this chapter is devoted to methods researchers use to generate new data, but they sometimes can take advantage of existing information.

We have already discussed several types of studies that rely on existing data. Meta-analyses and metasyntheses (see Chapter 7) are examples of studies that involve analyses of available data—that is, data from research reports. Historical research (Chapter 10) typically relies on available data in the form of written, narrative records of the past: diaries, letters, newspapers, minutes of meetings, and so forth. As we discussed in Chapter 11, researchers sometimes perform a secondary analysis, which is the use of data gathered in a previous study—often by other researchers—to test new hypotheses or address new research questions.

An important existing data source for nurse researchers is **records**. Hospital records, nursing charts, physicians' order sheets, and care plan statements all constitute rich data sources. Records are an economical and convenient source of information. Because the researchers were not responsible for collecting and recording information, however, they may be unaware of the records' limitations, biases, or incompleteness. If the records available for use are not the entire set of all possible records, investigators must deal with the issue of the records' representativeness. Existing records have been used in both qualitative and quantitative nursing studies.

Example of a study using records

Niederstadt (2004) conducted a study to determine the most appropriate time to begin analyzing activated clotting time levels for patients undergoing percutaneous coronary interventions. She used data from a retrospective chart audit of 44 patients.

CONSUMER TIP

Researchers describe their data collection plan in the method section of a research report. In a report for a quantitative study, the specific data collection methods are often described in a subsection labeled "Measures" or "Instruments." The actual steps taken to collect the data are sometimes described in a separate subsection with the heading "Procedures."

■

Major Types of Data for Nursing Studies

If existing data are unavailable or unsuitable for a research question, researchers must collect new data. In developing their data collection plan, researchers make many important decisions, including the decision about the basic type of data to gather. Three types have been used most frequently by nurse researchers: self-reports, observations, and biophysiologic measures. **Self-reports** are participants' responses to questions posed by the researcher, as in an interview. Direct **observation** of people's behaviors, characteristics, and circumstances is an alternative to self-reports for certain research questions. Nurses also use **biophysiologic measures** to assess important clinical variables. Sections of this chapter are devoted to these three major types of data collection.

In quantitative studies, researchers decide upfront how to operationalize their variables and how best to gather their data. Their data collection plans are almost always "cast in stone" before a single piece of data is collected. Self-reports are the most common data collection approach in quantitative nursing studies.

Qualitative researchers typically go into the field knowing the most likely sources of data, but they do not rule out other possible data sources that might come to light as data collection progresses. As in quantitative studies, the primary method of collecting qualitative data is through self-reports, that is, through interviews with study participants. Observation is often a part of many qualitative studies as well. Physiologic data are rarely collected in a naturalistic inquiry— except perhaps to describe participants' characteristics or to ascertain eligibility for the study.

Table 13-1 compares the types of data used by researchers in the three main qualitative traditions, as well as other aspects of the data collection process for each tradition. Ethnographers

TABLE 13.1	Data Collection in the Three Main Qualitative Traditions		
ISSUE	**ETHNOGRAPHY**	**PHENOMENOLOGY**	**GROUNDED THEORY**
Type of data	Primarily participant observation and interviews, plus documents, artifacts, maps, photographs, social network diagrams, genealogies	Primarily in-depth interviews, sometimes diaries, artwork, or other materials	Primarily individual interviews, sometimes group interviews, participant observations, journals
Unit of data collection	Cultural systems	Individuals	Individuals
Period of data collection	Extended period, many months or years	Typically moderate	Typically moderate
Salient field issues	Gaining entrée, determining a role, learning how to participate, encouraging candor, identification with group, premature exit	Bracketing one's views, building rapport, encouraging candor, listening intently while preparing next question, keeping "on track," handling personal emotions	Building rapport, encouraging candor, keeping "on track," listening intently while preparing next question, handling personal emotions

almost always triangulate data from various sources, with observation and interviews being the most important methods. Ethnographers also gather or examine products of the culture under study, such as documents, records, artifacts, photographs, and so on. Phenomenologists and grounded theory researchers rely primarily on in-depth interviews with individual participants, although observation also plays a role in some grounded theory studies.

Key Dimensions of Data Collection Methods

Regardless of the type of data collected in a study, data collection methods vary along several important dimensions:

▶ *Structure.* Research data can be collected in a highly structured manner: The same information is gathered from all participants in a comparable, prespecified way. Sometimes, however, it is more appropriate to be flexible and to allow participants to reveal relevant information in a naturalistic way.

▶ *Quantifiability.* Data that will be analyzed statistically must be gathered in such a way that they can be quantified. On the other hand, data that are to be analyzed qualitatively are collected in narrative form. Structured data collection approaches tend to yield data that are more easily quantified.

▶ *Obtrusiveness.* Data collection methods differ in terms of the degree to which people are aware of their status as study participants. If participants are fully aware of their role in a study, their behavior and responses might not be normal. When data are collected unobtrusively, however, ethical problems may emerge.

▶ *Objectivity.* Some data collection approaches require more subjective judgment than others. Quantitative researchers generally strive for methods that are as objective as possible. In qualitative research, however, the subjective judgment of the investigator is considered a valuable tool.

Sometimes, the research question dictates where on these four dimensions the data collection method will lie. For example, questions that are best suited for a phenomenological study tend to use methods that are low on structure, quantifiability, and objectivity, whereas research questions appropriate for a survey tend to require methods that are high on all four dimensions. However, researchers often have latitude in selecting or designing appropriate data collection plans.

CONSUMER TIP

Most data that are analyzed quantitatively actually begin as qualitative data. If a researcher asked respondents if they have been severely depressed, moderately depressed, somewhat depressed, or not at all depressed in the past week, they answer in words, not numbers. The words are transformed, through a coding process, into quantitative categories.

■

SELF-REPORT METHODS

A good deal of information can be gathered by directly questioning people. If, for example, we were interested in learning about patients' perceptions of hospital care, their preoperative fears, or their health-promoting activities, we would likely talk to them and ask them questions. For some research variables, alternatives to direct questioning exist, but the unique ability of humans to communicate verbally on a sophisticated level ensures that self-reports will always be a fundamental tool in nurse researchers' repertoire of data collection techniques.

Self-report techniques can vary in terms of structure. At one extreme are loosely structured methods that do not involve a formal written set of questions. At the other extreme are tightly structured methods involving the use of forms such as questionnaires. Some characteristics of different self-report approaches are discussed next.

Qualitative Self-Report Techniques

Self-report methods used in qualitative studies offer flexibility. When these unstructured methods are used, researchers do not have a set of questions that must be asked in a specific order and worded in a given way. Instead, they start with some general questions and allow respondents to tell their stories in a naturalistic, narrative fashion. In other words, unstructured or semi-structured self-reports, usually obtained in interviews, tend to be conversational in nature.

Unstructured interviews, which are used by researchers in all qualitative research traditions, encourage respondents to define the important dimensions of a phenomenon and to elaborate on what is relevant to them, rather than being guided by investigators' *a priori* notions of relevance. Unstructured interviews are the mode of choice when researchers do not have a clear idea of what it is they do not know.

TYPES OF QUALITATIVE SELF-REPORTS

There are several approaches to collecting qualitative self-report data. **Completely unstructured interviews** are used when researchers have no preconceived view of the content or flow of information to be gathered. Their aim is to elucidate respondents' perceptions of the world without imposing their own views. Typically, researchers begin by asking a broad **grand tour question** such as, "What happened when you first learned that you had AIDS?" Subsequent questions are more focused and are guided by initial responses. Ethnographic and phenomenological studies often use unstructured interviews.

Example of unstructured interviews

Cheung and Hocking (2004) explored the experience of spousal caregiving among people caring for spouses with multiple sclerosis. Data were collected from 10 caregivers through face-to-face unstructured interviews lasting between 1 and 2 hours. The leading question for each interview was, "What is it like for you to be caring for (name)?" Subsequent questions were based on participants' responses.

Semi-structured (or *focused*) **interviews** are used when researchers have a list of topics or broad questions that must be addressed in an interview. Interviewers use a written **topic guide** (or *interview guide*) to ensure that all question areas are covered. The interviewer's function is to encourage participants to talk freely about all the topics on the guide.

Example of semi-structured interviews

Paun (2004) conducted a phenomenological study to gain an in-depth understanding of the experience of Alzheimer's disease caregivers. She used a topic guide to ensure consistency. Examples of two of the questions in the guide are: "How do you make sense of the caregiving situation you are experiencing at the present time?" and "Have religious or spiritual values played a role in your decision to take care of your (husband)?"

Focus group interviews are interviews with groups of about five to 10 people whose opinions and experiences are solicited simultaneously. The interviewer (or *moderator*) guides the discussion according to a topic guide or set of questions. The advantages of a group format are that it is efficient and can generate a lot of dialogue. Some people, however, are uncomfortable expressing their views or describing their experiences in front of a group. Focus groups have been used by researchers in many qualitative research traditions and can play a particularly important role in feminist, critical theory, and participatory action research.

Example of focus group interviews

Abel and Painter (2003) explored factors that influence adherence to antiretroviral therapy in women with HIV disease. Women with HIV and health care providers participated in separate focus group interviews.

Life histories are narrative self-disclosures about individual life experiences. With this approach, researchers ask respondents to describe, often in chronologic sequence, their experiences regarding a specified theme, either orally or in writing. Some researchers have used this approach to obtain a total life health history.

Example of life histories

Haglund (2003) explored sexual abstinence from the perspective of abstinent African-American young women. Data were collected in two separate interviews with 14 adolescents using the life history method.

The **think aloud method** is a qualitative method that has been used to collect data about cognitive processes, such as thinking, problem-solving, and decision making. This method involves having people use audio-recording devices to talk about decisions as they are being made or while problems are being solved, over an extended period (e.g., throughout a shift). The method produces an inventory of decisions and underlying processes as they occur in a naturalistic context.

Example of the think-aloud method

Simmons, Lanuza, Fonteyn, Hicks, and Holm (2003) used the think aloud method to explore the clinical reasoning strategies of experienced nurses as they considered assessment findings of patients.

Personal **diaries** have long been used as a source of data in historical research. It is also possible to generate new data for a nonhistorical study by asking participants to maintain a diary or journal over a specified period. Diaries can be useful in providing an intimate description of a person's everyday life. The diaries may be completely unstructured; for example, individuals who have undergone an organ transplantation could be asked simply to spend 10 to 15 minutes a day jotting down their thoughts and feelings. Frequently, however, subjects are requested to make entries into a diary regarding some specific aspect of their experience, sometimes in a semi-structured format.

Example of narratives from diaries

Roberts and Mann (2003) explored, using the diary entries of 20 HIV-positive women, how and why women living with HIV or AIDS intentionally fail to adhere to their antiretroviral medications. The women made journal entries over a 1-month period.

The **critical incidents technique** is a method of gathering information about people's behaviors by examining specific incidents relating to the behavior under study. The technique focuses on a factual *incident*—an observable and integral episode of human behavior; *critical* means that the incident must have had a discernible impact on some outcome. The technique differs from other self-report approaches in that it focuses on something specific about which respondents can be expected to testify as expert witnesses. Generally, data on 100 or more critical incidents are collected, but this typically involves interviews with a much smaller number of people, because each participant can often describe multiple incidents.

Example of the critical incident technique

Cheek and Gibson (2003) used the critical incidents technique to explore issues that affect nurses' provision of residential care to older Australians. A purposive sample of 24 nurses completed interviews, which began with the initial prompt: "Think of something that has happened involving nursing care and older patients that you were part of or that you observed. It must be important to you and the quality of your nursing practice." The prompt was followed by a series of probing questions about the incident.

GATHERING QUALITATIVE SELF-REPORT DATA

Researchers gather narrative self-report data to develop a construction of a phenomenon that is consistent with that of participants. This goal requires researchers to take steps to overcome communication barriers and to enhance the flow of meaning. For example, researchers who study groups that use distinctive terms should strive before going into the field to understand those terms and their nuances.

Although qualitative interviews are conversational in nature, this does not mean that researchers enter into them casually. The conversations are purposeful ones that require advance thought and preparation. For example, the wording of questions should make sense to respondents and reflect their world view. In addition to being good questioners, researchers must be good listeners. Only by attending carefully to what respondents are saying can in-depth interviewers develop appropriate follow-up questions.

Unstructured interviews are typically long—sometimes lasting several hours. The issue of how best to record such abundant information is a difficult one. Some researchers take sketchy notes as the interview progresses, filling in the details after the interview is completed—but this method is risky in terms of data accuracy. Many prefer tape-recording the interviews for later transcription. Although some respondents are self-conscious when their conversation is recorded, they typically forget about the presence of recording equipment after a few minutes.

Quantitative Self-Report Techniques

Structured, quantitative approaches to collecting self-report data are appropriate when researchers know in advance exactly what they need to know and can, therefore, frame appropriate questions to obtain the needed information. Structured self-report data are usually collected by means of a formal, written document—an **instrument**. The instrument is known as an **interview schedule** when the questions are asked orally in either a face-to-face or telephone format and as a **questionnaire** when respondents complete the instrument themselves in writing or over the Internet.

QUESTION FORM

In a totally structured instrument, respondents are asked to respond to the same questions in the same order, and they are given the same set of options for their responses. **Closed-ended questions** (also called **fixed-alternative questions**) are ones in which the **response alternatives** are pre-specified by the researcher. The alternatives may range from a simple yes or no to complex expressions of opinion. The purpose of using questions with fixed alternatives is to ensure comparability of responses and to facilitate analysis.

Many structured instruments, however, also include some **open-ended questions**, which allow participants to respond to questions in their own words. When open-ended questions are included in questionnaires, respondents must write out their responses. In interviews, the interviewer writes down responses verbatim or uses a tape recorder for later transcription. Some examples of open-ended and closed-ended questions are presented in Box 13-1.

Both open-ended and closed-ended questions have strengths and weaknesses. Closed-ended questions are more difficult to construct than open-ended ones but easier to administer and, especially, to analyze. Furthermore, closed-ended questions are more efficient: People can complete more closed-ended questions than open-ended ones in a given amount of time. Also, respondents may be unwilling to compose lengthy written responses to open-ended questions in questionnaires.

The major drawback of closed-ended questions is that researchers might overlook some potentially important responses. Another concern is that closed-ended questions can be superficial; open-ended questions allow for richer and fuller information if the respondents are verbally expressive and cooperative. Finally, some respondents object to choosing from alternatives that do not reflect their opinions precisely.

INSTRUMENT CONSTRUCTION

In drafting (or borrowing) questions for a structured instrument, researchers must carefully monitor the wording of each question for clarity, sensitivity to respondents' psychological state, absence of bias, and (in questionnaires) reading level. Questions must be sequenced in a psychologically meaningful order that encourages cooperation and candor.

BOX 13.1   Examples of Question Types

Open-Ended

- What led to your decision to stop smoking?
- What did you do when you discovered you had AIDS?

Closed-Ended

1. Dichotomous Question

Have you ever been hospitalized?
- ❏ 1. Yes
- ❏ 2. No

2. Multiple-Choice Question

How important is it to you to avoid a pregnancy at this time?
- ❏ 1. Extremely important
- ❏ 2. Very important
- ❏ 3. Somewhat important
- ❏ 4. Not at all important

3. "Cafeteria" Question

People have different opinions about the use of hormone-replacement therapy for women in menopause. Which of the following statements best represents your point of view?
- ❏ 1. Hormone replacement is dangerous and should be totally banned.
- ❏ 2. Hormone replacement may have some undesirable side effects that suggests the need for caution in its use.
- ❏ 3. I am undecided about my views on hormone-replacement therapy.
- ❏ 4. Hormone replacement has many beneficial effects that merit its promotion.
- ❏ 5. Hormone replacement is a wonder cure that should be administered widely to menopausal women.

4. Rank-Order Question

People value different things about life. Below is a list of principles or ideals that are often cited when people are asked to name things they value most. Please indicate the order of importance of these values to you by placing a 1 beside the most important, 2 beside the next most important, and so forth.
- ❏ Career achievement/work
- ❏ Family relationships
- ❏ Friendships and social interaction
- ❏ Health
- ❏ Money
- ❏ Religion

5. Forced-Choice Question

Which statement most closely represents your point of view?
- ❏ 1. What happens to me is my own doing.
- ❏ 2. Sometimes I feel I don't have enough control over my life.

6. Rating Question

On a scale from 0 to 10, where 0 means extremely dissatisfied and 10 means extremely satisfied, how satisfied are you with the nursing care you received during your hospitalization?

Extremely dissatisfied   Extremely satisfied

0 1 2 3 4 5 6 7 8 9 10

Draft instruments are usually critically reviewed by peers or colleagues and then pretested with a small sample of respondents. A *pretest* is a trial run to determine whether the instrument is useful in generating desired information. In large studies, the development and pretesting of self-report instruments may take many months to complete.

INTERVIEWS VERSUS QUESTIONNAIRES

Researchers using structured self-reports must decide whether to use interviews or questionnaires. You should be aware of the limitations and strengths of these alternatives because the decision may affect the findings and the quality of the evidence. Questionnaires, relative to interviews, have the following advantages:

▶ Questionnaires are less costly and require less time and effort to administer; this is a particular advantage if the sample is geographically dispersed. Web-based questionnaires are especially economical.

▶ Questionnaires offer the possibility of complete anonymity, which may be crucial in obtaining information about illegal or deviant behaviors or about embarrassing traits.

▶ The absence of an interviewer ensures that there will be no biases reflecting respondents' reaction to the interviewer rather than to the questions themselves.

Example of mailed questionnaires

Cavendish and her colleagues (2004), as part of a multimethod study, mailed a questionnaire to 1000 randomly selected members of Sigma Theta Tau International. The questionnaire focused on the nurses' spirituality.

The strengths of interviews far outweigh those of questionnaires. These strengths include the following:

▶ The response rate tends to be high in face-to-face interviews. Respondents are less likely to refuse to talk to an interviewer than to ignore a questionnaire, especially a mailed questionnaire. Low response rates can lead to bias because respondents are rarely a random subset of those whom the researchers have sampled. In the mailed questionnaire study described earlier (Cavendish et al., 2004), the response rate was 55%.

▶ Many people simply cannot fill out a questionnaire; examples include young children, the blind, and the very elderly. Interviews are feasible with most people.

▶ Questions are less likely to be misinterpreted by respondents because interviewers can determine whether questions have been understood.

▶ Interviewers can produce additional information through observation of respondents' living situation, level of understanding, degree of cooperativeness, and so on—all of which can be useful in interpreting responses.

Most advantages of face-to-face interviews also apply to telephone interviews. Complicated or detailed instruments are not well suited to telephone interviewing, but for relatively brief instruments, the telephone interview combines relatively low costs with high response rates.

Example of in-person interviews

Resnick and Nigg (2003), who were studying factors that explained exercise behavior in older adults, conducted face-to-face interviews with men and women living independently in a retirement community. Of the 184 eligible people invited to participate, 179 completed an interview—a response rate of 97%.

Scales and Other Special Forms of Structured Self-Reports

Several special types of structured self-reports are used by nurse researchers. These include composite social-psychological scales, vignettes, and Q sorts.

SCALES

Social–psychological scales are often incorporated into a questionnaire or interview schedule. A **scale** is a device designed to assign a numeric score to people to place them on a continuum with respect to attributes being measured, like a scale for measuring weight. Social–psychological scales quantitatively discriminate among people with different attitudes, fears, motives, perceptions, personality traits, and needs.

The most common scaling technique is the **Likert scale**, which consists of several declarative statements (or *items*) that express a viewpoint on a topic. Respondents are asked to indicate how much they agree or disagree with the statement. Table 13-2 presents an illustrative, six-item Likert scale for measuring attitudes toward condom use. In this example, agreement with positively worded statements and disagreement with negatively worded statements are assigned higher scores. The first statement is positively phrased; agreement indicates a favorable attitude toward condom use. Because the item has five response alternatives, a score of 5 would be given to someone strongly agreeing, 4 to someone agreeing, and so forth. The responses of two hypothetical respondents are shown by a check or an X, and their item scores are shown in the right-hand columns. Person 1, who agreed with the first statement, has a score of 4, whereas person 2, who strongly disagreed, has a score of 1. The second statement is negatively worded, and so the scoring is reversed—a 1 is assigned to those who strongly agree, and so forth. This reversal is necessary so that a high score consistently reflects positive attitudes toward condom use. A person's total score is determined by summing item scores; hence, these scales are sometimes called **summated rating scales**. The total scores of the two respondents reflect a considerably more positive attitude toward condoms on the part of person 1 (score = 26) than person 2 (score = 11). Summing item scores makes it possible to make fine discriminations among people with different points of view. A single Likert question allows people to be put into only five categories. A six-item scale, such as the one in Table 13-2, permits much finer gradation—from a minimum possible score of 6 (6×1) to a maximum possible score of 30 (6×5).

Example of a Likert scale

Robbins, Pender, and Kazanis (2003) used a Likert scale in their study of perceived barriers to physical activity by adolescent girls. Examples of items include: "I am self-conscious about my looks when I exercise" and "I am not motivated to be active."

TABLE 13.2	Example of a Likert Scale to Measure Attitudes Toward Condoms							
		RESPONSES†					SCORE	
DIRECTION OF SCORING*	ITEM	SA	A	?	D	SD	PERSON 1 (✔)	PERSON 2 (✕)
+	1. Using a condom shows you care about your partner.		✔			✕	4	1
−	2. My partner would be angry if I talked about using condoms.			✕		✔	5	3
−	3. I wouldn't enjoy sex as much if my partner and I used condoms.		✕		✔		4	2
+	4. Condoms are a good protection against AIDS and other sexually transmitted diseases.			✔	✕		3	2
+	5. My partner would respect me if I insisted on using condoms.	✔				✕	5	1
−	6. I would be too embarrassed to ask my partner about using a condom.		✕			✔	5	2
	Total score						26	11

* Researchers would not indicate the direction of scoring on a Likert scale administered to subjects. The scoring direction is indicated in this table for illustrative purposes only.
† SA, strongly agree; A, agree; ?, uncertain; D, disagree; SD, strongly disagree.

Another technique for measuring attitudes is the **semantic differential** (SD). With the SD, respondents are asked to rate concepts (e.g., primary nursing, team nursing) on a series of *bipolar adjectives*, such as good/bad, strong/weak, effective/ineffective, important/unimportant. Respondents are asked to place a check at the appropriate point on a 7-point scale that extends from one extreme of the dimension to the other. An example of an SD

Example of a semantic differential

Phillips, Brewer, and deArdon (2001) developed the Elder Image Scale, a semantic differential instrument that measures a caregiver's mental image of an elder. Examples of adjective pairs include reasonable/unreasonable, even-tempered/hot-tempered, and considerate/abusive.

NURSE PRACTITIONERS

competent	7*	6	5	4	3	2	1	incompetent
worthless	1	2	3	4	5	6	7	valuable
important								unimportant
pleasant								unpleasant
bad								good
cold								warm
responsible								irresponsible
successful								unsuccessful

*The score values would not be printed on the form administered to actual subjects. The numbers are presented here solely for the purpose of illustrating how semantic differentials are scored.

FIGURE 13.1 Example of a semantic differential.

format is shown in Figure 13-1. The SD has the advantage of being flexible and easy to construct. The concept being rated can be virtually anything—a person, concept, controversial issue, and so on. The scoring procedure for SD responses is similar to that for Likert scales. Scores from 1 to 7 are assigned to each bipolar scale response, with higher scores generally associated with the positively worded adjective. Responses are then summed across the bipolar scales to yield a total score.

Another type of psychosocial measure is the **visual analog scale** (VAS), which can be used to measure subjective experiences, such as pain, fatigue, nausea, and dyspnea. The VAS is a straight line, the end anchors of which are labeled as the extreme limits of the sensation or feeling being measured. Participants are asked to mark a point on the line corresponding to the amount of sensation experienced. Traditionally, a VAS line is 100 mm in length, which makes it easy to derive a score from 0 to 100 by simply measuring the distance from one end of the scale to the mark on the line. An example of a VAS is presented in Figure 13-2.

Example of a visual analog scale

McCaffrey and Freeman (2003) conducted a clinical trial to determine the effectiveness of music on pain reduction in older people with osteoarthritis. A VAS was used to measure pain on days 1, 7, and 14 of the study.

Scales permit researchers to efficiently quantify subtle gradations in the strength or intensity of individual characteristics. A good scale can be useful both for group-level comparisons (e.g., comparing the stress levels of male versus female patients) and for making individual comparisons (e.g., predicting that patient X will not need as much emotional support as patient Y because of scores on a coping scale). Scales can be administered either verbally or in writing and thus are suitable for use with most people.

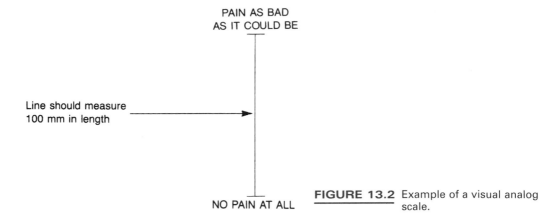

FIGURE 13.2 Example of a visual analog scale.

Scales are susceptible to several common problems, however, the most troublesome of which are referred to as **response set biases**. The most important biases include the following:

▶ *Social desirability response set bias*—a tendency to misrepresent attitudes or traits by giving answers that are consistent with prevailing social views
▶ *Extreme response set bias*—a tendency to consistently express attitudes or feelings in extreme responses (e.g., strongly agree), leading to distortions because extreme responses may not necessarily signify the greatest intensity of the trait being measured
▶ *Acquiescence response set bias*—a tendency to agree with statements regardless of their content by people who are referred to as *yea-sayers*. The opposite tendency for other people (*nay-sayers*) to disagree with statements independently of the question content is less common.

These biases can be reduced through such strategies as *counterbalancing* positively and negatively worded statements, developing sensitively worded questions, creating a permissive, nonjudgmental atmosphere, and guaranteeing the confidentiality of responses.

CONSUMER TIP

Most studies that collect self-report data involve one or more social–psychological scales. Typically, the scales are ones that were developed previously by other researchers.

■

VIGNETTES

Vignettes are brief descriptions of situations to which respondents are asked to react. The descriptions are structured to elicit information about respondents' perceptions, opinions, or knowledge about a phenomenon. The vignettes are usually written descriptions but can also be videotapes. The questions posed to respondents after the vignettes may be either open-ended (e.g., How would you recommend handling this situation?) or closed-ended (e.g., On the 7-point scale below, rate how well you think the nurse handled the situation).

Vignettes are an economical means of eliciting information about how people might behave in situations that would be difficult to observe in daily life. For example, we might want to assess how patients would react to or feel about nurses with different personal styles of interaction.

In clinical settings, it would be difficult to expose patients to many nurses, all of whom have been rated as having different interaction styles.

The principal problem with vignettes concerns the validity of responses. If respondents describe how they would react in a situation portrayed in the vignette, how accurate is that description of their actual behavior? Thus, although the use of vignettes can be profitable, the possibility of response biases should be recognized.

Example of vignettes

McDonald and her colleagues (2003) used vignettes to study how a patient's psychiatric diagnosis might affect nursing care for medical problems. Nurses read a vignette of a man admitted to an emergency department; some nurses were randomly assigned to read a vignette that described the man as being on medications used to treat schizophrenia.

Q SORTS

In a **Q sort**, participants are presented with a set of cards on which words, phrases, or statements are written. Participants are asked to sort the cards along a specified bipolar dimension, such as agree/disagree. Typically, there are between 60 and 100 cards to be sorted into nine or 11 piles, with the number of cards to be placed in each pile predetermined by the researcher.

The sorting instructions and objects to be sorted in a Q sort can vary. For example, personality can be studied by writing descriptions of personality traits on the cards; participants can then be asked to sort items on a continuum from "exactly like me" to "not at all like me." Other applications include asking patients to rate nursing behaviors on a continuum from least helpful to most helpful or asking cancer patients to rate various aspects of their treatment on a most distressing to least distressing continuum.

Q sorts can be a useful tool, but, like other data collection techniques, they also have drawbacks. On the positive side, Q sorts are versatile and can be applied to a wide variety of problems. Requiring people to place a predetermined number of cards in each pile eliminates many response biases that can occur in Likert scales. On the other hand, it is difficult and time-consuming to administer Q sorts to a large sample of people. Some critics argue that the forced distribution of cards according to researchers' specifications is artificial and excludes information about how participants would ordinarily distribute their responses.

Example of a Q sort

Snethen and Broome (2001) used Q sorts to explore the perceptions of adolescents living with end-stage renal disease. The statements on the cards described how the youths might view themselves (e.g., "I guess at my age, knowing about all of this stuff going on with my kidneys, I'm just kind of depressed a little"). Adolescents sorted 48 cards into 11 piles on a "most like me" to "most unlike me" continuum.

Evaluation of Self-Report Methods

Self-report techniques—the most common method of data collection in nursing studies—are strong with respect to their directness. If researchers want to know how people feel or what they believe, the most direct approach is to ask them. Moreover, self-reports frequently yield information that would be difficult, if not impossible, to gather by other means. Behaviors can be directly *observed*, but only if people are willing to engage in them publicly. It is usually impossible for researchers to observe such behaviors as contraceptive practices or drug use. Furthermore, observers can only observe behaviors occurring at the time of the study; self-report instruments can gather retrospective data about activities and events occurring in the past or about behaviors in which participants plan to engage in the future. Information about feelings, values, opinions, and motives can sometimes be inferred through observation, but people's actions do not always indicate their state of mind. Self-report instruments can be used to measure psychological characteristics through direct communication with participants.

Despite these advantages, self-report methods have some weaknesses. The most serious issue concerns the validity and accuracy of self-reports: How can we be sure that respondents feel or act the way they say they do? How can we trust the information that respondents provide, particularly if the questions ask them to admit to potentially undesirable traits? Investigators often have no alternative but to assume that most respondents have been frank. Yet, we all have a tendency to present ourselves in the best light, and this may conflict with the truth. When reading research reports, you should be alert to potential biases in self-reported data, particularly with respect to behaviors or feelings that society judges to be controversial or wrong.

You should also be familiar with the merits of unstructured and structured self-reports. In general, unstructured (qualitative) interviews are of greatest utility when a new area of research is being explored. A qualitative approach allows researchers to ascertain what the basic issues are, how sensitive or controversial the topic is, how individuals conceptualize and talk about a phenomenon, and what the range is of opinions or behaviors that are relevant to the topic. Qualitative methods may also help elucidate the underlying meaning of a pattern or relationship repeatedly observed in quantitative research.

Qualitative methods, however, are extremely time-consuming and demanding and are not appropriate for capturing the measurable aspects of a phenomenon, such as incidence (e.g., the percentage of women who experience post-partum depression or PPD); frequency (how often symptoms of PPD are experienced); duration (e.g., average time period during which PPD is present); or magnitude (e.g., degree of severity of PPD). Structured self-reports are also appropriate when researchers want to test hypotheses concerning relationships.

Critiquing Self-Reports

One of the first questions you should ask is whether the researcher made the right decision in obtaining the data by self-report rather than by an alternative method. Attention then should be paid to the adequacy of the actual methods used. Box 13-2 presents some guiding questions for critiquing self-reports.

It may be difficult to perform a thorough critique of self-report methods in studies reported in journals because researchers seldom include detailed descriptions of the data collection methods. What you can expect is information about the following aspects of the self-report data collection:

▶ The degree of structure used in the questioning
▶ Whether interviews or questionnaires (or variants such as a Q sort) were used
▶ How the instruments were administered (e.g., by telephone, in person, by mail, over the Internet)
▶ Where the interviews (if relevant) took place

BOX 13.2 Guidelines for Critiquing Self-Reports

1. Does the research question lend itself to a self-report method of data collection? Would an alternative method have been more appropriate?
2. Is the degree of structure consistent with the nature of the research question?
3. Given the research question and respondent characteristics, did the researcher use the best possible mode for collecting the data (i.e., personal interviews, telephone interviews, or self-administered questionnaires)?
4. Do the questions included in the instrument or topic guide adequately cover the complexities of the problem under investigation?
5. If a composite scale was used, does its use seem appropriate? Does the scale adequately capture the target research variable?
6. If a vignette or Q sort was used, does its use seem appropriate?

Degree of structure is especially important in your assessment of a data collection plan. The decision about an instrument's structure should be based on considerations that you can often evaluate. For example, respondents who are not very articulate are more receptive to instruments with many closed-ended questions than to questioning that forces them to compose lengthy answers. Other considerations include the amount of time available (structured instruments are more efficient); the expected sample size (open-ended questions and qualitative interviews are difficult to analyze with large samples); the status of existing information on the topic (in a new area of inquiry, a quantitative approach may not be warranted); and, most important, the nature of the research question.

CONSUMER TIP

In research reports, descriptions of data collection instruments are often brief; therefore, it is not always possible to evaluate the data collection plan thoroughly. For example, if a study involved the administration of a measure of depression (e.g., the Center for Epidemiological Studies Depression Scale, or CES-D), the research report most likely would not describe individual items on this scale—although the report should provide a reference to the appropriate source. Moreover, there is typically insufficient space in journals for the researcher to offer rationales (e.g., a rationale for why the CES-D was chosen instead of the Beck Depression Scale, or why depression was not measured through an approach other than structured self-report). Because of these facts, it may be difficult for you to undertake a detailed critique of the data collection plan.

▬

OBSERVATIONAL METHODS

For some research questions, direct observation of people's behavior is an alternative to self-reports. Within nursing research, observational methods have broad applicability, particularly for clinical inquiries. Nurses are in an advantageous position to observe, relatively unobtrusively, the behaviors and activities of patients, their families, and health care staff. Observational methods can be used to gather such information as the characteristics and conditions of individuals (e.g., the sleep–wake state of patients); verbal communication (e.g., exchange of information at change-of-shift report); nonverbal communication (e.g., body language); activities (e.g., geriatric patients' self-grooming activities); and environmental conditions (e.g., noise levels in nursing homes).

In observational studies, researchers have flexibility with regard to several important dimensions:

▶ *The focus of the observation.* The focus can be broadly defined events (e.g., patient mood swings), or it can be small, highly specific behaviors (e.g., gestures, facial expressions).

▶ *Concealment.* As discussed in Chapter 5, researchers do not always tell people they are being observed because awareness of being observed may cause people to behave abnormally, thereby jeopardizing the validity of the observations. The problem of behavioral distortions due to the known presence of an observer is called **reactivity**.

▶ *Duration of observation.* Some observations can be made in a short period of time, but others, particularly those in ethnographic and other field studies, may require months or years in the field.

▶ *Method of recording observations.* Observations can be made through the human senses and then recorded by paper-and-pencil methods, but they can also be done with sophisticated technical equipment (e.g., video equipment, specialized microphones and audio recording equipment, computers).

In summary, observational techniques can be used to measure a broad range of phenomena and are versatile along several key dimensions. Like self-report techniques, an important dimension for observational methods is degree of structure—that is, whether the observational data are amenable to qualitative or quantitative analysis.

Qualitative Observational Methods

Qualitative researchers collect observational data with a minimum of structure and researcher-imposed constraints. Skillful unstructured observation permits researchers to see the world as the study participants see it, to develop a rich understanding and appreciation of the phenomena of interest, to extract meaning from events and situations, and to grasp the subtleties of cultural variation.

Naturalistic observations often are made in field settings through a technique called **participant observation**. A participant observer participates in the functioning of the group or institution under study and strives to observe and record information within the contexts, experiences, and symbols that are relevant to the participants. By assuming a participating role, observers may have insights that would have eluded more passive or concealed observers. Not all qualitative observational studies use *participant* observation; some unstructured observations involve watching and recording unfolding behaviors without the observers' participation in activities. The great majority of qualitative observations, however, do involve some participation, particularly in ethnographic and grounded theory research.

Example of qualitative nonparticipant observation

Manias (2003) used unstructured observational methods to examine Australian nurses' management of postoperative patients' pain and anxiety—without participating in nursing activities. Nurses were observed during 2-hour observation sessions, during which time the observer made detailed notes on several broad topics (e.g., descriptions of "the evaluation undertaken by nurses following administration of medications to treat pain or anxiety," p. 587).

THE OBSERVER-PARTICIPANT ROLE IN PARTICIPANT OBSERVATION

In participant observation, the role observers play in the social group under study is important because their social position determines what they are likely to see. That is, the behaviors that are likely to be available for observation depend on the observers' position in a network of relations.

The extent of the observers' actual participation in a group is best thought of as a continuum. At one extreme of the continuum is complete immersion in the setting, with researchers assuming full participant status; at the other extreme is complete separation, with researchers assuming an onlooker status. Researchers may in some cases assume a fixed position on this continuum throughout the study. For example, researchers studying the stress and coping of parents whose infant has died of sudden infant death syndrome might spend time observing the parents' interactions with each other and with other family members in their homes, but they would not likely participate in the life of the family as an actual family member.

On the other hand, researchers' role as participants may evolve over the course of the field-work. A researcher may begin primarily as a bystander, with participation in group activities increasing over time. In other cases, it might be profitable to become immersed in a social setting quickly, with participation diminishing to allow more time for pure observation.

CONSUMER TIP

It is not unusual to find research reports that state that participant observation was used when in fact the description of the methods suggests that observation but not participation was involved. Some researchers appear to use the term "participant observation" to refer generally to unstructured observations conducted in the field.

Leininger (1985) has offered the following four-phase strategy as a possible model for participant observation: (1) primarily observation; (2) primarily observation with some participation; (3) primarily participation with some observation; and (4) reflective observation. In the initial phase, researchers observe and listen to those under study, allowing observers and participants to become acquainted and to get more comfortable in interacting. In phase 2, observation is enhanced by a modest degree of participation. As researchers participate more actively in the social group, the reactions of people to specific researcher behaviors can be more systematically studied. In phase 3, researchers strive to become more active participants, learning by the experience of doing rather than just watching and listening. In phase 4, researchers reflect on the total process of what transpired.

Observers must overcome at least two major hurdles in assuming a satisfactory role vis-à-vis participants. The first is to gain entrée into the social group under investigation; the second is to establish rapport and develop trust within that group. Without gaining entrée, the study cannot proceed; but without the trust of the group, the researcher will typically be restricted to "front stage" knowledge—that is, information distorted by the group's protective facades (Leininger, 1985). The goal of participant observers is to "get back stage"—to learn about the true realities of the group's experiences and behaviors. On the other hand, being a fully participating member does not *necessarily* offer the best perspective for studying a phenomenon—just as being an actor in a play does not offer the most advantageous view of the performance.

Example of a participant observation

McCarthy (2003) explored the influence of different care environments (acute, long-term, and community health care) on nurses' clinical reasoning related to the detection of acute confusion in older adults. Participant observation fieldwork was performed over a 3-month period. McCarthy attended intershift report sessions, attended multidisciplinary rounds, and observed nurse–patient, nurse–nurse, and nurse–physician interactions throughout the 24-hour workday on various units of the facilities. She also accompanied nurses on routine and on-call home visits.

GATHERING PARTICIPANT OBSERVATION DATA

Participant observers typically place few restrictions on the nature of the data collected, in keeping with the goal of minimizing observer-imposed meanings and structure. Nevertheless, participant observers often do have a broad plan for the types of information to be gathered. Among the aspects of an observed activity likely to be considered relevant are the following:

1. *The physical setting—"where" questions.* Where is the activity happening? What are the main features of the physical setting? What is the context within which human behavior unfolds?
2. *The participants—"who" questions.* Who is present? What are their characteristics? What are their roles? Who is given free access to the setting—who "belongs"? What brings these people together?
3. *Activities—"what" questions.* What is going on? What are participants doing? How do participants interact with one another? What methods do they use to communicate, and how frequently do they do so?
4. *Frequency and duration—"when" questions.* When did the activity begin and end? Is the activity a recurring one and, if so, how regularly does it recur?
5. *Process—"how" questions.* How is the activity organized? How are people interacting and communicating? How does the event unfold?
6. *Outcomes—"why" questions.* Why is the activity happening, or why is it happening in this manner? What kinds of things will ensue? What did not happen (especially if it ought to have happened) and why?

The next decision is to identify a way to sample observations and to select observational locations. Researchers generally use a combination of positioning approaches. *Single positioning* means staying in a single location for a period to observe transactions in that location. *Multiple positioning* involves moving around the site to observe behaviors from different locations. *Mobile positioning* involves following a person throughout a given activity or period.

Because participant observers cannot spend a lifetime in one site and cannot be in more than one place at a time, observation is usually supplemented with information from unstructured interviews or conversations. For example, informants may be asked to describe what went on in a meeting the observer was unable to attend, or to describe an event that occurred before the observer entered the field. In such cases, the informant functions as the observer's observer.

RECORDING OBSERVATIONS

The most common forms of record keeping in participant observation studies are logs and field notes, but photographs and videotapes may also be used. A **log** (or *field diary*) is a daily record of events and conversations. **Field notes** are much broader, more analytic, and more interpretive.

Field notes represent the observer's efforts to record information and also to synthesize and understand the data.

Field notes can be categorized according to their purpose. *Descriptive notes* (or *observational notes*) are objective descriptions of events and conversations. Descriptions of what has transpired must include enough contextual information about time, place, and actors to fully portray the situation. The term *thick description* is often used to characterize the goal of participation observers' descriptive notes.

A second broad class of field notes are called *reflective notes,* which document researchers' personal experiences, reflections, and progress while in the field. Reflective notes can serve a number of different purposes. *Theoretical notes* are interpretive attempts to attach meaning to observations. *Methodologic notes* are instructions or reminders about how subsequent observations will be made. *Personal notes* are comments about the researcher's own feelings during the research process. Box 13-3 presents examples of various types of field notes from Beck's (2002) study of mothering twins.

BOX 13.3   Example of Field Notes: Mothering Multiples Grounded Theory Study

Observational Notes: O.L. attended the mothers of multiples support group again this month but she looked worn out today. She wasn't as bubbly as she had been at the March meeting. She explained why she wasn't doing as well this month. She and her husband had just found out that their house has lead-based paint in it. Both twins do have increased lead levels. She and her husband are in the process of buying a new home.

Theoretical Notes: So far all the mothers have stressed the need for routine in order to survive the first year of caring for twins. Mothers, however, have varying definitions of routine. I.R. had the firmest routine with her twins. B.L. is more flexible with her routine, i.e., the twins are always fed at the same time but aren't put down for naps or bed at night at the same time. Whenever one of the twins wants to go to sleep is fine with her. B.L. does have a daily routine in regards to housework. For example, when the twins are down in the morning for a nap, she makes their bottles up for the day (14 bottles total).

Methodologic Notes: The first sign-up sheet I passed around at the Mothers of Multiples Support Group for women to sign up to participate in interviews for my grounded theory study only consisted of two columns: one for the mother's name and one for her telephone number. I need to revise this sign-up sheet to include extra columns for the age of the multiples, the town where the mother lives, and older siblings and their ages. My plan is to start interviewing mothers with multiples around 1 year of age so that the moms can reflect back over the process of mothering their infants for the first 12 months of their lives.

Right now I have no idea of the ages of the infants of the mothers who signed up to be interviewed. I will need to call the nurse in charge of this support group to find out the ages.

Personal Notes: Today was an especially challenging interview. The mom had picked the early afternoon for me to come to her home to interview her because that is the time her 2-year-old son would be napping. When I arrived at her house her 2-year-old ran up to me and said hi. The mom explained that he had taken an earlier nap that day and that he would be up during the interview. So in the living room with us during our interview were her two twin daughters (3 months old) swinging in the swings and her 2-year-old son. One of the twins was quite cranky for the first half hour of the interview. During the interview the 2-year-old sat on my lap and looked at the two books I had brought as a little present. If I didn't keep him occupied with the books, he would keep trying to reach for the microphone of the tape recorder.

From Beck, C. T. (2002). Releasing the pause button: Mothering twins during the first year of life. *Qualitative Health Research,* 12, 593–608.

The success of any participant observation study depends on the quality of the logs and field notes. It is clearly essential to record observations as quickly as possible, but participant observers cannot usually record information by openly carrying a clipboard or a tape recorder because this would undermine their role as ordinary participants of the group. Observers must develop the skill of making detailed mental notes that can later be written or tape-recorded. The use of laptop computers can greatly facilitate the recording and organization of notes in the field.

Quantitative Observational Methods

Structured observation for quantitative studies differs from unstructured techniques in the specificity of behaviors selected for observation, in the advance preparation of forms, and in the kinds of activity in which observers engage. The creativity of structured observation lies not in the observation itself but rather in the development of a system for accurately categorizing, recording, and encoding the observations and sampling the phenomena of interest.

CATEGORIES AND CHECKLISTS

The most common approach to making structured observations is to use a category system for classifying observed phenomena. A **category system** represents a method of recording in a systematic, quantitative fashion the behaviors and events of interest that transpire within a setting.

Some category systems are constructed so that *all* observed behaviors within a specified domain (e.g., all body positions and movements) can be classified into one and only one category. A contrasting technique is to develop a system in which only particular types of behavior (which may or may not be manifested) are categorized. For example, if we were studying autistic children's aggressive behavior, we might develop such categories as "strikes another child," "kicks or hits walls or floor," or "throws objects around the room." In this category system, many behaviors—all that are nonaggressive—would not be classified, and some children may exhibit *no* aggressive actions. Nonexhaustive systems are adequate for many purposes, but one risk is that resulting data might be difficult to interpret. When a large number of behaviors are not categorized, the investigator may have difficulty placing categorized behavior into perspective.

Example of a nonexhaustive checklist

Feldt (2001) created a checklist to capture the occurrence of nonverbal pain indicators. Observers indicate whether, during an observational session, subjects demonstrate such pain-related behaviors as nonverbal vocal complaints (e.g., moans, grunts, sighs); facial grimaces (e.g., furrowed brow, clenched teeth); and bracing (clutching onto side rails). Behaviors unrelated to pain are not captured.

One of the most important requirements of a category system is the careful and explicit operational definition of the behaviors and characteristics to be observed. Each category must be carefully explained, giving observers clear-cut criteria for assessing the occurrence of the phenomenon. Even with detailed definitions of categories, observers often are faced with making numerous on-the-spot inferences. Virtually all category systems require observer inference, to greater or lesser degree.

Example of moderate observer inference

Symanski, Hayes, and Akilesh (2002) examined premature infants' sleep–wake states before and after nursing interventions. The infants' behavioral states were measured with an observational category system applied to videotaped recordings of the infants. Within 3-minute intervals, observers categorized the infants' state into one of four categories: wake, drowse, quiet sleep, and active sleep. As an example, the definition of the "wake" state is: "The newborn's eyes are open, focused, and scanning the environment. State may include crying or fussing. Motor activity may be high or low. Respiration is regular and tracks motor activity" (p. 308).

After a category system has been developed, researchers typically construct a **checklist**, which is the instrument used to record observed phenomena. The checklist is generally formatted with the list of behaviors from the category system on the left and space for tallying their frequency or duration on the right. The task of the observer using an exhaustive category system (such as the one in the previous example) is to place *all* observed behaviors in one category for each integral unit of behavior (e.g., a sentence in a conversation, a time interval). Checklists based on exhaustive category systems tend to be demanding because the recording task is continuous. With nonexhaustive category systems, categories of behaviors that may or may not be manifested by participants are listed. The observer's tasks are to watch for instances of these behaviors and to record their occurrence. With this type of checklist, the observer does not classify all behaviors of the people being observed, but rather identifies the occurrence and frequency of particular behaviors.

RATING SCALES

Another approach to structured observations is to use a **rating scale**, which is a tool that requires observers to rate some phenomena in terms of points along a descriptive continuum. The observer may be required to make ratings of behavior at intervals throughout the observation or to summarize an entire event or transaction after observation is completed.

Rating scales can be used as an extension of checklists, in which the observer records not only the occurrence of some behavior but also some qualitative aspect of it, such as its magnitude or intensity. When rating scales are coupled with a category scheme in this fashion, considerably more information about the phenomena under investigation can be obtained. The disadvantage of this approach is that it places an immense burden on observers.

Example of observational ratings

The NEECHAM Confusion Scale is an observational measure designed for use by nurses to detect the presence and severity of acute confusion. The NEECHAM consists of three subscales—Processing, Behavior, and Physiologic Control. The first two subscales consist of several dimensions along which the observed elder is rated. For example, one rating in the Processing subscale concerns alertness/responsiveness, and the ratings are from 0 (responsiveness depressed) to 4 (full attentiveness). The NEECHAM has been used extensively for both clinical and research purposes. For example, Wakefield (2002) used the NEECHAM to study the relationship between admission risk factors and subsequent development of acute confusion in elderly hospitalized patients.

OBSERVATIONAL SAMPLING

Researchers must decide how and when structured observational systems will be applied. Observational sampling methods provide a mechanism for obtaining representative examples of the behaviors being observed. One system is **time sampling**, which involves the selection of time periods during which observations will occur. Time frames may be systematically selected (e.g., every 30 seconds at 2-minute intervals) or selected at random.

Event sampling selects integral behaviors or events for observation. Event sampling requires researchers to either have knowledge about the occurrence of events or be in a position to wait for or precipitate their occurrence. Examples of integral events that may be suitable for event sampling include shift changes of nurses in a hospital, cast removals of pediatric patients, and cardiac arrests in the emergency room. This sampling approach is preferable to time sampling when the events of interest are infrequent and may be missed if time sampling is used. When behaviors and events are relatively frequent, however, time sampling enhances the representativeness of the observed behaviors.

Evaluation of Observational Methods

The field of nursing is particularly well suited to observational research. Nurses are often in a position to watch people's behaviors and may, by training, be especially sensitive observers. Moreover, certain research questions are better suited to observation than to self-reports, such as when people cannot adequately describe their own behaviors. This may be the case when people are unaware of their own behavior (e.g., stress-induced behavior), when people are embarrassed to report their activities (e.g., aggressive or hostile actions), when behaviors are emotionally laden (e.g., grieving behavior), or when people are not capable of articulating their actions (e.g., young children or the mentally ill). Observational methods have an intrinsic appeal for directly capturing behaviors and events. Furthermore, observational methods can provide information of great depth and variety. With this approach, humans—the observers—are used as measuring instruments and provide a uniquely sensitive and intelligent (if fallible) tool.

Several of the shortcomings of the observational approach have already been mentioned. These include possible ethical difficulties and reactivity of the observed when the observer is conspicuous. However, one of the most pervasive problems is the vulnerability of observations to bias. A number of factors interfere with objective observations, including the following:

▶ Emotions, prejudices, and values of the observer may result in faulty inference.
▶ Personal interest and commitment may color what is seen in the direction of what the observer wants to see.
▶ Anticipation of what is to be observed may affect what is perceived.
▶ Hasty decisions before adequate information is collected may result in erroneous conclusions or classifications.

Observational biases probably cannot be eliminated, but they can be minimized through careful observer training.

Both unstructured and structured observational methods have advantages and disadvantages. Qualitative observational methods have the potential of yielding a richer understanding of human behaviors and social situations than is possible with structured procedures. Skillful participant observers can "get inside" a situation and get a more complete understanding of its complexities. Furthermore, qualitative observational approaches are inherently flexible and, therefore, permit observers freedom to reconceptualize the problem after becoming familiar with the situation. On the other hand, observer bias may pose a threat: once researchers begin to participate in a group's activities, the possibility of emotional involvement becomes a salient issue. Participant observers may develop a myopic view on issues of importance to the group. Another issue is that qualitative observational methods are highly dependent on the observational and interpersonal skills of the observer.

Researchers generally choose an approach that matches the research problem—and their paradigmatic orientation. Qualitative observational methods are especially profitable for in-depth research in which the investigator wishes to establish an adequate conceptualization of the important issues in a social setting or to develop hypotheses. Structured observation is better suited to formal hypothesis testing regarding measurable human behaviors.

Critiquing Observational Methods

As in the case of self-reports, the first question you should ask when critiquing an observational study is whether the data should have been collected by some other approach. The advantages and disadvantages of observational methods, discussed previously, should be helpful in considering the appropriateness of using observation.

Some additional guidelines for critiquing observational studies are presented in Box 13-4 A journal article should usually document the following aspects of the observational plan:

▶ The degree of structure in the observations
▶ The focus of the observations
▶ The degree to which the observer was concealed
▶ For qualitative studies, how entry into the observed group was gained, the relationship between the observer and those observed, the time period over which data were collected, and the method of recording data

---

BOX 13.4   Guidelines for Critiquing Observational Methods

1. Does the research question lend itself to an observational approach? Would an alternative method have been more appropriate?
2. Is the degree of structure consistent with the nature of the research question?
3. To what degree were observers concealed during data collection? If there was no concealment, what effect might the observers' presence have had on the behaviors being observed?
4. To what degree did the observer participate in activities with those being observed, and was this appropriate?
5. Where did the observations take place? To what extent did the setting influence the naturalness of the behaviors observed?
6. How were data actually recorded (e.g., on field notes, checklists)? Did the recording procedure appear appropriate?
7. What was the plan by which events or behaviors were sampled? Did this plan appear appropriate?
8. What steps were taken to minimize observer biases?

▶ For quantitative studies, a description of the category system or rating scales and the settings in which observations took place

▶ The plan for sampling events and behaviors to observe

BIOPHYSIOLOGIC MEASURES

One result of the trend toward clinical, patient-centered studies is greater use of biophysiologic and physical variables. Clinical nursing studies involve biophysiologic instruments both for creating independent variables (e.g., an intervention using biofeedback equipment) and for measuring dependent variables. For the most part, our discussion focuses on the use of biophysiologic measures as dependent (outcome) variables.

Most nursing studies in which biophysiologic measures have been used fall into one of six classes:

1. *Studies of basic biophysiologic processes that have relevance for nursing care.* These studies involve normal, healthy participants or an animal species.
2. *Descriptions of nursing actions and explorations of the ways in which nursing actions affect health outcomes.* These studies do not focus on specific interventions, but rather are designed to document standard procedures or to learn how standard nursing procedures affect patients.
3. *Evaluations of a specific nursing intervention.* These studies involve testing a new intervention, often in comparison with standard methods of care. Typically, these studies involve a hypothesis stating that the innovative nursing procedure will result in improved biophysiologic outcomes.
4. *Product assessments.* Some studies are designed to evaluate alternative products to enhance patient health or comfort, rather than to evaluate nursing actions.
5. *Studies to evaluate the measurement and recording of biophysiologic information gathered by nurses.* The accurate measurement of biophysiologic phenomena is crucial, and therefore some studies focus on improving clinical measurements.
6. *Studies of the correlates of physiologic functioning in patients with health problems.* Researchers study possible antecedents and consequences of biophysiologic indicators to gain insight into potential treatments or modes of care.

Example of evaluating measurement alternatives

Maxton, Justin, and Gillies (2004) conducted a study to determine which site most closely reflects core temperature in babies and children following cardiac surgery. They compared pulmonary artery temperature to the temperature measured at rectal, bladder, nasopharyngeal, axillary, and tympanic sites in 19 postoperative children in Sydney, Australia.

Types of Biophysiologic Measures

Biophysiologic measures include both *in vivo* and *in vitro* measures. *In vivo* measures are those performed directly within or on living organisms. Examples of *in vivo* measures include blood pressure, body temperature, and vital capacity measurement. *In vivo* instruments are available to measure all bodily functions, and technological advances continue to improve the ability to measure biophysiologic phenomena more accurately, conveniently, and rapidly.

Example of a study with in vivo measures

Using an experimental design, Waltman, Brewer, Rogers, and May (2004) compared the heart rates and oxygen saturation (SpO$_2$) levels of newborns who received oronasopharyngeal bulb suctioning at birth with those of newborns who did not.

With *in vitro* measures, data are gathered from participants by extracting some biophysiologic material from them and subjecting it to laboratory analysis. The analysis is normally done by specialized laboratory technicians. *In vitro* measures include chemical measures (e.g., the measurement of hormone, sugar, or potassium levels); microbiologic measures (e.g., bacterial counts and identification); and cytologic or histologic measures (e.g., tissue biopsies).

Example of a study with in vitro measures

Midthun, Paur, Lindseth, and VonDuvillard (2003) compared a new method of assessing bacteriuria in incontinent nursing home residents with the traditional clean-catch urine culture method. The new method used a urine dipstick applied to incontinence pads.

Evaluation of Biophysiologic Measures

Biophysiologic measures offer a number of advantages to nurse researchers, including the following:

▶ Biophysiologic measures are relatively accurate and precise, especially when compared with psychological measures, such as self-report measures of anxiety, pain, and so forth.
▶ Biophysiologic measures are objective. Two nurses reading from the same spirometer output are likely to record identical tidal volume measurements, and two different spirometers are likely to produce the same readouts. Patients cannot easily distort measurements of biophysiologic functioning deliberately.
▶ Biophysiologic instrumentation provides valid measures of the targeted variables: Thermometers can be depended on to measure temperature and not blood volume, and so forth. For nonbiophysiologic measures, there are typically concerns about whether an instrument is really measuring the target concept.
▶ Because equipment for obtaining biophysiologic measurements is available in hospital settings, nurse researchers may incur no or minimal costs for collecting biophysiologic data.

There are some potential drawbacks that may need to be considered:

▶ The measuring tool may affect the variables it is attempting to measure. For example, the presence of a sensing device (e.g., a transducer) located in a blood vessel partially blocks that vessel and, hence, alters the pressure-flow characteristics being measured.
▶ Energy must often be applied to the organism when taking the biophysiologic measurements; extreme caution must continually be exercised to avoid damaging cells by high-energy concentrations.

In summary, biophysiologic measures are plentiful, tend to be accurate and valid, and are extremely useful in clinical nursing studies. However, care must be exercised in using them with regard to practical, ethical, medical, and technical considerations.

BOX 13.5   **Guidelines for Critiquing Biophysiologic Methods**

1. Does the research question lend itself to a biophysiologic approach? Would an alternative method have been theoretically more appropriate?
2. Was the proper instrumentation used to obtain the biophysiologic measurements? Would an alternative instrument or method have been more appropriate?
3. Does the researcher appear to have the skills necessary for proper interpretation of the biophysiologic measures?

Critiquing Biophysiologic Measures

Biophysiologic measures offer nurse researchers many advantages, as discussed previously, and their shortcomings are relatively minor. As always, however, the most important consideration in evaluating a data collection strategy is the appropriateness of the measures for the research question. The objectivity, accuracy, and availability of biophysiologic measures are of little significance if an alternative method would have resulted in a better measurement of the key concepts. Stress, for example, could be measured in various ways: through self-report (e.g., through the use of a scale such as the State-Trait Anxiety Inventory); through direct observation of participants' behavior during exposure to stressful stimuli; or by measuring heart rate, blood pressure, or levels of adrenocorticotropic hormone in urine samples. The choice of which measure to use must be linked to the way that stress is conceptualized in the research problem.

Additional criteria for assessing the use of biophysiologic measures are presented in Box 13-5. The general questions to consider are these: Did the researcher select the correct biophysiologic measure? Was care taken in the collection of the data? Did the researcher competently interpret the data?

CONSUMER TIP

Many nursing studies—especially qualitative ones—integrate a variety of data collection approaches. Qualitative studies are especially likely to combine unstructured observations and self-reports. If multiple approaches are used in a quantitative study, structured self-reports combined with biophysiologic measures are most common.

IMPLEMENTING THE DATA COLLECTION PLAN

In addition to selecting methods for collecting data, researchers must develop and implement a plan for gathering their data. This involves decisions that could affect the quality of the data being collected.

One important decision concerns who will collect the data. Researchers often hire assistants to collect data rather than doing it personally. This is especially likely to be the case in large-scale quantitative studies. In other studies, nurses or other health care staff are asked to assist in the collection of data. From your perspective as a consumer, the critical issue is whether the people collecting data were able to produce valid and accurate data. In any research endeavor, adequate training of data collectors is essential.

> **BOX 13.6** **Guidelines for Critiquing Data Collection Procedures**
>
> 1. Who collected the research data? Were the data collectors qualified for their role, or is there something about them (e.g., their professional role, their relationship with study participants) that could undermine the collection of unbiased, high-quality data?
> 2. How were data collectors trained? Does the training appear adequate?
> 3. Where and under what circumstances were the data gathered? Were other people present during that data collection? Could the presence of others have created any distortions?
> 4. Did the collection of data place any undue burdens (in terms of time or stress) on participants? How might this have affected data quality?

Another issue concerns the circumstances under which data were gathered. For example, it may be critical to ensure total privacy to participants. In most cases, it is important for researchers to create a nonjudgmental atmosphere in which participants are encouraged to be candid or behave naturally. Again, you as a consumer must ask whether there is anything about the way in which the data were collected that could have created bias or otherwise affected data quality.

In evaluating the data collection plan of a study, then, you should critically appraise not only the actual methods chosen but also the procedures used to collect the data. Box 13-6 provides some specific guidelines for critiquing the procedures used to collect research data.

C H A P T E R   R E V I E W

Key new terms introduced in the chapter, together with a summary of major points, are presented in this section. In addition, Chapter 13 of the *Study Guide to Accompany Essentials of Nursing Research,* 6th edition offers various exercises and study suggestions for reinforcing the concepts presented in this chapter. For additional review, see the Student Self-Study Review Questions section of the Student Resource CD-ROM provided with this book.

K E Y   N E W   T E R M S

Biophysiologic measures
Category system
Checklist
Closed-ended question
Completely unstructured interview
Critical incidents technique
Diary
Event sampling
Field notes
Fixed-alternative question
Focus group interview
Grand tour question
Instrument
Interview schedule
Life history

Likert scale
Log
Observation
Open-ended question
Participant observation
Q sort
Questionnaire
Rating scale
Reactivity
Records
Response alternative
Response set bias
Scale
Self-reports
Semantic differential

Semi-structured interview
Summated rating scale
Think aloud method
Time sampling

Topic guide
Vignette
Visual analog scale

S U M M A R Y   P O I N T S

▷ Some researchers use existing data in their studies—for example, those doing historical research, meta-analyses, secondary analyses, or analyses of available **records**.

▷ Data collection methods vary along four dimensions: structure, quantifiability, researcher obtrusiveness, and objectivity.

▷ The three principal data collection methods for nurse researchers are self-reports, observations, and biophysiologic measures.

▷ Self-reports are the most widely used method of collecting data for nursing studies. Qualitative studies—especially ethnographies—are more likely than quantitative studies to triangulate data from different sources.

▷ **Self-report** data are collected by means of an oral interview or written questionnaire. Self-report methods are an indispensable means of collecting data but are susceptible to errors of reporting.

▷ Unstructured self-reports, used in qualitative studies, include **completely unstructured interviews**, which are conversational discussions on the topic of interest; **semi-structured** (or *focused*) **interviews**, using a broad **topic guide**; **focus group interviews**, which involve discussions with small groups; **life histories**, which encourage respondents to narrate their life experiences regarding some theme; the **think aloud method**, which involves having people talk about decisions as they are making them; **diaries**, in which respondents are asked to maintain daily records about some aspects of their lives; and the **critical incidents technique**, which involve probes about the circumstances surrounding a behavior or incident that is critical to an outcome of interest.

▷ Structured self-reports used in quantitative studies employ a formal **instrument**—a **questionnaire** or **interview schedule**—that may contain a combination of **open-ended questions** (which permit respondents to respond in their own words) and **closed-ended questions** (which offer respondents fixed alternatives from which to choose).

▷ Questionnaires are less costly than interviews, offer the possibility of anonymity, and run no risk of interviewer bias; however, interviews yield higher response rates, are suitable for a wider variety of people, and provide richer data than questionnaires.

▷ Social–psychological **scales** are self-report tools for quantitatively measuring the intensity of such characteristics as personality traits, attitudes, needs, and perceptions.

▷ **Likert scales** (or **summated rating scales**) present respondents with a series of *items* worded favorably or unfavorably toward some phenomenon; responses indicating level of agreement or disagreement with each statement are scored and summed into a composite score.

▷ The **semantic differential** (SD) technique consists of a series of scales with bipolar adjectives (e.g., good/bad) along which respondents rate their reactions toward phenomena.

▷ A **visual analog scale** (VAS) is used to measure subjective experiences (e.g., pain, fatigue) along a line designating a bipolar continuum.

▷ Scales are versatile and powerful but are susceptible to **response set biases**—the tendency of some people to respond to items in characteristic ways, independently of item content.

▷ **Vignettes** are brief descriptions of some event, person, or situation to which respondents are asked to react.

▷ With a **Q sort**, respondents sort a set of statements into piles according to specified criteria.

▷ Direct **observation** of phenomena, which includes both structured and unstructured procedures, is a technique for gathering data about behaviors and events.

▷ One type of unstructured observation is **participant observation**, in which the researcher gains entrée into the social group of interest and participates to varying degrees in its functioning while making in-depth observations of activities and events. **Logs** of daily events and **field notes** of the observer's experiences and interpretations constitute the major data collection instruments in unstructured observation.

▷ Structured observations for quantitative studies, which dictate what the observer should observe, often involve **checklists**—tools based on **category systems** for recording the appearance, frequency, or duration of prespecified behaviors or events. Alternatively, the observer may use **rating scales** to rate phenomena along a dimension of interest (e.g., energetic/lethargic).

▷ Structured observations often use a sampling plan (such as **time sampling** or **event sampling**) for selecting the behaviors, events, and conditions to be observed.

▷ Observational techniques are a versatile and important alternative to self-reports, but observational biases can pose a threat to the validity and accuracy of observational data.

▷ Data may also be derived from **biophysiologic measures**, which can be classified as either *in vivo* measurements (those performed within or on living organisms) or *in vitro* measurements (those performed outside the organism's body, such as blood tests). Biophysiologic measures have the advantage of being objective, accurate, and precise.

▷ In developing a data collection plan, the researcher must decide who will collect the data, how the data collectors will be trained, and what the circumstances for data collection will be.

RESEARCH EXAMPLES | Critical Thinking Activities

 EXAMPLE 1: Participant Observation and Focused Interviews

Aspects of an ethnographic study, featuring terms and concepts discussed in this chapter, are presented below, followed by some questions to guide critical thinking. (The full research report is available in *Qualitative Health Research, 14,* 61–77.)

Study

"Surfacing the life phases of a mental health support group" (Mohr, 2004)

Statement of Purpose

The purpose of this study was to explore how mental health advocacy or support groups start and develop, and what the challenges are that threaten their survival.

research examples continue on page 318

Method

Mohr undertook a 2½-year ethnographic study of a developing family support program that was associated with a system of care for children with emotional and behavioral disabilities. The group agreed to have Mohr function as a participating observer. Her family history (she had psychiatrically ill relatives) enhanced her acceptance and credibility with group members. Between 1999 and 2001, she attended 25 regular support group sessions and recorded field notes describing the meetings: who attended, where they sat, who came late or early, who presented, who asked questions, and who made comments. Observation also focused on the structure and content of group activities and on its processes. Then, in 2001, Mohr conducted focused interviews with five group leaders and seven other members of the group. The interviews were designed to help Mohr understand the informants' views on the support group's culture, the processes of formation and maintenance, and the role of the group in the informants' lives. The interviews were audiotaped and transcribed. In all, the data consisted of 703 pages of field notes, personal reflections, interview transcripts, and documents generated by the support group.

Key Findings

▶ The data revealed a dynamic pattern of group evolution that included several distinct sequential phases.

▶ The phases through which the support group evolved included exploring, shaping and shaking, structuring, turbulence, and maintenance.

Critical Thinking Suggestions*

*See the Student Resource CD-ROM for a discussion of these questions.

1. Answer the following questions, many of which are adapted from the critiquing guidelines presented in this chapter:
   a. How much structure did Mohr use in her data collection? Is the degree of structure she used consistent with the nature of the research question?
   b. Some of Mohr's data were gathered through observation; does the research question lend itself to an observational approach? If she had not undertaken observational work, would her findings likely be affected?
   c. How likely is it that Mohr's presence at group meetings affected the members' behaviors? Comment on Mohr's role as a participant observer; for example, how might Mohr's observations have been affected by her role as an active participant?
   d. Comment on the thoroughness of Mohr's observations; are there aspects of the meetings to which she appears not have attended?
   e. Some of Mohr's data were gathered through self-report; does the research question lend itself to a self-report approach? If she had not gathered self-report data, would her findings likely have been affected?
   f. Comment on her strategy of conducting the focused interviews toward the end of her fieldwork.

2. If the results of this study are trustworthy, what are some of the uses to which the findings might be put in clinical practice?

 EXAMPLE 2: Physiologic, Self-Report, and Observational Measures

Aspects of a quantitative nursing study, featuring terms and concepts discussed in this chapter, are presented below, followed by some questions to guide critical thinking. (The full research report is available in *Journal of Obstetric, Gynecologic, & Neonatal Nursing, 32,* 340–347.)

Study

"Co-bedding versus single-bedding premature multiple-gestation infants in incubators" (Byers, Yovaish, Lowman, & Francis, 2003)

Statement of Purpose

The study was designed to compare the physiologic stability and behavioral effects of co-bedding versus single-bedding premature multiple gestation infants in incubators, and to assess the psychological effects on their parents.

Method

A true experimental design was used in which multiple-gestation infants were assigned at random to a co-bedded group (16 infants) or to a single-bedded control group (22 infants). A wide range of data was gathered in the study, including data from records (demographic information, complication rates, blood cultures). Physiologic variables were measured using the heart rate, respiratory rate, and oxygen saturation information obtained from the infants' neonatal monitor. The infants' sleep–wake synchronicity and stress cue behaviors were measured through structured observation of the infants' behaviors by developmental specialists. Parental variables were measured via self-reports. For example, parental anxiety was measured using the "state" items from the State-Trait Anxiety Inventory. This scale consists of 20 items with a 4-point Likert-type scale. Parental attachment was measured using the Maternal Attachment Inventory, a 28-item measure with Likert-type items. Finally, parental satisfaction with care was measured with an 11-item parent satisfaction tool, which uses a 5-point Likert-type scale. The infants' physiologic and behavioral variables were recorded daily for 5 days and then averaged. Parental data were gathered at baseline (prior to random assignment) and then again 5 days later.

Key Findings

▶ Overall, the two groups of infants did not differ significantly in terms of physiologic stability and behavior.
▶ Sleep–wake synchronicity was significantly higher in the co-bedded than in the single-bedded group on days 1 and 3.
▶ Parental satisfaction, anxiety, and attachment were similar in the two groups.
▶ No adverse events (e.g., medication errors, infection) occurred in either group.

research examples continue on page 320

RESEARCH EXAMPLES *Continued*

Critical Thinking Suggestions

1. Answer the following questions, many of which are adapted from the critiquing guidelines presented in this chapter:

    a. How much structure did the researchers use in their data collection? Is the degree of structure they used consistent with the nature of the research question?

    b. Some of the researchers' outcome data were gathered through self-reports; does the research question lend itself to the use of self-report data? If they had not gathered self-report data, would their findings likely be affected?

    c. How do you think the self-report data were gathered (by interview or questionnaire)? What were the disadvantages or advantages of this approach?

    d. Some of the outcome data were gathered through observation; does the research question lend itself to an observational approach? If the researchers had not undertaken observational work, would the findings likely be affected?

    e. To what extent do you think the behavior of those being observed was affected by the presence of observers? Do you think that the risk of observational bias was high?

    f. Some of the researchers' outcome data were biophysiologic measures; is this compatible with the research question? Was this the best method to use?

    g. Comment on the researchers' overall data collection plan in terms of the timing of the data collection.

2. If the results of this study are valid and reliable, what are some of the uses to which the findings might be put in clinical practice?

▨ EXAMPLE 3: Structured Self-Reports

1. Read the method section from the Motzer et al. study ("Sense of Coherence") in Appendix A of this book, and then answer the relevant questions in Box 13-2.

2. Also consider the following targeted questions, which may further sharpen your critical thinking skills and assist you in assessing aspects of the study's merit:

    a. What would be the advantage of using the short-form of the SOCQ? What might be some of the disadvantages?

    b. Why do you think the researchers administered the Marlowe-Crowne Social Desirability index (SDI)?

EXAMPLE 4: Unstructured Self-Reports

Read the procedure section from Beck's study ("Birth Trauma") in Appendix B of this book, and then answer the relevant questions in Box 13-2. Also consider the following targeted questions, which may further sharpen your critical thinking skills and assist you in assessing aspects of the study:

    a. Comment on the potential added value of having some of the respondents' journals as a data source.

    b. Comment on the Beck's procedure of following up with further questions after she received the respondents' birth trauma stories.

SUGGESTED READINGS

Methodologic References

Frank-Stromberg, M. & Olsen, S. J. (Eds.). (2004). *Instruments for clinical health care.* Sudbury, MA: Jones & Bartlett Publishers.

Kerlinger, F. N., & Lee, H. B. (2000). *Foundations of behavioral research* (4th ed.). Orlando, FL: Harcourt College Publishers.

Leininger, M. M. (Ed.). (1985). *Qualitative research methods in nursing.* New York: Grune & Stratton.

Polit, D. F., & Beck, C. T. (2004). *Nursing research: Principles and methods* (7th ed.). Philadelphia: Lippincott Williams & Wilkins.

Rew, L., Bechtel, D., & Sapp, A. (1993). Self-as-instrument in qualitative research. *Nursing Research, 42,* 300–301.

Waltz, C. F., Strickland, O. L., & Lenz, E. R. (1991). *Measurement in nursing research* (2nd ed.). Philadelphia: F. A. Davis.

Studies Cited in Chapter 13

Abel, E., & Painter, L. (2003). Factors that influence adherence to HIV mediations: Perceptions of women and health care providers. *Journal of the Association of Nurses in AIDS Care, 14,* 61–69.

Byers, J. F., Yovaish, W., Lowman, L. B., & Francis, J. D. (2003). Co-bedding versus single-bedding premature multiple-gestation infants in incubators. *Journal of Obstetric, Gynecologic, & Neonatal Nursing, 32,* 340–347.

Cavendish, R., Luise, B. K., Russo, D., Mitzeliotis, C., Bauer, M., Bajo, M., et al. (2004). Spiritual perspectives of nurses in the United States relevant for education and practice. *Western Journal of Nursing Research, 26,* 196–212.

Cheek, J., & Gibson, T. (2003). Issues impacting on registered nurses providing care to older people in an acute care setting. *NT Research, 8,* 134–149.

Cheung, J. & Hocking, P. (2004). The experience of spousal carers of people with multiple sclerosis. *Qualitative Health Research, 14,* 153–166.

Feldt, K. S. (2001). Checklist of Nonverbal Pain Indicators. *Pain Management Nursing, 1,* 13–21.

Haglund, K. (2003). Sexually abstinent African American adolescent females' descriptions of abstinence. *Journal of Nursing Scholarship, 35,* 231–236.

Manias, E. (2003). Pain and anxiety management in the postoperative gastro-surgical setting. *Journal of Advanced Nursing, 41,* 585–594.

Maxton, F. J., Justin, L., & Gillies, D. (2004). Estimating core temperature in infants and children after cardiac surgery: A comparison of six methods. *Journal of Advanced Nursing, 45,* 214–222.

McCaffrey, R., & Freeman, E. (2003). Effect of music on chronic osteoarthritis pain in older people. *Journal of Advanced Nursing, 44,* 517–524.

McCarthy, M. C. (2003). Detecting acute confusion in older adults: Comparing clinical reasoning of nurses working in acute, long-term, and community health care environments. *Research in Nursing and Health, 26,* 203–212.

McDonald, D. D., Frakes, M., Apostolidis, B., Armstrong, B., Goldblatt, S., & Bernardo, D. (2003). Effect of a psychiatric diagnosis on nursing care for nonpsychiatric problems. *Research in Nursing & Health, 26,* 225–232.

Midthun, S. J., Paur, R. A., Lindseth, G., & VonDuvillard, S. P. (2003). Bacteriuria detection with a urine dipstick applied to incontinence pads of nursing home residents. *Geriatric Nursing, 24,* 206–209.

Mohr, W. K. (2004). Surfacing the life phases of a mental health support group. *Qualitative Health Report, 14,* 61–77.

Niederstadt, J. A. (2004). Frequency and timing of activated clotting time levels for sheath removal. *Journal of Nursing Care Quality, 19,* 34–38.

Paun, O. (2004). Female Alzheimer's patient caregivers share their strength. *Holistic Nursing Practice, 18,* 11–17.

Phillips, L. R., Brewer, B. B., & deArdon, E. T. (2001). The Elder Image Scale: A method for indexing history and emotion in family caregiving. *Journal of Nursing Measurement, 9,* 23–47.

Resnick, B., & Nigg, C. (2003). Testing a theoretical model of exercise behavior for older adults. *Nursing Research, 52,* 80–88.

Robbins, L. B., Pender, N. J., & Kazanis, A. S. (2003). Barriers to physical activity by adolescent girls. *Journal of Midwifery & Women's Health, 48,* 206–212.

Roberts, K. J., & Mann, T. (2003). Adherence to antiretroviral medications in HIV/AIDS care: A narrative exploration of one woman's foray into intentional nonadherence. *Health Care Women International, 24,* 552–564.

Simmons, B., Lanuza, D., Fonteyn, M., Hicks, F., & Holm, K. (2003). Clinical reasoning in experienced nurses. *Western Journal of Nursing Research, 25,* 701–719.

Snethen, J. A., & Broome, M. E. (2001). Adolescents' perception of living with end stage renal disease. *Pediatric Nursing, 27,* 159–167.

Symanski, M. E., Hayes, M. J., & Akilesh, M. K. (2002), Patterns of premature newborns'; sleep-wake states before and after nursing interventions on the night shift. *Journal of Obstetric, Gynecologic, and Neonatal Nursing, 31,* 305–313.

Wakefield, B. J. (2002). Risk for acute confusion on hospital admission. *Clinical Nursing Research, 11,* 153–172.

Waltman, P. S., Brewer, J. M., Rogers, B. P., & May, W. L. (2004). Building evidence for practice: A pilot study of newborn bulb suctioning at birth. *Journal of Midwifery & Women's Health, 49,* 32–38.

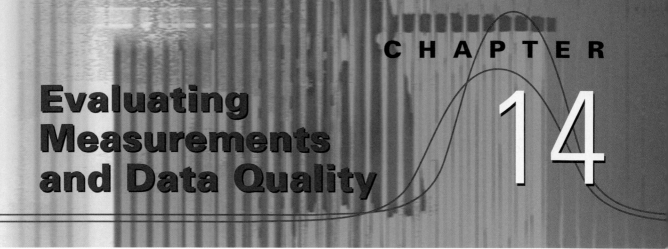

Evaluating Measurements and Data Quality

CHAPTER 14

STUDENT OBJECTIVES

On completing this chapter, you will be able to:

▌ Describe the major characteristics of measurement and identify major sources of measurement error
▌ Describe aspects of reliability and validity, and specify how each aspect can be assessed
▌ Interpret the meaning of reliability and validity coefficients
▌ Describe the four dimensions used in establishing the trustworthiness of qualitative data and identify methods of enhancing data quality in qualitative studies
▌ Evaluate the overall quality of a measuring tool or data collection approach used in a study
▌ Define new terms in the chapter

D ata collection methods vary in quality. An ideal data collection procedure is one that captures a phenomenon or concept in a way that is relevant, accurate, truthful, and sensitive. For most concepts of interest to nurse researchers, few, if any, data collection procedures match this ideal. In this chapter, we discuss criteria for evaluating the quality of data obtained in both quantitative and qualitative studies.

MEASUREMENT AND THE ASSESSMENT OF QUANTITATIVE DATA

Quantitative studies derive data through the measurement of variables. Before discussing the assessment of quantitative measures, we briefly discuss the concept of measurement.

Measurement

Measurement involves rules for assigning numeric values to *qualities* of objects to designate the *quantity* of the attribute. No attribute inherently has a numeric value; human beings invent rules to measure concepts. An often-quoted statement by an American psychologist, L. L. Thurstone, summarizes a position assumed by many quantitative researchers: "Whatever exists, exists in some amount and can be measured." The notion here is that attributes are not constant: They vary from day to day or from one person to another. This variability is capable of a numeric expression that signifies *how much* of an attribute is present. Quantification is used to communicate that amount. The purpose of assigning numbers is to differentiate among people who possess varying degrees of the critical attribute.

Measurement requires numbers to be assigned to objects according to rules rather than haphazardly. The rules for measuring temperature, weight, and other physical attributes are widely known and accepted. Rules for measuring many variables, however, have to be invented. What are the rules for measuring patient satisfaction? Pain? Depression? Whether the data are collected through observation, self-report, or some other method, researchers must specify the criteria according to which numeric values are to be assigned.

ADVANTAGES OF MEASUREMENT

A major strength of measurement is that it removes guesswork in gathering and communicating information. Consider how handicapped nurses and doctors would be in the absence of measures of body temperature, blood pressure, and so on. Because measurement is based on explicit rules, the information tends to be objective: Two people measuring a person's weight using the same scale would likely get identical results. Two people scoring responses to a self-report stress scale would likely arrive at identical scores. Not all quantitative measures are completely objective, but most incorporate rules for minimizing subjectivity.

Measurement also makes it possible to obtain reasonably precise information. Instead of describing Nathan as "rather tall," for example, we can depict him as a man who is 6 feet, 3 inches tall. If it were necessary, we could obtain even more precise height measurements. Such precision allows researchers to make fine distinctions among people who possess different amounts of an attribute.

Finally, measurement is a language of communication. Numbers are less vague than words and can thus communicate information to a broad audience. If a researcher reported that the average oral temperature of a sample of patients was "somewhat high," different readers might develop different conceptions about the sample's physiologic state. If the researcher reported an average temperature of 99.8°F, however, there is no ambiguity.

ERRORS OF MEASUREMENT

Researchers work with fallible measures. Values and scores from even the best measuring instruments have a certain amount of error. We can think of every piece of quantitative data as consisting of two parts: a true component and an error component. This can be written as an equation, as follows:

$$\text{Obtained score} = \text{True score} \pm \text{Error}$$

The **obtained** (or *observed*) **score** could be, for example, a patient's heart rate or score on an anxiety scale. The **true score** is the true value that would be obtained if it were possible to have an infallible measure of the target attribute. The true score is hypothetical; it can never be known because measures are not infallible. The **error of measurement**—the difference between true and obtained scores—reflects extraneous factors that affect the measurement and distort the results. Many factors contribute to errors of measurement. Among the most common are the following:

▶ *Situational contaminants.* Measurements can be affected by the conditions under which they are produced (e.g., people's awareness of an observer can affect their behavior; environmental factors such as temperature or time of day can be sources of measurement error).
▶ *Response set biases.* A number of relatively enduring characteristics of respondents can interfere with accurate measures of an attribute (see Chapter 13).
▶ *Transitory personal factors.* Temporary personal factors (e.g., fatigue, hunger, mood) can influence people's motivation or ability to cooperate, act naturally, or do their best.
▶ *Administration variations.* Alterations in the methods of collecting data from one person to the next can affect obtained scores (e.g., if some biophysiologic measures are taken before a feeding and others are taken postprandially).
▶ *Item sampling.* Errors can be introduced as a result of the sampling of items used to measure an attribute. For example, a student's score on a 100-item research methods test will be influenced to a certain extent by *which* 100 questions are included.

This list is not exhaustive, but it illustrates that data are susceptible to measurement error from a variety of sources.

Reliability

The reliability of a quantitative measure is a major criterion for assessing its quality. **Reliability** is the consistency with which an instrument measures the attribute. If a spring scale gave a reading of 120 lb for a person's weight one minute and a reading of 150 lb the next minute, we would naturally be wary of using such an unreliable scale. The less variation an instrument produces in repeated measurements of an attribute, the higher is its reliability.

Another way to define reliability is in terms of accuracy. An instrument is reliable if its measures accurately reflect true scores. A reliable measure is one that maximizes the true score component and minimizes the error component of an obtained score.

Three aspects of reliability are of interest to quantitative researchers: stability, internal consistency, and equivalence.

CONSUMER TIP

Many psychosocial scales contain two or more **subscales**, each of which tap distinct, but related, concepts (e.g., a measure of independent functioning might include subscales for motor activities, communication, and socializing). The reliability of each subscale is typically assessed and, if subscale scores are summed for a total score, the scale's overall reliability would also be assessed.

▬

STABILITY

The *stability* of a measure is the extent to which the same scores are obtained when the instrument is used with the same people on separate occasions. Assessments of stability are derived through **test–retest reliability** procedures. The researcher administers the same measure to a sample of people on two occasions, and then compares the scores.

Suppose, for example, we were interested in the stability of a self-report scale that measured self-esteem in adolescents. Because self-esteem is a fairly stable attribute that would not change markedly from one day to the next, we would expect a reliable measure of it to yield consistent scores on two separate tests. As a check on the instrument's stability, we arrange to administer the scale 3 weeks apart to a sample of teenagers. Fictitious data for this example are presented in Table 14-1.

On the whole, differences on the two tests are not large. Researchers compute a **reliability coefficient**, a numeric index of a measure's reliability, to objectively determine exactly how small the differences are. Reliability coefficients (designated as *r*) range from .00 to 1.00.* The higher the value, the more reliable (stable) is the measuring instrument. In the example shown in Table 14-1, the reliability coefficient is .95, which is quite high.

TABLE 14.1	**Fictitious Data for Test–Retest Reliability of Self-Esteem Scale**	
SUBJECT NUMBER	**TIME 1**	**TIME 2**
1	55	57
2	49	46
3	78	74
4	37	35
5	44	46
6	50	56
7	58	55
8	62	66
9	48	50
10	67	63

$r = .95$

* Computation procedures for reliability coefficients are not presented in this textbook, but formulas can be found in the references cited at the end of this chapter. Although reliability coefficients can technically be less than .00 (i.e., a negative value), they are almost invariably a number between .00 and 1.00.

CONSUMER TIP

For most purposes, reliability coefficients higher than .70 are satisfactory, but coefficients in the .85 to .95 range are far preferable. ■

The test–retest approach to estimating reliability has certain disadvantages. The major problem is that many traits of interest do change over time, independently of the instrument's stability. Attitudes, mood, knowledge, and so forth can be modified by experiences between two measurements. Thus, stability indexes are most appropriate for relatively enduring characteristics, such as personality and abilities. Even with such traits, test–retest reliability tends to decline as the interval between the two administrations increases.

Example of test–retest reliability

Needham, Abderhalden, Dassen, Haug, and Fischer (2004) developed and tested a short form of the Perception of Aggression Scale, which is designed to measure psychiatric nurses' attitudes toward, and perceptions of, patient aggression. To select items with the strongest stability, the researchers administered the full scale to three groups of psychiatric nurses twice: to one group after 4 days, to the second after 14 days, and to the third after 70 days. The 12 items selected for the short form had a test–retest reliability of .77.

INTERNAL CONSISTENCY

Scales that involve summing items are often evaluated for their internal consistency. Ideally, scales are composed of items that all measure the same critical attribute and nothing else. On a scale to measure empathy in nurses, it would be inappropriate to include an item that is a better measure of diagnostic competence than empathy. An instrument may be said to have **internal consistency** reliability to the extent that all its subparts measure the same characteristic. This approach to reliability assesses an important source of measurement error in multi-item measures: the sampling of items.

One of the oldest methods for assessing internal consistency is the *split-half technique*. In this approach, the items comprising a scale are split into two groups (usually, odd versus even items) and scored, and then scores on the two half-tests are used to compute a reliability coefficient. If the two half-tests are really measuring the same attribute, the reliability coefficient will be high. More sophisticated and accurate methods of computing internal consistency estimates are now in use, most notably, **Cronbach's alpha** (or **coefficient alpha**). This method gives an estimate of the split-half correlation for all possible ways of dividing the measure into two halves, not just odd versus even items. As with test–retest reliability coefficients, indexes of internal consistency range in value between .00 and 1.00. The higher the reliability coefficient, the more accurate (internally consistent) the measure.

Example of internal consistency reliability

Dobratz (2004) evaluated the Life Closure Scale (LCS), an instrument designed to measure psychological adaptation among end-of-life patients. The LCS had a total alpha of .87, and the alphas for the two subscales were .80 (self-reconciled subscale) and .82 (self-restructuring subscale).

EQUIVALENCE

The *equivalence* approach to estimating reliability—used primarily with observational instruments—determines the consistency or equivalence of the instrument by different observers or raters. As noted in Chapter 13, a potential weakness of direct observation is the risk for observer error. The degree of error can be assessed through **interrater** (or **interobserver**) **reliability**, which is estimated by having two or more trained observers make simultaneous, independent observations. The resulting data can then be used to calculate an index of equivalence or agreement. That is, a reliability coefficient can be computed to demonstrate the strength of the relationship between the observers' ratings. When two independent observers score some phenomenon congruently, the scores are likely to be accurate and reliable.

Example of interrater reliability

Kovach (2002) observed the behaviors of older persons with dementia over 30-minute observation sessions. Interrater reliability, calculated as percentage agreement between two raters, was .74 for the variable *activity*, .92 for *noxiousness*, and .84 for *agitation*.

INTERPRETATION OF RELIABILITY COEFFICIENTS

Reliability coefficients are an important indicator of an instrument's quality. A measure with low reliability prevents an adequate testing of research hypotheses. If data fail to confirm a hypothesis, one possibility is that the measuring tool was unreliable—not necessarily that the expected relationships do not exist. Knowledge about an instrument's reliability thus is critical in interpreting research results, especially if research hypotheses are not supported.

Reliability estimates vary according to the procedure used to obtain them. Estimates of reliability computed by different procedures for the same instrument are not identical.

Example of different forms of reliability

Gulick (2003) adapted the Postpartum Support Questionnaire (PSQ) for use with mothers with multiple sclerosis. She evaluated the adapted scale using both test–retest and internal consistency approaches. As an example of her findings, the coefficient alphas for the Emotional Support subscale were .90 and .91 at 1 and 3 months postpartum, respectively. The subscale's test–retest reliability over this 2-month period was .68.

In addition, reliability of an instrument is related to sample heterogeneity. The more homogeneous the sample (i.e., the more similar the scores), the lower the reliability coefficient will be. This is because instruments are designed to measure differences, and if sample members

CONSUMER TIP

If a research report provides information on the reliability of a quantitative scale without specifying the type of reliability measure used, it is probably safe to assume that internal consistency reliability was assessed by the Cronbach alpha method.

■

are similar to one another, it is more difficult for the instrument to discriminate reliably among those who possess varying degrees of the attribute. Finally, longer instruments (i.e., those with more items) tend to have higher reliability than shorter ones.

Validity

The second important criterion for evaluating a quantitative instrument is its validity. **Validity** is the degree to which an instrument measures what it is supposed to be measuring. When a researcher develops an instrument to measure patients' perceived susceptibility to illness, he or she should take steps to ensure that the resulting scores validly reflect this variable and not some other concept.

The reliability and validity of an instrument are not totally independent. A measuring device that is not reliable cannot possibly be valid. An instrument cannot validly be measuring the attribute of interest if it is erratic or inaccurate. An instrument can be reliable, however, without being valid. Suppose we had the idea to measure patients' anxiety by measuring the circumference of their wrists. We could obtain highly accurate, consistent, and precise measurements of wrist circumferences, but they would not be valid indicators of anxiety. Thus, the high reliability of an instrument provides no evidence of its validity; the low reliability of a measure *is* evidence of low validity.

CONSUMER TIP

Some methodologic studies are designed to evaluate the quality of instruments used by clinicians or researchers. In these **psychometric assessments**, information about the instrument's reliability and validity is carefully documented. ■

Like reliability, validity has a number of aspects and assessment approaches. One aspect is known as face validity. **Face validity** refers to whether the instrument looks as though it is measuring the appropriate construct.

Example of face validity

Shin and Colling (2000) undertook a cultural verification of the Profile of Mood States (POMS) scale for Korean elders. One part of the study involved an assessment of the translated scale's face validity, using a panel of Korean experts.

Although it is often useful for an instrument to have face validity, three other aspects of validity are of greater importance in assessments of an instrument: content validity, criterion-related validity, and construct validity.

CONTENT VALIDITY

Content validity is concerned with adequacy of coverage of the content area being measured. Content validity is crucial for tests of knowledge. In such a context, the validity question is: How representative are the questions on this test of the universe of all questions that might be asked on this topic?

Content validity is also relevant in measures of complex psychosocial traits. A person who wanted to develop a new instrument would begin by developing a thorough conceptualization of the construct of interest so that the measure would adequately capture the whole domain. Such a conceptualization might come from rich first-hand knowledge but is more likely to come from qualitative studies or from a literature review.

The content validity of an instrument is necessarily based on judgment. There are no totally objective methods for ensuring the adequate content coverage of an instrument. Experts in the content area are often called on to analyze the items' adequacy in representing the hypothetical content universe in the correct proportions. It is also possible to calculate a **content validity index** (CVI) that indicates the extent of expert agreement, but ultimately the experts' subjective judgments must be relied on.

Example of content validity

Wynd, Schmidt, and Schaefer (2003) used two alternative strategies for developing quantitative estimates of content validity for the Osteoporosis Risk Assessment Tool (ORAT). Both approaches relied on the judgments of a panel of eight experts, who were selected from nationally known clinicians and researchers with strong reputations in osteoporosis risk prevention and treatment.

CRITERION-RELATED VALIDITY

In **criterion-related validity** assessments, researchers seek to establish a relationship between scores on an instrument and some external criterion. The instrument, whatever abstract attribute it is measuring, is said to be valid if its scores correspond strongly with scores on some criterion. (One difficulty of criterion-related validation, however, is finding a criterion that is, in itself, reliable and valid.) After a criterion is established, validity can be estimated easily. A **validity coefficient** is computed by using a mathematic formula that correlates scores on the instrument with scores on the criterion variable. The magnitude of the coefficient indicates how valid the instrument is. These coefficients (r) range between .00 and 1.00, with higher values indicating greater criterion-related validity. Coefficients of .70 or higher are desirable.

Sometimes, a distinction is made between two types of criterion-related validity. **Predictive validity** refers to an instrument's ability to differentiate between people's performances or behaviors on some future criterion. When a school of nursing correlates students' incoming high school grades with their subsequent grade-point averages, the predictive validity of the high school grades for nursing school performance is being evaluated. **Concurrent validity** refers to an instrument's ability to distinguish among people who differ in their present status on some criterion. For example, a psychological test to differentiate between patients in a mental institution who could and could not be released could be correlated with current behavioral ratings of health care personnel. The difference between predictive and concurrent validity, then, is the difference in the timing of obtaining measurements on a criterion.

Example of predictive validity

Dennis (2003) developed a short form of the Breastfeeding Self-Efficacy Scale (BSES-SF), a scale to measure breastfeeding confidence. She determined the predictive validity of the scale by correlating mothers' scale scores with their method of infant feeding at 4 and 8 weeks postpartum.

CONSTRUCT VALIDITY

Validating an instrument in terms of **construct validity** is difficult and challenging. Construct validity is concerned with the following question: What construct is the instrument actually measuring? The more abstract the concept, the more difficult it is to establish the construct validity of the measure; at the same time, the more abstract the concept, the less suitable it is to use a criterion-related validation approach. What objective criterion is there for concepts such as empathy, grief, and separation anxiety?

Construct validation is addressed in several ways, but there is always an emphasis on testing relationships predicted on the basis of theoretical considerations. Researchers make predictions about the manner in which the construct will function in relation to other constructs.

One approach to construct validation is the **known-groups technique**. In this procedure, groups that are expected to differ on the critical attribute are administered the instrument, and group scores are compared. For instance, in validating a measure of fear of the labor experience, the scores of primiparas and multiparas could be contrasted. Women who had never given birth would likely experience more anxiety than women who had already had children; one might question the validity of the instrument if such differences did not emerge.

Another method of construct validation involves an examination of relationships based on theoretical predictions. Researchers might reason as follows: According to theory, construct X is related to construct Y; instrument A is a measure of construct X, and instrument B is a measure of construct Y. If scores on A and B are related to each other, as predicted by the theory, it can be inferred that A and B are valid measures of X and Y. This logical analysis is fallible, but it does offer supporting evidence.

Another approach to construct validation employs a statistical procedure known as **factor analysis**, which is a method for identifying clusters of related items on a scale. The procedure is used to identify and group together different measures of some underlying attribute and to distinguish them from measures of different attributes.

In summary, construct validation employs both logical and empirical procedures. Like content validity, construct validity requires a judgment pertaining to what the instrument is measuring. Construct validity and criterion-related validity share an empirical component, but, in the latter case, there is a pragmatic, objective criterion with which to compare a measure rather than a second measure of an abstract theoretical construct.

Example of construct validity

Creedy and her colleagues (2003) tested the Breastfeeding Self-Efficacy Scale (described earlier) with a sample of Australian women. They used a variety of techniques to assess cross-cultural construct validity, including a factor analysis and the known-groups technique (comparing multiparous women with prior breastfeeding experience with primiparous women). They also correlated scale scores with scores on a measure of perception of milk supply.

INTERPRETATION OF VALIDITY

Like reliability, validity is not an all-or-nothing characteristic of an instrument. An instrument cannot really be said to possess or lack validity; it is a question of degree. The testing of an instrument's validity is not proved but rather is supported by an accumulation of evidence.

Strictly speaking, researchers do not validate an instrument *per se* but rather some application of the instrument. A measure of anxiety may be valid for presurgical patients on the day before surgery but may not be valid for nursing students on the day of a final examination. Validation is a never-ending process: The more evidence that can be gathered that an instrument is measuring what it is supposed to be measuring, the greater the confidence researchers have in its validity.

CONSUMER TIP

In quantitative studies involving self-report or observational instruments, the research report usually provides validity and reliability information from an earlier study—often a study conducted by the person who developed the instrument. If the sample characteristics in the original study and the new study are similar, the citation provides valuable information about data quality in the new study. Ideally, researchers should also compute new reliability coefficients for the actual research sample. ▬

Sensitivity and Specificity

Reliability and validity are the two most important criteria for evaluating quantitative instruments, but researchers sometimes need to consider other qualities. In particular, for screening and diagnostic instruments, sensitivity and specificity need to be evaluated.

Sensitivity is the ability of an instrument to correctly identify a "case," that is, to correctly screen in or diagnose a condition. An instrument's sensitivity is its rate of yielding "true positives." **Specificity** is the instrument's ability to correctly identify non-cases, that is, to correctly screen *out* those without the condition. Specificity is an instrument's rate of yielding "true negatives." To determine an instrument's sensitivity and specificity, researchers need a reliable and valid criterion of "caseness" against which scores on the instrument can be assessed.

There is, unfortunately, a tradeoff between the sensitivity and specificity of an instrument. When sensitivity is increased to include more true positives, the number of true negatives declines. Therefore, a critical task is to develop the appropriate *cutoff point*, i.e., the score value used to distinguish cases and noncases. Instrument developers use sophisticated procedures to make such a determination.

Example of sensitivity and specificity

Curley, Razmus, Roberts, and Wypij (2003) adapted the Braden Scale—a scale for performing pressure ulcer risk assessments—for use with children (the Braden Q). At a cutoff score of 16, the researchers found that the sensitivity of the Braden Q was 88% and the specificity was 58%. After modifying the scale by eliminating subscales, the sensitivity at the cutoff score of 7 was increased to 92% and specificity was 59%.

THE ASSESSMENT OF QUALITATIVE DATA

The assessment procedures described thus far cannot be meaningfully applied to such qualitative materials as narrative responses in interviews or participant observers' field notes. This does not imply, however, that qualitative researchers are unconcerned with data quality. The central question underlying the concepts of validity and reliability is: Do the data reflect the truth? Certainly, qualitative researchers are as eager as quantitative researchers to have data reflecting the true state of human experience.

Nevertheless, there has been considerable controversy about the criteria to use for assessing the "truth value" of qualitative research. Whittemore, Chase, and Mandle (2001), who listed different criteria recommended by 10 influential authorities, noted that the difficulty in achieving universally accepted criteria (or even universally accepted labels for those criteria) stems in part from various tensions, such as the tension between the desire for rigor and the desire for creativity.

The criteria currently thought of as the "gold standard" for qualitative researchers are those outlined by Lincoln and Guba (1985). As noted in Chapter 2, these researchers have suggested four criteria for establishing the **trustworthiness** of qualitative data: credibility, dependability, confirmability, and transferability. It should be noted that these criteria go beyond an assessment of qualitative *data* alone, but rather are concerned with evaluations of interpretations and conclusions as well. These standards are often used by qualitative researchers in all major traditions.

CONSUMER TIP

Qualitative research reports are uneven in the amount of information they provide about data quality. Some do not address data quality issues at all, whereas others elaborate on the steps taken to assess trustworthiness. The absence of information makes it difficult for consumers to come to conclusions about the believability of qualitative findings. ■

Credibility

Careful qualitative researchers take steps to improve and evaluate data **credibility**, which refers to confidence in the truth of the data and interpretations of them. Lincoln and Guba note that the credibility of an inquiry involves two aspects: first, carrying out the investigation in a way that believability is enhanced, and second, taking steps to *demonstrate* credibility. Lincoln and Guba suggest various techniques for improving and documenting the credibility of qualitative data. A few that are especially relevant to the evaluation of qualitative studies are mentioned here.

PROLONGED ENGAGEMENT AND PERSISTENT OBSERVATION

Lincoln and Guba recommend activities that increase the likelihood of producing credible data and interpretations. A first and very important step is **prolonged engagement**—the investment of sufficient time in data collection activities to have an in-depth understanding of the culture, language, or views of the group under study and to test for misinformation. Prolonged engagement may also be essential for building trust and rapport with informants.

Credible data collection also involves **persistent observation**, which refers to the researcher's focus on the aspects of a situation that are relevant to the phenomena being studied. As Lincoln and Guba note, "If prolonged engagement provides scope, persistent observation provides depth" (1985, p. 304).

Example of prolonged engagement and persistent observation

Beck (2002) conducted a grounded theory study of mothering twins during the first year of life. In addition to prolonged engagement for 10 months of fieldwork, she engaged in persistent observation. After interviewing mothers in their homes, Beck often stayed and helped them with their twins, using the time for persistent observation of the mothers' caretaking (e.g., details of how the mothers talked to their twins and what they said).

TRIANGULATION

Triangulation can also enhance credibility. As previously noted, triangulation refers to the use of multiple referents to draw conclusions about what constitutes truth. The aim of triangulation is to "overcome the intrinsic bias that comes from single-method, single-observer, and single-theory studies" (Denzin, 1989, p. 313). It has also been argued that triangulation helps to capture a more complete and contextualized portrait of the phenomenon under study—a goal shared by researchers in all qualitative traditions. Denzin (1989) identified four types of triangulation:

1. *Data source triangulation*: using multiple data sources in a study (e.g., interviewing diverse key informants such as nurses and patients about the same topic)
2. *Investigator triangulation*: using more than one person to collect, analyze, or interpret a set of data
3. *Theory triangulation:* using multiple perspectives to interpret a set of data
4. *Method triangulation:* using multiple methods to address a research problem (e.g., observations plus interviews)

Triangulation provides a basis for convergence on the truth. By using multiple methods and perspectives, researchers strive to distinguish true information from information with errors.

Example of data source and method triangulation

MacDonald and Callery (2004) studied the meaning of respite care to parents of children with complex conditions, and to respite providers. The researchers collected data from 19 mothers, seven fathers, 13 nurses, and four social workers in the United Kingdom. Data sources included in-depth interviews, participant observation, and document review.

EXTERNAL CHECKS: PEER DEBRIEFING AND MEMBER CHECKS

Two other techniques for establishing credibility involve external checks on the inquiry. **Peer debriefing** is a session held with objective peers to review and explore various aspects of the inquiry. Peer debriefing exposes investigators to the searching questions of others who are experienced in either qualitative research or in the phenomenon being studied, or both. These sessions can also be useful to researchers interested in testing some working hypotheses or in exploring new avenues in the emergent research design.

Member checks involve soliciting study participants' reactions to preliminary findings and interpretations. Member checking can be carried out both informally in an ongoing way as data are being collected and more formally after data have been collected and analyzed. Lincoln and Guba consider member checking the most important technique for establishing the credibility of qualitative data. However, not all qualitative researchers use member checking to ensure credibility. For example, member checking is not a component of Giorgi's method of descriptive phenomenology. Giorgi (1989) argued that asking participants to evaluate the researcher's psychological interpretation of their own descriptions exceeds the role of participants.

Example of peer debriefing and member checking

Navon and Morag (2003) studied advanced prostate cancer patients' ways of coping with the hormonal therapy's effect on their body and their sexuality. Their grounded theory study was based on in-depth interviews with 15 patients in Israel. The researchers discussed their preliminary findings with three study participants and two physicians and two nurses involved in treating patients with prostate cancer.

SEARCHING FOR DISCONFIRMING EVIDENCE

Data credibility can be enhanced by researchers' systematic search for data that challenge an emerging conceptualization or descriptive theory. The search for **disconfirming evidence** occurs through purposive sampling but is facilitated through other processes already described here, such as prolonged engagement and peer debriefings. The sampling of individuals who can offer conflicting viewpoints can greatly strengthen a comprehensive description of a phenomenon.

Lincoln and Guba (1985) refer to a similar activity of **negative case analysis**—a process by which researchers revise their hypotheses through the inclusion of cases that appear to disconfirm earlier hypotheses. The goal of this procedure is to refine a hypothesis or theory continuously until it accounts for all cases without exception.

Example of negative case analysis

Hauck and Irurita (2003) explored the process of managing breastfeeding and weaning in their grounded theory study with a sample of families in western Australia. Data were collected in interviews with mothers, questionnaires from fathers, field notes, and other sources. During the ongoing sampling of participants, potential negative cases were sought in an attempt to test or challenge the researchers' initial categories.

RESEARCHER CREDIBILITY

Another aspect of credibility discussed by Patton (2001) is **researcher credibility**, the faith that can be put in the researcher. In qualitative studies, researchers *are* the data collecting instruments—as well as creators of the analytic process—and, therefore, the researchers' training, qualifications, and experience are important in establishing confidence in the data.

From your point of view as consumer, the research report ideally should contain information about the researchers, including information about credentials and about any personal connections the researchers had to the people, topic, or community under study. For example, it is relevant for a reader of a report on AIDS patients' coping mechanisms to know that the researcher is HIV positive. Patton argues that the researcher should report "any personal and professional information that may have affected data collection, analysis and interpretation—negatively or positively. . ." (2002, p. 566).

 Example of researcher credibility

Mohr (2000) studied the experiences of families with children under care in mental health care settings. In a section of her report labeled "Reflexive Notes," Mohr presented her credentials as a nurse (various nursing roles in psychiatric hospitals), her personal background (her mother was schizophrenic), and her strong advocacy activities (involvement with the National Alliance for the Mentally Ill). A brief biography establishing her credentials also was included at the end of the report, a common feature in the journal *Qualitative Health Research*. Mohr's more recent study (2004) of mental health support groups, described as the research example at the end of Chapter 13, similarly documented her personal and professional credentials to undertake the research.

Dependability

The **dependability** of qualitative data refers to data stability over time and over conditions. It might be said that credibility (in qualitative studies) is to validity (in quantitative studies) what dependability is to reliability. Like the reliability–validity relationship in quantitative research, there can be no credibility in the absence of dependability.

One approach to assessing data dependability is to undertake a **stepwise replication**. This approach, which is conceptually similar to a split-half technique, involves having several researchers who can be divided into two teams. These teams deal with data sources separately and conduct, essentially, two independent inquiries through which data and conclusions can be compared.

Another technique relating to dependability is the **inquiry audit**. An inquiry audit involves a scrutiny of the data and relevant supporting documents by an external reviewer, an approach that also has a bearing on data confirmability, as we discuss next.

 Example of dependability

Williams, Schutte, Evers, and Holkup (2000) used a stepwise replication and inquiry audit in their study of coping with normal results from predictive gene testing for neurodegenerative disorders. Ten participants were interviewed three times. Three researchers read through transcripts of the first set of interviews and made marginal notes for coding. The three researchers compared their codes and revised them until agreement was reached. All transcripts from the remaining interviews were coded independently, and the researchers met periodically to compare codes and reach a consensus. Once coding was completed, a qualitative nurse researcher reviewed the entire set of transcribed interviews and validated the findings with the three researchers.

Confirmability

Confirmability refers to the objectivity or neutrality of the data, that is, the potential for congruence between two or more independent people about the data's accuracy, relevance, or meaning. Bracketing (in phenomenological studies) and maintaining a reflexive journal are methods that can enhance confirmability, although these strategies do not actually document that it has been achieved.

Inquiry audits can be used to establish both the dependability and confirmability of the data. In an inquiry audit, the investigator develops an **audit trail**, which is a systematic collection of documentation that allows an independent auditor to come to conclusions about the data. After the audit trail materials are assembled, the inquiry auditor proceeds to audit, in a fashion analogous to a financial audit, the trustworthiness of the data and the meanings attached to them. Six classes of records are important in creating an adequate audit trail: (1) raw data (e.g., field notes, interview transcripts); (2) data reduction and analysis products (e.g., theoretical notes, documentation on working hypotheses); (3) process notes (e.g., methodologic notes, notes from member check sessions); (4) materials relating to intentions and dispositions (e.g., personal notes on intentions); (5) instrument development information (e.g., pilot topic guides); and (6) data reconstruction products (e.g., drafts of the final report).

Researchers can also enhance the **auditability** of their inquiry (i.e., the degree to which an outside person can follow the researchers' methods, decisions, and conclusions) by maintaining an adequate **decision trail**. A decision trail articulates the researchers' decision rules for categorizing data and making inferences in the analysis. When researchers share decision trail information in their research report, readers are in a better position to evaluate the soundness of the decisions and to draw conclusions about the trustworthiness of the study.

Example of confirmability

In her research on mothering twins, Beck (2002) developed a four-phased grounded theory entitled, "Life on hold: Releasing the pause button." In her report, Beck presented a partial audit trail for Phase III, which she called "striving to reset."

Transferability

In Lincoln and Guba's (1985) framework, **transferability** refers to the extent to which the findings from the data can be transferred to other settings or groups and is thus similar to the concept of generalizability. This is, to some extent, an issue relating to sampling and design rather than to the soundness of the data *per se*. As Lincoln and Guba note, however, a researcher's responsibility is to provide sufficient descriptive data in the research report for consumers to evaluate the applicability of the data to other contexts: "Thus the naturalist cannot specify the external validity of an inquiry; he or she can provide only the thick description necessary to enable someone interested in making a transfer to reach a conclusion about whether transfer can be contemplated as a possibility" (1985, p. 316). **Thick description** refers to a rich, thorough description of the research setting, and the transactions and processes observed during the inquiry. Thus, if there is to be transferability, the burden of proof rests with researchers to provide sufficient information to permit judgments about contextual similarity.

Example of transferability

In their ethnographic study, Banister, Jakubec, and Stein (2003) explored Canadian adolescent girls' health concerns in their dating relationships. Four 90-minute focus group sessions were held with four groups of young women. To achieve ethnic and socioeconomic diversity and enhance transferability, five sites were used to recruit participants. To assess the transferability of their results, the researchers showed the findings "to a number of practitioners at various sites in the community, who perceived them as congruent with their practice experiences" (p. 22).

CONSUMER TIP

Because the process of assessing data quality in qualitative studies may be inextricably linked to data analysis, discussions of data quality are sometimes included in the results section rather than the method section of the report. In some cases, the text will not explicitly point out that data quality issues are being discussed. Readers may have to be alert to evidence of triangulation or other verification techniques in such statements as, "Informants' reports of experiences of serious illness were supported by discussions with three public health nurses."

CRITIQUING DATA QUALITY

If data are seriously flawed, the study cannot contribute useful evidence. Therefore, it is important for you as a consumer to consider whether researchers have taken appropriate steps to collect data that accurately reflect reality. In both qualitative and quantitative studies, you have the right—indeed, the obligation—to ask: Can I trust the data? Do the data accurately reflect the true state of the phenomenon under study?

In quantitative studies, you should expect some discussion of the reliability and validity of the measures—preferably, information collected directly with the sample under study (rather than evidence from other studies). You should be wary about the results of quantitative studies when the report provides no information about data quality or when it suggests unfavorable reliability or validity. Also, data quality deserves special scrutiny when the research hypotheses are not confirmed. There may be many reasons that hypotheses are not supported by data (e.g., too small a sample or a faulty theory), but the quality of the measures is an important area of concern. When hypotheses are not supported, one possibility is that the instruments were not good measures of the research constructs. Box 14-1 provides some guidelines for critiquing data quality in quantitative studies.

Information about data quality is equally important in qualitative studies. You should be particularly alert to information on data quality when a single researcher has been responsible for collecting, analyzing, and interpreting all the data, as is frequently the case. Some guidelines for critiquing the trustworthiness of data in qualitative studies are presented in Box 14-2.

CONSUMER TIP

The amount of detail about data quality in a research report varies considerably. Some articles have virtually no information. Sometimes such information is not needed (e.g., when biophysiologic instrumentation with a proven and widely known record for accuracy is used). Most research reports, however, should provide some evidence that data quality was sufficiently high to answer the research questions. Information about data quality normally is presented in the method section of the report.

BOX 14.1   **Guidelines for Evaluating Data Quality in Quantitative Studies**

1. Is there congruence between the research variables as conceptualized (i.e., as discussed in the introduction of the report) and as operationalized (i.e., as described in the method section)?
2. If operational definitions (or scoring procedures) are specified, do they clearly indicate the rules of measurement? Do the rules seem sensible? Were data collected in such a way that measurement errors were minimized?
3. Does the report offer evidence of the reliability of measures? Does the evidence come from the research sample itself, or is it based on other studies? If the latter, is it reasonable to conclude that data quality would be similar for the research sample as for the reliability sample (e.g., are sample characteristics similar)?
4. If reliability is reported, which estimation method was used? Was this method appropriate? Should an alternative or additional method of reliability appraisal have been used? Is the reliability sufficiently high?
5. Does the report offer evidence of the validity of the measures? Does the evidence come from the research sample itself, or is it based on other studies? If the latter, is it reasonable to believe that data quality would be similar for the research sample as for the validity sample (e.g., are the sample characteristics similar)?
6. If validity information is reported, which validity approach was used? Was this method appropriate? Does the validity of the instrument appear to be adequate?
7. If there is no reliability or validity information, what conclusion can you reach about the quality of the data in the study?
8. If a diagnostic or screening tool was used, is information provided about its sensitivity and specificity, and were these qualities adequate?
9. Were the research hypotheses supported? If not, might data quality play a role in the failure to confirm the hypotheses?

BOX 14.2   **Guidelines for Evaluating Data Quality in Qualitative Studies**

1. Does the report discuss efforts to enhance or evaluate the trustworthiness of the data? If so, is the description sufficiently detailed and clear? If not, is there other information that allows you to conclude that data are of high quality?
2. Which techniques (if any) did the researcher use to enhance and appraise the credibility of the data? Was the investigator in the field for an adequate amount of time? Was triangulation used, and if so, of what type? Did the researcher search for disconfirming evidence? Were there peer debriefings and/or member checks? Do the researcher's qualifications enhance the credibility of the data?
3. Which techniques (if any) did the researcher use to enhance and appraise the dependability, confirmability, and transferability of the data?
4. Given the efforts to enhance data quality, what can you conclude about the trustworthiness of the data? In light of this assessment, how much faith can be placed in the results of the study?

CHAPTER REVIEW

Key new terms introduced in the chapter, together with a summary of major points, are presented in this section. In addition, Chapter 14 of the *Study Guide to Accompany Essentials of Nursing Research,* 6th edition offers various exercises and study suggestions for reinforcing the concepts presented in this chapter. For additional review, see the Student Self-Study Review Questions section of the Student Resource CD-ROM provided with this book.

KEY NEW TERMS

Audit trail
Auditability
Coefficient alpha
Concurrent validity
Confirmability
Construct validity
Content validity
Content validity index
Credibility
Criterion-related validity
Cronbach's alpha
Decision trail
Dependability
Disconfirming evidence
Error of measurement
Face validity
Factor analysis
Inquiry audit
Internal consistency
Interobserver reliability
Interrater reliability
Known-groups technique
Measurement

Member check
Negative case analysis
Obtained score
Peer debriefing
Persistent observation
Predictive validity
Prolonged engagement
Psychometric assessment
Reliability
Reliability coefficient
Researcher credibility
Sensitivity
Specificity
Stepwise replication
Test–retest reliability
Thick description
Transferability
Triangulation
True score
Trustworthiness
Validity
Validity coefficient

SUMMARY POINTS

▷ **Measurement** involves a set of rules according to which numeric values are assigned to objects to represent varying degrees of some attribute.

▷ Few quantitative measuring instruments are infallible. Sources of measurement error include situational contaminants, response set biases, and transitory personal factors, such as fatigue.

▷ **Obtained scores** from an instrument consist of a **true score** component—the value that would be obtained if it were possible to have a perfect measure of the attribute—and an error component, or **error of measurement**, that represents measurement inaccuracies.

◦ **Reliability** is the degree of consistency or accuracy with which an instrument measures an attribute. The higher the reliability of an instrument, the lower the amount of error in the obtained scores.

◦ There are different methods for assessing an instrument's reliability and for computing a **reliability coefficient**. The *stability* aspect, which concerns the extent to which the instrument yields the same results on repeated administrations, is evaluated by **test–retest procedures**.

◦ The **internal consistency** aspect of reliability, which refers to the extent to which all the instrument's items are measuring the same attribute, is assessed using either the *split-half reliability technique* or, more likely, **Cronbach's alpha** method.

◦ When the focus of a reliability assessment is on establishing *equivalence* between observers in rating or coding behaviors, estimates of **interrater (or interobserver) reliability** are obtained.

◦ **Validity** is the degree to which an instrument measures what it is supposed to be measuring.

◦ **Face validity** refers to whether an instrument appears, on the face of it, to be measuring the appropriate construct.

◦ **Content validity** is concerned with the sampling adequacy of the content being measured.

◦ **Criterion-related validity** focuses on the correlation between the instrument and an outside criterion.

◦ **Construct validity** refers to the adequacy of an instrument in measuring the construct of interest. One construct validation method is the **known-groups technique**, which contrasts the scores of groups that are presumed to differ on the attribute; another is **factor analysis**, a statistical procedure for identifying unitary clusters of items or measures.

◦ Sensitivity and specificity are important criteria for evaluating screening and diagnostic instruments. **Sensitivity** is the instrument's ability to correctly identify a case, i.e., its rate of yielding true positives. **Specificity** is the instrument's ability to correctly identify a noncase, i.e., its rate of yielding true negatives.

◦ Qualitative researchers evaluate the **trustworthiness** of their data using the criteria of credibility, dependability, confirmability, and transferability.

◦ **Credibility**, roughly analogous to validity in a quantitative study, refers to the believability of the data. Techniques to improve the credibility of qualitative data include **prolonged engagement**, which strives for adequate scope of data coverage, and **persistent observation**, which is aimed at achieving adequate depth.

◦ **Triangulation** is the process of using multiple referents to draw conclusions about what constitutes the truth. The four major forms are *data source triangulation, investigator triangulation, theoretical triangulation,* and *method triangulation.*

◦ Two important tools for establishing credibility are **peer debriefings**, wherein the researcher obtains feedback about data quality and interpretation from peers, and **member checks**, wherein informants are asked to comment on the data and the researcher's interpretations.

◦ **Dependability** of qualitative data refers to the stability of data over time and over conditions and is somewhat analogous to the concept of reliability in quantitative studies.

◦ **Confirmability** refers to the objectivity or neutrality of the data. Independent **inquiry audits** by external auditors can be used to assess and document dependability and confirmability.

◦ The **auditability** of a study is enhanced when researchers maintain and share portions of an **audit trail** and **decision trail** in their reports.

◦ **Transferability** is the extent to which findings from the data can be transferred to other settings or groups. Transferability can be enhanced through **thick descriptions** of the context of the data collection.

RESEARCH EXAMPLES   Critical Thinking Activities

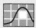 **EXAMPLE 1: Quantitative Research**

Aspects of two related psychometric assessments, featuring terms and concepts discussed in this chapter, are presented below, followed by some questions to guide critical thinking. (The two research reports are available in (1) *Nursing Research, 49,* 272–282 and (2) *Nursing Research, 50,*155–164.)

Study

(1) "Postpartum Depression Screening Scale: Development and psychometric testing" (Beck & Gable, 2000) and (2) "Further validation of the Postpartum Depression Screening Scale" (Beck & Gable, 2001)

Statement of Purpose

The two methodologic studies involved developing and testing the quality of a new scale to screen women for postpartum depression (PPD).

Background

Beck had studied PPD in a series of qualitative studies, using both a phenomenological approach (1992, 1996) and a grounded theory approach (1993). Based on her in-depth understanding of PPD, she began in the late 1990s to develop a scale that could be used to screen for PPD, the Postpartum Depression Screening Scale (PDSS). Working with Gable, an expert psychometrician, Beck refined and evaluated the PDSS. (Psychometric testing of the Spanish version of the PDSS was reported in Beck and Gable, 2003).

Content Validity

Content validity was enhanced by using direct quotes from the qualitative studies as items on the Likert-type scale (e.g., "I felt like I was losing my mind"). A pilot version of the PDSS was subjected to ratings by a panel of five content experts. This content validity effort led to some modifications.

Construct Validity

The PDSS was administered to a sample of 525 new mothers in six states (Beck & Gable, 2000). Preliminary analyses resulted in the deletion of several items. The PDSS was finalized as a 35-item scale with seven subscales, each with 5 items. This version of the PDSS was subjected to factor analyses, which indicated that the items mapped well onto underlying constructs. In their subsequent study, Beck and Gable (2001) administered the PDSS and other scales to 150 new mothers. To further validate their scale, they tested theoretically driven hypotheses about how scores on the PDSS would correlate with scores on other scales.

research examples continue on page 342

RESEARCH EXAMPLES *Continued*

Criterion-Related Validity

In the second study, Beck and Gable correlated scores on the PDSS with an expert clinician's diagnosis of PPD for each woman. The validity coefficient was .70.

Internal Consistency Reliability

In both studies, Beck and Gable evaluated the internal consistency reliability of the PDSS and its subscales. Reliability for the subscales ranged from .83 to .94 in the first study and from .80 to .91 in the second study.

Sensitivity and Specificity

In the second study, Beck and Gable used the expert diagnosis of PPD to establish a cutoff score and evaluate the scale's sensitivity and specificity. Based on their analyses, Beck and Gable recommended a cutoff score of 80 for major postpartum depression. This cutoff accurately screened in 94% of true PPD cases and mistakenly screened in 2% who did not have the mood disorder.

Critical Thinking Suggestions*

*See the Student Resource CD-ROM for a discussion of these questions.

1. Answer questions 3–6 and 8 from Box 14-1 regarding this study.
2. Also consider the following targeted questions, which may assist you in further assessing aspects of the study:
   a. Was the criterion-related validity effort an example of concurrent or predictive validity?
   b. The researchers determined that there should be seven subscales to the PDSS. Why do you think this might be the case?
   c. Each item on the PDSS is scored on a 5-point scale from 1 to 5. What is the range of possible scores on the scale (and what is the range of scores on each subscale)? Comment on where the cutoff score of 80 falls on the total scale.
   d. Comment on the researchers' credentials for undertaking this study together, and on the appropriateness of their overall effort.
3. What might be some of the uses to which the scale could be put in clinical practice?

 EXAMPLE 2: Qualitative Research

Aspects of a qualitative nursing study, featuring terms and concepts discussed in this chapter, are presented below, followed by some questions to guide critical thinking. (The research report is available in *Qualitative Health Research, 11,* 58–68.)

Study

"Pediatric lung transplantation: Families' need for understanding" (Stubblefield & Murray, 2001)

RESEARCH EXAMPLES *Continued*

Statement of Purpose

The purpose of the study was to explore how parents whose children had undergone lung transplantation perceived their relationships with others before, during, and after the transplantation.

Method

Stubblefield and Murray, both of whom have a clinical specialty in psychiatric–mental health nursing, interviewed 15 parents of 12 children who had undergone lung transplantation. Each parent was interviewed at least three times, with the main interviews ranging in length from 45 minutes to 2½ hours. Interviews were audio-taped and later transcribed. The researchers used several strategies to enhance the trustworthiness of the study findings.

Credibility

Prolonged engagement was one method of increasing credibility: The researchers were in contact with the parents over a 9-month period, which facilitated their understanding of what it was like to live with a lung transplant situation. Investigator triangulation and peer debriefings were additional techniques used to increase credibility. The investigators discussed their descriptive categories as they were developing them with each other and with a peer who was an expert in qualitative research. Member checks were done by returning to the parents for a final validating step. Parents were asked how the findings compared to their experiences with the transplant situation. Data saturation (i.e., obtaining redundant information) was yet another method used to enhance credibility.

Dependability and Confirmability

Stubblefield and Murray maintained an audit trail that identified the analytical decisions made during data collection and data analysis.

Transferability

Transferability was facilitated through rich description of the parents' experiences with their children's lung transplantation. Also, the sample was selected to reflect various educational and socioeconomic levels. The report included information about the demographic characteristics of the parents and children, which could be used to determine transferability of the study findings.

Key Findings

Some parents perceived a sense of diminished support from family and friends as they coped with living with the transplant, which they attributed, in part, to a lack of understanding. Although the parents described professional counseling as an important source of support, many were hesitant to seek it.

Critical Thinking Suggestions

1. Answer the questions from Box 14-2 regarding this study.

research examples continue on page 344

RESEARCH EXAMPLES *Continued*

2. Also consider the following targeted questions, which may assist you in further assessing aspects of the study:
   a. Can you think of other types of triangulation that the researchers could have used?
   b. Explain how investigator triangulation and peer debriefings could affect confirmability as well as credibility in this study.
   c. How did audio-taping and transcription enhance the trustworthiness of the data?
3. If the results of this study are trustworthy, what are some of the uses to which the findings might be put in clinical practice?

 EXAMPLE 3: Quantitative Research

1. Read the introduction and method sections from the study ("Sense of Coherence") in Appendix A of this book, and then answer the relevant questions in Box 14-1.
2. Also consider the following targeted questions, which may further sharpen your critical thinking skills and assist you in assessing aspects of the study:
   a. In this study, both the short form and long form of the SOC were administered. The internal consistency of these scales was .88 and .92, respectively. Why do you think the internal consistency was not the same for the two forms?
   b. If the internal consistency reliability for the SOC and QOL scales were computed separately for just the women in the sample with IBS, do you think the reliability coefficient would be higher, lower, or the same as for the whole sample?
   c. Suggest some "known groups" that could be used to validate the SOC and QOL scales.

 EXAMPLE 4: Qualitative Research

1. Read the method section from Beck's study ("Birth Trauma") in Appendix B of this book, and then answer the relevant questions in Box 14-2.
2. Also consider the following targeted questions, which may assist you in assessing aspects of the study's merit:
   a. Beck is a mother of two children. She herself has not experienced birth trauma, but she has interacted with pregnant women and new mothers extensively both clinically and in her research. Discuss how Beck's background has relevance for this study.
   b. Give one or two examples of additional (or alternative) steps Beck could have taken to address issues of trustworthiness on her study.

SUGGESTED READINGS

Methodologic References

Denzin, N. K. (1989). *The research act* (3rd ed.). New York: McGraw-Hill.

Giorgi, A. (1989). Some theoretical and practical issues regarding the psychological and phenomenological method. *Saybrook Review, 7,* 71–85.

Hall, J. M., & Stevens, P. E. (1991). Rigor in feminist research. *Advances in Nursing Science, 13,* 16–29.

Kerlinger, F. N., & Lee, H. B. (2000). *Foundations of behavioral research* (4th ed.). Orlando, FL: Harcourt College Publishers.

Lincoln, Y. S., & Guba, E. G. (1985). *Naturalistic inquiry.* Newbury Park, CA: Sage Publications.

Morse, J. M. (1999). Myth # 93: Reliability and validity are not relevant to qualitative inquiry. *Qualitative Health Research, 9,* 717–718.

Nunnally, J., & Bernstein, I. H. (1994). *Psychometric theory* (3rd ed.). New York: McGraw-Hill.

Patton, M. Q. (2002). *Qualitative evaluation and research methods* (3rd ed.). Thousand Oaks, CA: Sage Publications.

Whittemore, R., Chase, S. K., & Mandle, C. L. (2001). Validity in qualitative research. *Qualitative Health Research, 11,* 522–537.

Studies Cited in Chapter 14

Banister, E. M., Jakubec, S. L., & Stein, J. A. (2003). "Like, what am I supposed to do?": Adolescent girls' health concerns in their dating relationships. *Canadian Journal of Nursing Research, 35,* 16–33.

Beck, C. T. (1992). The lived experience of postpartum depression. *Nursing Research, 41,* 166–170.

Beck, C. T. (1993). Teetering on the edge: A substantive theory of postpartum depression. *Nursing Research, 42,* 42–48.

Beck, C. T. (1996). Postpartum depressed mothers interacting with their children. *Nursing Research, 45,* 98–104.

Beck, C. T. (2002). Releasing the pause button: Mothering twins during the first year of life. *Qualitative Health Research, 12,* 593–608.

Beck, C. T., & Gable, R. K. (2000). Postpartum Depression Screening Scale: Development and psychometric testing. *Nursing Research, 49,* 272–282.

Beck, C. T., & Gable, R. K. (2001). Further validation of the Postpartum Depression Screening Scale. *Nursing Research, 50,* 155–164.

Beck, C. T., & Gable, R. K. (2003). Postpartum Depression Screening Scale: Spanish version. *Nursing Research, 52,* 296–306.

Creedy, D. K., Dennis, C., Blyth, R., Moyle, W., Pratt, J., & DeVries, S. M. (2003). Psychometric characteristics of the Breastfeeding Self-Efficacy Scale: Data from an Australian sample. *Research in Nursing & Health, 26,* 143–152.

Curley, M. A. Q., Razmus, I. S., Roberts, K. E., & Wypij, D. (2003). Predicting pressure ulcer risk in pediatric patients. *Nursing Research, 52,* 22–31.

Dennis, C. (2003). The Breastfeeding Self-Efficacy Scale: Psychometric assessment of the short form. *Journal of Obstetric, Gynecologic, & Neonatal Nursing, 32,* 734–744.

Dobratz, M. C. (2004). The Life Closure Scale: Additional psychometric testing of a tool to measure psychological adaptation in death and dying. *Research in Nursing & Health, 27,* 52–62.

Gulick, E. E. (2003). Adaptation of the Postpartum Support Questionnaire for mothers with multiple sclerosis. *Research in Nursing and Health, 26,* 30–39.

Hauck, Y. L., & Irurita, V. F. (2003). Incompatible expectations: The dilemma of breastfeeding mothers. *Health Care for Women International, 24,* 62–78.

Kovach, C. R., & Wells, T. (2002). Pacing of activity as a predictor of agitation. *Journal of Gerontological Nursing, 28,* 28–35.

MacDonald, H., & Callery, P. (2004). Different meanings of respite: A study of parents, nurses, and social workers caring for children with complex needs. *Child Care & Health Development, 30,* 279–288.

Mohr, W. K. (2000). Rethinking professional attitudes in mental health settings. *Qualitative Health Research, 10,* 595–611.

Mohr, W. K. (2004). Surfacing the life phases of a mental health support group. *Qualitative Health Research, 14,* 61–77.

Navon, L., & Morag, A. (2003). Advanced prostate cancer patients' ways of coping with the hormonal therapy's effect on body, sexuality, and spousal ties. *Qualitative Health Research, 13,* 1378–1392.

Needham, I., Abderhalden, C., Dassen, T., Haug, H. J., & Fischer, J. E. (2004). The perception of aggression by nurses: Psychometric scale testing and derivation of a short instrument. *Journal of Psychiatric and Mental Health Nursing, 11,* 36–42.

Shin, Y., & Colling, K. B. (2000). Cultural verification and application of the Profile of Mood States (POMS) with Korean elders. *Western Journal of Nursing Research, 22,* 68–83.

Stubblefield, C., & Murray, R. L. (2001). Pediatric lung transplantation: Families' need for understanding. *Qualitative Health Research, 11,* 58–68.

Williams, J. K., Schutte, D. L., Evers, C., & Holkup, P. A. (2000). Redefinition: Coping with normal results from predictive gene testing for neurodegenerative disorders. *Research in Nursing & Health, 23,* 260–269.

Wynd, C. A., Schmidt, B., & Schaefer, M. A. (2003). Two quantitative approaches for estimating content validity. *Western Journal of Nursing Research, 25,* 508–518.

Data
Analysis

Analyzing Quantitative Data

STUDENT OBJECTIVES

On completing this chapter, you will be able to:

▶ Identify the four levels of measurement and compare their characteristics
▶ Describe the characteristics of frequency distributions and identify and interpret various descriptive statistics
▶ Describe the logic and purpose of tests of statistical significance and describe hypothesis testing procedures
▶ Specify the appropriate applications for t-tests, analysis of variance, chi-squared tests, and correlation coefficients
▶ Describe the applications and principles of multiple regression and analysis of covariance
▶ Understand the results of simple statistical procedures described in a research report
▶ Define new terms in the chapter

T he data collected in a study do not by themselves answer research questions or test research hypotheses. Data need to be systematically analyzed so that trends and patterns can be detected. This chapter describes procedures for analyzing quantitative data, and Chapter 16 discusses the analysis of qualitative data.

LEVELS OF MEASUREMENT

A quantitative measure can be classified according to its **level of measurement**. This classification system is important because the analyses that can be performed on data depend on their measurement level. There are four major classes, or levels, of measurement:

1. **Nominal measurement,** the lowest level, involves using numbers simply to categorize attributes. Examples of variables that are nominally measured include gender and blood type. The numbers assigned in nominal measurement do not have quantitative meaning. If we coded males as 1 and females as 2, the numbers would not have quantitative implications—the number 2 does not mean "more than" 1. Nominal measurement provides information only about categorical equivalence and nonequivalence and so the numbers cannot be treated mathematically. It is nonsensical, for example, to compute the average gender of the sample by adding the numeric values of the codes and dividing by the number of participants.

Example of nominal measurement

Stastny, Ichinose, Thayer, Olson, and Keens (2004) studied infant sleep positioning by mothers and nursery staff in newborn hospital nurseries. Infant sleep positioning was a nominal measure with the following categories: prone, side only, side or supine, and supine only.

2. **Ordinal measurement** ranks objects based on their relative standing on an attribute. If a researcher rank-orders people from heaviest to lightest, this is ordinal measurement. As another example, consider this ordinal coding scheme for measuring ability to perform activities of daily living: 1 = completely dependent; 2 = needs another person's assistance; 3 = needs mechanical assistance; and 4 = completely independent. The numbers signify incremental ability to perform activities of daily living independently. Ordinal measurement does not, however, tell us how much greater one level is than another. For example, we do not know

Example of ordinal measurement

Champion, Piper, Holden, Korte, and Shain (2004) studied risk for pelvic inflammatory disease in a sample of women with sexually transmitted diseases. They created a set of variables to measure genitourinary symptoms, several of which were ordinal measures. For example, abdominal pain was coded as "none," "intermediate," or "pathologic," based on the women's report about the type, severity, and frequency of abdominal pain.

if being completely independent is twice as good as needing mechanical assistance. As with nominal measures, the mathematic operations permissible with ordinal-level data are restricted.

3. **Interval measurement** occurs when researchers can specify the ranking of objects on an attribute *and* the distance between those objects. Most educational and psychological tests are based on interval scales. For example, the Stanford-Binet Intelligence Scale—a standardized intelligence (IQ) test used in many countries—is an interval measure. A score of 140 on the Stanford-Binet is higher than a score of 120, which, in turn, is higher than 100. Moreover, the difference between 140 and 120 is presumed to be equivalent to the difference between 120 and 100. Interval scales expand analytic possibilities: Interval-level data can be averaged meaningfully, for example. Many sophisticated statistical procedures require interval measurements.

Example of interval measurement

Aronowitz and Morrison-Beedy (2004) studied the role of mother–daughter connectedness in the daughters' resilience to risk-taking behaviors among poor young African-American women. *Maternal caring,* a component of the construct "connectedness," was measured with a 5-item scale whose scores could range from 0 to 25. A score of 0 on this scale clearly does not reflect a total absence of maternal caring, and a score of 20 does not mean twice as much maternal caring as a score of 10.

4. **Ratio measurement** is the highest level of measurement. Ratio scales, unlike interval scales, have a rational, meaningful zero and therefore provide information about the absolute magnitude of the attribute. The Fahrenheit scale for measuring temperature (interval measurement) has an arbitrary zero point. Zero on the thermometer does not signify the absence of heat; it would not be appropriate to say that 60°F is twice as hot as 30°F. Many physical measures, however, are ratio measures with a real zero. A person's weight, for example, is a ratio measure. It is acceptable to say that someone who weighs 200 lb is twice as heavy as someone who weighs 100 lb. The statistical procedures suitable for interval data are also appropriate for ratio-level data.

Example of ratio measurement

Melkus and colleagues (2004) developed and tested a culturally competent intervention for African-American women with type 2 diabetes mellitus. Several of the physiologic outcome variables were ratio-level measures. Examples include weight (in pounds) and fasting blood glucose (in milligrams per deciliter).

Researchers usually strive to use the highest levels of measurement possible—especially for their dependent variables—because higher levels yield more information and are amenable to more powerful analysis than lower levels.

HOW-TO-TELL TIP

How can you tell the measurement level of a variable? A variable is *nominal* if the values could be interchanged (e.g., 1 = male, 2 = female OR 1 = female, 2 = male—the codes are arbitrary). A variable is usually *ordinal* if there is a quantitative ordering of values AND if there are only a small number of values (e.g., very important, important, not too important, unimportant). A variable is usually considered *interval* if it is measured with a composite scale or psychological test. A variable is *ratio*-level if it makes sense to say that one value is twice as much as another (e.g., 100 mg is twice as much as 50 mg).

■

DESCRIPTIVE STATISTICS

Statistical procedures enable researchers to organize, interpret, and communicate numeric information. Statistics are either descriptive or inferential. **Descriptive statistics** are used to synthesize and describe data. Averages and percentages are examples of descriptive statistics. When such indexes are calculated on data from a population, they are called **parameters**. A descriptive index from a sample is a **statistic**. Most scientific questions are about parameters; researchers calculate statistics to estimate them.

Frequency Distributions

Data that are not analyzed or organized are overwhelming. It is not even possible to discern general trends in the data without some structure. Consider the 60 numbers in Table 15-1. Let us assume that these numbers are the scores of 60 pre-operative patients on a 6-item measure of anxiety—scores that we will consider to be on an interval scale. Visual inspection of the numbers in this table provides little insight on students' anxiety levels.

Frequency distributions are a method of imposing order on numeric data. A **frequency distribution** is a systematic arrangement of numeric values from the lowest to the highest, together with a count (or percentage) of the number of times each value was obtained. The 60 anxiety scores are presented as a frequency distribution in Table 15-2. This arrangement makes it convenient to see at a glance the highest and lowest scores, the most common score, where the scores clustered, and how many patients were in the sample (total sample size is typically designated as *N* in research reports). None of this was easily discernible before the data were organized.

Some researchers display frequency data graphically in a *frequency polygon* (Figure 15-1). In such graphs, scores are on the horizontal line, with the lowest value on the left, and frequency

TABLE 15.1   Patients' Anxiety Scores

22	27	25	19	24	25	23	29	24	20
26	16	20	26	17	22	24	18	26	28
15	24	23	22	21	24	20	25	18	27
24	23	16	25	30	29	27	21	23	24
26	18	30	21	17	25	22	24	29	28
20	25	26	24	23	19	27	28	25	26

TABLE 15.2	Frequency Distribution of Patients' Anxiety Scores	
SCORE	**FREQUENCY**	**PERCENTAGE**
15	1	1.7
16	2	3.3
17	2	3.3
18	3	5.0
19	2	3.3
20	4	6.7
21	3	5.0
22	4	6.7
23	5	8.3
24	9	15.0
25	7	11.7
26	6	10.0
27	4	6.7
28	3	5.0
29	3	5.0
30	2	3.3
	$N = 60$	100.0

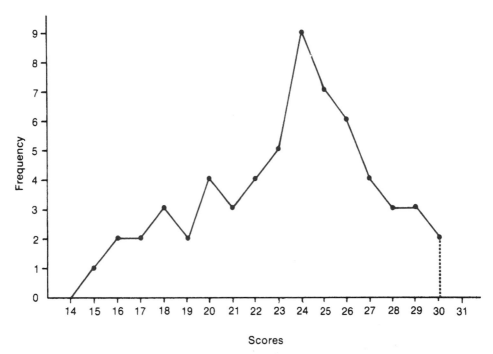

FIGURE 15.1 Frequency polygon of patients' anxiety scores.

A.   B.

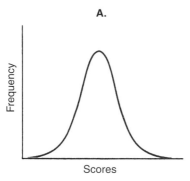 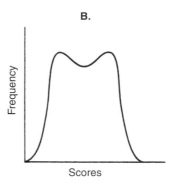

FIGURE 15.2 Examples of symmetric distributions.

counts or percentages are on the vertical line. Data distributions can be described by their shapes. **Symmetric distribution** occurs if, when folded over, the two halves of a frequency polygon would be superimposed (Figure 15-2). In an asymmetric or **skewed distribution**, the peak is off center, and one tail is longer than the other. When the longer tail is pointed toward the right, the distribution has a **positive skew**, as in the first graph of Figure 15-3. Personal income is an example of a positively skewed attribute. Most people have moderate incomes, with only a few people with high incomes at the right end of the distribution. If the longer tail points to the left, the distribution has a **negative skew**, as in the second graph in Figure 15-3. Age at death is an example of a negatively skewed attribute. Here, the bulk of people are at the far right end of the distribution, with relatively few people dying at an early age.

Another aspect of a distribution's shape concerns how many peaks or high points it has. A *unimodal distribution* has one peak (graph A, Figure 15-2), whereas a *multimodal distribution* has two or more peaks—that is, two or more values of high frequency. A multimodal distribution with two peaks is a *bimodal distribution,* illustrated in graph B of Figure 15-2.

A distribution of particular interest is the **normal distribution** (sometimes called *a bell-shaped curve*). A normal distribution is symmetric, unimodal, and not very peaked, as illustrated in graph A of Figure 15-2. Many human attributes (e.g., height, intelligence) approximate a normal distribution.

Example of frequency information

Table 15-3 presents distribution information on sample characteristics from a study of callers who used telephone advice nursing (Moscato et al., 2003). This table shows, for selected background characteristics, both the frequency (N) and percentage of sample members in various categories. For example, 71 subjects (86.6%) were women and 16 (13.4%) were men. Most subjects (67.6%) never or rarely used the Internet to obtain information on health.

Central Tendency

For variables on an interval or ratio scale, a distribution of values is usually of less interest than an overall summary. Researchers ask such questions as: What was the patients' average postintervention blood pressure? and How depressed was the typical mother after childbirth? These

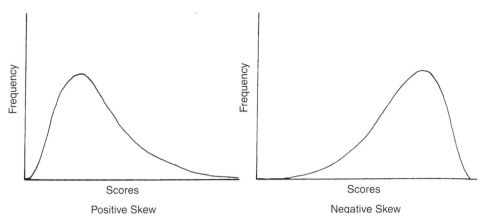

FIGURE 15.3 Examples of skewed distributions.

questions seek a single number that best represents the whole distribution. Such indexes of typicalness are measures of **central tendency**. To lay people, the term *average* is normally used to designate central tendency. There are three commonly used kinds of averages, or measures of central tendency: the mode, the median, and the mean.

▶ **Mode:** The mode is the number that occurs most frequently in a distribution. In the following distribution, the mode is 53:

50 51 51 52 53 53 53 53 54 55 56

The value of 53 occurred four times, a higher frequency than for other numbers. The mode of the patients' anxiety scores in Table 15-2 was 24. The mode, in other words, identifies the most popular value. The mode is used most often to describe typical or high-frequency values for nominal measures. For example, in the study by Moscato and co-researchers (see Table 15-3), we could make the following statement: The typical (modal) caller was a female, between the ages of 19 and 40, and had some post-high school education.

▶ **Median:** The median is the point in a distribution that divides scores in half. Consider the following set of values:

2 2 3 3 4 5 6 7 8 9

The value that divides the cases in half is midway between 4 and 5, and thus 4.5 is the median. For the patient anxiety scores, the median is 24, the same as the mode. An important characteristic of the median is that it does not take into account individual values and is thus insensitive to extremes. In the above set of numbers, if the value of 9 were changed to 99, the median would remain 4.5. Because of this property, the median is the preferred index of central tendency to describe a highly skewed distribution. In research reports, the median may be abbreviated as *Md* or *Mdn*.

▶ **Mean:** The mean is equal to the sum of all values divided by the number of participants —what people refer to as the average. The mean of the patients' anxiety scores is 23.4 (1405 + 60). As another example, here are the weights of eight people:

85 109 120 135 158 177 181 195

TABLE 15.3   Example of Table With Frequency Information: Characteristics of Callers Using Telephone Advice Nursing

CALLER CHARACTERISTIC	NUMBER OF RESPONDENTS ($N = 87$)	PERCENT OF RESPONDENTS
Age		
≤18 years	3	3.7
19–40 years	36	43.9
41–64 years	29	35.4
65+ years	14	17.1
Gender		
Female	71	86.6
Male	16	13.4
Educational status		
High school or less	20	24.4
Some college/technical school	32	39.0
College graduate	19	23.2
Some graduate education	11	13.4
Use of computer for information on health		
Never or rarely	54	67.6
Occasionally	16	20.0
Often	10	12.5

Adapted from Moscato, S. R., et al. (2003). Tool development for measuring caller satisfaction and outcome with telephone advice nursing. *Clinical Nursing Research, 12*, 266–281.

In this example, the mean is 145. Unlike the median, the mean is affected by the value of every score. If we were to exchange the 195-lb person for one weighing 275 lb, the mean weight would increase from 145 lb to 155 lb. A substitution of this kind would leave the median unchanged. In research reports, the mean is often symbolized as *M* or *X* (e.g., $\overline{X} = 145$).

For interval-level or ratio-level measurements, the mean, rather than the median or mode, is usually the statistic reported. Of the three indexes, the mean is the most stable: if repeated samples were drawn from a population, the means would fluctuate less than the modes or medians. Because of its stability, the mean usually is the best estimate of a population central tendency. When a distribution is highly skewed, however, the mean does not characterize the center of the distribution; in such situations, the median is preferred. For example, the median is a better central tendency measure of family income than the mean because income is positively skewed.

Variability

Two sets of data with identical means could be quite different with respect to how spread out the data are (i.e., how different people are from one another on an attribute). The **variability** of two distributions could be different even when the means are identical. Consider the distributions in Figure 15-4, which represent hypothetical scores of students from two schools on the Stanford-Binet IQ test. Both distributions have an average score of 100, but the two groups of students are clearly different. In school A, there is a wide range of scores—from scores below 70 to some above 130. In school B, on the other hand, there are few low scorers but also few

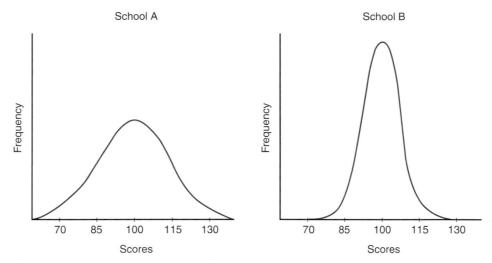

FIGURE 15.4 Two distributions of different variability.

outstanding performers. School A is more heterogeneous (i.e., more variable) than school B, whereas school B is more homogeneous than school A.

Researchers compute an index of variability to summarize the extent to which scores in a distribution differ from one another. Several such indexes have been developed, the most important of which are the range and the standard deviation.

▷ **Range:** The range is the highest score minus the lowest score in a distribution. In the example of the patients' anxiety scores, the range is 15 (30 − 15). In the distributions in Figure 15-4, the range for school A is about 80 (140 − 60), whereas the range for school B is about 50 (125 − 75). The chief virtue of the range is its ease of computation. Because it is based on only two scores, however, the range is unstable: From sample to sample drawn from the same population, the range tends to fluctuate considerably. Moreover, the range ignores score variations between the two extremes. In school B of Figure 15-4, if a single student obtained a score of 60 and another obtained a score of 140, the range of both schools would then be 80—despite large differences in heterogeneity. For these reasons, the range is used largely as a gross descriptive index.

▷ **Standard deviation:** The most widely used variability index is the standard deviation. Like the mean, the standard deviation is calculated based on every value in a distribution. The standard deviation summarizes the *average* amount of deviation of values from the mean. In the anxiety scale example, the standard deviation is 3.725.[1] In research reports, the standard deviation is often abbreviated as *s* or *SD*. Occasionally, the standard deviation is simply shown in relation to the mean without a formal label, such as M = 4.0 (1.5) or M = 4.0 ± 1.5, where 4.0 is the mean and 1.5 is the standard deviation.[2]

---

[1] Formulas for computing the standard deviation, as well as other statistics discussed in this chapter, are not shown in this textbook. The emphasis here is on helping you to understand statistical applications. References at the end of the chapter can be consulted for computation formulas.

[2] Research reports occasionally refer to an index of variability known as the **variance.** The variance is simply the value of the standard deviation squared. In the example of the patients' anxiety scores, the variance is 3.725^2, or 13.88.

A standard deviation is more difficult to interpret than the range. With regard to the SD of the anxiety scores, you might ask, 3.725 *what?* What does the number mean? We can answer these questions from several angles. First, as discussed, the SD is an index of how variable scores in a distribution are. If male and female nursing students had means of 23 on the anxiety scale, but females had an SD of 7 and males had an SD of 3, we would immediately know that the males were more homogeneous (i.e., their scores were more similar to one another).

The standard deviation represents the *average* of deviations from the mean. The mean tells us the single best point for summarizing an entire distribution, and a standard deviation tells us how much, on average, the scores deviate from that mean. In the anxiety scale example, they deviated by an average of just under four points. A standard deviation might thus be interpreted as an indication of our degree of error when we use a mean to describe an entire sample.

In normal and near-normal distributions, there are roughly three standard deviations above and below the mean. Suppose we had a normal distribution with a mean of 50 and an SD of 10 (Figure 15-5). In such a distribution, a fixed percentage of cases fall within certain distances from the mean. Sixty-eight percent of all cases fall within 1 SD above and below the mean. Thus, in this example, nearly seven of 10 scores are between 40 and 60. In a normal distribution, 95% of the scores fall within 2 SDs from the mean. Only a handful of cases—about 2% at each extreme—lie more than 2 SDs from the mean. Using this figure, we can see that a person with a score of 70 achieved a higher score than about 98% of the sample.

Example of means and SDs

Table 15-4 presents descriptive statistics from a nursing study that examined predictors of physical functioning among elderly cancer patients (Given, Given, Azzouzz, & Stommel, 2001). The table shows the means, SDs, and medians of physical functioning scores, using the SF-36 scale, for four types of cancer patients before diagnosis and then 6–8 weeks after diagnosis. According to these data, physical functioning deteriorated in all groups (i.e., mean scores were lower after diagnosis), especially among lung cancer patients. Variability was constant over time except for prostate cancer patients, who became more heterogeneous after diagnosis.

Bivariate Descriptive Statistics

So far, our discussion has focused on *univariate* (one-variable) *descriptive statistics*. The mean, mode, standard deviation, and so forth are used to describe one variable at a time. *Bivariate* (two-variable) *descriptive statistics* describe relationships between two variables.

CONTINGENCY TABLES

A **contingency table** is a two-dimensional frequency distribution in which the frequencies of two variables are **cross-tabulated**. Suppose we had data on patients' gender and whether they are nonsmokers, light smokers (<1 pack of cigarettes a day), or heavy smokers (≥1 pack a day). The question is whether there is a tendency for the men to smoke more heavily than the women or *vice versa*. Some fictitious data on these two variables are shown in a contingency table in

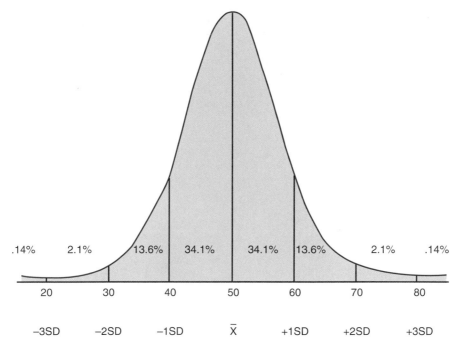

FIGURE 15.5 Standard deviations in a normal distribution.

Table 15-5. Six cells are created by using one variable (gender) for columns and the other variable (smoking status) for rows. After all subjects are allocated to the appropriate cells, percentages can be computed. This simple procedure allows us to see at a glance that, in this sample, women were more likely than men to be nonsmokers (45.4% versus 27.3%) and less likely to be heavy smokers (18.2% versus 36.4%). Contingency tables usually are used with nominal data or

TABLE 15.4	**Example of Descriptive Statistics: Physical Functioning Scores (SF-36) of Elderly Cancer Patients***			
	BEFORE DIAGNOSIS		**6–8 WEEKS AFTER DIAGNOSIS**	
	Mean (SD)	**Median**	**Mean (SD)**	**Median**
Patients with breast cancer	80 (24)	90	68 (24)	70
Patients with colon cancer	85 (27)	95	61 (27)	65
Patients with lung cancer	72 (28)	85	44 (28)	35
Patients with prostate cancer	88 (19)	100	76 (26)	85

*Adapted from Given, B., Given, C., Azzouzz, F., & Stommel, M. (2001). Physical functioning of elderly cancer patients prior to diagnosis and following initial treatment. *Nursing Research, 50,* 222–232.

TABLE 15.5 Contingency Table for Gender and Smoking Status Relationship

	GENDER					
	Female		Male		Total	
SMOKING STATUS	*n*	%	*n*	%	*n*	%
Nonsmoker	10	45.4	6	27.3	16	36.4
Light smoker	8	36.4	8	36.4	16	36.4
Heavy smoker	4	18.2	8	36.4	12	27.3
TOTAL	22	50.0	22	50.0	44	100.0

ordinal data that have few levels or ranks. In the present example, gender is a nominal measure, and smoking status is an ordinal measure.

Example of a contingency table

Table 15-6 presents a contingency table from an actual study that examined the relationship between frequency of religious attendance and importance of religion in a sample of patients with a life-threatening illness (Kub et al., 2003). Overall, 69.6% of the sample said that religion was very important, but fewer than half (44.6%) attended a religious service once a week or more. Almost all the patients (96.0%) who attended at least weekly said that religion was very important.

A comparison of Tables 15-5 and 15-6 illustrates that cross-tabulated data can be presented two ways: Percentages for each cell can be computed on the basis of either row totals or column totals. In Table 15-5, the number 10 in the first cell (female nonsmokers) was divided by the column total (i.e., by the total number of females—22) to arrive at the percentage (45%) of females who were nonsmokers. The table could have shown 63% in this cell (10 + 16)—the percentage of nonsmokers who were female. In Table 15-6, the number 8 in the first cell (patients who never attended services and rated religion as not important) was divided by the row total of 15 (i.e., by the number of patients who never attended) to yield the percentage of 53.3%. Computed the other way, the researchers would have gotten 66.7%—the percentage of

CONSUMER TIP

You may need to spend an extra minute when examining contingency tables to determine which total—row or column—was used as the basis for calculating percentages.

■

TABLE 15.6	Example of a Contingency Table: Frequency of Religious Attendance by Importance of Religion In Patients with a Life-Threatening Illness

	IMPORTANCE OF RELIGION							
FREQUENCY OF ATTENDANCE	**Not important**		**Somewhat important**		**Very important**		**Total**	
	N	**%**	**N**	**%**	**N**	**%**	**N**	**%**
Never	8	53.3	3	20.0	4	26.7	15	13.4
Once or twice/year	4	14.3	13	46.4	11	39.3	28	25.0
Once a month	0	0.0	4	21.1	15	78.9	19	17.0
Once a week or more	0	0.0	2	4.0	48	96.0	50	44.6
Total	12	10.7	22	19.6	78	69.6	112	100.0

Adapted from Kub, J. E., et al. (2003). Religious importance and practices of patients with a life-threatening illness: Implications for screening protocols. *Applied Nursing Research, 16*, 196–200.

patients rating religion as not important who never attended services. Either approach is acceptable, although the former is often preferred because then the percentages in a column add up to 100%.

CORRELATION

Relationships between two variables are usually described through **correlation** procedures. The correlation question is: To what extent are two variables related to each other? For example, to what degree are anxiety scores and blood pressure measures related? This question can be answered quantitatively by calculating a **correlation coefficient**, which describes the *intensity* and *direction* of a relationship.

Two variables that are related are height and weight: Tall people tend to weigh more than short people. The relationship between height and weight would be a *perfect relationship* if the tallest person in a population was the heaviest, the second tallest person was the second heaviest, and so on. The correlation coefficient summarizes how "perfect" a relationship is. The possible values for a correlation coefficient range from −1.00 through .00 to +1.00. If height and weight were perfectly correlated, the correlation coefficient expressing this would be 1.00 (the actual correlation coefficient is in the vicinity of .50 to .60 for a general population). Height and weight have a **positive relationship** because greater height tends to be associated with greater weight.

When two variables are unrelated, the correlation coefficient is zero. One might anticipate that women's shoe size is unrelated to their intelligence. Women with large feet are as likely to perform well on IQ tests as those with small feet. The correlation coefficient summarizing such a relationship would presumably be in the vicinity of .00. Correlation coefficients running between .00 and −1.00 express a **negative**, or *inverse*, **relationship**. When two variables are inversely related, increments in one variable are associated with decrements in the second. For example, there is a negative correlation between depression and self-esteem. This means that, on average, people with *high* self-esteem tend to be *low* on depression. If the relationship were perfect (i.e., if the person with the highest self-esteem score had the lowest depression score and so on), then the correlation coefficient would be -1.00. In actuality, the relationship between depression and self-esteem is moderate—usually in the vicinity of $-.40$ or $-.50$. Note that the higher the *absolute value* of the coefficient (i.e., the value disregarding the sign), the stronger the relationship. A correlation of $-.80$, for instance, is much stronger than a correlation of $+.20$.

The most commonly used correlation index is the **product–moment correlation coefficient** (also referred to as **Pearson's r**), which is computed with interval or ratio measures. The correlation index often used for ordinal measures is **Spearman's rank-order correlation** (r_s), sometimes referred to as **Spearman's rho**.

It is difficult to offer guidelines on what should be interpreted as strong or weak relationships, because it depends on the nature of the variables. If we were to measure patients' body temperature both orally and rectally, a correlation (r) of .70 between the two measurements would be low. For most psychosocial variables (e.g., stress and severity of illness), however, an r of .70 would be rather high. Perfect correlations ($+1.00$ and -1.00) are extremely rare.

In research reports, correlation coefficients are often reported in tables displaying a two-dimensional **correlation matrix**, in which variables are displayed in both rows and columns. To read a correlation matrix, one finds the row for one variable and reads across until the row intersects with the column for another variable.

Example of a correlation matrix

Heinrich (2003) conducted a study to examine interrelationships between hope, spirituality, uncertainty in illness, and perceptions of health among HIV seropositive men. Table 15-7, adapted from the research report, presents the correlation matrix for key study variables. This table lists, on the left, four variables: the men's perceived health (variable 1), hope (2), spirituality (3), and uncertainty in illness (4). The numbers in the top row, from 1 to 4, correspond to the four variables: 1 is perceived health, and so on. The correlation matrix shows, in column 1, the correlation coefficient between perceived health with all four variables. At the intersection of row 1, column 1, we find 1.00, which simply indicates that perceived health scores are perfectly correlated with themselves. The next entry in the first column is the value of r between perceived health and hope. The value of .56 (which can be read as $+.56$) indicates a moderate, positive relationship between these two variables: Men who perceived their health more positively tended to be more hopeful. Looking down at the last row in this table, we see that scores on the uncertainty in illness scale were negatively correlated with all other variables. In other words, the lower the uncertainty, the greater the perceived health, hope, and spirituality.

INTRODUCTION TO INFERENTIAL STATISTICS

Descriptive statistics are useful for summarizing data, but researchers usually do more than simply describe. **Inferential statistics,** which are based on the *laws of probability*, provide a means for drawing conclusions about a population, given data from a sample.

Sampling Distributions

When using a sample to estimate population characteristics, it is important to obtain a sample that is representative, and random sampling is the best means of securing such samples. Inferential

TABLE 15.7	Example of a Correlation Matrix: Study of Perceived Health of HIV Seropositive Men			
VARIABLE	**1**	**2**	**3**	**4**
1 Perceived health	1.00			
2 Hope	.56	1.00		
3 Spirituality	.31	.63	1.00	
4 Uncertainty in illness	−.65	−.54	−.28	1.00

Adapted from Heinrich, C. R. (2003). Enhancing the perceived health of HIV seropositive men. *Western Journal of Nursing Research, 25,* 367–382.

statistics are based on the assumption of random sampling from populations—although this assumption is widely violated.

Even with random sampling, however, sample characteristics are seldom identical to those of the population. Suppose we had a population of 30,000 nursing school applicants whose mean score on a standardized entrance exam was 500 with a standard deviation of 100. Now suppose that we do not know these parameters but that we must estimate them based on scores from a random sample of 25 applicants. Should we expect a mean of exactly 500 and a standard deviation of 100 for the sample? It would be improbable to obtain identical values. Let us suppose that the sample mean was 505. If a completely new random sample of 25 students was drawn and another mean computed, we might obtain a value of 497. Sample statistics fluctuate and are unequal to the population parameter because of sampling error. Researchers need a way to determine whether sample statistics are good estimates of population parameters.

To understand the logic of inferential statistics, we must perform a mental exercise. Consider drawing a sample of 25 students from the population of applicants, calculating a mean test score, replacing the students, and drawing a new sample. Each mean is considered one datum. If we drew 5000 samples of 25 applicants, we would have 5000 means (data points) that could be used to construct a frequency polygon (Figure 15-6). This distribution is called a **sampling distribution of the mean**. A sampling distribution is a theoretical rather than an actual distribution because in practice no one draws consecutive samples from a population and plots their means. Statisticians have demonstrated that (1) sampling distributions of means follow a normal distribution and (2) the mean of a sampling distribution for an infinite number of sample means equals the population mean. In our example, the mean of the sampling distribution is 500, the same as the population mean.

Remember that when scores are normally distributed, 68% of the cases fall between +1 SD and −1 SD from the mean. Because a sampling distribution of means is normally distributed, the probability is 68 out of 100 that any randomly drawn sample mean lies between +1 SD and −1 SD of the population mean. The problem is to determine the standard deviation of the sampling distribution—which is called the **standard error of the mean** (SEM). The word *error* signifies that the sample means contain some error as estimates of the population mean. The smaller the standard error (i.e., the less variable the sample means), the more accurate are the means as estimates of the population value.

Because no one actually constructs a sampling distribution, how can its standard deviation be computed? Fortunately, there is a formula for estimating the SEM from data from a

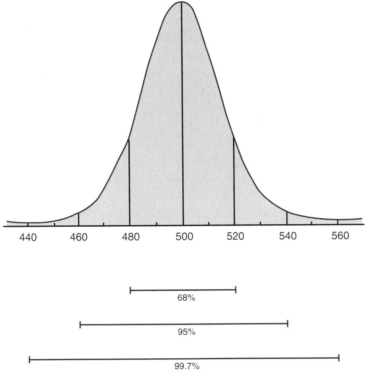

FIGURE 15.6 Sampling distribution of a mean.

single sample, using two pieces of information: the sample's standard deviation and its size. In the present example, the SEM has been calculated as 20, as shown in Figure 15-6. This statistic is an estimate of how much sampling error there would be from one sample mean to another in an infinite number of samples of 25 nursing school applicants.

We can now estimate the probability of drawing a sample with a certain mean. With a sample size of 25 and a population mean of 500, the chances are about 95 out of 100 that a sample mean would fall between the values of 460 and 540—2 SDs above and below the mean. Only 5 times out of 100 would the mean of a randomly selected sample of 25 applicants be greater than 540 or be less than 460. In other words, only 5 times out of 100 would we be likely to draw a sample whose mean deviates from the population mean by more than 40 points.

Because the SEM is partly a function of sample size, we need only increase sample size to increase the accuracy of our estimate. Suppose that instead of using a sample of 25 applicants to estimate the population mean, we used a sample of 100. With this many students, the standard error of the mean would be 10, not 20—and the probability would be about 95 in 100 that a sample mean would be between 480 and 520. The chances of drawing a sample with a mean very different from that of the population are reduced as sample size increases because large numbers promote the likelihood that extreme cases will cancel each other out.

You may be wondering why you need to learn about these abstract statistical notions. Consider, though, that what we are talking about concerns how likely it is that a researcher's results are accurate. As an intelligent consumer, you need to evaluate critically how believable research evidence is so that you can decide whether to incorporate it into your nursing practice. The concepts underlying the standard error are important in such an evaluation and are related to issues we stressed in Chapter 12 on sampling. First, the more homogeneous the population is on the critical attribute (i.e., the smaller the standard deviation), the more likely it is that results calculated from a sample will be accurate. Second, the larger the sample size, the greater is the likelihood of accuracy. The concepts discussed in this section are the basis for statistical hypothesis testing.

Hypothesis Testing

Statistical inference consists of two major techniques: estimation of parameters and hypothesis testing. **Estimation procedures** are used to estimate a single population characteristic, such as a mean value (e.g., the mean temperature of presurgical patients). Estimation procedures, however, are not common because researchers typically are more interested in relationships between variables than in estimating the accuracy of a single sample value. For this reason, we focus on hypothesis testing.

Statistical **hypothesis testing** provides objective criteria for deciding whether research hypotheses should be accepted as true or rejected as false. Suppose we hypothesized that maternity patients exposed to a teaching film on breastfeeding would breastfeed longer than mothers who did not see the film. We find that the mean number of days of breastfeeding is 131.5 for 25 experimental subjects and 125.1 for 25 control subjects. Should we conclude that the hypothesis has been supported? True, group differences are in the predicted direction, but perhaps in another sample the group means would be nearly identical.

Two explanations for the observed outcome are possible: (1) the film is truly effective in encouraging breastfeeding or (2) the difference in this sample was due to chance factors (e.g., differences in the characteristics of the two groups even before the film was shown, reflecting a selection bias).

The first explanation is the researcher's *research hypothesis*, and the second is the *null hypothesis*. The null hypothesis, it may be recalled, states that there is no relationship between the independent and dependent variables. Statistical hypothesis testing is basically a process of disproof or rejection. It cannot be demonstrated directly that the research hypothesis is correct. But it is possible to show, using theoretical sampling distributions, that the null hypothesis has a high probability of being incorrect, and such evidence lends support to the research hypothesis. Hypothesis testing helps researchers to make objective decisions about study results—that is, to decide which results are likely to reflect chance differences in the sample and which are likely to reflect true hypothesized effects.

The rejection of the null hypothesis, then, is what researchers seek to accomplish through **statistical tests**. Although null hypotheses are accepted or rejected on the basis of sample data, the hypothesis is made about population values. The real interest in testing hypotheses, as in all statistical inference, is to use a sample to draw conclusions about a population.

TYPE I AND TYPE II ERRORS

Researchers decide whether to accept or reject the null hypothesis by determining how probable it is that observed group differences are due to chance. Because information about the population is not available, it cannot be asserted flatly that the null hypothesis is or is not true.

The researcher calculates a test statistic and decides that the null hypothesis is:	The actual situation is that the null hypothesis is: True	False
True (Null accepted)	Correct decision	Type II error
False (Null rejected)	Type I error	Correct decision

FIGURE 15.7 Outcomes of statistical decision making.

Researchers must be content to say that hypotheses are either *probably* true or *probably* false. Statistical inferences are based on incomplete information; hence, there is always a risk of making an error.

A researcher can make two types of error: (1) rejection of a true null hypothesis or (2) acceptance of a false null hypothesis. Figure 15-7 summarizes the possible outcomes of a researcher's decision. An investigator makes a **Type I error** by rejecting the null hypothesis when it is, in fact, true. For instance, if we concluded that the film was effective in promoting breastfeeding when, in fact, group differences were due to sampling error, we would have made a Type I error—a false positive conclusion. In the reverse situation, we might conclude that observed differences in breastfeeding were due to random sampling fluctuations when the film actually did have an effect. Acceptance of a false null hypothesis is called a **Type II error**—a false negative conclusion.

LEVEL OF SIGNIFICANCE

Researchers do not know when an error in statistical decision making has been committed. The validity of a null hypothesis could only be ascertained by collecting data from the population, in which case there would be no need for statistical inference. Researchers control the degree of risk in making a Type I error by selecting a **level of significance**. Level of significance is the term used to signify the probability of making a Type I error. The two most frequently used levels of significance (referred to as **alpha** or $\boldsymbol{\alpha}$) are .05 and .01. With a .05 significance level, we accept the risk that out of 100 samples, a true null hypothesis would be wrongly rejected five times. In 95 out of 100 cases, however, a true null hypothesis would be correctly accepted. With a .01 significance level, the risk of making a Type I error is lower: In only one sample out of 100 would we wrongly reject the null hypothesis. By convention, the minimal acceptable alpha level for scientific research is .05.

Naturally, researchers would like to reduce the risk of committing both types of error. Unfortunately, lowering the risk of a Type I error increases the risk of a Type II error. The stricter the criterion for rejecting a null hypothesis, the greater the probability of accepting a false null hypothesis. However, researchers can reduce the risk of a Type II error simply by increasing their sample size.

The probability of committing a Type II error, referred to as **beta** (β), can be estimated through *power analysis,* the same procedure we mentioned in Chapter 12 in connection with sample size. *Power* refers to the ability of a statistical test to detect true relationships, and is the complement of beta (that is, power $= 1 - \beta$). The standard criterion for an acceptable risk for a Type II error is .20, and thus researchers ideally use a sample size that gives them a minimum power of .80.

CONSUMER TIP

In many studies, the risk of a Type II error is high because of small sample size, suggesting a need for greater use of power analysis among nurse researchers. If a research report indicates that a research hypothesis was not supported by the data, consider whether a Type II error might have occurred as a result of inadequate sample size.

TESTS OF STATISTICAL SIGNIFICANCE

Researchers testing hypotheses use study data to compute a **test statistic**. For every test statistic, there is a theoretical sampling distribution, analogous to the sampling distribution of means. Hypothesis testing uses theoretical distributions to establish *probable* and *improbable* values for the test statistics, which are, in turn, used as a basis for accepting or rejecting the null hypothesis.

A simple (if contrived) example will illustrate the process. Suppose we wanted to test the hypothesis that the average entrance examination score for students applying to nursing schools in New York state is higher than that for applicants in all states, whose mean score is 500. The null hypothesis is that there is no difference in the mean population scores of students applying to nursing schools in New York versus elsewhere. Let us say that the mean score for a sample of 100 nursing school applicants in New York is 525, with a standard deviation of 100. Using statistical procedures, we can test the hypothesis that the mean of 525 is not merely a chance fluctuation from the population mean of 500.

In hypothesis testing, researchers assume that the null hypothesis is true and then gather evidence to disprove it. Assuming a mean of 500 for the entire nursing school applicant population, a sampling distribution can be constructed with a mean of 500 and a standard deviation equal to 10. In this example, 10 is the standard error of the mean, calculated from a formula that used the sample standard deviation of 100 for a sample of 100 students. This is shown in Figure 15-8. Based on normal distribution characteristics, we can determine probable and improbable values of sample means from the New York nursing school applicant population. If, as is assumed according to the null hypothesis, the population mean for New York applicants is 500, 95% of all sample means would fall between 480 and 520 because 95% of the cases are within 2 SDs of the mean. The obtained sample mean of 525 lies in the region considered *improbable* if the null hypothesis were correct, assuming that our criterion of improbability is an alpha level of .05. The improbable range beyond 2 SDs corresponds to only 5% (100% $-$ 95%) of the sampling distribution. We would thus reject the null hypothesis that the mean of the New York applicant population equals 500. We would not be justified in saying that we have proved the research hypothesis because the possibility of having made a Type I error remains.

Researchers reporting the results of hypothesis tests state whether their findings are **statistically significant**. The word *significant* should not be read as important or meaningful. In statistics, the term *significant* means that obtained results are not likely to have been due to chance, at

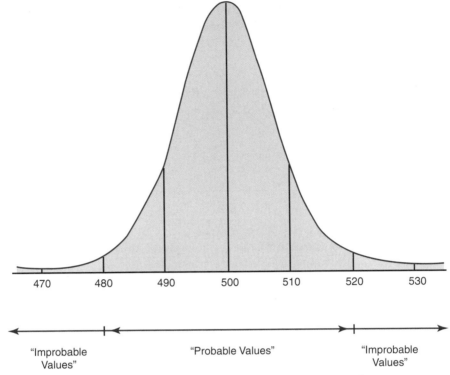

470   480   490   500   510   520   530

"Improbable   "Probable Values"   "Improbable
Values"   Values"

FIGURE 15.8 Sampling distribution for hypothesis test example of entrance
examination scores.

some specified level of probability. A **nonsignificant result** means that any observed difference or relationship could have been the result of a chance fluctuation.

CONSUMER TIP

Inferential statistics are usually more difficult to understand than descriptive statistics. It may help to keep in mind that inferential statistics are just a tool to help us evaluate whether the results are likely to be real and replicable, or simply spurious. As recommended in Chapter 4, you can overcome much of the obscurity of the results section by translating the basic thrust of research findings into everyday language.

■

PARAMETRIC AND NONPARAMETRIC TESTS

The bulk of the tests that we discuss in this chapter—and also most tests used by researchers—are **parametric tests**. Parametric tests have three attributes: (1) they focus on population parameters; (2) they require measurements on at least an interval scale; and (3) they involve other assumptions about the variables under consideration, such as the assumption that the variables are normally distributed in the population.

Nonparametric tests, by contrast, do not estimate parameters and involve less restrictive assumptions about the shape of the distribution of the critical variables. Nonparametric tests are usually applied when the data have been measured on a nominal or ordinal scale.

Parametric tests are more powerful than nonparametric tests and are generally preferred when variables are measured on at least the interval scale. Nonparametric tests are most useful when the data under consideration cannot be construed as interval measures or when the data distribution is markedly skewed.

OVERVIEW OF HYPOTHESIS TESTING PROCEDURES

In the next section, a few statistical procedures for testing research hypotheses are discussed. The emphasis is on explaining applications of statistical tests and on interpreting their meaning rather than on explaining computations.

Each statistical test has a particular application and can be used only with certain kinds of data; however, the overall process of testing hypotheses is basically the same for all tests. The steps that researchers take are the following:

1. *Selecting an appropriate test statistic.* Researchers select a test based on such factors as whether a parametric test is justified, which levels of measurement were used, and, if relevant, how many groups are being compared.
2. *Selecting the level of significance.* An α level of .05 is usually chosen, but sometimes the level is set more stringently at .01.
3. *Computing a test statistic.* Researchers then calculate a test statistic based on the collected data.
4. *Determining degrees of freedom.* The term **degrees of freedom** *(df)* is used throughout hypothesis testing to refer to the number of observations free to vary about a parameter. The concept is too complex for full elaboration here, but computing degrees of freedom is easy.
5. *Comparing the test statistic to a tabled value.* Theoretical distributions have been developed for all test statistics, and values for these distributions are available in tables for specified degrees of freedom and level of significance. The *tabled* value enables researchers to determine whether the *computed* value of the statistic is beyond what is probable if the null hypothesis is true. If the absolute value of the computed statistic is larger than the tabled value, the results are statistically significant; if the computed value is smaller, the results are nonsignificant.

When a computer is used for the analysis, researchers follow only the first step and then give the necessary commands to the computer. The computer calculates the test statistic, degrees of freedom, and the *actual* probability that the relationship being tested is due to chance. For example, the computer may print that the probability (p) of an experimental group doing better on a measure of postoperative recovery than the control group on the basis of chance alone is .025. This means that fewer than 3 times out of 100 (or only 25 times out of 1000) would a group difference of the size observed occur by chance. This computed probability can then be compared with the desired level of significance. In the present example, if the significance level were .05, the results would be significant because .025 is more stringent than .05. If .01 was the significance level, the results would be nonsignificant (sometimes abbreviated *NS*). Any computed probability level greater than .05 (e.g., .20) indicates a nonsignificant relationship (i.e., one that could have occurred on the basis of chance in more than 5 out of 100 samples).

BIVARIATE STATISTICAL TESTS

Researchers use a variety of statistical tests to make inferences about the validity of their hypotheses. The most frequently used bivariate tests are briefly described and illustrated below.

t-Tests

A common research situation is the comparison of two scores on a dependent variable for groups of people. The procedure used to test the statistical significance of a difference between the means of two groups is the parametric test called the ***t*-test**.

Suppose we wanted to test the effect of early discharge of maternity patients on their perceived maternal competence. We administer a scale of perceived maternal competence 1 week after delivery to 10 primiparas who were discharged early (i.e., within 24 hours of delivery) and to 10 others who remained in the hospital for longer periods. Some hypothetical data for this example are presented in Table 15-8. The mean scores for the two groups are 19.0 and 25.0, respectively. Is this difference a true population difference—is it likely to be replicated in other samples of early-discharge and later-discharge mothers? Or is the group difference just the result of chance fluctuations in this sample? The 20 scores—10 for each group—vary from one person to another. Some variability reflects individual differences in perceived maternal competence. Some variability might be due to measurement error (e.g., the scale's low reliability), some could result from participants' moods on a particular day, and so forth. The research question is: Can a significant portion of the variability be attributed to the independent variable—time of discharge from the hospital? The *t*-test allows us to answer this question objectively.

The formula for the *t* statistic uses group means, variability, and sample size to calculate a value for *t*. The computed value of *t* for the data in Table 15-8 is 2.86. Next, degrees of freedom are calculated. Here, the degrees of freedom are equal to the total sample size minus 2 ($df = 20 - 2 = 18$). Then, the tabled value for *t* with 18 degrees of freedom is ascertained. For an α level of .05, the tabled value of *t* is 2.10. *This value establishes an upper limit to what is probable if the null hypothesis is true.* Thus, the calculated *t* of 2.86, which is larger than the tabled value of the statistic, is improbable (i.e., statistically significant). We are now in a position to say that the primiparas discharged early had significantly lower perceptions of maternal competence than those who were not discharged early. The group difference in perceived maternal competence is sufficiently large that it is unlikely to reflect merely chance fluctuations. In fewer than 5 out of 100 samples would a difference in means this great be found by chance alone.

The situation we just described calls for an *independent groups t-test*: Mothers in the two groups were different people, independent of each other. There are situations for which this type of *t*-test is not appropriate. For example, if means for a single group of people measured

Example of a *t*-test

Tsay and Hung (2004) tested the effectiveness of an empowerment program on the empowerment level and depression of Taiwanese patients with end-stage renal disease, using an experimental design. The results indicated that patients in the experimental group had significantly higher empowerment scores ($t = 6.54$, $df = 48$, $p < .001$) and significantly lower depression scores ($t = 2.49$, $df = 48$, $p < .05$) than those in the control group.

TABLE 15.8	Fictitious Data for *t*-Test Example: Scores on a Perceived Maternal Competence Scale for Two Groups of Mothers

REGULAR-DISCHARGE MOTHERS	EARLY-DISCHARGE MOTHERS
23	30
17	27
22	25
18	20
20	24
26	32
16	17
13	18
21	28
14	29
Mean = 19.0	Mean = 25.0
$t = 2.86$; $df = 18$; $p < .05$	

before and after an intervention were being compared, researchers would compute a *paired t-test* (also called a *dependent groups t-test*), using a different formula.

Analysis of Variance

Analysis of variance (ANOVA) is a parametric procedure used to test mean group differences of three or more groups. The statistic computed in an ANOVA is the **F ratio**. ANOVA decomposes the variability of a dependent variable into two components: variability attributable to the independent variable (i.e., group status) and variability due to all other sources (e.g., individual differences, measurement error). Variation *between* groups is contrasted with variation *within* groups to yield an *F* ratio.

Suppose we wanted to compare the effectiveness of different instructional techniques to teach high school students about AIDS. One group of students is exposed to an interactive Internet course on AIDS, a second group is given three special lectures, and a third control group receives no special instruction. The dependent variable is the student's score on an AIDS knowledge test after the intervention. The null hypothesis is that the group population means for AIDS knowledge test scores are the same, whereas the research hypothesis predicts that they are different.

Test scores for 60 students are shown in Table 15-9, according to treatment group. As this table shows, there is variation from one student to the next within a group, and there are also group differences. The mean test scores are 25.35, 24.75, and 20.35 for groups A, B, and C, respectively. These means are different, but are they significantly different—or do the differences reflect random fluctuations?

An ANOVA applied to these data yields an *F* ratio of 18.64. Two types of degrees of freedom are calculated in ANOVA: between groups (number of groups minus 1) and within groups (total number of subjects minus the number of groups). In this example, $df = 2$ and 57. In a table of values for a theoretical *F* distribution, we would find that the value of *F* for 2 and 57 *df*, with an alpha of .05, is 3.16. Because our obtained *F* value of 18.64 exceeds 3.16, we reject the null hypothesis that the population means are equal. The observed group differences in mean test scores would

TABLE 15.9	Fictitious Data for One-Way ANOVA: Effects of Instructional Mode on AIDS Knowledge Test Scores

INTERNET GROUP (A)		LECTURE GROUP (B)		CONTROL GROUP (C)	
26	25	22	24	15	22
20	29	24	25	26	19
16	30	27	21	24	20
25	27	23	27	18	22
25	29	23	25	20	18
23	28	26	21	20	24
26	26	22	24	19	18
25	25	24	29	21	23
24	27	24	28	17	20
23	28	30	26	17	24
Mean 25.35		24.75		20.35	

$$F = 18.64; df = 2.57; p < .001$$

be obtained by chance in fewer than 5 samples out of 100. (Actually, the probability of achieving an F of 18.64 by chance is less than 1 in 1000.)

The data in our example support the hypothesis that the instructional interventions affected students' knowledge about AIDS, but we cannot tell from these results whether treatment A was significantly more effective than treatment B. Statistical analyses known as **multiple comparison procedures** (also called *post hoc* **tests**) are needed. The function of these procedures is to isolate the differences between group means that are responsible for rejecting the overall ANOVA null hypothesis. Note that it is *not* appropriate to use a series of t-tests (group A versus B, A versus C, and B versus C) in this situation because this would increase the risk of a Type I error.

ANOVA also can be used to test the effect of two (or more) independent variables on a dependent variable (e.g., when a factorial experimental design has been used). Suppose we wanted to determine whether the two instructional techniques discussed previously (Internet versus lecture) were equally effective in helping male and female students acquire knowledge about AIDS. We could set up a design in which males and females would be randomly assigned, separately, to the two modes of instruction. Some hypothetical data, shown in Table 15-10, reveal the following about two *main effects*: On average, people in the Internet group scored higher than those in the lecture group (25.35 versus 24.75), and female students scored higher than male students (26.20 versus 23.90). In addition, there is an *interaction effect:* Females scored higher when exposed to the Internet course, whereas males scored higher when exposed to the lecture. By performing a *two-way ANOVA* on these data, it would be possible to ascertain the statistical significance of these differences.

A type of ANOVA known as **repeated measures ANOVA** is often used when the means being compared are means at different points in time (e.g., mean blood pressure at 2, 4, and 6 hours after surgery). This is analogous to a paired t-test, extended to three or more points of data collection, because it is the same people being measured multiple times. When two or more groups are measured several times, a repeated measures ANOVA provides information about a main effect for time (do the measures change significantly over time, irrespective of group?); a main effect for groups (do the group means differ significantly, irrespective of time?); and an interaction effect (do the groups differ more at certain times?).

Example of ANOVA

Holditch-Davis, Cox, Miles, and Belyea (2003) observed three groups of infants interacting with their mothers for 1 hour: (1) medically fragile full-term infants, (2) medically fragile premature infants, and (3) premature infants without chronic illness. The researchers used ANOVA to compare the three groups in terms of maternal activities and behaviors and infant states and behaviors. The groups were similar on many outcomes, but significant differences emerged for others, such as infant sleeping time. The mean time spent sleeping was 15.1, 9.4, and 1.7 minutes for the three groups, respectively ($F = 4.33$, $df = 2, 86$, $p = .02$). A multiple comparison test indicated that the group difference accounting for this significant F value was for the nonchronically ill premature versus the medically fragile full-term infants.

CONSUMER TIP

Experimental crossover or repeated measures designs (see Chapter 9) call for either a dependent groups t-test or a repeated measures ANOVA because the same people are measured more than once after being randomly assigned to a different ordering of treatments. Repeated measures ANOVA can also be used in studies that do not involve an experimental crossover design (e.g., in one-group pre-experimental designs) if outcomes are measured more than once and the hypothesis concerns changes over time.

TABLE 15.10	Fictitious Data for Two-Way (2 x 2) ANOVA Example: Instructional Mode and Gender in Relation to Test Scores				
	INSTRUCTIONAL MODE				
YEAR IN SCHOOL	**Internet**		**Lecture**		
Male	26 20 16 25 25 23 26 25 24 23	$\bar{X} = 23.3$	22 24 27 33 23 26 22 24 24 30	$\bar{X} = 24.5$	Male mean = 23.90
Female	25 29 30 27 29 28 26 25 27 28	$\bar{X} = 27.4$	24 25 21 27 27 25 21 24 28 26	$\bar{X} = 25.0$	Female mean = 26.20
Internet group mean	25.35	Lecture group mean	24.75		Grand mean = 25.05

TABLE 15.11	Observed Frequencies for a Chi-Squared Example on Patient Compliance		
	EXPERIMENTAL	**CONTROL**	**TOTAL**
Compliant	60	30	90
Noncompliant	40	70	110
TOTAL	100	100	200

$\chi^2 = 18.18$; $df = 1$; $p < .001$.

Chi-Squared Test

The **chi-squared** (χ^2) **test** is a nonparametric procedure used to test hypotheses about the proportion of cases that fall into various categories, as in a contingency table. Suppose we were interested in studying the effect of planned nursing instruction on patients' compliance with a medication regimen. The experimental group is instructed by nurses who are implementing a new instructional approach based on Orem's Self-Care Model. Control group patients are cared for by nurses using their usual mode of instruction. The research hypothesis is that a higher proportion of people in the experimental than in the control group will comply with the regimen. Some hypothetical data for this example are presented in Table 15-11.

The chi-squared statistic is computed by summing differences between the *observed frequencies* in each cell and the *expected frequencies*—the frequencies that would be expected if there were no relationship between the two variables. In this example, the value of the χ^2 statistic is 18.18, which we can compare with the value from a theoretical chi-squared distribution. For the chi-squared statistic, the degrees of freedom are equal to the number of rows minus 1 times the number of columns minus 1. In the present case, $df = 1 \times 1$, or 1. With 1 df, the value that must be exceeded to establish significance at the .05 level is 3.84. The obtained value of 18.18 is substantially larger than would be expected by chance. Thus, we can conclude that a significantly larger percentage of patients in the experimental group (60%) than in the control group (30%) were compliant.

Example of a chi-squared test

Buist, Morse, and Durkin (2003) conducted a longitudinal study of first-time fathers in Melbourne, Australia, and examined factors related to their level of distress from mid-pregnancy to 4 months postpartum. Men were classified as distressed or nondistressed based on their scores on a depression scale. One of the findings was that men who had been in their relationship for less than 2 years were significantly more likely to be distressed postpartum than men who were in longer-term relationships ($\chi^2 = 4.0$, $df = 1$, $p < .05$).

Correlation Coefficients

Pearson's r is both descriptive and inferential. As a descriptive statistic, r summarizes the magnitude and direction of a relationship between two variables. As an inferential statistic, r tests hypotheses about population correlations; the null hypothesis is that there is no relationship between two variables.

Suppose we were studying the relationship between patients' self-reported level of stress (higher scores imply more stress) and the pH level of their saliva. With a sample of 50 patients, we find that $r = -.29$. This value indicates a tendency for people with high stress scores to have lower pH levels than those with low stress scores. But we need to ask whether this finding can be generalized to the population. Does the coefficient of $-.29$ reflect a random fluctuation, observed only in this particular sample, or is the relationship significant? Degrees of freedom for correlation coefficients are equal to the number of participants minus 2, which is 48 in this example. The tabled value for r with $df = 48$ and $\alpha = .05$ is .282. Because the absolute value of the calculated r is .29 and thus larger than .282, the null hypothesis can be rejected. There is a modest but significant relationship between patients' self-reported level of stress and the acidity of their saliva.

Example of correlation coefficients

Suen, Morris, and McDougall (2004) studied correlates of memory function among older Taiwanese Americans. The correlations between memory function and three independent variables (sleep quality, physical activity, and depression) were modest and nonsignificant ($r = -.18, .11,$ and $-.13$, respectively). However, the older the age, the lower the memory function score was ($r = -.54, p < .001$). Memory function scores were positively and significantly correlated with years of education ($r = .46, p < .001$).

Guide to Bivariate Statistical Tests

The selection of a statistical test depends on several factors, such as the number of groups and the levels of measurement of the research variables. To aid you in evaluating the appropriateness of statistical tests used in studies, a chart summarizing the major features of several tests is presented in Table 15-12. This table does not include every test you may encounter in research reports, but it does include the bivariate statistical tests most often used by nurse researchers, including a few not discussed in this book.

CONSUMER TIP

Every time a report presents information about statistical tests such as those described in this section, it means that the researcher was testing hypotheses—whether those hypotheses were formally stated in the introduction or not.

■

MULTIVARIATE STATISTICAL ANALYSIS

Nurse researchers have become increasingly sophisticated, and many now use complex **multivariate statistics** to analyze their data. We use the term *multivariate* to refer to analyses dealing with at least three—but usually more—variables simultaneously. This evolution has resulted in

TABLE 15.12	Guide to Widely Used Bivariate Statistical Tests				
				MEASUREMENT LEVEL*	
NAME	TEST STATISTIC	PURPOSE		IV	DV
PARAMETRIC TESTS					
t-test for independent groups	t	To test the difference between two independent group means		Nominal	Interval, ratio
t-test for dependent group	t	To test the difference between two dependent group means		Nominal	Interval, ratio
Analysis of variance (ANOVA)	F	To test the difference among the means of three or more independent groups, or of more than one independent variable		Nominal	Interval, ratio
Repeated measures ANOVA	F	To test the difference among means of three or more related groups or sets of scores		Nominal	Interval, ratio
Pearson's r	r	To test the existence of a relationship between two variables		Interval, ratio	Interval, ratio
NONPARAMETRIC TESTS					
Chi-squared test	χ^2	To test the difference in proportions in two or more independent groups		Nominal	Nominal
Mann-Whitney U-test	U	To test the difference in ranks of scores of two independent groups		Nominal	Ordinal
Kruskal-Wallis test	H	To test the difference in ranks of scores of three or more independent groups		Nominal	Ordinal
Wilcoxon signed ranks test	$T(Z)$	To test the difference in ranks of scores of two related groups		Nominal	Ordinal
Friedman test	χ^2	To test the difference in ranks of scores of three or more related groups		Nominal	Ordinal
Phi coefficient	ϕ	To test the magnitude of a relationship between two dichotomous variables		Nominal	Nominal
Spearman's rank-order correlation	r_s	To test the existence of a relationship between two variables		Ordinal	Ordinal

*Measurement level of the independent variable (IV) and dependent variable (DV).

increased rigor and better-quality evidence in nursing studies, but one unfortunate side effect is that it has become more challenging for novice consumers to understand research reports.

Given the introductory nature of this text and the fact that many of you are not proficient with even simple statistical tests, it is not possible to describe in detail the complex analytic procedures that now appear in nursing journals. However, we present some basic information that might assist you in reading reports in which two commonly used multivariate statistics are used: multiple regression and analysis of covariance (ANCOVA).

Multiple Regression

Correlations enable researchers to make predictions. For example, if the correlation between secondary school grades and nursing school grades were .60, nursing school administrators could make predictions—albeit imperfect predictions—about applicants' future academic performance. Because two variables are rarely perfectly correlated, researchers often strive to improve their ability to predict a dependent variable by including more than one independent variable in the analysis.

As an example, we might predict that infant birth weight is related to the amount of maternal prenatal care. We could collect data on birth weight and number of prenatal visits and then compute a correlation coefficient to determine whether a significant relationship between the two variables exists (i.e., whether prenatal care would help predict infant birth weight). Birth weight is affected by many other factors, however, such as gestational period and mothers' smoking behavior. Many researchers, therefore, perform an analysis called **multiple regression analysis** (or *multiple correlation analysis*) that allows them to use more than one independent variable to explain or predict a dependent variable. In multiple regression, the dependent variables are interval- or ratio-level variables. Independent variables (also called **predictor variables** in multiple regression) are either interval- or ratio-level variables or dichotomous nominal-level variables, such as male/female.

When several independent variables are used to predict a dependent variable, the resulting statistic is the **multiple correlation coefficient**, symbolized as R. Unlike the bivariate correlation coefficient r, R does not have negative values. R varies from .00 to 1.00, showing the *strength* of the relationship between several independent variables and a dependent variable, but not *direction*.

There are several ways of evaluating R. One is to determine whether R is statistically significant—that is, whether the overall relationship between the independent variables and the dependent variable is likely to be real or the result of chance sampling fluctuations. This is done through the computation of an F statistic that can be compared with tabled F values.

A second way of evaluating R is to determine whether the addition of new independent variables adds further predictive power. For example, we might find that the R between infant birth weight on the one hand and maternal weight and prenatal care on the other is .30. By adding a third independent variable—let's say maternal smoking behavior—R might increase to .36. Is the increase from .30 to .36 statistically significant? In other words, does knowing whether the mother smoked during her pregnancy improve our understanding of the birth weight outcome, or does the larger R value simply reflect factors peculiar to this sample? Multiple regression provides a way of answering this question.

The magnitude of the R statistic is also informative. Researchers would like to predict a dependent variable perfectly. In the birth weight example, if it were possible to identify all the factors that lead to differences in infants' weight, we could collect the relevant data to obtain an R of 1.00. Usually, the value of R in nursing studies is much smaller—seldom higher than .70. An interesting feature of the R statistic is that, when squared, it can be interpreted as the proportion of the variability in the dependent variable accounted for or explained by the independent variables. In predicting infant birth weight, if we achieved an R of .60 ($R^2 = .36$), we could say that the independent variables accounted for just over one third (36%) of the variability in infants' birth weights. Two thirds of the variability, however, was caused by factors not identified or measured. Researchers usually report multiple correlation results in terms of R^2 rather than R.

Example of multiple regression

Anderson, Issel, and McDaniel (2003) examined the relationship between various nursing home characteristics and management practices on the one hand and nursing home residents' outcomes on the other. Using multiple regression, they found, for example, that communication openness and the nursing director's years of experience as director were significant predictors of restraint use. Overall, the R^2 between predictor variables and restraint use was .16, $p < .001$.

We will use this study by Anderson and her colleagues, with some findings summarized in Table 15-13, to illustrate some additional features of multiple regression analysis. First, multiple regressions yield information about whether each independent variable is related significantly to the dependent variable. In Table 15-13, the first column shows that the analysis used eight independent variables to predict the average prevalence of restraint use in 152 nursing homes. The next column shows the values for b, which are the *regression coefficients* associated with each predictor.

TABLE 15.13	Example of Multiple Regression Analysis: Average Prevalence of Restraint Use for Nursing Home Residents, Regressed on Nursing Home Characteristics, Manager Characteristics, and Management Practices				
PREDICTOR VARIABLE	**b**	**SE**	**BETA (β)**	**p**	
Number of beds	−2.10	.61	−.29	<.001	
Ownership type (profit vs. non-profit)	1.29	.72	.14	NS	
Director of nursing tenure in current position	−.41	.18	−.19	<.05	
Years of experience as director of nursing	−.48	.22	−.18	<.05	
Communication openness	−1.59	.61	−.23	<.05	
RN participation in decision-making	−.06	.24	−.02	NS	
Relationship-oriented leadership	−.32	.53	−.05	NS	
Formalization of rules and procedures	.21	.62	.03	NS	

N = 152 nursing homes

$F = 4.70$ $df = 8,143$ $p < .001$ $R^2 = .21$ Adjusted $R^2 = .16$

Adapted from Anderson, R. A., Issel, L. M., & McDaniel, R. R. (2003). Nursing homes as complex adaptive systems: Relationship between management practice and resident outcomes (Table 3). *Nursing Research, 52,* 12–21.

These coefficients, which were computed from the raw study data, could be used to actually predict restraint use in other nursing homes—but they are not values you need to be concerned with in interpreting a regression table. The next column shows the standard error (SE) of the regression coefficients. When the regression coefficient (b) is divided by the standard error, the result is a value for the t statistic, which can be used to determine the significance of individual predictors. In this table, the t values are not shown, but many regression tables in reports *do* present them. We can compute them, though, from information in the table; for example, the value of t for the predictor *number of beds* would be -3.44 ($-2.10 \div .61 = -3.44$). This is highly significant, as shown in the last column: The probability (p) is less than 1 in 1000 that the relationship between number of beds in a nursing home and the use of restraints is spurious. The table indicates that as the number of beds in a nursing home increases, the use of restraints *decreases*, as indicated by the negative regression coefficient. Three other predictor variables were significantly related to restraint use: the more experienced the director of nursing, the longer his or her tenure in the position, and the greater the communication openness in the nursing home, the lower the use of restraints. Other predictors in the analysis (e.g., whether the nursing home was for-profit or not-for-profit) was not related significantly to restraint use (shown as *NS*) once other factors were taken into consideration.

You should recognize that multiple regression analysis indicates whether an independent variable is significantly related to the dependent variable *even after* the other predictor variables are controlled—a concept we explain more fully in the next section. In this example, number of beds in a nursing home was a significant predictor of restraint use, even with the other seven variables controlled. Thus, multiple regression, like analysis of covariance (discussed next), is a means of controlling extraneous variables statistically.

The fourth column of Table 15-13 shows the value of the *beta* (β) *coefficients* for each predictor. Although it is beyond the scope of this textbook to explain beta coefficients, suffice it to say that, unlike the b regression coefficients, betas are all in the same measurement units and their absolute values are sometimes used to compare the relative importance of predictors. In this particular sample, and with these particular predictors, the variable *number of beds* was the best predictor of restraint use ($\beta = -.29$), and the variable *communication openness* was the second best predictor ($\beta = -.23$).

At the bottom of the table, we see that the value of F for the overall regression equation, with eight and 143 df, was highly significant, $p < .001$. The value of R^2 is .21, but after adjustments are made for sample size and number of predictors, the value is reduced to .16. Thus, 16% of the variance in restraint use is explained by the combined effect of the eight predictors. The remaining 84% of variation is explained by other factors, including characteristics of the residents themselves.

Analysis of Covariance

Analysis of covariance (ANCOVA), which is essentially a combination of ANOVA and multiple regression, is used to control extraneous variables statistically. This approach can be especially valuable in certain research situations, such as when a nonequivalent control group design is used. The initial equivalence of the experimental and comparison groups in these studies is always questionable and so researchers must consider whether the results reflect preexisting group differences. When control through randomization is lacking, ANCOVA offers the possibility of *post hoc* statistical control.

Because the concept of statistical control may mystify you, we will explain the underlying principle with a simple illustration. Suppose we were interested in testing the effectiveness of a special training program on physical fitness, using employees of two companies as subjects. Employees of one company receive the physical fitness intervention, and those of the second company do not. The employees' score on a physical fitness test is the dependent variable. The research question is: Can some of the group difference in performance on the physical fitness test be attributed to participation in the special program? Physical fitness is also related to other, extraneous characteristics of the study participants (e.g., their age)—characteristics that might differ between the two intact groups.

Figure 15-9 illustrates how ANCOVA works. The large circles represent total variability (i.e., the total extent of individual differences) in physical fitness scores for both groups. A certain amount of variability can be explained by age differences: Younger people tend to perform better on the test than older people. This relationship is represented by the overlapping small circle on the left in part A of Figure 15-9. Another part of the variability can be explained by participation in the physical fitness program, represented here by the overlapping small circle on the right. In part A, the fact that the two small circles (age and program participation) themselves overlap indicates that there is a relationship between these two variables. In other words, people in the experimental group are, on average, either older or younger than those in the comparison group. Because of this relationship, which could distort the results of the study, age should be controlled.

ANCOVA can do this by statistically removing the effect of the extraneous variable (age) on physical fitness. This is designated in part A of Figure 15-9 by the darkened area of the large circle. Part B illustrates that the analysis would examine the effect of program participation on fitness scores *after* removing the effect of age (called a **covariate**). With the variability

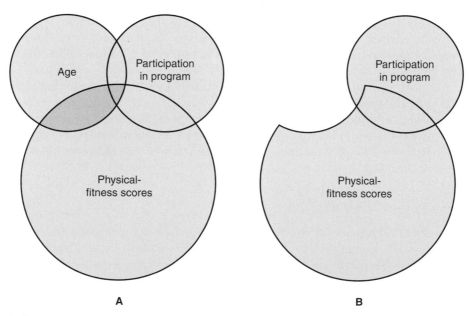

A   B

FIGURE 15.9 Schematic diagram illustrating the principle of analysis of covariance.

associated with age removed, we get a more precise estimate of the training program's effect on physical fitness. Note that even after removing variability resulting from age, there is still individual variability not associated with program participation (the bottom half of the large circle) that is not explained. This means that analytic precision could be further enhanced by controlling additional extraneous variables (for example, nutritional habits, smoking status). ANCOVA can accommodate multiple extraneous variables.

Analysis of covariance tests the significance of differences between group means after adjusting scores on the dependent variable to eliminate the effect of the covariates. This adjustment uses regression procedures. The ANCOVA procedure produces *F* statistics—one for evaluating the significance of the covariates and another for evaluating the significance of group differences—that can be compared with tabled values of *F* to determine whether to accept or reject the null hypothesis.

ANCOVA, like multiple regression analysis, is an extremely powerful and useful analytic technique for controlling extraneous or confounding influences on dependent measures. ANCOVA can be used in conjunction with true experimental designs, because randomization can never guarantee that groups are totally equivalent. In such situations, baseline measures of the dependent variables make particularly good covariates.

Example of ANCOVA

Schaeffer and Tian (2004) tested the effectiveness of a theory-based asthma education intervention. They used ANCOVA to test for differences between the experimental and control group on pharmacy-verified adherence 6 months after the intervention, controlling for baseline adherence.

Other Multivariate Techniques

Other multivariate techniques increasingly are being used in nursing studies. We mention a few techniques briefly to acquaint you with terms you might encounter in the research literature.

DISCRIMINANT FUNCTION ANALYSIS
In multiple regression analysis, the dependent variable being predicted is a measure on either the interval or ratio scale. **Discriminant function analysis** is used to make predictions about membership in groups—that is, about a dependent variable measured on the nominal scale. For example, a researcher might wish to use multiple independent variables to predict membership in such groups as: compliant versus noncompliant cancer patients; obese versus non-obese people; or patients with or without decubiti. In discriminant function analysis, as in multiple regression, the predictor variables and any covariates are either interval- or ratio-level measures or dichotomous nominal variables (e.g., smoker versus nonsmoker).

LOGISTIC REGRESSION
Logistic regression (or *logit analysis*) analyzes the relationships between multiple independent variables and a nominal-level dependent variable. It is thus used in situations similar to discriminant function analysis, but it employs a different statistical estimation procedure that many prefer for nominal-level dependent variables. Logistic regression transforms the probability of an event

occurring (e.g., that a woman will practice breast self-examination or not) into its *odds* (i.e., into the ratio of one event's probability relative to the probability of a second event). After further transformations, the analysis examines the relationship of the independent variables to the transformed dependent variable. For each predictor, the logistic regression yields an **odds ratio** (OR), which is the factor by which the odds change for a unit change in the predictors.

Example of logistic regression

Tang (2003) conducted a study to identify some of the determinants of using hospice services among terminally ill cancer patients in the United States. Tang used data from a sample of 127 cancer patients who died, about half of whom had used hospice home care. The logistic regression analysis revealed that being female and having home as a preferred place of death were significant predictors. For example, the odds of using hospice care was more than five times higher among patients who preferred to die at home than among other patients (OR = 5.58, $p < .05$).

FACTOR ANALYSIS

Factor analysis is widely used by researchers seeking to develop, refine, or validate complex instruments. The major purpose of factor analysis is to reduce a large set of variables into a smaller, more manageable set. Factor analysis disentangles complex interrelationships among variables and identifies which variables go together as unified concepts or factors. For example, suppose we developed 50 Likert statements to measure men's attitudes toward a vasectomy. It would not be appropriate to combine all 50 items to form a scale score because there are various dimensions, or themes, to men's attitudes toward vasectomy. One dimension may relate to the issue of masculinity and virility, another may concern the loss of ability to reproduce, and so on. These various dimensions should serve as the basis for scale construction, and factor analysis offers an objective, empirical method for doing so.

Example of factor analysis

Bray, Nash, and Froman (2003) developed a scale designed to measure young adolescents' perceptions of self-efficacy for physical and emotional health. They administered 28 items to a sample of 354 students, whose responses were factor analyzed. The analysis revealed three underlying factors: interpersonal concerns, preventive health, and potential for substance abuse.

MULTIVARIATE ANALYSIS OF VARIANCE

Multivariance analysis of variance (MANOVA) is the extension of ANOVA to more than one dependent variable. This procedure is used to test the significance of differences between the means of two or more groups on two or more dependent variables, considered simultaneously. For instance, if we wanted to compare the effect of two alternative methods of exercise treatment on both blood pressure and heart rate, then a MANOVA would be appropriate. Covariates can also be included, in which case the analysis would be called a **multivariate analysis of covariance (MANCOVA)**.

CAUSAL MODELING

Causal modeling involves the development and statistical testing of a hypothesized explanation of the causes of a phenomenon, usually with nonexperimental data. **Path analysis**, which is based on multiple regression, is a widely used approach to causal modeling. Alternative methods of testing causal models are also being used by nurse researchers, the most important of which is **linear structural relations analysis**, more widely known as **LISREL**. Both LISREL and path analysis are highly complex statistical techniques whose utility relies on a sound underlying causal theory.

Guide to Multivariate Statistical Analyses

In selecting a multivariate analysis, researchers must attend to such issues as the number of independent variables, the number of dependent variables, the measurement level of all variables, and the desirability of controlling extraneous variables. Table 15-14 is an aid to help you evaluate the appropriateness of multivariate statistics used in research reports. This chart includes the major multivariate analyses used by nurse researchers.

READING AND UNDERSTANDING STATISTICAL INFORMATION

Statistical findings are communicated in the results section of research reports and are reported in the text as well as in tables (or, less frequently, figures). This section provides some assistance in reading and interpreting statistical information.

Tips on Reading Text With Statistical Information

There are usually three types of statistical information reported in the results section of a research report. First, there are descriptive statistics (such as those shown in Table 15-4), which typically provide readers with a basic overview of participants' characteristics. Information about the subjects' background characteristics enables readers to draw conclusions about the groups to which the findings might be generalized. Second, some researchers provide statistical information for evaluating the extent of any biases. For example, researchers sometimes compare the characteristics of people who did and did not agree to participate in the study (e.g., using t-tests). Or, in a quasi-experimental design, evidence of the preintervention comparability of the experimental and comparison groups might be presented so that readers can evaluate the study's internal validity. Finally, inferential statistics relating to the research questions or hypotheses are presented. Supplementary analyses are sometimes presented to help unravel the meaning of the results.

The text of research reports normally provides certain information about the statistical tests, including (1) which test was used, (2) the actual value of the calculated statistic, (3) the degrees of freedom, and (4) the level of statistical significance. Examples of how the results of various statistical tests would likely be reported in the text are shown below.

1. t-test: $t = 1.68$; $df = 160$; $p = .09$
2. Chi-squared: $\chi^2 = 16.65$; $df = 2$; $p < .001$
3. Pearson's r: $r = .36$; $df = 100$; $p < .01$
4. ANOVA: $F = 0.18$; $df = 1, 69$, NS

TABLE 15.14 Guide to Widely Used Multivariate Statistical Analyses

NAME	PURPOSE	MEASUREMENT LEVEL* IV	DV	COV	NUMBER OF: IVs	DVs	COVs
Multiple correlation, regression	To test the relationship between two or more IVs and one DV; to predict a DV from two or more IVs	N, I, R	I, R		2+	1	
Analysis of covariance (ANCOVA)	To test the difference between the means of two or more groups, while controlling for one or more covariate	N	I, R	N, I, R	1+	1	1+
Multivariate analysis of variance (MANOVA)	To test the difference between the means of two or more groups for two or more DVs simultaneously	N	I, R		1+	2+	
Multivariate analysis of covariance (MANCOVA)	To test the difference between the means of two or more groups for two or more DVs simultaneously, while controlling for one or more covariate	N	I, R	N, I, R	1+	2+	1+
Factor analysis	To determine the dimensionality or structure of a set of variables						
Discriminant analysis	To test the relationship between two or more IVs and one DV; to predict group membership; to classify cases into groups	N, I, R	N		2+	1	
Logistic regression	To test the relationship between two or more IVs and one DV; to predict the probability of an event, to estimate relative risk (odds ratios)	N, I, R	N		2+	1	

*Measurement level of the independent variable (IV), dependent variable (DV), and covariates (COV): N = nominal, I = interval, R = ratio.

Note that the significance level is sometimes reported as the *actual* computed probability that the null hypothesis is correct, as in example 1. In this case, the observed group differences could be found by chance in 9 out of 100 samples; thus, this result is not statistically significant because the differences have an unacceptably high chance of being spurious. The probability level is sometimes reported simply as falling below or above the researchers' significance criterion, as in examples 2 and 3. In both cases, the results are statistically significant because the probability of obtaining such results by chance alone is less than 1 in 100. Note that you need to be careful to read the symbol that follows the *p* **value** (the probability value) correctly: The symbol $<$ means less than—that is, the results are statistically significant; the symbol $>$ means greater than—that is, the results are not statistically significant. When results do not achieve statistical significance at the desired level, researchers simply may indicate that the results were not significant (NS), as in example 4.

Statistical information usually is noted parenthetically in a sentence describing the findings, as in the following example: The patients in the experimental group had a significantly lower rate of infection than those in the control group ($\chi^2 = 7.99$, $df = 1$, $p < .01$). In reading research reports, it is not important to absorb numeric information for the actual test statistic. For example, the actual value of χ^2 has no inherent interest. What is important is to grasp whether the statistical tests indicate that the research hypotheses were accepted as probably true (as demonstrated by significant results) or rejected as probably false (as demonstrated by nonsignificant results).

Tips on Reading Statistical Tables

The use of tables allows researchers to condense a considerable amount of statistical information into a compact space and also prevents redundancy. Consider, for example, putting information from a correlation matrix (see Table 15-7) into the text: "The correlation between perceived health and hope was .56; the correlation between perceived health and spirituality was .31...."

Unfortunately, although tables are efficient, they may be daunting and difficult to decipher. Part of the problem is the lack of standardization in table preparation. There is no universally accepted method of presenting *t*-test information, for example, and so each table may present a new challenge. Another problem is that some researchers try to include an enormous amount of information in their tables; we deliberately used tables of relative simplicity and clarity as examples in this chapter.

We know of no magic solution for helping you to comprehend tables in research reports, but we have a few suggestions. First, read the text and the tables simultaneously because the text may help to unravel what the table is trying to communicate. Second, before trying to understand the numbers in a table, try to glean as much information as possible from the accompanying words. Table titles and footnotes often communicate critical pieces of information. The table headings should be carefully reviewed because these indicate what the variables in the analyses are (often listed in the far left-hand column of the table as row labels) and what statistical information is included (often specified in the top row as the column headings). Third, you may find it helpful to consult the glossary of symbols in Box 15-1 to determine the meaning of a statistical symbol included in a report table. Note that not all symbols in Box 15-1 were described in this chapter; therefore, it may be necessary to refer to a statistics textbook, such as that of Polit (1996), for further information. We recommend that you devote some extra time to making sure you have grasped what the tables are conveying and that, for each table, you write out a sentence or two that summarizes some of the tabular information in "plain English."

BOX 15.1　GLOSSARY OF SELECTED STATISTICAL SYMBOLS

This list contains some commonly used symbols in statistics. The list is in approximate alphabetical order, with English and Greek letters intermixed. Nonletter symbols have been placed at the end.

a	Regression constant, the intercept
α	Greek alpha; significance level in hypothesis testing, probability of Type I error
b	Regression coefficient, slope of the line
β	Greek beta, probability of a Type II error; also, a standardized regression coefficient (beta weights)
χ^2	Greek chi squared, a test statistic for several nonparametric tests
CI	Confidence interval around estimate of a population parameter
df	Degrees of freedom
η^2	Greek eta squared, index of variance accounted for in ANOVA context
f	Frequency (count) for a score value
F	Test statistic used in ANOVA, ANCOVA, and other tests
H_0	Null hypothesis
H_1	Alternative hypothesis; research hypothesis
λ	Greek lambda, a test statistic used in several multivariate analyses (Wilks' lambda)
μ	Greek mu, the population mean
M	Sample mean (alternative symbol for $\bar{X}$)
MS	Mean square, variance estimate in ANOVA
n	Number of cases in a subgroup of the sample
N	Total number of cases or sample members
p	Probability that observed data are consistent with null hypothesis
r	Pearson's product–moment correlation coefficient for a sample
r_s	Spearman's rank-order correlation coefficient
R	Multiple correlation coefficient
R^2	Coefficient of determination, proportion of variance in *dependent variable* attributable to *independent variables*
R_c	Canonical correlation coefficient
ρ	Greek rho, population correlation coefficient
SD	Sample standard deviation
SEM	Standard error of the mean
σ	Greek sigma (lowercase), population standard deviation
Σ	Greek sigma (uppercase), sum of
SS	Sum of squares
t	Test statistics used in t-tests (sometimes called Student's t)
U	Test statistic for the Mann-Whitney U-test
$\bar{X}$	Sample mean
x	Deviation score
Y'	Predicted value of Y, dependent variable in regression analysis
z	Standard score in a normal distribution
$\|\ \|$	Absolute value
$\leq$	Less than or equal to
$\geq$	Greater than or equal to
$\neq$	Not equal to

CONSUMER TIP

In tables, probability levels associated with the significance tests are sometimes presented directly (e.g., $p < .05$), as in Table 15-13. Here, the significance of each test is indicated in the last column, headed "p". However, researchers often indicate significance levels in tables through asterisks placed next to the value of the test statistic. By convention, one asterisk usually signifies $p < .05$, two asterisks signify $p < .01$, and three asterisks signify $p < .001$ (there is usually a key at the bottom of the table that indicates what the asterisks mean). Thus, a table might show: $t = 3.00$, $p < .01$ or $t = 3.00.$** The absence of an asterisk would signify a nonsignificant result.

CRITIQUING QUANTITATIVE ANALYSES

For novice research consumers, it is often difficult to critique statistical analyses. We hope this chapter has helped to demystify what statistics are all about, but we also recognize the limited scope of this presentation. Although it would be unreasonable to expect you to now be adept at evaluating statistical analyses, there are certain things you should routinely look for in reviewing research reports. Some specific guidelines are presented in Box 15-2.

One aspect of the critique should focus on the analyses included in the report. Researchers generally perform many more analyses than can be reported in a short journal article. You should determine whether the reported statistical information adequately describes the sample and reports the results of statistical tests for all hypotheses. You might also wish to consider whether the author included statistical information that was not really needed, given the

---

BOX 15.2   GUIDELINES FOR CRITIQUING QUANTITATIVE ANALYSES

1. Does the report include any descriptive statistics? Do these statistics sufficiently describe the major characteristics of the researcher's data set?
2. Were the correct descriptive statistics used? (e.g., Were percentages reported when a mean would have been more informative?)
3. Does the report include any inferential statistical tests? If not, should it have (e.g., were groups compared without information on the statistical significance of group differences)?
4. Was a statistical test performed for each of the hypotheses or research questions?
5. Do the selected statistical tests appear to be appropriate (e.g., are the tests appropriate for the level of measurement of key variables)?
6. Were any multivariate procedures used? If not, should multivariate analyses have been conducted—would the use of a multivariate procedure strengthen the internal validity of the study?
7. Were the results of any statistical tests significant? Nonsignificant? What do the tests tell you about the plausibility of the research hypotheses? Can you draw any conclusions about the possibility that Type I or Type II errors were committed?
8. Was an appropriate amount of statistical information reported? Were important analyses omitted, or were unimportant analyses included?
9. Were tables used judiciously to summarize statistical information? Is information in the text and tables totally redundant? Are the tables clear, with a good title and carefully labeled headings?
10. Is the researcher sufficiently objective in reporting the results?

stated aims of the study. Another presentational issue concerns the researcher's judicious use of tables to summarize statistical information.

A thorough critique also addresses whether researchers used the appropriate statistics. Tables 15-12 and 15-14 provide summaries of the most frequently used statistical tests—although we do not expect that you will readily be able to determine the appropriateness of the tests used in a study without further statistical instruction. The major issues to consider are the number of independent and dependent variables, the levels of measurement of the research variables, the number of groups (if any) being compared, and the appropriateness of using a parametric test.

If researchers did not use a multivariate technique, you should consider whether the bivariate analysis adequately tests the relationship between the independent and dependent variables. For example, if a *t*-test or ANOVA was used, could the internal validity of the study have been enhanced through the statistical control of extraneous variables, using ANCOVA? The answer will almost always be "yes, even when an experimental design was used."

Finally, you can be alert to possible exaggerations or subjectivity in the reported results. Researchers should never claim that the data proved, verified, confirmed, or demonstrated that the hypotheses were correct or incorrect. Hypotheses should be described as being *supported* or *not supported, accepted* or *rejected.*

The main task for beginning consumers in reading a results section of a research report is to understand the meaning of the statistical tests. What do the quantitative results indicate about the researcher's hypothesis? How believable are the findings? The answer to such questions form the basis for interpreting the research results, a topic discussed in Chapter 17.

C H A P T E R   R E V I E W

Key new terms introduced in the chapter, together with a summary of major points, are presented in this section. In addition, Chapter 15 of the *Study Guide to Accompany Essentials of Nursing Research,* 6th edition offers various exercises and study suggestions for reinforcing the concepts presented in this chapter. For additional review, see the Student Self-Study Review Questions section of the Student Resource CD-ROM provided with this book.

K E Y   N E W   T E R M S

Alpha (α)	Degrees of freedom (df)
Analysis of covariance (ANCOVA)	Descriptive statistics
Analysis of variance (ANOVA)	Discriminant function analysis
Beta (β)	Estimation procedures
Causal modeling	*F* ratio
Central tendency	Factor analysis
Chi-squared test	Frequency distribution
Contingency table	Hypothesis testing
Correlation	Inferential statistics
Correlation coefficient	Interval measurement
Correlation matrix	Level of measurement
Covariate	Level of significance
Cross-tabulation	Linear structural relations analysis (LISREL)

Logistic regression
Mean
Median
Mode
Multiple comparison procedures
Multiple correlation coefficient (R)
Multiple regression analysis
Multivariate analysis of covariance
    (MANCOVA)
Multivariate analysis of variance
    (MANOVA)
Multivariate statistics
N
Negative relationship
Negative skew
Nominal distribution
Nominal measurement
Nonsignificant result (NS)
Nonparametric test
Odds ratio
Ordinal measurement
p value
Parameter
Parametric test
Path analysis
Pearson's r
Positive relationship

Positive skew
Post hoc test
Predictor variable
Product–moment correlation
    coefficient
r
R
R^2
Range
Ratio measurement
Repeated measures ANOVA
Sampling distribution of the mean
Skewed distribution
Spearman's rank-order correlation
Spearman's rho
Standard deviation
Standard error of the mean (SEM)
Statistics
Statistical test
Statistically significant
Symmetric distribution
Test statistic
t-test
Type I error
Type II error
Variability
Variance

S U M M A R Y   P O I N T S

▷ There are four major **levels of measurement:** (1) **nominal measurement**—the classification of characteristics into mutually exclusive categories; (2) **ordinal measurement**—the ranking of objects based on their relative standing on an attribute; (3) **interval measurement**—indicating not only the ranking of objects but also the distance between them; and (4) **ratio measurement**—distinguished from interval measurement by having a rational zero point.

▷ **Descriptive statistics** enable researchers to synthesize and summarize quantitative data.

▷ In a **frequency distribution**, numeric values are ordered from lowest to highest, together with a count of the number (or percentage) of times each value was obtained; *frequency polygons* display frequency information graphically.

▷ A set of data for a variable can be completely described in terms of the shape of its distribution, central tendency, and variability.

▷ The shape of a distribution can be **symmetric** or **skewed**, with one tail longer than the other; it can also be unimodal with one peak (i.e., one value of high frequency), or multimodal with more than one peak.

▷ A **normal distribution** (bell-shaped curve) is symmetric, unimodal, and not too peaked.

▷ Measures of **central tendency** represent the average or typical value of a variable. The **mode** is the value that occurs most frequently in the distribution; the **median** is the point on a scale above which and below which 50% of the cases fall; and the **mean** is the arithmetic average of all scores. The mean is usually the preferred measure of central tendency because of its stability.

▷ Measures of **variability**—how spread out the data are—include the range and standard deviation. The **range** is the distance between the highest and lowest scores, and the **standard deviation** indicates how much, on average, scores deviate from the mean.

▷ A **contingency table** is a two-dimensional frequency distribution in which the frequencies of two nominal- or ordinal-level variables are **cross-tabulated**.

▷ **Correlation coefficients** describe the direction and magnitude of a relationship between two variables. The values range from -1.00 for a perfect negative correlation, to .00 for no relationship, to $+1.00$ for a perfect positive correlation. The most frequently used correlation coefficient is the **product–moment correlation coefficient (Pearson's r)**, used with interval- or ratio-level variables.

▷ **Inferential statistics**, which are based on *laws of probability*, allow researchers to make inferences about a population based on data from a sample; they offer a framework for deciding whether the sampling error that results from sampling fluctuation is too high to provide reliable population estimates.

▷ The **sampling distribution of the mean** is a theoretical distribution of the means of an infinite number of same-sized samples drawn from a population. Sampling distributions are the basis for inferential statistics.

▷ The **standard error of the mean (SEM)**—the standard deviation of this theoretical distribution—indicates the degree of average error of a sample mean; the smaller the standard error, the more accurate are the estimates of the population value based on the sample mean.

▷ **Hypothesis testing** through statistical tests enables researchers to make objective decisions about relationships between variables.

▷ The *null hypothesis* states that no relationship exists between the variables and that any observed relationship is due to chance or sampling fluctuations; rejection of the null hypothesis lends support to the research hypothesis.

▷ A **Type I error** occurs if a null hypothesis is incorrectly rejected (false positives). A **Type II error** occurs when a null hypothesis that should be rejected is accepted (false negatives).

▷ Researchers control the risk of making a Type I error by establishing a **level of significance** (or **alpha** level), which specifies the probability that such an error will occur. The .05 level means that in only 5 out of 100 samples would the null hypothesis be rejected when it should have been accepted.

▷ The probability of committing a Type II error, referred to as **beta** (β), can be estimated through *power analysis*. *Power,* the ability of a statistical test to detect true relationships, is the complement of beta (i.e., power equals $1 - \beta$). The standard criterion for an acceptable level of power is .80.

▷ Results from hypothesis tests are either significant or nonsignificant; **statistically significant** means that the obtained results are not likely to be due to chance fluctuations at a given probability level (*p* **value**).

▷ **Parametric tests** involve the estimation of at least one parameter, the use of interval- or ratio-level data, and an assumption of normally distributed variables; **nonparametric tests** are used when the data are nominal or ordinal and the normality of the distribution cannot be assumed.

▷ Two common statistical tests are the *t*-test and **analysis of variance (ANOVA)**, both of which can be used to test the significance of the difference between group means; ANOVA is used when there are more than two groups.

▷ The most frequently used nonparametric test is the **chi-squared test**, which is used to test hypotheses about differences in proportions.

▷ Pearson's *r* can be used to test whether a correlation is significantly different from zero.

▷ **Multivariate statistics** are increasingly being used in nursing research to untangle complex relationships among three or more variables.

▷ **Multiple regression analysis**, or *multiple correlation*, is a method for understanding the effect of two or more **predictor** (independent) **variables** on a dependent variable. The **multiple correlation coefficient *(R)***, can be squared to estimate the proportion of variability in the dependent variable accounted for by the predictors.

▷ **Analysis of covariance (ANCOVA)** permits researchers to control extraneous variables (called **covariates**) before determining whether group differences are statistically significant.

▷ Other multivariate procedures used by nurse researchers include discriminant function analysis, logistic regression, factor analysis, multivariate analysis of variance (MANOVA), multivariate analysis of covariance (MANCOVA), path analysis, and LISREL.

RESEARCH EXAMPLES **Critical Thinking Activities**

 EXAMPLE 1: Descriptive, Bivariate, and Multivariate Statistics

Aspects of a quantitative nursing study, featuring terms and concepts discussed in this chapter, are presented below, followed by some questions to guide critical thinking. (The full research report is available in *Nursing Research, 52,* 361–369.)

Study

"Hispanic chronic disease self-management: A randomized community-based outcome trial" (Lorig, Ritter, & Gonzalez, 2003).

Statement of Purpose

The purpose of the study was to evaluate the health and health care utilization outcomes of a 6-week community-based program for Spanish speakers with chronic diseases (heart disease, lung disease, or type 2 diabetes).

Intervention

Tomando Control de su Salud (Taking Control of Your Health) is a 14-hour community-based health program given in 2½ hour sessions over a 6-week period. Two trained peer leaders taught the program material in a variety of community settings (e.g., churches, clinics) to classes of 10 to 15 people. Program participants also received other material for self-instruction (texts, audio exercise tapes, etc.)

research examples continue on page 392

RESEARCH EXAMPLES | *Continued*

Research Design

Spanish-speaking adults with a chronic illness were recruited into the study and randomly assigned (on a 3:2 ratio) to either the treatment group or the control (usual care) group. Control group members were in a delay-of-treatment situation, wherein they could participate in the Tomando intervention after being wait-listed for 4 months. Data on a wide range of health status, health behavior, and health care utilization variables were measured at baseline and again 4 months later. A total of 443 subjects completed two rounds of data collection. Some 271 participants from both groups were then followed up after 1 year, at which point everyone had been exposed to the intervention.

Descriptive Statistics

The researchers reported means, SDs, and percentages to describe the baseline characteristics of the sample. For example, participants were mostly female (79%), married (57%), foreign-born (94%), not working (70%), middle-aged (mean age = 57, SD = 14), and with just under two chronic disease conditions (mean = 1.9, SD = .8).

Bivariate Inferential Statistics

To evaluate the effectiveness of randomization, the researchers compared the background characteristics of those in the treatment and control groups using *t*- tests and chi-squared tests. There were no significant group differences on any demographic variables, but the treatment group had a significantly higher number of chronic diseases at baseline than the control group. Bivariate tests (paired *t*-tests) were also used to determine whether changes between baseline and the 1-year follow-up for the sample as a whole were significant. Significant changes were observed for 11 of the 13 outcome variables. For example, mean scores on a scale of fatigue improved from 4.77 at baseline to 3.43 1 year later ($p < .001$).

Multivariate Analyses

Analysis of covariance was used to test hypotheses that health outcomes would improve more in the treatment group than in the control group 4 months after random assignment. Table 15-15 shows the group means and SDs for five selected outcomes, for baseline scores and changes 4 months later. In these analyses, 4-month scores on the outcomes were the dependent variables and treatment group status was the independent variable; the covariates were age, gender, education, acculturation, number of chronic conditions, and baseline scores on the respective outcome measure. As the table shows, for the majority of outcomes examined, the treatment group had significantly better outcomes at the 4-month follow-up than the control group. In Table 15-15, the group difference for only one outcome (number of physician visits) was not statistically significant at conventional levels ($p = .057$), just narrowly missing it. Note that in this table *lower* scores indicate better outcomes.

Conclusions

The researchers concluded that the Tomando program has the potential to improve the lives of Hispanics with chronic illness.

TABLE 15.15   Selected Health Outcomes at Baseline and 4-Month Change for Treatment and Control Groups

HEALTH OUTCOME	TREATMENT GROUP ($n = 265$)		CONTROL GROUP ($n = 178$)		
	Baseline Mean (SD)	4-Month Change Mean (SD)	Baseline Mean (SD)	4-Month Change Mean (SD)	p
Self-reported health*	3.80 (.8)	−.39 (1.0)	3.80 (.8)	−.03 (.8)	<.0001
Health distress*	2.33 (1.4)	−.74 (1.6)	2.27 (1.4)	−.07 (1.6)	<.0001
Physical discomfort*	4.82 (3.5)	−1.26 (3.6)	4.68 (3.6)	−.46 (4.0)	.014
Minutes of exercise/wk	106.0 (123)	63.7 (172)	96.2 (103)	31.0 (132)	.001
No. of physician visits, past 4 months	2.78 (2.7)	−.48 (2.8)	2.69 (2.3)	−.03 (2.4)	.057

*The lower the score, the better the outcome

Adapted from Lorig, K. R., Ritter, P. L., & Gonzalez, V. M. (2003). Hispanic chronic disease self-management: A randomized community-based outcome trial (Table 2). *Nursing Research, 52*, 361–369.

RESEARCH EXAMPLES   *Continued*

*Critical Thinking Suggestions**

*See the Student Resource CD-ROM for a discussion of these questions.

1. Answer the questions from Box 15-2 regarding this study.
2. Also consider the following targeted questions, which may assist you in further assessing aspects of the study:
   a. What were the actual mean scores of the treatment and control group members at the 4-month follow-up on the self-reported health scale?
   b. Comment on the difference in variability between the two groups on the "minutes of exercise per week" variable.
   c. Which outcomes have the least likelihood of spurious group differences?
   d. In all cases, the changes for the control group were in the same direction as those for the treatment group. Why might this have happened? Did this threaten the internal validity of the study? How would you assess the study's internal validity?
   e. If one of the outcome variables had been *"did versus did not visit the emergency room in the past 4 months,"* what analysis could have been used to test group differences?
3. If the results of this study are valid and reliable, what are some of the uses to which the findings might be put in clinical practice?

 EXAMPLE 2: Descriptive and Inferential Statistics

1. Read the results section from the study ("Sense of Coherence") in Appendix A of this book, and then answer the relevant questions in Box 15-2.

research examples continue on page 394

RESEARCH EXAMPLES *Continued*

2. Also consider the following targeted questions, which may further sharpen your critical thinking skills and assist you in assessing aspects of the study:

a. Table 1 presents demographic characteristics of the two groups of women. Statistical tests were used to determine how, if at all, the two groups (IBS and non-IBS) differed in terms of these characteristics. Which statistical tests would have been appropriate to use for the following variables: age; currently has/does not have health insurance; and scores on the SDI scale? What is the level of measurement of these three variables?

b. The text indicates that the two groups were significantly different with regard to which demographic characteristic?

c. Does Table 2 present descriptive or inferential statistics? What is the level of measurement of the variable "severity of abdominal pain"? What is the mode of this variable for the two groups?

d. In Table 3, differences between the two groups were tested using independent groups *t*-tests. Could paired-groups *t*-tests have been used? Why or why not?

e. Which multivariate analysis could have been used with the bivariate results shown in Table 4?

SUGGESTED READINGS

Methodologic References

Jaccard, J., & Becker, M. A. (2001). *Statistics for the behavioral sciences* (4th ed.). Belmont, CA: Wadsworth.

McCall, R. B. (2000). *Fundamental statistics for behavioral sciences* (8th ed.). Belmont, CA: Wadsworth.

Polit, D. F. (1996). *Data analysis and statistics for nursing research.* Stamford, CT: Appleton & Lange.

Welkowitz, J., Ewen, R. B., & Cohen, J. (2000). *Introductory statistics for the behavioral sciences* (5th ed.). New York: Harcourt College Publishers.

Studies Cited in Chapter 15

Anderson, R. A., Issel, L. M., & McDaniel, R. R. (2003). Nursing homes as complex adaptive systems: Relationship between management practice and resident outcomes. *Nursing Research, 52,* 12–21.

Aronowitz, T., & Morrison-Beedy, D. (2004). Resilience to risk-taking behaviors in impoverished African American girls: The role of mother-daughter connectedness. *Research in Nursing & Health, 27,* 29–39.

Bray, C. O., Nash, K., & Froman, R. D. (2003). Validation of measures of middle-schoolers' self-efficacy for physical and emotional health, and academic tasks. *Research in Nursing & Health, 26,* 376–386.

Buist, A., Morse, C. A., & Durkin, S. (2003). Men's adjustment to fatherhood. *Journal of Obstetric, Gynecologic, & Neonatal Nursing, 32,* 172–180.

Champion, J. D., Piper, J., Holden, A., Korte, J., & Shain, R. N. (2004). Abused women and risk for pelvic inflammatory disease. *Western Journal of Nursing Research, 26,* 176–191.

Given, B., Given, C., Azzouzz, F., & Stommel, M. (2001). Physical functioning of elderly cancer patients prior to diagnosis and following initial treatment. *Nursing Research, 50,* 222–232.

Heinrich, C. R. (2003). Enhancing the perceived health of HIV seropositive men. *Western Journal of Nursing Research, 25,* 367–382.

Holditch-Davis, D., Cox, M. F., Miles, M. S., & Belyea, M. (2003). Mother-infant interactions of medically fragile infants and non-chronically ill premature infants. *Research in Nursing & Health, 26,* 300–311.

Kub, J. E., Nolan, M. T., Hughes, M. T., Terry, P. B., Sulmasy, D. P., Astrow, A., & Forman, J. H. (2003). Religious importance and practices of patients with a life-threatening illness: Implications for screening protocols. *Applied Nursing Research, 16,* 196–200.

Lorig, K. R., Ritter, P. L., & Gonzalez, V. M. (2003). Hispanic chronic disease self-management: A randomized community-based outcome trial. *Nursing Research, 52,* 361–369.

Melkus, G. D., Spollett, G., Jefferson, V., Chyun, D., Tuohy, B., Robinson, T., & Kaisen, A. (2004). A culturally competent intervention of education and care for black women with type 2 diabetes. *Applied Nursing Research, 17,* 10–20.

Moscato, S. R., David, M., Valanis, B., Gullion, C. M., Tanner, C., Shapiro, S., Izumi, S., & Mayo, A. (2003). Tool development for measuring caller satisfaction and outcome with telephone advice nursing. *Clinical Nursing Research, 12,* 266–281.

Schaffer, S. D., & Tian, L. (2004). Promoting adherence: Effects of theory-based asthma education. *Clinical Nursing Research, 13,* 69–89.

Stastny, P. F., Ichinose, T. Y., Thayer, S. D., Olson, R. J., & Keens, T. G. (2004). Infant sleep positioning by nursery staff and mothers in newborn hospital nurseries. *Nursing Research, 53,* 122–129.

Suen, L. W., Morris, D., & McDougall, G. J. (2004). Memory functions of Taiwanese American older adults. *Western Journal of Nursing Research, 26,* 222–241.

Tang, S. T. (2003). Determinants of hospice home care use among terminally ill cancer patients. *Nursing Research, 52,* 217–225.

Tsay, S. L., & Hung, L. O. (2004). Empowerment of patients with end-stage renal disease—a randomized controlled trial. *International Journal of Nursing Studies, 41,* 59–65.

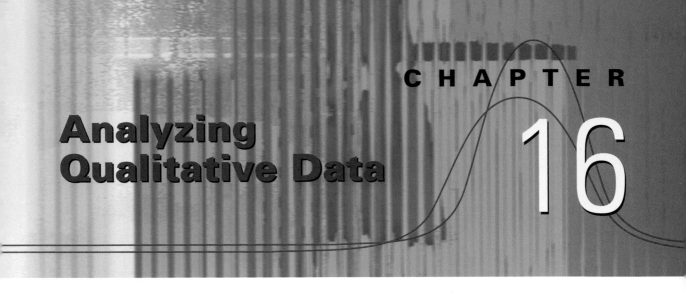

Analyzing Qualitative Data

STUDENT OBJECTIVES

On completing this chapter, you will be able to:

▸ Distinguish prototypical qualitative analysis styles and describe the intellectual processes that can play a role in qualitative analysis
▸ Describe activities that qualitative researchers perform to manage and organize their data
▸ Discuss the procedures used to analyze qualitative data, including both general procedures and those used in grounded theory, phenomenological, and ethnographic research
▸ Assess the quality of researchers' descriptions of their analytic procedures and evaluate the adequacy of those procedures
▸ Define new terms in the chapter

A s we saw in Chapter 13, qualitative data are derived from narrative materials such as verbatim transcripts from in-depth interviews, field notes from participant observation, or personal diaries. This chapter describes methods for analyzing such qualitative data.

INTRODUCTION TO QUALITATIVE ANALYSIS

Qualitative analysis is a labor-intensive activity that requires creativity, conceptual sensitivity, and sheer hard work. Qualitative analysis is more complex and difficult to do well than quantitative analysis because it is less formulaic. In this section, we discuss some general issues relating to qualitative analysis.

Qualitative Analysis: General Considerations

The purpose of data analysis, regardless of the type of data or the underlying research tradition, is to organize, provide structure to, and elicit meaning from the data. Data analysis is particularly challenging for qualitative researchers, for three major reasons. First, there are no universal rules for analyzing and summarizing qualitative data. The absence of standard analytic procedures makes it difficult to present findings in such a way that their validity is apparent. Some of the procedures described in Chapter 14 (e.g., member checking and investigator triangulation) are important tools for enhancing the trustworthiness not only of the data themselves but also of the analyses and interpretation of those data.

The second challenge of qualitative analysis is the enormous amount of work required. The qualitative analyst must organize and make sense of pages and pages of narrative materials. In a recent multimethod study by one of us (Polit), the qualitative data consisted of transcribed, unstructured interviews with about 25 to 30 low-income women in four cities discussing life stressors and health problems over a 3-year period. The transcriptions ranged from 30 to 50 pages in length, resulting in thousands of pages that had to be read and reread and then organized, integrated, and interpreted.

The final challenge comes in reducing the data for reporting purposes. Quantitative results can often be summarized in two or three tables. Qualitative researchers, by contrast, must balance the need to be concise to adhere to journal requirements with the need to maintain the richness and evidentiary value of their data.

CONSUMER TIP

Qualitative analyses are often more difficult to do than quantitative ones, but qualitative findings are generally easier to understand than quantitative findings because the stories are often told in everyday language. However, qualitative analyses are harder to evaluate critically than quantitative analyses because readers cannot know first-hand if researchers adequately captured thematic patterns in the data. ▬

Analysis Styles

Crabtree and Miller (1999) observed that there are nearly as many qualitative analysis strategies as there are qualitative researchers. However, they have identified three major analysis styles that fall along a continuum. At one extreme is a style that is more systematic and standardized, and at the other is a style that is more intuitive, subjective, and interpretive. The three prototypical styles are described as follows:

▶ **Template analysis style.** In this style, researchers develop a *template*—a category and analysis guide for sorting the narrative data. Although researchers usually begin with a rudimentary template before collecting data, the template undergoes constant revision as the data are gathered and analyzed. This style is most likely to be adopted by researchers whose research tradition is ethnography, ethology, discourse analysis, or ethnoscience.

▶ **Editing analysis style.** Researchers using an editing style act as interpreters who read through texts in search of meaningful segments. Once segments are identified and reviewed, researchers develop a category scheme and corresponding codes that can be used to sort and organize the data. The researchers then search for the patterns and structures that connect the thematic categories. Researchers whose research tradition is grounded theory, phenomenology, hermeneutics, or ethnomethodology use procedures that fall within the editing analysis pattern.

▶ **Immersion/crystallization analysis style.** This style involves the analyst's total immersion in and reflection of the text materials, resulting in an intuitive crystallization of the data. This interpretive and subjective style is exemplified in personal case reports of a semianecdotal nature and is less frequently encountered in the nursing research literature than the other two styles.

Researchers seldom use terms like template analysis style or editing style in their reports—these terms are *post hoc* characterizations of styles that are adopted. However, King (1998) has described the process of undertaking a template analysis, and his approach has been adopted by some nurse researchers undertaking descriptive qualitative studies.

Example of a template analysis

King, Carroll, Newton, and Dornan (2002) used a template analysis process to analyze transcripts of 22 in-depth interviews focusing on the experience of adaptation to diabetic renal disease. Their template, developed in draft at the outset, included four main categories (immediate reactions to diagnosis; explanations of renal disease; living with renal disease; and hopes, fears, and expectations for the future). Categories and subcategories in the template were refined in the course of the analysis.

The Qualitative Analysis Process

The analysis of qualitative data is an active and interactive process. Qualitative researchers typically scrutinize their data carefully and deliberatively. Insights and theories cannot spring forth from the data unless the researchers are completely familiar with those data, and so they often read their narrative data over and over in search of meaning. Morse and Field (1995) note that qualitative analysis is "a process of fitting data together, of making the invisible obvious, of linking and attributing consequences to antecedents. It is a process of conjecture and verification, of correction and modification, of suggestion and defense" (p. 126). Morse and Field identified four cognitive processes that play a role in qualitative analysis:

▶ *Comprehending.* Early in the analytic process, qualitative researchers strive to make sense of the data and to learn "what is going on." When comprehension is achieved, researchers are able to prepare a thorough description of the phenomenon under study, and new data do not add much to that description. Thus, comprehension is completed when saturation has been attained.

▶ *Synthesizing.* Synthesizing involves a "sifting" of the data and inductively putting pieces together. At this stage, researchers get a sense of what is typical with regard to the phenomenon and what variation is like. At the end of the synthesis process, researchers can make some generalized statements about the phenomenon and about study participants.

▶ *Theorizing.* Theorizing involves a systematic sorting of the data. During the theorizing process, researchers develop alternative explanations of the phenomenon under study and then hold these explanations up to determine their "fit" with the data. The theorizing process continues to evolve until the best and most parsimonious explanation is obtained.

▶ *Recontextualizing.* The process of *recontextualization* involves the further development of the theory such that its applicability to other settings or groups is explored. In qualitative inquiries whose ultimate goal is theory development, it is the theory that must be recontextualized and generalized.

Although the intellectual processes in qualitative analysis are not linear in the same sense that quantitative analysis is, these four processes follow a rough progression over the course of the study. Comprehension occurs primarily while in the field. Synthesis begins in the field but may continue well after the fieldwork has been completed. Theorizing and recontextualizing are processes that are difficult to undertake before synthesis has been completed.

Example of cognitive processes in qualitative analysis

Daggett (2002) conducted a phenomenological study of the lived experience of middle-aged men facing spousal bereavement. Here is how she described the four processes: "The process of comprehending began with my transcribing and coding interview audiotapes. Recurring words, phrases, or themes were organized into meaningful clusters. During the process of synthesizing, interpretations of the data were made and concepts linked. I considered various theoretical explanations to determine which best described the phenomenon. During recontextualization, I developed a theoretical model of bereavement in light of the new findings" (p. 629).

QUALITATIVE DATA MANAGEMENT AND ORGANIZATION

The intellectual processes of qualitative analysis are supported and facilitated by early tasks that help to organize and manage the masses of narrative data.

Developing a Category Scheme

Qualitative researchers begin their analysis by organizing their data. The main organizational task is developing a method to classify and index the data. Researchers must design a means of gaining access to parts of the data, without having to repeatedly re-read the data set in its entirety. This phase of data analysis is essentially reductionist—data must be converted to smaller, more manageable units that can be retrieved and reviewed.

The most widely used procedure is to develop a category scheme and then to code the data according to the categories. A category system (or template) is sometimes drafted before data collection, but more typically the qualitative analyst develops categories based on a scrutiny of the actual data.

There are, unfortunately, no straightforward or easy guidelines for this task. The development of a high-quality category scheme for qualitative data involves a careful reading of the data, with an eye to identifying underlying regularities, concepts, and clusters of concepts. Depending on the aims of the study, the nature of the categories may vary in level of detail or specificity as well as in level of abstraction.

Researchers whose aims are primarily descriptive tend to use concrete categories. The category scheme may focus on actions or events or on different phases in a chronologic unfolding of an experience. In developing a category scheme, related concepts are often grouped together to facilitate the coding process.

Example of a descriptive category scheme

The category scheme used by Polit, London, and Martinez (2000) to categorize data relating to food insecurity and hunger in low-income families is an example of a system that was concrete and descriptive. For example, one major coding category was "Strategies used to avoid hunger." The subcategories used to code the interview transcripts included eight strategies, such as "Stretching food, eating smaller portions" and "Eating old or unsafe food."

Studies designed to develop a theory are more likely to develop abstract and conceptual categories. In designing conceptual categories, researchers must break the data into segments, closely examine them, and compare them to other segments for similarities and dissimilarities to determine what type of phenomena are reflected in them and what the meaning of those phenomena are. Researchers ask questions about discrete events, incidents, or thoughts, such as the following:

▶ What is this?
▶ What is going on?
▶ What does it stand for?
▶ What else is like this?
▶ What is this distinct from?

Important concepts that emerge from close examination of the data are then given a label that forms the basis for a categorization scheme. These category names are necessarily abstractions, but the labels are generally sufficiently graphic that the nature of the material to which it refers is clear—and often provocative. Strauss and Corbin (1998) advise qualitative researchers as follows: "This is very important—that the conceptual name or label should be suggested by the context in which an event is located" (p. 106).

Example of a conceptual category scheme

Box 16-1 shows the category scheme developed by Beck (2004) to categorize data from her Internet interviews on birth trauma (see Appendix B). The coding scheme included four major thematic categories with subcodes. For example, an excerpt that described a mother's feelings of humiliation would be coded under category 1B (i.e., being stripped of her dignity).

BOX 16.1   Beck's (2004) Coding Scheme for Birth Trauma

Theme 1. To care for me: Was that too much to ask?
A. Feeling abandoned and alone
B. Stripped of dignity
C. Lack of interest in a woman as a unique person
D. Lack of support and reassurance

Theme 2. To communicate with me: Why was this neglected?
A. Labor and delivery staff failed to communicate with the patients.
B. Labor and delivery staff spoke as if the woman in labor was not present.
C. Clinicians failed to communicate among themselves.

Theme 3. To provide safe care: You betrayed my trust and I felt powerless.
A. Perceived unsafe care
B. Feared for their own safety and that of their unborn infants
C. Felt powerless

Theme 4. The end justifies the means: At whose expense? At what price?
A. Traumatic deliveries were glossed over.
B. Successful outcome of the baby took center stage.
C. The mother was made to feel guilty.
D. No one wanted to listen to the mother.

CONSUMER TIP

A good category scheme is crucial to the analysis of qualitative data. Without a high-quality category system, researchers cannot retrieve the narrative information that has been collected. Unfortunately, research reports rarely present the category scheme for readers to review, but they may provide information about its development. This, in turn, may help you evaluate its adequacy (e.g., researchers may say that the scheme was reviewed by peers or developed and independently verified by two or more researchers). ■

Coding Qualitative Data

Once a category scheme has been developed, the data are then read in their entirety and coded for correspondence to or exemplification of the identified categories. The process of coding qualitative material is seldom an easy one. Researchers may have difficulty in deciding which code is most appropriate or they may not fully comprehend the underlying meaning of some aspect of the data. It may take a second or third reading of the material to grasp its nuances.

Moreover, researchers often discover in going through the data that the initial category system was incomplete or inadequate. It is not unusual for some themes to emerge that were not initially conceptualized. When this happens, it is risky to assume that the topic failed to appear in previously coded materials. That is, a concept might not be identified as salient until it has emerged a third or fourth time in the data. In such a case, it would be necessary to reread all previously coded material to have a truly complete grasp of that category.

Another issue is that narrative materials are generally not linear. For example, paragraphs from transcribed interviews may contain elements relating to three or four different categories, embedded in a complex fashion.

Example of coding qualitative data

An example of a multitopic segment of an interview from Beck's (2004) phenomenological study of birth trauma is shown in *Figure 16-1*. The codes in the margin represent codes from the scheme presented in *Box 16-1*.

Manual Methods of Organizing Qualitative Data

A variety of procedures have traditionally been used to organize and manage qualitative data. Before the advent of computer programs for managing qualitative data, the most usual procedure was the development of **conceptual files**. This approach involves creating a physical file for each category, and then cutting out and inserting into the file all of the materials relating to that category.

"At some point a fetal scalp monitor was introduced then what seemed to be very shortly after that, my own OB came in and said my baby was in fetal distress and that a c-section was probably needed given that I was only 6 cms. This floored me in every imaginable way-emotionally, physically, and mentally. I'd labored in what I thought was "well mannered" for 12 hours. NO ONE had told me they were monitoring my baby. NO ONE told me they suspected she was in distress. Then BOOM, my baby is in trouble and my almost picture-perfect labor is gone. After that point, things became blurry because I can only see them through what I describe as an emotional fog. I lost it in front of everybody which I rarely do.   **2 A**

2 A   As they wheeled me into the theatre, I asked again where was my husband. They said he was on his way. They wheeled me in and told me to curl my back for the epidural. There were a few nurses there and I remember them talking about me as if I wasn't   **2 B**

2 A   there. Didn't they realize that I could hear them? The needle must have gone in 4 or 5 times. I was crying. I was scared and the epidural hurt a bloody lot. Some one please help me. I felt all alone. And I was thinking that I don't want another baby and go through this again. I recall thinking how much more pain do I have to put up with? Was my baby going to be all right? I needed reassurance but none was given.   **1 D**

Then another man took over the epidural and asked me to sit up and bend over while he put the needle in. I started to feel numb below my waist. I felt a pin prick and felt my tummy being pulled apart. It was awful as I couldn't see or feel anything.

1 A   So my trauma was a result of that emergency caesarean. It happened so fast. Of feeling so scared and alone and having to go through it all alone with out my husband there. The nurses didn't tell me anything about what was going on. I felt powerless.

3 C   I also felt the hospital staff could have given me some indication that I may have   **2 A**
had to have an emergency caesarean instead of letting me think that I was going to have a natural labor. I also wished that the doctor herself could have come to see

1 C   how I was doing afterwards. I think it would have helped me a lot if she had come and talked about how I was doing and how I felt and why I had to have an emer-   **2 A**
gency c-section.

4 B   All people kept telling me after my daughter was born was how lucky I was and that I could have lost her. I know I was lucky but telling that does not help how I felt. With them telling me that, I felt guilty for feeling the way I did. I wanted some attention too. I wanted to be looked after and listened to. I tried several times to bring up how   **4 C**

4 D   I felt but it was brushed away with the "I've been through that before and so what response." I really felt like I was in the wrong to feel the way I did because I had a healthy baby."

FIGURE 16.1 Coded excerpt from Beck's (2004) Study.

Researchers can then retrieve all of the content on a particular topic by reviewing the applicable file folder.

The creation of such conceptual files is clearly a cumbersome and labor-intensive task. This is particularly true when segments of the narrative materials have multiple codes (e.g., the excerpt shown in Figure 16-1). In such a situation, there would need to be 3 copies of the last paragraph—one for each file corresponding to the 3 codes used. Researchers must also be sensitive to the need to provide enough context that the cut-up material can be understood. Thus, it is often necessary to include material preceding or following the directly relevant materials.

Computer Programs for Managing Qualitative Data

Traditional manual methods of organizing qualitative data have a long and respected history, but sophisticated computer programs for managing qualitative data are now widely used. These programs permit the entire data file to be entered onto the computer, each portion of an interview or observational record coded, and then portions of the text corresponding to specified codes retrieved and printed (or shown on a screen) for analysis. The current generation of programs also has features that go beyond simple indexing and retrieval—they offer possibilities for actual analysis and integration of the data.

Example of manual organization of qualitative data

Manns and Chad (2001) explored quality of life among persons with a quadriplegic or paraplegic spinal cord injury. The transcribed interviews with 15 informants were then read several times. Here is how the researchers described their next steps: "The process of unitizing was then performed, which involved working with the data to find units of information that came directly from the transcripts and included phrases, sentences, or entire paragraphs. The next stage...involved the formation of categories. The units of information gathered from the unitizing process were grouped into provisional categories when the units seemed to relate to the same or similar content. In this investigation, the file folder method was used; following placement of the similar units of information into the file folders, researchers began to look for themes..." (p. 798).

Computer programs remove the drudgery of cutting and pasting pages and pages of narrative material. However, some people prefer manual indexing because it allows them to get closer to the data. Others have raised concerns about using programs for the analysis of qualitative data, objecting to having a process that is basically cognitive turned into an activity that is mechanical and technical. Despite these issues, some qualitative researchers have switched to computerized data management because it frees up their time and permits them to pay greater attention to more important conceptual issues.

Example of using computers to manage qualitative data

Fletcher (2004) studied health care providers' views on spirituality and barriers to discussing spiritual issues with patients. Data came from five focus group interviews with a wide array of providers (nurses, physicians, psychologists, chaplains) at two veterans' hospitals. Transcribed interviews from the focus group sessions were entered into a computer program called "NVivo" for coding and sorting. One researcher used the software while another used manual review.

CONSUMER TIP

A good category system is of little utility if the actual coding is not done with care. There is, of course, no way for you as a reader to know whether coding was diligently performed. However, you can have more confidence if the report mentions that two or more people were involved in coding the data, or at least portions of it, to ensure intercoder reliability.

■

ANALYTIC PROCEDURES

Data *management* tasks in qualitative research are typically reductionist in nature because they convert large masses of data into smaller, more convenient units. By contrast, qualitative data *analysis* tasks are constructionist: They involve putting segments together into a meaningful conceptual pattern. Although there are several approaches to qualitative data analysis, some elements are common to several of them. We provide some general guidelines, followed by a description of the procedures used by ethnographers, phenomenologists, and grounded theory researchers.

It should be noted that qualitative researchers who conduct studies that are not based in a specific research tradition sometimes say that a **content analysis** was performed. Qualitative content analysis is the analysis of the content of narrative data to identify prominent themes and patterns among the themes—primarily using an analysis style that can be characterized as either template analysis or editing analysis.

Example of a content analysis

McDonald and her colleagues (2003) conducted interviews with 119 community-dwelling adults that focused on discussions they had had with others about their end-of-life preferences. Content analysis was used to examine the content, discussions, and communication processes employed by respondents in these end-of-life discussions.

A General Analytic Overview

The analysis of qualitative materials generally begins with a search for recurring regularities or themes. DeSantis and Ugarriza (2000), in their thorough review of the way in which the term **theme** is used among qualitative researchers, offer this definition: "A theme is an abstract entity that brings meaning and identity to a current experience and its variant manifestations. As such, a theme captures and unifies the nature or basis of the experience into a meaningful whole" (p. 362).

Themes emerge from the data. They often develop within categories of data (i.e., within categories of the coding scheme used for indexing materials) but sometimes cut across them. For example, in Beck's (2004) study (see Box 16-1) one theme that emerged was the clinicians' neglect of communication, including failure to communicate with their patients in labor and delivery (code 2A) and failure to communicate amongst themselves (code 2C).

The search for themes involves not only the discovery of commonalities across participants but also a search for natural variation. Themes that emerge are never universal. Researchers must attend not only to what themes arise but also to how they are patterned. Does the theme apply only to certain subsets of participants? In certain types of communities or organizations? In certain contexts? At certain periods? What are the conditions that precede the observed phenomenon, and what are the apparent consequences of it? In other words, the qualitative analyst must be sensitive to *relationships* within the data.

CONSUMER TIP

Major themes are often the subheadings used by qualitative researchers in the results section of their reports. For example, in their feminist study of Korean women's attitudes toward physical activity, Im and Choe (2004) identified five main themes that were used to organize their results section. The five themes were: "A holistic view of physical activity," "Death as the opposite of physical activity," "Exercise differentiated from physical activity," "Exercise related to health," and "Lack of exercise because of a busy daily life."

Researchers' search for themes, regularities, and patterns in the data can sometimes be facilitated by charting devices that enable them to summarize the evolution of behaviors, events, and processes. For example, for qualitative studies that focus on dynamic experiences (e.g., decision making), it is often useful to develop flow charts or time-lines that highlight time sequences, major decision points, or events.

Example of a time-line

In Beck's (2002) grounded theory study of mothering twins during the first year of life, time-lines that highlighted mothers' 24-hour schedule were helpful. Figure 16-2 presents an example for a 23-year-old mother of twins who had been born premature and were in the NICU for 2 months. At the time of the interview, the twins had recently been discharged from the hospital. Until they were 3 months old, the mother fed them on the same schedule they had been on in the hospital—every 3 hours. The time-line illustrates a typical 24-hour period for this mother during the 4 weeks after hospital discharge.

A further step involves validation to determine whether the themes inferred are an accurate representation of the phenomenon. Several validation procedures can be used, as discussed in Chapter 14. If more than one researcher is working on the study, sessions in which the themes are reviewed and specific cases discussed can be highly productive. Investigator triangulation cannot ensure thematic validity, but it can minimize idiosyncratic biases. It is also useful to undertake member checks—that is, to present the preliminary thematic analysis to some informants, who can be encouraged to offer comments to support or contradict the analysis.

At this point, some researchers introduce **quasi-statistics**—a tabulation of the frequency with which certain themes, relations, or insights are supported by the data. The frequencies cannot be interpreted in the same way as frequencies generated in survey studies because of imprecision in the sampling of cases and enumeration of the themes. Nevertheless, as Becker (1970) pointed out,

> *Quasi-statistics may allow the investigator to dispose of certain troublesome null hypotheses. A simple frequency count of the number of times a given phenomenon appears may make untenable the null hypothesis that the phenomenon is infrequent. A comparison of the number of such instances with the number of negative cases—instances in which some*

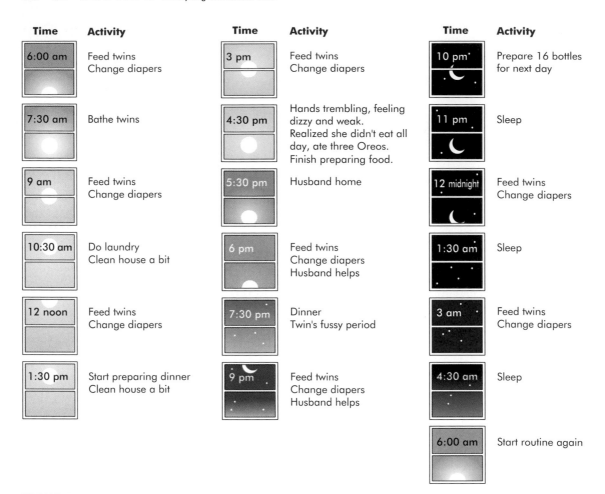

FIGURE 16.2 Example of a timeline for mothering multiples study.

alternative phenomenon that would not be predicted by his theory appears—may make possible a stronger conclusion, especially if the theory was developed early enough in the observational period to allow a systematic search for negative cases (p. 81).

Example of tabulating qualitative data

Wilde (2003) studied the lived experiences of long-term users of indwelling urinary catheters. She tabulated various aspects of the participants' acceptance of the catheter and their experience of stigma and vulnerability in living with a catheter in two "theme grids." For example, many of the 14 study participants noted that they considered the catheter to be "part of me" (64%). A majority also explicitly mentioned that one of their coping mechanisms was to hide the catheter (57%).

In the final analysis stage, researchers strive to weave the thematic pieces together into an integrated whole. The various themes need to be interrelated to provide an overall structure (such as a theory or integrated description) to the data. The integration task is a difficult one because it demands creativity and intellectual rigor if it is to be successful.

CONSUMER TIP

Research reports vary in the amount of detail provided about qualitative analytic procedures. At one extreme are researchers who say little more than that their data were analyzed qualitatively. At the other extreme are researchers who describe the steps they took to analyze their data and validate the emerging themes. Most studies fall between the two extremes, but limited detail is more prevalent than abundant detail.

■

These general analytic procedures provide an overview of how qualitative researchers make sense of their data and distill from them insights into processes and behaviors operating in naturalistic settings. However, variations in the goals and philosophies of qualitative researchers also lead to variations in analytic strategies. The next section describes data analysis in ethnographic studies.

Analysis of Ethnographic Data

Analysis in ethnography begins from the moment the researcher sets foot in the field. Ethnographers are continually looking for *patterns* in the behavior and thoughts of the participants, comparing one pattern against another, and analyzing many patterns simultaneously (Fetterman, 1989). As they analyze patterns of everyday life, ethnographers acquire a deeper understanding of the culture being studied. They analyze key events (e.g., social events) because these events provide a lens through which to view a culture. Maps, flowcharts, and organizational charts are also useful analytic tools that help to crystallize and illustrate the data being collected. Matrices (two-dimensional displays) can also help to highlight a comparison graphically, to cross-reference categories, and to discover emerging patterns.

Spradley's (1979) developmental research sequence is one method that is often used for data analysis in an ethnographic study. His method is based on the premise that language is the primary means that relates cultural meaning in a culture. The task of ethnographers is to describe cultural symbols and to identify their coding rules. His sequence of 12 steps, which includes both data collection and data analysis, is as follows:

1. Locating an informant
2. Interviewing an informant
3. Making an ethnographic record
4. Asking descriptive questions
5. Analyzing ethnographic interviews
6. Making a domain analysis
7. Asking structural questions
8. Making a taxonomic analysis
9. Asking contrast questions

10. Making a componential analysis
11. Discovering cultural themes
12. Writing the ethnography

Thus, in Spradley's method there are four levels of data analysis: domain, taxonomic, componential, and theme. *Domain analysis* is the first level of analysis. **Domains**, which are units of cultural knowledge, are broad categories that encompass smaller categories. There is no pre-established number of domains to be uncovered in an ethnographic study. During this first level of data analysis, ethnographers identify relational patterns among terms in the domains that are used by members of the culture. Ethnographers focus on the cultural meaning of terms and symbols (objects and events) used in a culture, and their interrelationships.

In *taxonomic analysis*, the second level of data analysis, ethnographers decide how many domains the data analysis will encompass. Will only one or two domains be analyzed in depth, or will a number of domains be studied less intensively? After making this decision, a **taxonomy**—a system of classifying and organizing terms—is developed to illustrate the internal organization of a domain and the relationship among the subcategories of the domain.

In *componential analysis*, multiple relationships among terms in the domains are examined. Ethnographers analyze data for similarities and differences among cultural terms in a domain. Finally, in *theme analysis*, cultural themes are uncovered. Domains are connected in cultural themes, which help to provide a holistic view of the culture being studied. The discovery of cultural meaning is the outcome.

Example of a study using Spradley's method

Tzeng and Lipson (2004) investigated experiences of patients and family members after a suicide attempt within the cultural context of Taiwan. Their analysis of data from interviews and participant observations was ongoing from the beginning of data collection. The analysis began with the coding of categories and terms, which they "associated into higher order domains" (p. 348). They also undertook a componential analysis by conducting "a back and forth process to establish different categories: searching for contrasts among these domains, grouping some together as dimensions, and combining related dimensions" (p. 348). The postsuicide stigma suffered by patients and their families reflected such cultural themes as "Suicide is bu-hsiao" (nonfilial piety).

Other approaches to ethnographic analysis have also been developed. For example, in her ethnonursing research method, Leininger (2001) provided ethnographers with a data analysis guide to help systematically analyze large amounts of data from their fieldwork. There are four phases to

---

Example of a study using Leininger's ethnonursing method

Miller and Petro-Nustas (2002) studied Jordanian women's health and care patterns in the political context of their homeland. Using Leininger's ethnonursing research method the researchers interviewed 15 Jordanian women and undertook participant observation. Data analysis involved coding the data, identifying descriptors, discerning patterns, and developing the following five themes: "Culture of caring connectedness," "Caring for family honor: the agony and the ecstasy," "Islam as the foundation of feminist thought," "Political care for women: tribal, religious, state influences," and "Reviving Rufaida: return to community care" (Rufaida was the first Islamic nurse in 624 AD).

Leininger's ethnonursing data analysis guide. In the first phase ethnographers collect, describe, and record data. The second phase involves identifying and categorizing descriptors. In phase 3, data are analyzed to discover repetitive patterns in their context. The fourth and final phase involves abstracting major themes and presenting findings.

Phenomenological Analysis

Schools of phenomenology have developed different approaches to data analysis. Three frequently used methods of data analysis for descriptive phenomenology are the methods of Colaizzi (1978), Giorgi (1985), and Van Kaam (1966), all of whom are from the Duquesne school of phenomenology, based on Husserl's philosophy. Table 16-1 presents a comparison of the steps involved in these three methods of analysis. The basic outcome of all three methods is the description of the meaning of an experience, often through the identification of essential themes. The phenomenologist searches for common patterns shared by particular instances. However, there are some important differences among these three approaches. Colaizzi's method, for example, is the only one that calls for a final validation of the results by returning to study participants (i.e., member checking). Giorgi's analysis relies solely on the researcher. His view is that it is inappropriate to either return to the participants to validate the findings or to use external judges to review the analysis. Van Kaam's method requires that intersubjective agreement be reached with other expert judges.

Example of a study using Colaizzi's method

Anderson and Spencer (2002) studied AIDS patients' cognitive representations of their illness. Interviews with 58 men and women with AIDS were analyzed using Colaizzi's phenomenological method. First, all transcripts were read several times to obtain an overall "feel" for the narratives. Then, significant phrases or sentences pertaining to the lived experience of AIDS were identified. Meanings were then formulated from significant statements. As an example, one significant statement was, "AIDS is a disease that has no cure. Meaning of dread and doom and you got to fight it the best way you can. You got to fight it with everything you can to keep going." The formulated meaning for this was, "AIDS is a dangerous disease that requires every fiber of your being to fight so you can live" (p. 1343). The meanings were clustered into themes. The results were integrated into an in-depth description of the phenomenon, which was validated through member checking.

A second school of phenomenology is the Utrecht School. Phenomenologists using this Dutch approach combine characteristics of descriptive and interpretive phenomenology. Van Manen's (1990) method is an example of this combined approach in which researchers try to grasp the essential meaning of the experience being studied. In reflecting on lived experience, researchers analyze the thematic aspects of that experience. According to Van Manen, themes can be uncovered or isolated from participants' descriptions of an experience by three different means: (1) the holistic approach, (2) the selective or highlighting approach, and (3) the detailed or line-by-line approach. In the *holistic approach*, researchers view the text as a whole and try to capture its meanings. In the *selective approach*, researchers underline, highlight, or pull out statements or phrases that seem essential to the experience under study. In the *detailed approach*, researchers analyze every sentence. Once the themes have been identified, they become the objects of reflecting and interpreting through follow-up interviews with participants. Through this process, the essential themes are discovered. In addition to identifying themes from participants' descriptions, Van Manen's method also encourages gleaning thematic descriptions from artistic sources (e.g., from poetry, novels, and other art forms).

TABLE 16.1	Comparison of Three Phenomenologic Methods	
COLAIZZI (1978)	**GIORGI (1985)**	**VAN KAAM (1966)**
1. Read all protocols to acquire a feeling for them.	1. Read the entire set of protocols to get a sense of the whole.	1. List and group preliminarily the descriptive expressions, which must be agreed upon by expert judges. Final listing presents percentages of these categories in that particular sample.
2. Review each protocol and extract significant statements.	2. Discriminate units from participants' description of phenomenon being studied.	2. Reduce the concrete, vague, and overlapping expressions of the participants to more descriptive terms. (Intersubjective agreement among judges needed.)
3. Spell out the meaning of each significant statement (i.e., formulate meanings).	3. Articulate the psychological insight in each of the meaning units.	3. Eliminate elements not inherent in the phenomenon being studied or that represent blending of two related phenomena.

4. Organize the formulated meanings into clusters of themes.
  a. Refer these clusters back to the original protocols to validate them.
  b. Note discrepancies among or between the various clusters, avoiding the temptation of ignoring data or themes that do not fit.
	4. Synthesize all of the transformed meaning units into a consistent statement regarding participants' experiences (referred to as the "structure of the experience"); can be expressed on a specific or general level.	4. Write a hypothetical identification and description of the phenomenon being studied.

5. Integrate results into an exhaustive description of the phenomenon under study.		5. Apply hypothetical description to randomly selected cases from the sample. If necessary, revise the hypothesized description, which must then be tested again on a new random sample.
6. Formulate an exhaustive description of the phenomenon under study in as unequivocal a statement of identification as possible.		6. Consider the hypothesized identification as a valid identification and description once preceding operations have been carried out successfully.
7. Ask participants about the findings thus far as a final validating step.		

Example of a study using Van Manen's method

As noted earlier, Wilde (2002, 2003) conducted a phenomenological study of living with a urinary catheter. She described in detail how Van Manen's approach was used to analyze data from interviews with 14 adults. Phenomenological reflection and writing were used iteratively "to create an internal dialogue between me and the text.... Through this dialectical process I was able to engage perspectives broader than my own, enrich data analysis, and deepen my understanding of the experience of living with a catheter.... As understandings grew, my writing began to incorporate meanings of participants and imagery in the descriptions to invoke an appreciation of what it is like to live with a catheter. For example, writing about 'urine flowing like water' required prolonged reflection as gradually I began to notice the richness of the water metaphor in the textual descriptions" (2002, pp. 18–19).

As this example illustrates, some qualitative researchers—especially phenomenologists—use *metaphors* as an analytic strategy. A metaphor, a figurative comparison, can be a powerfully creative and expressive tool for qualitative analysts. As a literary device, metaphors can permit greater insight and understanding in qualitative data analysis in addition to helping link together parts to the whole. One researcher, who studied adolescent mothers' depression after giving birth, described the integration of a storm metaphor (which emerged from the adolescents' descriptions of their experiences) into her analysis.

Example of a metaphor

"Data had been collected over the cold winter months and the researcher felt the intensity of the participants' descriptions translate into a powerful visual image. Their experience of feeling depressed as an adolescent mother following the birth of their babies was like being faced with a sudden storm. While some storm patterns are merely a nuisance—something you deal with—others have the potential to cripple entire regions of a country. Nor'easters in particular are strange weather systems that suddenly pop out of nowhere. It was this image that emerged from the participants' descriptions and is presented here as a metaphor to frame the thematic structure" (Clemmens, 2002, p. 556).

The third school of phenomenology is an interpretive approach called Heideggerian hermeneutics. Central to analyzing data in a hermeneutic study is the notion of the **hermeneutic circle**. The circle signifies a methodologic process in which, to reach understanding, there is continual movement between the parts and the whole of the text that is being analyzed. To interpret a text is to understand the possibilities that can be revealed by the text. Gadamer (1975) stressed that to interpret a text, researchers cannot separate themselves from the meanings of the text. Ricoeur (1981) broadened this notion of text to include not just the written text but any human action or situation.

Diekelmann, Allen, and Tanner (1989) have proposed a seven-stage process of data analysis in hermeneutics that involves collaborative effort by a team of researchers. The goal of this process is to describe shared practices and common meanings. Diekelmann and colleagues' stages include the following:

1. Reading all interviews or texts for an overall understanding
2. Preparing interpretive summaries of each interview
3. Analyzing selected transcribed interviews or texts by a research team
4. Resolving any disagreements on interpretation by going back to the text

5. Identifying recurring themes that reflect common meanings and shared practices of everyday life by comparing and contrasting the texts
6. Identifying emergent relationships among themes
7. Presenting a draft of the themes, along with exemplars from texts, to the team; incorporating responses and suggestions into the final draft

According to Diekelmann and colleagues, the discovery in step 6 of a **constitutive pattern**—a pattern that expresses the relationships among relational themes and is present in all the interviews or texts—forms the highest level of hermeneutical analysis. A situation is constitutive when it gives actual content or style to a person's self-understanding or to a person's way of being in the world.

Example of Diekelmann's hermeneutic analysis

Cheung and Hocking (2004) used Diekelmann's method to explore spousal caregivers' experience of caring for victims of multiple sclerosis. First, the researchers read all transcripts from their interviews with 10 spousal caregivers in Australia to gain an overall understanding. Then they read and re-read the transcripts in search of similar categories and themes. Next, they analyzed data for relational themes that cut across all texts. Finally, they examined the data to identify a constitutive pattern that described the ways in which participants' experiences of caring for their partner had changed their way of living and their personal meanings. The constitutive pattern that emerged from the data was called "Weaving Through a Web of Paradoxes."

Another data analytic approach for hermeneutic phenomenology is offered by Benner (1994). Her interpretive analysis consists of three interrelated processes: the search for paradigm cases, thematic analysis, and analysis of exemplars. **Paradigm cases** are "strong instances of concerns or ways of being in the world" (Benner, 1994, p.113). Paradigm cases are used early in the analytic process as a strategy for gaining understanding. Thematic analysis is done to compare and contrast similarities across cases. Lastly, paradigm cases and thematic analysis can be enhanced by *exemplars* that illuminate aspects of a paradigm case or theme. The presentation of paradigm cases and exemplars in research reports allows readers to play a role in consensual validation of the results by deciding whether the cases support the researchers' conclusions.

Example of Benner's hermeneutic analysis

Raingruber and Kent (2003) conducted an interpretive phenomenological study of faculty and student experiences with sensations and perceptions experienced during traumatic clinical events. The researchers interviewed students and faculty in nursing and social work as well as psychiatrists. Using Benner's interpretive analysis, one paradigm case and 12 exemplars were described in support of their conclusion that faculty and students experienced strong physical sensations during traumatic situations in their practice. In the paradigm case, "Trina, a social work student, described suddenly feeling like her body was 'a ripe apple ready to drop from the tree when a little boy surprised her by calling her momma'" (p. 455).

Grounded Theory Analysis

As noted in Chapter 10, there are two major approaches to substantive grounded theory analysis. One grounded theory approach was developed by Glaser and Strauss (1967), and another by Strauss and Corbin (1998).

GLASER AND STRAUSS'S GROUNDED THEORY METHOD

Grounded theory in both systems of analysis uses the **constant comparative method** of data analysis. This method involves a comparison of elements present in one data source (e.g., in one interview) with those identified in another. The process is continued until the content of each source has been compared to the content in all sources. In this fashion, commonalities are identified.

The concept of fit is an important element in Glaser and Strauss's grounded theory analysis. **Fit** is the process of identifying characteristics of one piece of data and comparing them with the characteristics of another datum to determine if they are similar. In the analytic process, fit is used to sort and reduce data. Fit enables the researcher to determine if data can be placed in the same category or if they can be related to one another—but data should not be forced or distorted to fit the developing category. Glaser and Strauss (1967) talked about fit as an important issue when grounded theory is applied elsewhere: The theory must closely "fit" the substantive area where it will be used.

Coding in Glaser and Strauss's grounded theory approach is used to conceptualize data into patterns or concepts. The substance of the topic being studied is conceptualized though **substantive codes** while **theoretical codes** provide insights into how the substantive codes relate to each other.

In the Glaser and Strauss approach, there are two types of substantive codes: open and selective. **Open coding**, used in the first stage of the constant comparative analysis, captures what is going on in the data. Open codes may be the actual words used by the participants. Through open coding, data are broken down into incidents and their similarities and differences are examined. During open coding, researchers ask "What category or property of a category does this incident indicate?" (Glaser, 1978, p. 57).

There are three different levels of open coding that vary in level of abstraction. **Level I codes** (sometimes called *in vivo codes*) are derived directly from the language of the substantive area. They have vivid imagery and "grab." Table 16-2 presents five level I codes from interviews in Beck's (2002) grounded theory study on mothering twins, and excerpts associated with those codes.

As researchers constantly compare new level I codes with previously identified ones, they condense them into broader categories—**level II codes**. For example, in Table 16-2, Beck's five level I codes were collapsed into the level II code, "Reaping the Blessings." **Level III codes** (or theoretical constructs) are the most abstract level of codes. These constructs "add scope beyond local meanings" (Glaser, 1978, p. 70) to the generated theory. Collapsing level II codes aids in identifying constructs.

Example of open codes in grounded theory analysis

Knobf (2002) studied responses to chemotherapy-induced premature menopause in women with early-stage breast cancer. Figure 1 in Knobf's article, on the Student Resource CD-ROM, shows how 20 level I codes were collapsed into three level II codes (Relying on Self; Structured Silence; and Being Prepared), These, in turn, were integrated in the theoretical construct (level III code), Facing Uncertainty.

Open coding ends when the core category is discovered, and then selective coding begins. The **core category** is a pattern of behavior that is relevant and/or problematic for study participants. In **selective coding** (which can also have three levels of abstraction) researchers

| TABLE 16.2 | Collapsing Level I Codes Into the Level II Code of *"REAPING THE BLESSINGS"* (Beck, 2002) | |

QUOTE	LEVEL I CODE
I enjoy just watching the twins interact so much. Especially now that they are mobile. They are not walking yet but they are crawling. I will tell you they are already playing. Like one will go around the corner and kind of peek around and they play hide and seek. They crawl after each other.	Enjoying Twins
With twins it's amazing. She was sick and she had a fever. He was the one acting sick. She didn't seem like she was sick at all. He was. We watched him for like 6–8 hours. We gave her the medicine and he started calming down. Like WOW! That is so weird. 'Cause you read about it but it's like, Oh come on! You know that doesn't really happen and it does. It's really neat to see.	Amazing
These days it's really neat 'cause you go to the store or you go out and people are like, "Oh, they are twins, how nice." And I say, "Yeah they are. Look, look at my kids."	Getting Attention
I just feel blessed to have two. I just feel like I am twice as lucky as a mom who has one baby. I mean that's the best part. It's just that instead of having one baby to watch grow and change and develop and become a toddler and school age child you have two.	Feeling Blessed
It's very exciting. It's interesting and it's fun to see them and how the twin bond really is. There really is a twin bond. You read about it and you hear about it but until you experience it, you just don't understand. One time they were both crying and they were fed. They were changed and burped. There was nothing wrong. I couldn't figure out what was wrong. So I said to myself, "I am just going to put them together and close the door." I put them in my bed together and they patty caked their hands and put their noses together and just looked at each other and went right to sleep.	Twin Bonding

code only those data that are related to the core variable. One kind of core variable can be a **basic social process (BSP)** that evolves over time in two or more phases. All BSPs are core variables, but not all core variables have to be BSPs.

Glaser (1978) provided nine criteria to help researchers decide on a core category:

1. It must be central, meaning that it is related to many categories.
2. It must reoccur frequently in the data.
3. It takes more time to saturate than other categories.
4. It relates meaningfully and easily to other categories.
5. It has clear and grabbing implications for formal theory.
6. It has considerable carry-through.
7. It is completely variable.
8. It is a dimension of the problem.
9. It can be any kind of theoretical code.

Theoretical codes help the grounded theorist to weave the broken pieces of coded data back together again. Glaser (1978) proposed 18 families of theoretical codes that researchers can use to conceptualize how substantive codes relate to each other. Four examples of the 18 families include the following:

❱ Process: stages, phases, passages, transitions
❱ Strategy: tactics, techniques, maneuverings
❱ Cutting point: boundaries, critical junctures, turning points
❱ The six C's: causes, contexts, contingencies, consequences, covariances, and conditions

Throughout coding and analysis, grounded theory researchers document their ideas about the data, categories, and emerging conceptual scheme in *memos*. Memos preserve ideas that may initially not seem productive but may later prove valuable once further developed. Memos also encourage researchers to reflect on and describe patterns in the data, relationships between categories, and emergent conceptualizations.

Glaser and Strauss's grounded theory method is concerned with the *generation* of categories, properties, and hypotheses rather than testing them. The product of the typical grounded theory analysis is a conceptual or theoretical model that endeavors to explain a pattern of behavior that is both relevant and problematic for the people in the study. Once the basic problem emerges, the grounded theorist goes on to discover the process these participants experience in coping with or resolving this problem.

Example of a Glaser and Strauss grounded theory analysis

Figure 16-3 presents the model developed by Beck (2002) in her grounded theory study that conceptualized "Releasing the Pause Button" as the core category and the process through which mothers of twins progressed as they attempted to resume their lives after giving birth. According to this model, the process involves four phases: Draining Power, Pausing Own Life, Striving to Reset, and Resuming Own Life. Beck used 10 of the 18 coding families in her theoretical coding for the Releasing the Pause Button process. The family *cutting point* provides an illustration. Three months seemed to be the turning point for mothers, when life started to become more manageable. Here is an excerpt from an interview that Beck coded as a cutting point: "Three months came around and the twins sort of slept through the night and it made a huge, huge difference."

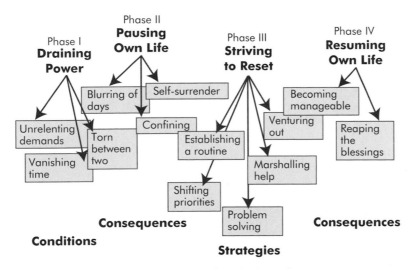

FIGURE 16.3 Beck's (2002) model of mothering twins.

TABLE 16.3　　**Comparison of Glaser's and Strauss/Corbin's Methods**

	GLASER	STRAUSS & CORBIN
Initial data analysis	Breaking down and conceptualizing data involves comparison of incident to incident so patterns emerge	Breaking down and conceptualizing data includes taking apart a single sentence, observation, and incident
Types of coding	Open, selective, theoretical	Open, axial, selective
Connections between categories	18 coding families	Paradigm model (conditions, contexts, action/interactional strategies, and consequences)
Outcome	Emergent theory (discovery)	Conceptual description (verification)

STRAUSS AND CORBIN'S GROUNDED THEORY METHOD

The Strauss and Corbin (1998) approach to grounded theory analysis differs from the original Glaser and Strauss method with regard to method and outcomes. Table 16-3 summarizes major analytic differences between these two grounded theory analysis methods.

Glaser (1978) stressed that to generate a grounded theory, the basic problem must emerge from the data—it must be discovered. The theory is, from the very start, grounded in the data, rather than starting with a preconceived problem. Strauss and Corbin, however, argued that the research itself is only one of four possible sources of the research problem. Research problems can, for example, come from the literature or from researchers' personal and professional experience.

The Strauss and Corbin method involves three types of coding: open, axial, and selective coding. In **open coding**, data are broken down into parts and compared for similarities and differences. Similar actions, events, and objects are grouped together as more abstract concepts, which are called categories. In open coding the researcher focuses on generating categories and their properties and dimensions. In **axial coding**, the analyst systematically develops categories and links them with subcategories. Strauss and Corbin (1998) term this process of relating categories and their subcategories as "axial because coding occurs around the axis of a category, linking categories at the level of properties and dimensions" (p. 123). What is called the *paradigm* is used to help identify linkages among categories. The basic components of the paradigm include conditions, actions/interactions, and consequences. **Selective coding** is a process in which the findings are integrated and refined. The first step in integrating the findings is to decide on the **central category** (sometimes called the core category), which is the main pattern or category of the research. Recommended techniques to facilitate identifying the central category are writing the storyline, using diagrams, and reviewing and organizing memos.

The outcome of the Strauss and Corbin approach is a full conceptual description. The original grounded theory method (Glaser & Strauss, 1967), by contrast, generates a theory that explains how a basic social problem that emerged from the data is processed in a social setting.

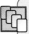

Example of a Strauss and Corbin grounded theory analysis

O'Brien, Evans, and White-McDonald (2002) used the Strauss and Corbin method in their descriptive–exploratory study of women's coping with severe nausea and vomiting during pregnancy. Interviews with 24 women admitted to a large tertiary care hospital in western Canada were read and coded by at least two researchers. Lines, paragraphs, and words were coded and emerging categories were discussed and finalized by consensus. "Data were then reconstructed by linking categories and subcategories within a set of relationships so that the context in which the experience occurred could be described (axial coding). A concept (i.e., core category) around which all emerging categories could be related was selected" (p. 304). The core category was the process (diagrammed in Figure 16-4) of increasingly complete isolation to cope with unrelenting and severe symptoms.

CRITIQUING QUALITATIVE ANALYSES

The task of evaluating a qualitative analysis is not an easy one, even for researchers with experience in doing qualitative research. The problem stems, in part, from the lack of standardized procedures for data analysis, but the difficulty lies mainly in the fact that readers must accept largely on faith that researchers exercised good judgment and critical insight in coding the narrative materials, developing a thematic analysis, and integrating the materials into a meaningful whole. This is because researchers are seldom able to include more than a handful of examples of actual data in a research report published in a journal and because the process of inductively abstracting meaning from the data is difficult to describe.

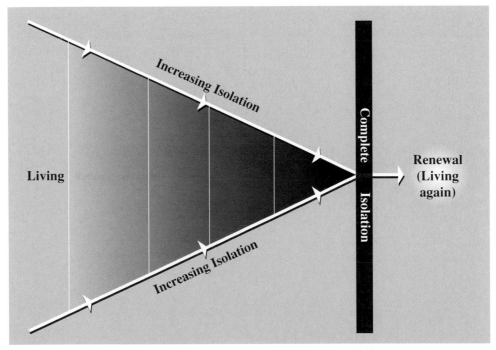

FIGURE 16.4 Isolated from living: process of coping with severe nausea, vomiting, and/or retching of pregnancy. (O'Brien, Evans, & White-McDonald, 2002)

In a critique of qualitative analysis, a primary task usually is determining whether researchers took sufficient steps to validate inferences and conclusions. A major focus of a critique of qualitative analyses, then, is whether the researchers have adequately documented the analytic process. The report should provide information about the approach used to analyze the data. For example, a report for a grounded theory study should indicate whether the researchers used the Glaser and Strauss or the Strauss and Corbin method.

Quantitative analyses can be evaluated in terms of the adequacy of specific analytic decisions (e.g., Did the researcher use the appropriate statistical test?). Critiquing analytic decisions is substantially less clear-cut in a qualitative study. For example, it typically would be inappropriate to critique a phenomenological analysis for following Giorgi's approach rather than Colaizzi's approach. Both are respected methods of conducting a phenomenological study and analyzing the resulting data (although phenomenologists themselves may have cogent reasons for preferring one approach over the other).

One aspect of a qualitative analysis that *can* be critiqued, however, is whether the researchers have documented that they have used one approach consistently and have been faithful to the integrity of its procedures. Thus, for example, if researchers say they are using the Glaser and Strauss approach to grounded theory analysis, they should not also include elements from the Strauss and Corbin method. An even more serious problem occurs when, as sometimes happens, the researchers "muddle" traditions. For example, researchers who describe their study as a grounded theory study should not have a presentation of *themes*, because grounded theory analysis does not yield themes. Furthermore, researchers who

---

BOX 16.2   Guidelines for Critiquing Qualitative Analyses

1. Given the nature of the data, was the data analysis approach appropriate for the research design?
2. Is the category scheme described? If so, does the scheme appear logical and complete? Does there seem to be unnecessary overlap or redundancy in the categories?
3. Were manual methods used to index and organize the data, or was a computer program used?
4. Does the report adequately describe the process by which the actual analysis was performed? Does the report indicate whose approach to data analysis was used (e.g., Glaser & Strauss or Strauss & Corbin, in grounded theory studies)? Was this method consistently and appropriately applied?
5. What major themes or processes emerged? If excerpts from the data are provided, do the themes appear to capture the meaning of the narratives—that is, does it appear that the researcher adequately interpreted the data and conceptualized the themes? Is the analysis parsimonious—could two or more themes be collapsed into a broader and perhaps more useful conceptualization?
6. What evidence does the report provide that the analysis is accurate and replicable?
7. Were data displayed in a manner that allows you to verify the researcher's conclusions? Was a conceptual map, model, or diagram effectively displayed to communicate important processes?
8. Was the context of the phenomenon adequately described? Does the report give you a clear picture of the social or emotional world of study participants?
9. Did the analysis yield a meaningful and insightful picture of the phenomenon under study? Is the resulting theory or description trivial or obvious?

attempt to blend elements from two traditions may not have a clear grasp of the analytic precepts of either one. For example, a researcher who claims to have undertaken an ethnography using a grounded theory approach to analysis may not be well-informed about the underlying goals and philosophies of these two traditions.

Some further guidelines that may be helpful in evaluating qualitative analyses are presented in Box 16-2.

CHAPTER REVIEW

Key new terms introduced in the chapter, together with a summary of major points, are presented in this section. In addition, Chapter 16 of the *Study Guide to Accompany Essentials of Nursing Research,* 6th edition offers various exercises and study suggestions for reinforcing the concepts presented in this chapter. For additional review, see the Student Self-Study Review Questions section of the Student Resource CD-ROM provided with this book.

KEY NEW TERMS

Axial coding
Basic social process (BSP)
Category scheme
Central category
Conceptual file
Constant comparative method
Constitutive pattern
Content analysis
Core category
Domain
Editing analysis style
Fit
Hermeneutic circle

Immersion/crystallization analysis style
Level I codes
Level II codes
Level III codes
Open coding
Paradigm case
Quasi-statistics
Selective coding
Substantive code
Taxonomy
Template analysis style
Theme
Theoretical code

SUMMARY POINTS

▷ Qualitative analysis is a challenging, labor-intensive activity, guided by few standardized rules.

▷ Although there are no universal strategies, three prototypical analytic styles have been identified: (1) a **template analysis style** that involves the development of an analysis guide (*template*) to sort the data; (2) an **editing analysis style** that involves an interpretation of the data on which a **category scheme** is based; and (3) an **immersion/crystallization style** that is characterized by the analyst's total immersion in and reflection of text materials.

▷ Qualitative analysis typically involves four intellectual processes: comprehending, synthesizing, theorizing, and recontextualizing (exploration of the developed theory vis-á-vis its applicability to other settings or groups).

▷ The first major step in analyzing qualitative data is to organize and index the data for easy retrieval, typically by coding the content according to a category scheme.

▷ Traditionally, researchers have organized their coded data by developing **conceptual files**, which are physical files in which excerpts of data relevant to specific categories are placed.

Now, however, computer programs are widely used to perform basic indexing functions and to facilitate data analysis.

▷ The actual analysis of data begins with a search for patterns, regularities, or **themes** in the data, which involves not only the discovery of commonalities across subjects, but also of natural variation in the data.

▷ Another analytic step generally involves a validation of the thematic analysis. Some researchers use **quasi-statistics**, which involves a tabulation of the frequency with which certain themes or relations are supported by the data.

▷ In a final analytic step, analysts try to weave thematic strands together into an integrated picture of the phenomenon under investigation.

▷ In ethnographies, analysis begins as the researcher enters the field. Ethnographers continually search for *patterns* in the behavior and expressions of study participants.

▷ One approach to analyzing ethnographic data is Spradley's method, which involves four levels of data analysis: *domain analysis* (identifying **domains**, or units of cultural knowledge); *taxonomic analysis* (selecting key domains and constructing **taxonomies** or systems of classification); *componential analysis* (comparing and contrasting terms in a domain); and *theme analysis* (to uncover cultural themes).

▷ Leininger's method to ethnonursing research involves four phases: collecting and recording data; categorizing descriptors; searching for repetitive patterns; and abstracting major themes.

▷ There are various approaches to phenomenological analysis, including the descriptive methods of Colaizzi, Giorgi, and Van Kaam, in which the goal is to find common patterns of experiences shared by particular instances.

▷ In Van Manen's approach, which involves efforts to grasp the essential meaning of the experience being studied, researchers search for themes, using either a *holistic approach* (viewing text as a whole); a *selective approach* (pulling out key statements and phrases); or a *detailed approach* (analyzing every sentence).

▷ Central to analyzing data in a hermeneutic study is the notion of the **hermeneutic circle**, which signifies a methodologic process in which there is continual movement between the parts and the whole of the text under analysis.

▷ In hermeneutics there are several choices for data analysis. Diekelmann's method calls for the discovery of a **constitutive pattern** which expresses the relationships among themes. Benner's approach to interpretive analysis consists of three processes: searching for **paradigm cases**, thematic analysis, and analysis of *exemplars*.

▷ Grounded theory uses the **constant comparative method** of data analysis.

▷ One approach to grounded theory is the Glaser and Strauss method, in which there are two broad types of codes: **substantive codes** (in which the empirical substance of the topic is conceptualized) and **theoretical codes** (in which the relationships among the substantive codes are conceptualized).

▷ Substantive coding involves **open coding** to capture what is going on in the data, and then **selective coding**, (in which only variables relating to a core category is coded). The **core category**, a behavior pattern that has relevance for participants, is sometimes a **basic social process (BSP)** that involves an evolutionary process of coping or adaptation.

▷ In the Glaser and Strauss method, open codes begin with **level I** *(in vivo)* **codes**, which are collapsed into a higher level of abstraction in **level II codes**. Level II codes are then used to formulate **level III codes**, which are theoretical constructs.

▷ The Strauss and Corbin method is an alternative grounded theory method whose outcome is a full conceptual description. This approach to grounded theory analysis involves three types of coding: open (in which categories are generated), **axial coding** (where categories are linked with subcategories), and selective (in which the findings are integrated and refined).

▷ Some researchers identify neither a specific approach nor a specific research tradition; rather, they might say that they used qualitative **content analysis** as their analytic method.

RESEARCH EXAMPLES **Critical Thinking Activities**

 EXAMPLE 1: Analysis in a Grounded Theory Study

Aspects of a grounded theory study, featuring terms and concepts discussed in this chapter, are presented below, followed by some questions to guide critical thinking. (The full research report is available in *Western Journal of Nursing Research, 25,* 725–741.)

Study

"Reworking professional nursing identity" (MacIntosh, 2003)

Statement of Purpose

The purpose of this study was to explore experienced nurses' perceptions of how they became professional.

Method

MacIntosh used Glaser and Strauss's grounded theory methods to explore how experienced nurses interpreted their professional development and how they addressed problems in that development. She conducted interviews with 21 nurses who had from 3 to 34 years of nursing experience working in urban and rural communities in eastern Canada. Each interview was transcribed and analyzed before the next interview was conducted, providing MacIntosh with information for theoretical sampling and the framing of appropriate questions with subsequent participants. Data collection ended when saturation was achieved.

Analysis

Data analysis was ongoing as new interviews were conducted. Constant comparison among concepts and incidents was used to identify relevant processes, connections, and contextual conditions. Both substantive and theoretical coding of the data occurred. When doing substantive coding, MacIntosh chose words from the verbatim transcripts to represent each line of data, comparing these words with other codes and then clustering those with similar meanings into initial categories. At the theoretical level, MacIntosh sorted categories by similarities and differences, examined relationships among the categories, and asked questions of the data to "elevate them to a conceptual level" (p. 729). One of the families of theoretical codes that she used was the "strategy" family. For example, one of the strategies nurses used in the final stage of professionalization was mentoring other nurses. MacIntosh noted that she kept copious memos to record thoughts, insights, and questions. Her analysis was validated through several means, including member checks (second interviews with a sample of participants) and discussions of the analytic process with another researcher experienced in grounded theory analysis.

research examples continue on page 422

RESEARCH EXAMPLES *Continued*

Key Findings

▶ The data revealed a three-stage process among nurses in addressing the problematic issue of dissonance between expectations and experiences as they became and sustained being professional. The process was called "Reworking Professional Identity."

▶ The first stage was "Assuming Adequacy," which involved two processes: neglecting reflection and concentrating on technical tasks.

▶ The second stage, "Realizing Practice," also involved two processes: becoming aware of discrepancies and feeling dissonance, and attempting balance.

▶ In the final stage, "Developing a Reputation," the processes were establishing practice patterns, choosing standards, and helping to advance nursing. Mentoring other nurses was a strategy used in this stage, as exemplified by the following quote: "And once you have seen, or once it's opened for you to have advanced, you want to go around opening all the doors for everyone" (p. 736).

Critical Thinking Suggestions*

*See the Student Resource CD-ROM for a discussion of these questions.

1. Answer questions 1–9 from Box 16-2 regarding this study.

2. Also answer the following targeted questions, which may assist you in further assessing aspects of this study:

    a. In the description of her analytic procedures, MacIntosh cited both Glaser and Strauss and Strauss and Corbin. Comment on this.

    b. MacIntosh analyzed data from interviews with experienced nurses in this study. What other data sources could have been used to augment and validate her understandings?

3. If the results of this study are trustworthy, what are some of the uses to which the findings might be put in clinical practice?

 EXAMPLE 2: Analysis in an Ethnographic Study

Aspects of an ethnographic nursing study, featuring terms and concepts discussed in this chapter, are presented below, followed by some questions to guide critical thinking. (The full research report is available in *Advances in Nursing Science, 26,* 215–226, and in Appendix D of the associated *Study Guide to Accompany Essentials of Nursing Research*, 6th edition.)

Study

"'The people know what they want': An empowerment process of sustainable, ecological community health" (Bent, 2003).

Statement of Purpose

The purpose of this study was to explore the relationships among health, environment, and culture from the cultural context of one community.

RESEARCH EXAMPLES *Continued*

Context

This study was a critical ethnography of the low-income urban *barrio* (a Spanish-speaking neighborhood) of San José in Albuquerque, New Mexico. Because of a heavy concentration of toxic waste sites, two locales in San José were listed on a national priority list for environmental cleanup efforts (Superfund site status). The previously prosperous agricultural community had become a high poverty neighborhood marred not only by industrial emissions but also by drugs and high crime rates. A grassroots organization (the Awareness Council), formed in 1988 in response to environmental health hazards, brought dramatic remediation and improvements. San José was selected as a site for the study because it was a culturally and ethnically diverse community that used grassroots political action to focus on sustainable solutions to health problems.

Method

Data were collected during 10 months of fieldwork. Data sources included interviews, participant observations, photographs, artifacts, and existing documents. A sample of 33 key informants was purposively sampled, including government officials, members of the Awareness Council, and other community residents. Each key informant was interviewed up to four times for approximately 1 hour at each interview. Questions were originally broad (e.g., "Is San José a healthy place to live?") but became more focused over time (e.g., "How are issues of growth related to health in San José?"). Participant observation included attendance at church services, public meetings, Awareness Council meetings, neighborhood fairs, and events of daily life.

Analysis

Interview transcripts and field notes were entered into a computer program called NUD*IST© for subsequent coding and analysis. Analytic activities began with reflecting, reading, and re-reading the data, and coding the data into categories that were created for such aspects of the data as events, processes, emotions, and characteristics. Categories were analyzed for central ideas; when categories were grouped for similarities, cultural domains (locally specific symbols of shared meaning) emerged. Following the identification of cultural domains, the data were analyzed for cultural themes. A number of approaches (prolonged engagement, member checks, peer debriefing) were used to enhance the credibility of the data and the analysis.

Key Findings

▶ From the analysis, five cultural domains, four cultural themes, and one integrative theme about community experiences of health, environment, culture, and health policy emerged. (The article focused on themes and did not indicate the domains.)
▶ The integrative theme was that in San José, sustainable community health embodied and reflected an empowerment process.
▶ One supporting cultural theme was that there is a persistent sense of community in San José: People held an abiding view about the "essence" of San José, in which the community was grounded in the people and the culture.

research examples continue on page 424

RESEARCH EXAMPLES *Continued*

Critical Thinking Suggestions

1. Answer questions 1–9 from Box 16-2 regarding this study.

2. Also answer the following targeted questions, which may assist you in further assessing aspects of this study:

  a. Comment on the amount of data that had to be analyzed in this study.

  b. What parts of Spradley's analytic method appear to have been followed?

3. If the results of this study are valid and reliable, what are some of the uses to which the findings could be put in clinical practice?

 EXAMPLE 3: Analysis in a Phenomenological Study

1. Read the method and results section from the Beck study ("Birth Trauma") in Appendix B of this book, and then answer the relevant questions in Box 16-2.

2. Also consider the following targeted questions, which may further sharpen your critical thinking skills and assist you in assessing aspects of the study's merit:

  a. Comment on the amount of data that had to be analyzed in this study.

  b. If Beck had used Giorgi's method of phenomenological data analysis instead of Colaizzi's, would it have been appropriate for her to return to the mothers who participated in the study to validate the findings?

SUGGESTED READINGS

Methodologic References

Beck, C. T. (2004). Grounded theory. In J. Fain (Ed.), *Reading, understanding, and applying nursing research* (2nd ed.). Philadelphia: F. A. Davis.

Becker, H. S. (1970). *Sociological work*. Chicago: Aldine.

Benner, P. (1994). The tradition and skill of interpretive phenomenology in studying health, illness, and caring practices. In P. Benner (Ed.), *Interpretive phenomenology*. Thousand Oaks, CA: Sage Publications.

Colaizzi, P. (1978). Psychological research as the phenomenologist views it. In R. Valle & M. King (Eds.), *Existential phenomenological alternatives for psychology*. New York: Oxford University Press.

Crabtree, B. F., & Miller, W. L. (Eds.). (1999). *Doing qualitative research* (2nd ed.). Newbury Park, CA: Sage Publications.

DeSantis, L., & Ugarriza, D. N. (2000). The concept of theme as used in qualitative nursing research. *Western Journal of Nursing Research, 22*, 351–372.

Diekelmann, N., Allen, D., & Tanner, C. (1989). *The NLN criteria for appraisal of baccalaureate programs: A critical hermeneutic analysis*. New York: NLN Press.

Fetterman, D. M. (1989). *Ethnography: Step by step*. Newbury Park, CA: Sage Publications.

Gadamer, H. G. (1975). *Truth and method*. (G. Borden & J. Cumming, Trans.). London: Sheed and Ward.

Giorgi, A. (1985). *Phenomenology and psychological research*. Pittsburgh, PA: Duquesne University Press.

Glaser, B. G. (1978*). Theoretical sensitivity: Advances in the methodology of grounded theory*. Mill Valley, CA: Sociology Press.

Glaser, B. G., & Strauss, A. L. (1967). *The discovery of grounded theory: Strategies for qualitative research*. Chicago: Aldine.

King, N. (1998). Template analysis. In C. Cassell & G. Symon (Eds.), *Qualitative methods and analysis in organizational research*. London: Sage Publications.

Leininger, M. (2001). *Culture care diversity and universality: A theory of nursing*. Boston: Jones and Bartlett.

Morse, J. M., & Field, P. A. (1995). *Qualitative research methods for health professionals* (2nd ed.). Thousand Oaks, CA: Sage Publications.

Ricoeur, P. (1981). *Hermeneutics and the social sciences.* (J. Thompson, Ed. & Trans.). New York: Cambridge University Press.

Spradley, J. P. (1979). *The ethnographic interview.* New York: Holt, Rinehart, and Winston.

Strauss, A., & Corbin, J. (1998). *Basics of qualitative research: Techniques and procedures for developing grounded theory* (2nd ed.). Thousand Oaks, CA: Sage Publications.

Van Kaam, A. (1966). *Existential foundations of psychology.* Pittsburgh, PA: Duquesne University Press.

Van Manen, M. (1990). *Researching lived experience.* New York: State University of New York.

Studies Cited in Chapter 16

Anderson, E. H., & Spencer, M. H. (2002). Cognitive representation of AIDS: A phenomenological study. *Qualitative Health Research, 12,* 1338–1352.

Beck, C. T. (2002). Releasing the pause button: Mothering twins during the first year of life. *Qualitative Health Research, 12,* 593–608.

Beck, C. T. (2004). Birth trauma: In the eye of the beholder. *Nursing Research, 53,* 28–35.

Bent, K. N. (2003). "The people know what they want." An empowerment process of sustainable, ecological community health. *Advances in Nursing Science, 26,* 215–226.

Cheung, J., & Hocking, P. (2004). The experience of spousal carers of people with multiple sclerosis. *Qualitative Health Research, 14,* 153–166.

Clemmens, D. A. (2002). Adolescent mothers' depression after the birth of their babies: Weathering the storm. *Adolescence, 37,* 551–565.

Daggett, L. M. (2002). Living with loss: Middle-aged men face spousal bereavement. *Qualitative Health Research, 12,* 625–639.

Fletcher, C. E. (2004). Health care providers' perceptions of spirituality while caring for veterans. *Qualitative Health Research, 14,* 546–561.

Im, E., & Choe, M. (2004). Korean women's attitudes toward physical activity. *Research in Nursing & Health, 27,* 4–18.

King, N., Carroll, C., Newton, P., & Dornan, T. (2002). "You can't cure it so you have to endure it": The experience of adaptation to diabetic renal disease. *Qualitative Health Research, 12,* 329–346.

Knobf, M. T. (2002). Carrying on: The experience of premature menopause in women with early stage breast cancer. *Nursing Research, 51,* 9–17.

Manns, P. J., & Chad, K. E. (2001). Components of quality of life for persons with a quadriplegic and paraplegic spinal cord injury. *Qualitative Health Research, 11,* 795–811.

McDonald, D. D., Deloge, J., Josline, N., Petow, W., Severson, J., Votino, R., Shea, M., Drenga, J., Brennan, M., Moran, A., & Del Signore, E. (2003). Communicating end-of-life preferences. *Western Journal of Nursing Research, 25,* 652–666.

MacIntosh, J. (2003). Reworking professional nursing identity. *Western Journal of Nursing Research, 25,* 725–741.

Miller, J. E., & Petro-Nustas, W. (2002). Context of care for Jordanian women. *Journal of Transcultural Nursing, 13,* 228–236.

O'Brien, B., Evans, M., & White-McDonald, E. (2002). Isolation from "being alive": Coping with severe nausea and vomiting of pregnancy. *Nursing Research, 51,* 302–308.

Polit, D. F., London, A., & Martinez (2000). *Food security and hunger in poor, mother-headed families in four U.S. cities.* New York: MDRC, Inc.

Raingruber, B., & Kent, M. (2003). Attending to embodied responses: A way to identify practice based and human meanings associated with secondary trauma. *Qualitative Health Research, 13,* 449–468.

Tzeng, W., & Lipson, J. G. (2004). The cultural context of suicide stigma in Taiwan. *Qualitative Health Research, 14,* 345–358.

Wilde, M. H. (2002). Urine flowing: A phenomenological study of living with a urinary catheter. *Research in Nursing & Health, 25,* 14–24.

Wilde, M. H. (2003). Life with an indwelling urinary catheter: The dialectic of stigma and acceptance. *Qualitative Health Research, 13,* 1189–1204.

Critical Appraisal and Utilization of Nursing Research

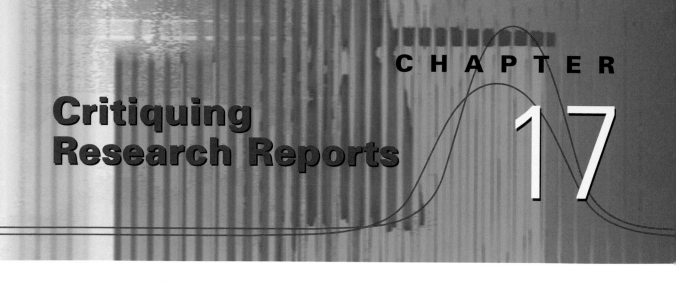

CHAPTER 17

Critiquing Research Reports

STUDENT OBJECTIVES

On completion of this chapter, the student will be able to:

▸ Describe aspects of a study's findings important to consider in developing an interpretation of quantitative and qualitative studies
▸ Evaluate researchers' interpretation of their results
▸ Describe the purposes and dimensions of a research critique
▸ Conduct a comprehensive critique of a qualitative or quantitative research report
▸ Define new terms in the chapter

Throughout this book, we have provided questions and suggestions for critiquing various aspects of nursing research reports. This chapter describes the purposes of a research critique and offers further tips on how to evaluate research reports. One important aspect of a research critique involves the reviewer's interpretation of the study findings. Therefore, we begin this chapter by offering some suggestions on interpreting research results.

INTERPRETING STUDY RESULTS

The analysis of research data provides the *results* of the study. These results need to be evaluated and interpreted, which is often a challenging task. *Interpretation* should take into consideration the study's aims, its theoretical underpinnings, the existing body of related research knowledge, and the limitations of the adopted research methods. The interpretive task involves a consideration of the following aspects of the study findings:

▶ The credibility and accuracy of the results
▶ The meaning of the results
▶ The importance of the results
▶ The extent to which the results can be generalized or have potential for use in other contexts
▶ The implications for practice, theory, or research

In this section, we review issues relating to these interpretive aspects for quantitative and qualitative research reports.

Interpreting Quantitative Results

Quantitative research results often offer the consumer more interpretive opportunities than qualitative ones—in large part, because a quantitative report summarizes most of the study data in statistical tables, whereas qualitative reports contain only illustrative examples of the data. When reading quantitative reports, you will need to give careful thought to the possible meaning behind the numbers. Your interpretations can then be compared with those of the researchers, who discuss their views on the meaning and implications of the study results in the Discussion section of their reports.

THE CREDIBILITY OF QUANTITATIVE RESULTS

One of the first tasks you will face in interpreting quantitative results is assessing their accuracy. A thorough assessment of the credibility of the results relies on critical thinking skills and on your understanding of research methods. The evaluation should be based on an analysis of evidence, not on personal opinions and "gut feelings." Both external and internal evidence can be brought to bear. External evidence comes primarily from the body of prior research. If the results are consistent, the credibility of the findings is enhanced. If the results are inconsistent with prior research, possible reasons for the discrepancy should be sought. What was different about the way the data were collected, the sample was selected, key variables were operationalized, extraneous variables were controlled, and so on? You should also consider whether the findings are consistent with common sense and with your own clinical experiences.

Internal evidence for the accuracy of the findings comes from an evaluation of the methods used. You will need to evaluate carefully all the major methodologic decisions made in planning and executing the study to determine whether alternative decisions might have yielded different results. This issue is discussed in greater detail later in this chapter.

A critical analysis of the research methods and conceptualization and an examination of various types of external and internal evidence almost inevitably indicate some limitations. These limitations must be taken into account in interpreting the results, and in contrasting your interpretation with that of the researchers themselves.

THE MEANING OF QUANTITATIVE RESULTS

In quantitative studies, the results are usually in the form of test statistic values and probability levels, which do not in and of themselves confer meaning. The statistical results must be translated conceptually and interpreted. In this section, we discuss the interpretation of research outcomes within a statistical hypothesis testing context.

CONSUMER TIP

Many research reports do not formally specify hypotheses, but rather present research questions or purpose statements (see Chapter 6). However, every time researchers use an inferential statistic (e.g., a *t*-test or chi-squared test), they are using statistics to test a hypothesis. The research hypothesis being tested almost invariably is that, in the population, the groups being compared are different or that variables are truly related. When hypotheses are not stated but statistical tests are performed, you may have to infer the hypotheses.

Interpreting Hypothesized Significant Results

When statistical tests support the researcher's hypotheses, the task of interpreting the results may be straightforward because the rationale for the hypotheses typically offers an explanation of what the findings mean. However, hypotheses can be correct even when the researcher's explanation of what is going on is not. As a reviewer, you will need to evaluate whether the researchers went beyond the data in interpreting the results. For example, suppose a nurse researcher hypothesized that a relationship exists between a pregnant woman's level of anxiety about the labor and delivery experience and the number of children she has already borne. The study data reveal that a negative relationship between anxiety levels and parity does exist ($r = -.40$; $p < .05$). The researcher concludes that childbirth experience reduces anxiety. Is this conclusion supported by the data? The conclusion seems logical, but, in fact, there is nothing within the data that leads to this interpretation. An important, indeed critical, research precept is: Correlation does not prove causation. The finding that two variables are related offers no evidence about which of the two variables—if either—caused the other. Alternative explanations for the findings should always be considered. If competing interpretations can be excluded on the basis of the data or previous research findings, so much the better, but interpretations should always be given adequate competition.

Throughout the interpretation process, you should bear in mind that the support of research hypotheses through statistical testing never constitutes proof of their veracity. Hypothesis testing is probabilistic, and it is always possible that obtained relationships were due to chance. Also, if there are reasons to question the study's credibility, there may also be reasons to challenge the findings.

Example of corroboration of a hypothesis

Harrison, Stuifbergen, Adachi, and Becker (2004) hypothesized that the stability of a marital relationship would influence the ability of people with multiple sclerosis to accept their disability. Consistent with the hypothesis, the researchers found in their longitudinal study of 399 participants (all of whom were married at the outset) that people who had remained married over the 6-year period had a higher acceptance of their disability at the end of the study than people whose marriages ended through separation, divorce, or widowhood. A further analysis revealed that the relationship was significant for men, but not for women.

This study is actually a good example of the challenges of interpreting quantitative findings in nonexperimental studies. There are several possible explanations for the pattern of findings. The researchers' interpretation was that marriage confers psychosocial benefits, a conclusion that they support with evidence from other studies. However, there is nothing in their data that would rule out the possibility that a person's difficulty accepting his or her disabilities led to marital discord. Another possibility is that the type of person who is most vulnerable to having trouble accepting the disability is also less capable than others of sustaining a relationship in the face of a stressful circumstance.

Interpreting Nonsignificant Results

Nonsignificant results pose interpretive problems. Standard statistical procedures are geared toward disconfirmation of the null hypothesis. Failure to reject a null hypothesis (i.e., obtaining results indicating no relationship between the independent and dependent variables) could occur for either of two reasons: (1) because the null hypothesis is true (i.e., there really is no relationship among research variables) or (2) because the null hypothesis is false (i.e., a true relationship exists but the data failed to reveal it). Neither you nor the researchers can know which of these situations prevails. In the first situation (a true null hypothesis), the problem is likely to be in the logical reasoning or the conceptualization that led the researcher to posit the hypotheses. The second situation (a false null hypothesis), by contrast, generally reflects methodologic limitations, such as internal validity problems, a small or atypical sample, or a weak statistical procedure. Thus, the interpretation must consider both substantive and methodologic reasons for nonsignificant results. Whatever the underlying cause, there is never justification for interpreting a retained null hypothesis as proof of a lack of relationship among variables. The safest interpretation is that nonsignificant findings represent a lack of evidence for either truth or falsity of the hypothesis.

Note, however, that there is a decided bias against publishing the results of studies in which the results are nonsignificant. This may reflect beliefs among those making publication decisions that nonsignificant results are likely to reflect methodologic limitations.

Example of nonsignificant results

Schultz, Andrews, Goran, Mathew, and Sturdevant (2003) compared treatments for reducing postoperative nausea and vomiting in gynecologic surgery patients. Subjects were randomly assigned to one of four groups (droperidol and acupressure bands; droperidol and placebo bands; placebo drug and acupressure bands; and placebo drugs and bands). It was hypothesized that fewer women in the combined modality group than in other groups would experience moderate to severe nausea and vomiting, but this hypothesis was not supported in this sample of 103 women.

Because statistical procedures are designed to provide support for the *rejection* of null hypotheses, they are not well-suited for testing actual research hypotheses about the *absence* of relationships between variables or about *equivalence* between groups. Yet sometimes this is exactly what researchers want to do—and this is especially true in clinical situations in which the goal is to determine if one practice is just as effective as another. When the actual *research* hypothesis is null (i.e., a prediction of no group difference or no relationship), stringent additional strategies must be used to provide supporting evidence. For one thing, it is imperative to perform a power analysis to demonstrate that the risk of a Type II error is small. There may also be clinical standards that can be used to corroborate that nonsignificant—but predicted—results can be accepted as consistent with the research hypothesis.

Example of nonsignificant results supporting a hypothesis

Medves and O'Brien (2004) conducted a clinical trial to test the hypothesis that thermal stability would be comparable for infants bathed for the first time by a parent and for those bathed by a nurse. As predicted, there was no difference in temperature change between newborns bathed by nurses or parents. The researchers provided additional support for concluding that heat loss is not associated with who bathes the newborn by indicating that a power analysis had been used to determine sample size needs. They noted that the parents for the two groups of infants were comparable demographically at the outset. Also, although the prebath temperatures of the infants in the two groups were significantly different, the researchers used initial temperature as a covariate to control these differences. Finally, they made an *a priori* determination that a change in temperature of 1° C would be clinically significant; at four points in time after the bath, the group differences in temperature were never this large; thus, the differences were clinically insignificant.

Interpreting Unhypothesized Significant Results

Although this does not often happen, there are situations in which researchers obtain significant results that are the opposite of the research hypothesis—that is, *unhypothesized significant results*. For example, a researcher might predict a negative relationship between patient satisfaction with nursing care and the length of stay in the hospital, but a significant *positive* relationship might be found. In such cases, it is less likely that the methods are flawed than that the reasoning or theory is incorrect. In attempting to explain such findings, you should pay particular attention to the results of previous research and alternative theories. It is also useful to consider, however, whether there is anything unusual about the sample that might have led participants to behave or respond atypically.

Example of unhypothesized significant results

Provencher, Perreault, St.-Onge, and Rousseau (2003) studied predictors of psychological distress in Canadian family caregivers of family members with psychiatric disabilities. Contrary to their hypothesis that social support would be beneficial, the researchers found that caregivers who perceived more support from friends experienced a higher level of distress than those who perceived less support. Also contrary to their predictions, relatives who had more contact with their relatives' primary mental health providers were more distressed than those with less contact.

Interpreting Mixed Results

The interpretive process is often complicated by *mixed results*: some hypotheses are supported by the data, whereas others are not. Or a hypothesis may be accepted when one measure of the dependent variable is used but rejected with a different measure. When only some results run counter to a theoretical position or conceptual scheme, the research methods are the first aspect of the study deserving critical scrutiny. Differences in the validity and reliability of the various measures may account for such discrepancies, for example. On the other hand, mixed results may suggest that a theory needs to be qualified, or that certain constructs within the theory need to be reconceptualized.

Example of mixed results

Stark (2003) used a strong quasi-experimental design to test whether an intervention—spending increased time in the natural environment—would improve concentration for women in the third trimester of pregnancy. She compared the scores of 29 women in the experimental group with those of 28 women in the comparison group on six tests of directed attention that required concentration skill. The hypothesis regarding the effectiveness of the intervention was supported for one test, but the groups were not significantly different on the other five.

THE IMPORTANCE OF QUANTITATIVE RESULTS

In quantitative studies, results supporting the hypotheses are described as being significant. A careful analysis of study results involves an evaluation of whether, in addition to being statistically significant, they are important.

The fact that statistical significance was attained in testing the hypothesis does not necessarily mean the results were of value. Statistical significance indicates that the results were unlikely to be a function of chance. This means that the observed group differences or observed relationships were probably real—but not necessarily important. With large samples, even modest relationships are statistically significant. For instance, with a sample of 500 subjects, a correlation coefficient of .10 is significant at the .05 level, but a relationship of this magnitude might have little practical value. As a reviewer, therefore, you should pay attention to the numeric values obtained in an analysis in addition to the significance level when assessing the implications of the findings.

Conversely, the absence of statistically significant results does not mean that the results are unimportant—although, because of problems in interpreting nonsignificant results, the case is more complex. Suppose we compared two methods of making a clinical assessment (e.g., pain) and retained the null hypothesis (i.e., found no statistically significant differences between the two methods). If the study involved a small sample, the nonsignificant results would be ambiguous. If a very large sample was used, however, the probability of a Type II error would be low. It might then reasonably be concluded that the two procedures yield equally accurate assessments. If one of these procedures were more efficient, less stressful, or less costly than the other, the nonsignificant findings could, indeed, be clinically important.

Another criterion for assessing the importance of quantitative research results concerns whether the findings are trivial or obvious. If the findings do little more than confirm common sense, their contribution to knowledge may be marginal.

It should be noted that, especially in an evidence-based practice environment, research findings need not necessarily reveal new information to be consequential. To build a strong base of knowledge upon which practice decisions will be made, replicated findings are quite important.

THE GENERALIZABILITY OF QUANTITATIVE RESULTS

Another aspect of quantitative results that you should assess is their generalizability. Researchers are not interested in discovering relationships among variables for a specific group of people at a specific point in time. The aim of most nursing research is to develop evidence for use in nursing practice. Therefore, an important interpretive question is whether the intervention will work or whether the observed relationships will hold in other settings, with other people. Part of the interpretive process involves asking the question: To what groups, environments, and conditions can the results of the study be applied?

THE IMPLICATIONS OF QUANTITATIVE RESULTS

After you have formed conclusions about the accuracy, meaning, importance, and generalizability of the results, you are ready to draw inferences about their implications. You might consider the implications of the findings with respect to future research (What should other researchers working in this area do—what is the right "next step"?) or theory development (What are the implications for nursing theory?). However, you are most likely to consider the implications for nursing practice (How, if at all, should the results be used by other nurses in their practice—or by me in my own work as a nurse?). Of course, if you have reached the conclusion that the results have limited credibility or importance, they may be of little utility to your practice.

Interpreting Qualitative Results

It is usually difficult for readers of a qualitative research report to interpret qualitative findings thoroughly because the researchers have necessarily had to be selective in the amount and types of data included for perusal. Nevertheless, you should strive to consider the same five interpretive dimensions for a qualitative study as for a quantitative one.

THE CREDIBILITY OF QUALITATIVE RESULTS

As with the case of quantitative reports, you should question whether the results of a qualitative inquiry are believable. It is reasonable to expect authors of qualitative reports to provide evidence of the credibility of the findings, as described in Chapter 14—although this does not always happen. Because readers of qualitative reports are exposed to only a portion of the data, they must rely on researchers' efforts to corroborate findings through such mechanisms as peer debriefings, member checks, audits, and triangulation.

CONSUMER TIP

Even when peer debriefings or member checks have been undertaken, you should realize that they do not unequivocally establish proof that the results are believable. For example, member checks may not always be effective in illuminating flaws. Perhaps some participants are too polite to disagree with the researcher's interpretations. Or perhaps they become intrigued with a conceptualization they themselves would never have developed on their own—a conceptualization that is not necessarily accurate. ▄

In thinking about the believability of qualitative results—as with quantitative results—it is advisable to adopt the posture of a person who needs to be persuaded about the researcher's conceptualization and to expect the researcher to marshal solid evidence with which to persuade you. It is also appropriate to consider whether the researcher's conceptualization of the phenomenon is consistent with common experiences and with your own clinical insights.

THE MEANING OF QUALITATIVE RESULTS

In qualitative studies, interpretation and analysis of the data occur virtually simultaneously. That is, researchers interpret the data as they categorize them, develop a thematic analysis, and integrate the themes into a unified whole. Efforts to validate the qualitative analysis are necessarily efforts to validate interpretations as well. Thus, unlike quantitative analyses, the meaning of the data flows from qualitative analysis.

Nevertheless, prudent qualitative researchers hold their interpretations up for closer scrutiny—self-scrutiny as well as review by peers and outside reviewers. Thus, for qualitative researchers as well as quantitative researchers, it is important to consider possible alternative explanations for the findings and to take into account methodologic or other limitations that could have affected study results.

Example of seeking alternative explanations

Cheek and Ballantyne (2001) studied family members' selection process for a long-term-care facility for elderly patients being discharged from an acute setting. In describing their methods, they explicitly noted that "attention throughout was paid to looking for rival or competing themes or explanations" (p. 225). In their analysis, they made a conscious effort to weigh alternatives.

THE IMPORTANCE OF QUALITATIVE RESULTS

Qualitative research is especially productive when it is used to describe and explain poorly understood phenomena. But the amount of prior research on a topic is not a sufficient barometer for deciding whether the findings can make a contribution to nursing knowledge. The phenomenon must be one that merits rigorous scrutiny. For example, some people prefer the color green and others like red. Color preference may not, however, be a sufficiently important topic for an in-depth inquiry. Thus, you must judge whether the topic under study is important or trivial.

In a critical evaluation of a study's importance, you should also consider whether the findings themselves are trivial. Perhaps the topic is worthwhile, but you may feel after reading the report that nothing has been learned beyond what is common sense or everyday knowledge—which can result when the data are too "thin" or when the conceptualization is shallow. Qualitative researchers often attach catchy labels to their themes and processes, but you should ask yourself whether the labels have really captured an insightful construct that goes beyond common knowledge.

THE TRANSFERABILITY OF QUALITATIVE RESULTS

Although qualitative researchers do not strive for generalizability, the application of the results to other settings and contexts must be considered. If the findings are only relevant to the people who participated in the study, they cannot be useful to nursing practice. Thus, in interpreting qualitative results, you should consider how transferable the findings are. In what other types of settings and contexts would you expect the phenomena under study to be manifested in a similar fashion? Of course, to make such an assessment, the author of the report must have described in sufficient detail the context in which the data were collected. Because qualitative studies are context bound, it is only through a careful analysis of the key parameters of the study context that the transferability of results can be assessed.

THE IMPLICATIONS OF QUALITATIVE RESULTS

If the findings are judged to be believable and important, and if you are satisfied with the interpretation of the meaning of the results, you can begin to consider what the implications of the findings might be. As with quantitative studies, the implications can be multidimensional. First, you can consider the implications for further research: Should a similar study be undertaken in a new setting? Can the study be expanded (or circumscribed) in meaningful or productive ways? Do the results suggest that an important construct has been identified that merits the development of a formal measuring instrument? Does the emerging theory suggest hypotheses that could be tested through controlled quantitative research? Second, do the findings have implications for nursing practice? For example, could the health care needs of a subculture (e.g., the homeless) be identified and addressed more effectively as a result of the study? Finally, do the findings shed light on fundamental processes that are incorporated into nursing theory?

RESEARCH CRITIQUES

If nursing practice is to be based on research evidence, the worth of studies appearing in the nursing literature must be critically appraised. Sometimes, consumers mistakenly believe that if a research report was accepted for publication, the study must be sound. Unfortunately, this is not necessarily the case. Indeed, most studies have limitations and weaknesses, and, for this reason, no single study can provide definitive answers to research questions. Nevertheless, the methods of disciplined inquiry continue to provide us with the best possible means of answering certain questions. Evidence is accumulated not by an individual researcher conducting a single, isolated study but rather through the conduct of several studies addressing the same or similar questions and through the subsequent critical appraisal of these studies by others. Thus, consumers who can thoughtfully critique research reports also play a role in the advancement of nursing knowledge.

Purposes of a Research Critique

A research **critique** is not just a summary of a study but rather a careful appraisal of its merits and flaws. Regardless of the scope or purpose of a critique, its function is not to hunt dogmatically for and expose mistakes. A good critique objectively identifies areas of adequacy and inadequacy, virtues as well as faults. Sometimes, the need for this balance is obscured by the terms *critique* and *critical appraisal*, which connote unfavorable observations. The merits of a study are as important as its limitations in coming to conclusions about the worth of its findings. Therefore, a research critique should reflect a thoughtful, objective, and balanced consideration of the study's validity and significance. Critiques can vary in scope, length, and form, depending on the underlying purpose. Three main types of critiques that are relevant to nursing research include critiques that are:

▶ undertaken by students to demonstrate their skills;
▶ conducted by other researchers (**peer reviewers**) to assist journal editors with publication decisions; and

▶ conducted by researchers whose intent is to evaluate the strength of evidence of related studies as part of an integrative review (including meta-analyses and metasyntheses).

There are other types of critiques, of course, some written and others more informal. For example, nurses are sometimes involved in journals clubs that convene to discuss and critique studies informally. Researchers are sometimes invited to prepare a written commentary for publication in a journal along with the report itself. For example, the *Western Journal of Nursing Research* often publishes several commentaries in each issue. However, these commentaries tend to be brief and selective, emphasizing a few key issues.

In this chapter we focus primarily on the type of critique that students undertake. We briefly describe the two other main types of critiques, however, because although you are developing skills now that are used primarily in student critiques, you may one day be part of an integrative review team or be called upon to be a peer reviewer.

The three types of critiques we consider here vary in terms of the salience of different types of questions. For example, all three types attach great importance to whether the study focused on a problem of importance to the nursing profession. Yet other aspects of a study are of more concern to some types of critiques than to others. For example, a meta-analyst would not be as concerned about the ethical aspects of a study (e.g., Was informed consent obtained?) as a student conducting a comprehensive critique. The emphases in a critique depend to a great degree on the overall purpose of conducting it.

STUDENT CRITIQUES

As a student, you are likely to be asked to prepare a critique of a research report as part of the course requirement. Such critiques are usually expected to be thorough and comprehensive, with attention paid to all five of the major dimensions of a report (substantive and theoretical; methodologic; ethical; interpretive; and presentational). The purpose of such a critique is to cultivate critical thinking, to induce you to use newly acquired skills in research methods, to obtain documentation of those skills, and to prepare you for a rewarding professional nursing career in which research will almost surely play a role. Writing research critiques is an important first step on the path to developing an evidence-based practice.

Although student critiques are comprehensive, involving the evaluation of all aspects of a report, there are a few critiquing questions that are typically less relevant for students than for others. For example, students are typically not required to be sufficiently knowledgeable about the substantive content of a report that they would be able to critically evaluate the thoroughness of its literature review. In other words, students would usually not be expected to have in-depth knowledge about the topic under study. Students also may not be expected to evaluate the qualifications of a research team, an issue that might have greater salience in other types of critiques.

Much of the remainder of this chapter presents materials that are relevant to comprehensive reviews such as those you are likely to undertake. The Student Resource CD-ROM—which contains a quantitative and qualitative research report, respectively—also includes comprehensive critiques that you can use as models.

PEER REVIEWS

Most nursing journals that publish research reports have a policy of independent, anonymous (sometimes referred to as **blind**) **reviews** by two or more peers who are experts in the field. By anonymous, we mean that the peer reviewers do not know the identity of the authors, and authors do not learn the identity of reviewers. Journals that have such a policy are **refereed journals**, and are generally more prestigious than **nonrefereed journals**. The journals *Nursing Research* and *Nursing in Research & Health* and many other journals cited in this book are refereed journals. Peer reviewers develop written critiques and make a recommendation about whether or not to publish the report.

Example of categories of recommendation for peer reviewers

The journal *Research in Nursing and Health* asks reviewers to make one of six recommendations to the editorial staff: (1) Highly recommend; few revisions needed; (2) Publish if suggested revisions are satisfactorily completed; (3) Major revisions needed; revised version should be re-reviewed; (4) May have potential; encourage resubmission as a new manuscript; (5) Reject; do not encourage resubmission; and (6) Not appropriate for journal; send to another type of journal.

Peer reviewers' critiques can address a wide array of concerns, but they typically are brief and focus primarily on key substantive and methodologic issues. However, reviewers also are expected to comment on prominent presentational deficiencies (for example, a confusing table or faulty organization) and noteworthy ethical issues. Peer reviewers' comments may be written in narrative, essay form or may take the form of a bulleted list of the study's strengths and weaknesses. Researchers typically revise their manuscripts based on the critiques that peer reviewers prepare, addressing to the extent possible the reviewers' suggestions for improvement.

Example of peer review comments

One of the authors (Polit), who is a regular reviewer for peer-reviewed nursing journals, was asked by one journal to review and critique a manuscript for a mixed-method study on a vulnerable population. Although the specifics of the study have been omitted to safeguard the identity of the researchers, a few of Polit's comments on the manuscript are presented in Table 17-1. Polit recommended that major revisions be undertaken before publication.

CONSUMER TIP

To help potential authors understand more fully the peer review process, the journal *Nursing Research* has taken steps to open the peer review process. On the *Nursing Research* website, an original manuscript by one of this book's authors (Beck) is posted, along with its reviews and the revised manuscript. Correspondence from the author and editor are also posted. See Open Manuscript Review highlighted on the journal's home page at http://sonweb.unc.edu/nursing-research-editor.

CRITIQUES FOR ASSESSING A BODY OF LITERATURE

Critiques of individual studies are sometimes undertaken as part of a formal, systematic evaluation of multiple studies on a topic. Such reviews are often undertaken with the aim of developing practice guidelines or drawing conclusions about the state of knowledge on which practice can be based. As described in Chapter 7, there are various ways of integrating findings on a topic from the research literature, including meta-analyses (for quantitative research) and metasyntheses (for qualitative

TABLE 17.1	Selected Comments from a Peer Review of a Manuscript on a Vulnerable Group

This manuscript describes a study about a very important population, namely (blank).* This is not only an important population, but one that is difficult to study, so the overall effort is commendable. Methodologically, the study had a number of strong points. I particularly liked the collection and analysis of both qualitative and quantitative data. However, the study has a number of flaws...

Substantive/theoretical:
▶ The paper states (p. 4) that a framework of (blank) guided this study. If it did, the guidance seems to be somewhat superficial. The...framework should have suggested some hypotheses, but none were offered. Similarly, the framework...should have been the centerpiece of the discussion of the findings...

▶ There are some peculiarities about the variables themselves. Why, for example, was *perceived* health the focus of the inquiry rather than actual health? Perhaps there is a good reason, but it should be made explicit. It would also be useful to know if... there is a correlation between actual and perceived health (i.e., does the perceived health status measure have validity).

Methodologic:
▶ The notion of triangulation is very appealing. But while the researchers collected both qualitative and quantitative data, the data were not integrated in any meaningful way. That is, the authors do not use the qualitative findings to illustrate correlations detected in the quantitative analysis, do not use the quantitative results to validate the themes from the qualitative analysis, etc. The findings need to be knit together in a more purposeful way.

▶ It was commendable that both the researcher and research associate independently analyzed the content of the qualitative materials.

▶ The quantitative results are impossible to interpret as they are presented because there is no context or comparative information. As but one example, the authors indicate on page 9 that the mean score on the (blank) scale was 26.97. What does this mean? Is it high or low? Are there any norms for this scale, or is there evidence from a study of a less vulnerable population regarding their scores?

* Specific names of variables, scales, frameworks, and so on have been purged to protect the authors' anonymity.

ones). In both cases, reviewers must draw conclusions about what is known about a topic or phenomenon, and most consider the quality of the studies included in the review.

Chapter 18, which focuses on the utilization of nursing research for evidence-based practice, discusses the important role of systematic, integrative reviews. These reviews, rather than being comprehensive, are highly focused on the methodologic dimension of studies and on the study findings. A person undertaking an integrative review as part of an EBP effort is not typically concerned with, for example, the thoroughness of the literature review in the individual reports, because it has no bearing on the quality of study's *evidence*.

Integrative reviews of a body of research typically do not involve narrative, written critiques of individual studies. More often, the people doing such reviews use a formal instrument for evaluating each study, often with quantitative ratings of different aspects of the study, so that appraisals across studies ("scores") can be compared and summarized. Many such instruments have been developed for use with quantitative research, as we discuss in Chapter 18. Each instrument uses somewhat different criteria for drawing conclusions about the worth of a study's evidence.

Although less has been done to develop formal scoring systems and checklists for evaluating the quality of evidence in qualitative research, work in this area has begun. One example is the system developed by Cesario, Morin, and Santa-Donato (2002) as part of a project to develop clinical guidelines by the Association of Women's Health, Obstetric, and Neonatal Nurses (AWHONN). Another tool is the Primary Research Appraisal Tool, which was developed for determining an individual study's eligibility for a metasynthesis (Paterson, Thorne, Canam, & Jillings, 2001).

Dimensions of a Research Critique

This section is designed to offer guidance primarily to those preparing a comprehensive and detailed written critique, such as the ones that students prepare in research courses. The goal of such critiques is to evaluate thoroughly the decisions the researcher made in conceptualizing, designing, and executing the study and in interpreting and communicating the results. Each study tends to have its own peculiar flaws because each researcher, in addressing the same or a similar research question, makes different decisions about how the study should be done. It is not uncommon for researchers who have made different *methodologic decisions* to arrive at different answers to the same research question. It is precisely for this reason that you as a consumer must be knowledgeable about research methods. You must be able to evaluate research decisions so that you can determine how much faith should be put in the study findings. You must ask: What other approaches could have been used to study this research problem? and, If another approach had been used, would the results have been more reliable, credible, or replicable? In other words, you need to evaluate the impact of the researcher's decisions on the study's ability to reveal the truth.

Much of this book has been designed to acquaint you with a range of methodologic options for the conduct of research—options on how to design a study, collect and analyze data, select a sample, and so on. We hope a familiarity with these options will provide you with the tools to challenge a researcher's decisions when it is appropriate to do so.

As previously noted, a comprehensive review involves an appraisal of five dimensions of a research report, each of which is discussed below. Specific critiquing guidelines for quantitative and qualitative studies are presented later in the chapter.

SUBSTANTIVE AND THEORETICAL DIMENSION

In preparing a critique, you need to determine whether the study was important in terms of the significance of the problem, the soundness of the conceptualizations, the appropriateness of the theoretical framework, and the insightfulness of the analysis and interpretation. The research problem should have obvious relevance to some aspect of nursing. It is not enough that a problem be interesting if it offers no possibility of contributing to nursing knowledge or improving nursing practice.

Another issue that has both substantive and methodologic implications is the congruence between the study question and the methods used to address it. There must be a good fit between the research problem on the one hand and the overall study design, data collection methods, and analytic approach on the other. Questions that deal with poorly understood phenomena, with processes, with the dynamics of a situation, or with in-depth description, for example, are usually best addressed with flexible designs, unstructured methods of data collection, and qualitative analysis. Questions that involve the measurement of well-defined variables, cause-and-effect relationships, or the effectiveness of some specific intervention, however, are usually better suited to more structured, quantitative approaches using designs that maximize research control.

A final issue to consider is whether the researcher has appropriately placed the research problem into a larger theoretical context. As we stressed in Chapter 8, researchers do little to enhance the value of a study if the connection between the research problem and a conceptual framework is contrived. But a research problem that is genuinely framed as a part of a larger intellectual problem can often make an especially important contribution to nursing knowledge.

METHODOLOGIC DIMENSION

Researchers make a number of important decisions regarding how best to answer their research questions or test their research hypotheses. It is your job as consumer to evaluate critically the consequences of those decisions. In fact, the heart of a research critique lies in the appraisal of the researchers' methodologic decisions. The quality of evidence that a study yields is inextricably linked to the researchers' choice of methods and strategies for study design and for collecting and analyzing data.

One thing to keep in mind in assessing a study's methods is that, because of practical constraints, researchers almost always make compromises between what is ideal and what is feasible. For example, a quantitative researcher might ideally like to have a sample of 500 subjects, but resources may prohibit a sample larger than 200. A qualitative researcher might recognize that 3 years of fieldwork would yield an especially rich and deep understanding of the culture or group under study, but cannot afford to devote this much time to the effort. In doing a critique, you cannot realistically demand that researchers always attain methodologic ideals, but you must evaluate how much damage has been done by failure to achieve them.

ETHICAL DIMENSION

In performing a comprehensive critique, you should consider whether there is evidence of ethical violations. If there are any potential ethical problems, you will need to consider the impact of those problems on the scientific merit of the study as well as on the subjects' well-being.

Sometimes ethical transgressions are inadvertent. For example, privacy and confidentiality can sometimes be compromised when interviews are conducted in participants' homes and other family members are nearby. In other cases, researchers are aware of potential ethical problems but consciously decide that the violation is minor in relation to the knowledge gained. For example, researchers may decide not to obtain informed consent from the parents of minor children attending a family planning clinic because such consent might discourage participation in the study and lead to a biased sample of clinic users; it could also violate the minors' right to confidential treatment at the clinic. When researchers knowingly elect not to follow the ethical principles outlined in Chapter 5, the decision itself, the researchers' rationale, and the likely effect of the decision on the study's rigor should be evaluated.

CONSUMER TIP

Sometimes ethical transgressions actually strengthen the methodologic rigor of a study, and so you may need to "pit" one dimension of the critique against another.

INTERPRETIVE DIMENSION

Research reports almost always conclude with a discussion, conclusions, or implications section. In this final section, researchers offer an interpretation of the findings, consider whether the findings are congruent with a conceptual framework or earlier research, and discuss what the findings might imply for nursing.

As a reviewer, you should be somewhat wary if the discussion section fails to point out any limitations. Researchers are in the best position to detect and assess the impact of sampling deficiencies, practical constraints, data quality problems, and so on, and it is a professional responsibility to alert readers to these difficulties. Moreover, when researchers note methodologic shortcomings, readers know that these limitations were considered in interpreting the results.

Example of researcher-noted limitations

Zalon (2004) conducted a study to examine the recovery patterns of older adults who have had major abdominal surgery. Data were collected from a sample of over 100 adults aged 60 or older. Zalon found that pain, depression, and fatigue were related to patients' self-perception of recovery and their functional status. She discussed some of the study limitations: "The group investigated in this study was not a random sample of abdominal surgery patients. Patients not discharged directly to a home setting were excluded. Some patients who declined participation or dropped out of the study indicated that they were 'too sick' to participate.... Thus, the participants in this study may have been relatively well as compared with abdominal surgery patients in general....A limitation of this study is that baseline data were not available because the participants did not complete the instruments preoperatively. Therefore, additional research including baseline data is recommended to describe the impact of surgery on recovery" (p. 105).

Of course, researchers are unlikely to note all relevant shortcomings of their own work. Thus, the inclusion of comments about study limitations in the discussion section, although important, does not relieve you of the responsibility of appraising methodologic and analytic decisions. Your task as reviewer is to contrast your own interpretation and assessment of limitations with those of the researchers, to challenge conclusions that do not appear to be warranted by the results, and to indicate how the study's evidence could have been enhanced.

It may be especially difficult for you to determine the validity of qualitative researchers' interpretations. To help readers understand the lens from which they interpreted their data, qualitative researchers ideally should mention whether they kept field notes or a journal of their actions and emotions during the investigation, discuss their own behavior and experiences in relation to the participants' experiences, and acknowledge any effects of their presence on data quality. You should look for such information in critiquing qualitative reports and drawing conclusions about the interpretations.

In addition to contrasting your interpretation with that of the researchers (when this is possible), your critique should also draw conclusions about the stated implications of the study. Some

CONSUMER TIP

Researchers are more likely to note limitations in their discussion section when their hypotheses are not supported or when their findings are inconsistent with findings from other studies. However, even when hypotheses are confirmed there are likely to be a number of limitations that should be considered in interpreting the findings and drawing conclusions from them.

■

BOX 17.1   **Guidelines for Critiquing the Discussion Section of a Research Report**

Interpretation of the Findings

1. Are all important results discussed? If not, what is the likely explanation for omissions?
2. Does the report discuss the limitations of the study and possible effects of the limitations on the results?
3. Are interpretations consistent with results? Do the interpretations take limitations into account? Do the interpretations suggest distinct biases?
4. What types of evidence are offered in support of the interpretation, and is that evidence persuasive? Are results interpreted in light of findings from other studies? Are results interpreted in terms of the study hypotheses and the conceptual framework?
5. In qualitative studies, are the findings interpreted within an appropriate social or cultural context?
6. Are alternative explanations for the findings mentioned, and is the rationale for their rejection presented?
7. In quantitative studies, does the interpretation distinguish between practical and statistical significance?
8. Are any unwarranted interpretations of causality made?
9. Are generalizations made that are not warranted?

Implications of the Findings and Recommendations

10. Do the researchers discuss the study's implications for clinical practice, nursing education, nursing administration, or nursing theory, or make specific recommendations?
11. If yes, are the stated implications appropriate, given the study's limitations and given the body of evidence from other studies? Are there important implications that the report neglected to include?

---

researchers make grandiose claims or offer unfounded recommendations on the basis of modest results. Some guidelines for evaluating researchers' interpretation and implications, which are typically included in the report's discussion section, are offered in Box 17-1.

PRESENTATION AND STYLISTIC DIMENSION

Although the worth of the study is primarily reflected in the dimensions discussed thus far, the manner in which the information is communicated in the research report is also fair game in a comprehensive critical appraisal. Box 17-2 summarizes points that should be taken into account in evaluating the presentation of a research report.

An important consideration is whether the research report has provided sufficient information for a thoughtful critique of the other dimensions. For example, if the report does not describe how participants were selected, reviewers cannot comment on the adequacy of the sample, but they can criticize the report's failure to include information on sampling. When vital pieces of information are missing, researchers leave readers little choice but to assume the worst because this would lead to the most cautious interpretation of the worth of the evidence.

The writing in a research report, as in any published document, should be clear, grammatical, concise, and well organized. Unnecessary jargon should be minimized. Inadequate organization is another presentation flaw in some research reports: Continuity and logical thematic development are critical to good communication of scientific information. Tables and figures should highlight key points and should be capable of "standing alone," without forcing readers

---

Box 17.2   Guidelines for Critiquing the Presentation of a Research Report

1. Does the report include a sufficient amount of detail to permit a thorough critique of the study's substantive, methodologic, ethical, and interpretive dimensions? Does the report neglect to include key aspects of the study's methods?
2. Is the report understandable to those with moderate research skills, or is it unnecessarily abstruse? Is research jargon or clinical jargon used when simpler language could have improved communication to a broad audience of nurses?
3. Does the report suggest any overt biases on the part of the researcher? Does the researcher convey the tentative nature of research findings (e.g., avoiding words liked "demonstrated" or "proved")?
4. Is the report well-organized, or is the presentation confusing? Is there a logical, orderly presentation of ideas? Are transitions smooth, and is the report characterized by continuity of thought and expression?
5. Is the report well-written and grammatical?
6. Does the report avoid sexist language? Does the report suggest any insensitivity to racial, ethnic, or cultural groups?
7. Does the report title adequately capture key concepts and the target population? Does the abstract adequately summarize the research problem, study methods, and key findings?

---

to scrutinize the text to grasp what they mean. Styles of writing do differ for qualitative and quantitative reports, and it is unreasonable to apply the standards considered appropriate for one paradigm to the other. Quantitative research reports are typically written in a more formal, impersonal fashion, using either the third person or passive voice to connote objectivity. Qualitative studies are likely to be written in a more literary style, using the first or second person and active voice to connote proximity and intimacy with the data and the phenomenon under study. Regardless of style, however, you should, as a reviewer, be alert to indications of overt biases, unwarranted exaggerations, emotionally laden comments, or melodramatic language.

In summary, the research report is meant to be an account of how and why a problem was studied and what results were obtained. The report should be accurate, clearly written, cogent, and concise. It should reflect scholarship, but not pedantry, and it should be written in a manner that piques the reader's interest and curiosity.

GUIDELINES FOR CRITIQUING RESEARCH REPORTS

Most chapters in this text have presented guidelines for evaluating various research decisions and aspects of written research reports. The guidelines presented a series of detailed questions, whose primary function was to encourage you to read particular sections of research reports carefully and critically. Hopefully, these thorough questions helped to reinforce the methodologic content of this book. However, you would seldom be expected to answer all of these questions in an overall critique of a research report. If you did this, the critique would be far longer than the report itself!

This section presents an abridged set of critiquing questions to assist you in evaluating quantitative and qualitative reports. We can begin by offering a few general suggestions. First, you will need to read the report you are critiquing at least twice, and you may need to read parts

> **Box 17.3   General Guidelines for Conducting a Written Research Critique**
>
> 1. The function of a critique is not to *describe* a study or to *summarize* the content of the report. A research critique should provide an appraisal of the worth of the study itself and the merits of the report.
> 2. Be sure to comment on the study's strengths *and* weaknesses. The critique should be a balanced analysis of the study's value, noting positive as well as negative aspects.
> 3. Avoid vague generalizations—give specific examples of the study's strengths and limitations, providing direct references or quotes with page numbers.
> 4. Justify your criticisms. Offer a rationale for how a limitation affected the quality of the study, and suggest an alternative approach that could have eliminated the problem—but be sure that your suggestions are practical.
> 5. Be as objective as possible. Try not to be overly critical of a study simply because, for example, your world view is inconsistent with the underlying paradigm or because your field of specialization is different from that of the researchers.
> 6. If you are writing a critique that the report authors themselves will receive, be sensitive to your tone and the sharpness of your criticisms, and avoid sarcasm.

of it several times. It may be helpful to skim the section titled "Reading and Summarizing Research Reports" in Chapter 4 of this book, which offers suggestions on how to carefully and actively read research reports. Obviously, the first step in preparing a critique is to understand what the report is saying.

It is sometimes helpful to create a preliminary list of the aspects of the study that you thought were well-done and those you viewed as problematic, without worrying too much initially about the organization of your thoughts. Once you have a preliminary list, you can organize it by arranging the items or bullets into a structure corresponding to the major sections of the report. You can then revise and augment your list by using the guidelines we provide later in this section.

When you are ready to do the actual write-up of the critique, it may be useful to begin by preparing an abstract or introductory summary that will give you—and the person reading your critique—an overall "road map." The abstract should succinctly state what your final conclusions are about the merits of the study and the degree of confidence that can be placed in the study findings. Then in the body of the critique, you will need to document the specific features that led you to those conclusions.

An important thing to remember is that it is appropriate to assume the posture of a skeptic when you are critiquing a report. Just as a careful clinician seeks evidence from research findings that certain practices are or are not effective, you as a reviewer should demand evidence from the report that the researchers' substantive and methodologic decisions were suitable.

Some additional broad tips for preparing a formal, written research critique are presented in Box 17-3.

Critiquing Quantitative Reports

Table 17-2 presents guidelines for critiquing quantitative research reports. The guidelines are organized using the IMRAD format, following the structure of most research reports (i.e., Introduction, Method, Results, and Discussion). The first column identifies the section of the

TABLE 17.2	Guide to an Overall Critique of a Quantitative Research Report	

ASPECT OF THE REPORT	DETAILED CRITIQUING GUIDELINES	BASIC QUESTIONS FOR A CRITIQUE
Title		▶ Was the title a good one, suggesting the research problem and the study population?
Abstract		▶ Does the abstract clearly and concisely summarize the main features of the report?
Introduction Statement of the problem	Box 6-1, page 126	▶ Is the problem stated unambiguously and is it easy to identify? ▶ Does the problem statement make clear the concepts and the population under study? ▶ Does the problem have significance for nursing? ▶ Is there a good match between the research problem and the paradigm and methods used? Is a quantitative approach appropriate?
Literature review	Box 7-1, page 146	▶ Is the literature review thorough, up-to-date, and based mainly on primary sources? ▶ Does the review summarize knowledge on the dependent and independent variables and the relationship between them? ▶ Does the literature review lay a solid basis for the new study?
Conceptual/ theoretical framework	Box 8-1, page 166	▶ Are key concepts adequately defined conceptually? ▶ Is there a conceptual/theoretical framework and is it appropriate? If not, is the absence of one justified?
Hypotheses or research questions	Box 6-1, page 126	▶ Are research questions and/or hypotheses explicitly stated? If not, is their absence justified? ▶ Are questions and hypotheses appropriately worded? ▶ Are the questions/hypotheses consistent with the literature review and the conceptual framework?
Method Research design	Box 9-1, page 202	▶ Was the most rigorous possible design used, given the study purpose? ▶ Were appropriate comparisons made to enhance interpretability of the findings? ▶ Was the number of data collection points appropriate? ▶ Did the design minimize threats to the internal and external validity of the study?
Population and sample	Box 12-1, page 277	▶ Was the population identified and described? Was the sample described in sufficient detail? ▶ Was the best possible sampling design used to enhance the sample's representativeness? ▶ Was the sample size adequate? Was a power analysis used to estimate sample size needs?

table continues on page 448

TABLE 17.2		**Guide to an Overall Critique of a Quantitative Research Report** (continued)

ASPECT OF THE REPORT	DETAILED CRITIQUING GUIDELINES	BASIC QUESTIONS FOR A CRITIQUE
Data collection and measurement	Box 13-2, page 303; Box 13-4, page 311; Box 13-5, page 314; Box 14-1, page 338	▶ Are the operational and conceptual definitions congruent? ▶ Were key variables operationalized using the best possible method (e.g., interviews, observations, and so on)? ▶ Were the specific instruments adequately described and were they good choices? ▶ Did the report provide evidence that the data collection methods yielded data that were high on reliability and validity?
Procedures	Box 13-6, page 315; Box 5-3, page 101	▶ If there was an intervention, was it adequately described and was it properly implemented? ▶ Were data collected in a manner that minimized bias? Were data collection staff appropriately trained? ▶ Were appropriate procedures used to safeguard the rights of study participants?
Results Data analysis	Box 15-2, page 387	▶ Were analyses undertaken to address each research question or test each hypothesis? ▶ Were appropriate statistical methods used, given the level of measurement of the variables, number of groups being compared, and so on? ▶ Was the most powerful analytic method used? (e.g., Did the analysis help to control for extraneous variables)?
Findings	Box 15-2, page 388	▶ Were the findings adequately summarized, with good use of tables and figures? ▶ Do the findings provide strong evidence regarding the research questions? Were Type I and Type II errors minimized?
Discussion Interpretation of the findings	Box 17-1, page 444	▶ Are all major findings interpreted and discussed within the context of prior research and/or the study's conceptual framework? ▶ Are the interpretations consistent with the results and with the study's limitations? ▶ Does the report address the issue of the generalizability of the findings?
Implications/ recommendations	Box 17-1, page 444	▶ Do the researchers discuss the implications of the study for clinical practice or further research—and are those implications reasonable and complete?
Global Issues Presentation	Box 17-2, page 445	▶ Was the report well-written, well-organized, and sufficiently detailed for critical analysis? ▶ Were you able to understand the study? Was the report written in a manner that makes the findings accessible to practicing nurses?

TABLE 17.2	**Guide to an Overall Critique of a Quantitative Research Report** (continued)	
ASPECT OF THE REPORT	**DETAILED CRITIQUING GUIDELINES**	**BASIC QUESTIONS FOR A CRITIQUE**
Summary assessment		▶ Despite any identified limitations, do the study findings appear to be valid—do you have confidence in the *truth* value of the results? ▶ Does the study contribute any meaningful evidence that can be used in nursing practice or that is useful to the nursing discipline?

report for which the questions are relevant. The next column provides cross-references to the more detailed guidelines in the earlier chapters of the book. And the final column lists some key critiquing questions that have broad applicability to quantitative studies.

A few comments about these guidelines are in order. First, the wording of the questions calls for a yes or no answer (although for some, it may well be that your answer will be "Yes, *but...*"). In all cases, the desirable answer is "yes"; that is, a "no" suggests a possible limitation and a "yes" suggests a strength. Therefore, the more "yeses" a study gets, the stronger it is likely to be. Thus, these guidelines can cumulatively suggest a global assessment: A report that has 25 "yeses" is likely to be superior to one that has only 10.

However, it is also important to realize that not all "yeses" and "nos" are equal. Some elements are far more important in drawing conclusions about the rigor of the study than others. For example, the inadequacy of a literature review is far less damaging to the validity of the study findings than the use of a design with internal validity problems. In general, the questions addressing the researchers' methodologic decisions (i.e., the questions under "Method," as well as questions relating to the statistical analysis) are especially important in evaluating the integrity of a study's evidence.

Although the questions in Table 17-2 elicit yes or no responses, your critique will obviously need to do more than point out what the study did and did not do. Each relevant issue needs to be discussed—and you will need to supply supporting evidence for your conclusions. For example, if you answered "no" to the question about whether the design minimized threats to the internal validity of the study, your critique should elaborate on why you said this—for example, by pointing out that the design was vulnerable to self-selection bias, and that the groups being compared might not have been comparable at the outset. Each time you answered one of the questions negatively, it might be profitable to review the more detailed questions presented in earlier chapters of the book.

CONSUMER TIP

There are many questions in these guidelines for which there are no totally objective answers. Even experts sometimes disagree about what the best methodologic strategies for a study are. Thus, you should not be afraid to "stick out your neck" to express an evaluative opinion—but do be sure that your comments have some basis in methodologic principles discussed in this book.

We must acknowledge that our simplified guidelines have a number of shortcomings. In particular, the guidelines are generic despite the fact that critiquing cannot really use a one-size-fits-all list of questions. Critiquing questions that are relevant to certain types of studies (e.g., experiments) do not fit into a set of general questions for all quantitative studies. For example, we have not included a question about whether subjects or research staff were blinded to experimental treatments because this question would not be relevant to most studies, which are nonexperimental. As another example, the issue of internal validity is not especially relevant for a purely descriptive study. Furthermore, many supplementary questions would be needed to thoroughly assess certain types of research—for example, mixed method studies. Thus, you will need to use some judgment about whether the guidelines are sufficiently comprehensive for the type of study you are critiquing.

Another word of caution is that we developed these guidelines based on our years of experience as researchers and research methodologists. They do not represent a formal, rigorously developed set of questions that can be used for a formal EBP-type critique. They should, however, facilitate your beginning efforts to critically appraise nursing studies.

Critiquing Qualitative Reports

Table 17-3 presents guidelines for you to use in critiquing qualitative research reports. These guidelines, like the ones in Table 17-2, are organized using the IMRAD format. Although qualitative reports are somewhat less likely than quantitative ones to follow this format, many of them do. In any event, it would still be possible to organize your critique using this structure, regardless of how the report is organized. Table 17-3 also presents, for each section, a series of questions and cross-references to more in-depth critiquing questions.

The comments about the guidelines for quantitative studies presented in the previous section are also relevant for critiquing qualitative ones. In particular, the difficulty with a "one-size-fits-all" approach is also salient for critiques of qualitative studies. Supplementary questions may be needed to fully critique studies within specific qualitative research traditions. Additional questions would be relevant for comprehensive critiques of, say, grounded theory studies (e.g., Did the categories describe the full range of the continuum of the process?)

In undertaking a critique of a qualitative study, you should keep in mind that richness and thoroughness of description are especially important. Rich detail is required in the description of the methods in part because of the lack of standardization in qualitative studies—readers need to have sufficient information with which to judge the researchers' approach. For example, in a quantitative study, it might be sufficient to say that the data analysis involved a series of *t*-tests, while in a qualitative report it is important to know, for example, how the data were coded, how coding categories were combined, who did the coding, whether there was intercoder agreement, and so on. Vivid description is also needed in presenting results in qualitative studies, because without descriptive clarity and eloquence, readers cannot grasp the nuances and complexities of the phenomenon under study. Qualitative studies can be a "gold mine for clinical insights" (Kearney, 2001, p. 146) only when the presentation is richly detailed and powerfully narrated.

As noted earlier, formal systems have been proposed to evaluate the quality of evidence in qualitative studies, and these approaches are typically not organized according to sections of a report but rather according to a number of cross-cutting themes. For example, Cesario and her colleagues (2002), who were involved with the AWHONN practice guideline

TABLE 17.3	Guide to an Overall Critique of a Qualitative Research Report	
ASPECT OF THE REPORT	**DETAILED CRITIQUING GUIDELINES**	**BASIC QUESTIONS FOR A CRITIQUE**
Title		▶ Was the title a good one, suggesting the key phenomenon and the group or community under study?
Abstract		▶ Does the abstract clearly and concisely summarize the main features of the report?
Introduction Statement of the problem	Box 6-1, page 126	▶ Is the phenomenon of interest clearly identified? ▶ Is the problem stated unambiguously and is it easy to identify? ▶ Does the problem have significance for nursing? ▶ Is there a good match between the research problem and the paradigm and methods used? Is a qualitative approach appropriate?
Literature review	Box 7-1, page 146	▶ Does the report summarize the existing body of knowledge related to the problem or phenomenon of interest? ▶ Is the literature review adequate? ▶ Does the literature review lay a solid basis for the new study?
Conceptual underpinnings	Box 8-1, page 166	▶ Are key concepts adequately defined conceptually? ▶ Is the philosophical basis, underlying tradition, conceptual framework, or ideological orientation made explicit and is it appropriate for the problem?
Research questions	Box 6-1, page 126	▶ Are research questions explicitly stated? If not, is their absence justified? ▶ Are the questions consistent with the study's philosophical basis, underlying tradition, conceptual framework, or ideological orientation?
Method Research design and research tradition	Box 10-1, page 228	▶ Is the identified research tradition (if any) congruent with the methods used to collect and analyze data? ▶ Was an adequate amount of time spent in the field or with study participants? ▶ Did the design unfold in the field, allowing researchers to capitalize on early understandings? ▶ Was there evidence of reflexivity in the design? ▶ Was there an adequate number of contacts with study participants?
Sample and setting	Box 12-2, page 278	▶ Was the group or population of interest adequately described? Were the setting and sample described in sufficient detail? ▶ Was the approach used to gain access to the site or to recruit participants appropriate? ▶ Was the best possible method of sampling used to enhance information richness and address the needs of the study? ▶ Was the sample size adequate? Was saturation achieved?

table continues on page 452

TABLE 17.3	**Guide to an Overall Critique of a Qualitative Research Report** (continued)	

ASPECT OF THE REPORT	DETAILED CRITIQUING GUIDELINES	BASIC QUESTIONS FOR A CRITIQUE
Data collection	Box 13-2, page 303; Box 13-4, page 311	▶ Were the methods of gathering data appropriate? Were data gathered through two or more methods to achieve triangulation? ▶ Did the researcher ask the right questions or make the right observations, and were they recorded in an appropriate fashion? ▶ Was a sufficient amount of data gathered? Was the data of sufficient depth and richness?
Procedures	Box 13-6, page 315; Box 5-3, page 101	▶ Were data collection and recording procedures adequately described and do they appear appropriate? ▶ Were data collected in a manner that minimized bias or behavioral distortions? Were data collection staff appropriately trained? ▶ Were appropriate procedures used to safeguard the rights of study participants?
Enhancement of rigor	Box 14-2, page 338	▶ Were methods used to enhance the trustworthiness of the data (and analysis), and was the description of those methods adequate? ▶ Were the methods used to enhance credibility appropriate and sufficient? ▶ Did the researcher document research procedures and decision processes sufficiently that findings are auditable and confirmable?
Results Data analysis	Box 16-1, page 401	▶ Were the data management (e.g., coding) and data analysis methods sufficiently described? ▶ Was the data analysis strategy compatible with the research tradition and with the nature and type of the data gathered? ▶ Did the analysis yield an appropriate "product" (e.g., a theory, taxonomy, thematic pattern, etc.)? ▶ Did the analytic procedures suggest the possibility of biases?
Findings	Box 16-1, page 401	▶ Were the findings effectively summarized, with good use of excerpts? ▶ Do the themes adequately capture the meaning of the data? Does it appear that the researcher satisfactorily conceptualized the themes or patterns in the data? ▶ Did the analysis yield an insightful, provocative, and meaningful picture of the phenomenon under investigation?
Theoretical integration	Box 16-1, page 401	▶ Are the themes or patterns logically connected to each other to form a convincing and integrated whole? ▶ Were figures, maps, or models used effectively to summarize conceptualizations? ▶ If a conceptual framework or ideological orientation guided the study, are the themes or patterns linked to it in a cogent manner?

TABLE 17.3	Guide to an Overall Critique of a Qualitative Research Report (continued)	
ASPECT OF THE REPORT	**DETAILED CRITIQUING GUIDELINES**	**BASIC QUESTIONS FOR A CRITIQUE**
Discussion Interpretation of the findings	Box 17-1, page 444	▶ Are the findings interpreted within an appropriate social or cultural context? ▶ Are major findings interpreted and discussed within the context of prior studies? ▶ Are the interpretations consistent with the study's limitations? ▶ Does the report address the issue of the transferability of the findings?
Implications/ recommendations	Box 17-1, page 444	▶ Do the researchers discuss the implications of the study for clinical practice or further inquiry—and are those implications reasonable?
Global Issues Presentation	Box 17-2, page 445	▶ Was the report well-written, well-organized, and sufficiently detailed for critical analysis? ▶ Was the description of the methods, findings, and interpretations sufficiently rich and vivid?
Summary assessment		▶ Do the study findings appear to be trustworthy—do you have confidence in the *truth* value of the results? ▶ Does the study contribute any meaningful evidence that can be used in nursing practice or that is useful to the nursing discipline?

development project, used five broad categories that were suggested by Burns (1989) for rating the quality of qualitative studies: descriptive vividness, methodologic congruence, analytic precision, theoretical connectedness, and heuristic relevance. Our guidelines cover most of the same issues and questions as were included in this rating system, but we think students may have an easier time using our less abstract structure.

CHAPTER REVIEW

Key new terms introduced in the chapter, together with a summary of major points, are presented in this section. In addition, Chapter 17 of the *Study Guide to Accompany Essentials of Nursing Research,* 6th edition offers various exercises and study suggestions for reinforcing the concepts presented in this chapter. For additional review, see the Student Self-Study Review Questions section of the Student Resource CD-ROM provided with this book.

KEY NEW TERMS

Blind review Peer reviewers
Critique Refereed journal
Nonrefereed journal

SUMMARY POINTS

◊ The *interpretation* of research findings is a search for the broader meaning and implications of the results of an investigation.

◊ Interpretation of both qualitative and quantitative results typically involves: (1) analyzing the credibility of the results; (2) determining their meaning; (3) considering their importance; (4) determining the generalizability or transferability of the findings; and (5) assessing the implications in regard to theory, nursing practice, and future research.

◊ A research **critique** is a careful, critical appraisal of the strengths and limitations of a study to draw conclusions about the worth of the evidence and its significance to nursing.

◊ Critiques are done for a variety of purposes, including comprehensive critiques by students to demonstrate their research skills; assessments by **peer reviewers** to assist journal editors with publication decisions; and critiques done as part of an integrated review.

◊ Peer reviewers who critique studies for a **refereed journal** often do **blind reviews** in which the reviewers do not learn the identity of the researchers, and vice versa.

◊ Critiques of individual studies done in an effort to come to conclusions about a body of literature (e.g., those done by a meta-analyst) often involve the use of a structured instrument or scale to rate aspects of study quality.

◊ A reviewer preparing a comprehensive review should consider five major dimensions of the study: the substantive and theoretical, methodologic, ethical, interpretive, and presentation and stylistic dimensions.

◊ Researchers designing a study must make a number of important *methodologic decisions* that affect the quality and integrity of the research. Consumers preparing a critique must evaluate the decisions the researchers made to determine how much faith can be placed in the results.

◊ When undertaking a critique, it is appropriate to assume the posture of a skeptic who demands evidence from the report that the conclusions are credible and significant.

RESEARCH EXAMPLES | **Critical Thinking Activities**

 EXAMPLE 1: Interpretation of Quantitative Findings

1. Read the Discussion section from Motzer et al.'s study ("Sense of Coherence") in Appendix A of this book, and then answer the relevant questions in Box 17-1.

2. Also consider the following targeted questions, which may further sharpen your critical thinking skills and assist you in assessing aspects of the report's merit:

   a. Comment on the following sentence in the report (fifth paragraph in the Discussion): "Holistic QOL is significantly lower for women aged 19–49 with IBS compared to control women."

   b. If you were making a recommendation for how a future study on this topic should be designed, what would you suggest in terms of research design, sampling, data collection, and analysis?

   c. Can you think of potential clinical implications for the study (assuming that the results have both internal and external validity)?

 EXAMPLE 2: Interpretation of Qualitative Findings

1. Read the Discussion section from Beck's study ("Birth Trauma") in Appendix B of this book, and then answer the relevant questions in Box 17-1.

RESEARCH EXAMPLES *Continued*

2. Also consider the following targeted questions, which may further sharpen your critical thinking skills and assist you in assessing aspects of the study's merit:

    a. Suggest two future studies that researchers could conduct based on the findings of Beck's birth trauma study. One study should be quantitative and one study should be qualitative.

    b. Suggest a qualitative study that would increase the transferability of Beck's findings.

 EXAMPLE 3: Critique of a Quantitative Study

Read the full study "Beneficial Effects of Noetic Therapies," on the Student Resource CD-ROM, and then address the following activities and questions.

1. Before reading our critique, which accompanies the full report on the CD-ROM, either write your own critique or prepare a list of what you think are the major strengths and weaknesses of the study. Then contrast your critique or list with ours. Remember that you (or your instructor) do not necessarily have to agree with all of the points made in our critique and that you may identify strengths and weaknesses that we overlooked.

2. Using the guidelines in Table 17-2, how many "yes" ratings would you give the study? Compare your "score" with that of other classmates.

3. In selecting studies to include in this textbook, we avoided choosing a poor-quality study—which would have been much easier to critique. We did not, however, wish to create a publicly embarrassing situation for any member of the nursing research community. In the questions below, we offer some "pretend" scenarios in which the researchers for the first study on the CD-ROM made different methodologic decisions than the ones they in fact did make. Write a paragraph or two critiquing these "pretend" decisions, pointing out how these alternatives would have affected the quality of the study.

    a. Pretend that the researchers had been unable to randomize subjects to treatments and had also been unable to get preintervention ratings of subjects' moods. The design, in other words, would be a posttest-only quasi-experiment, with treatments administered to groups of patients who were not in a treatment on a random basis.

    b. Pretend that the researchers had administered only seven VASs—everything except "worry."

    c. Pretend that the researchers had used ANOVA rather than ANCOVA to analyze their data

 EXAMPLE 4: Critique of a Qualitative Study

Read the full study ("Carrying On"), on the Student Resource CD-ROM, and then address the following activities and questions.

1. Before reading our critique, which accompanies the full report on the CD-ROM, either write your own critique or prepare a list of what you think are the major strengths and weaknesses of the study. Then contrast your critique or list with ours. Remember that you (or your instructor) do not necessarily have to agree with all of the points made in our critique and that you may identify strengths and weaknesses that we overlooked.

2. Using the guidelines in Table 17-3, how many "yes" ratings would you give the study? Compare your "score" with that of other classmates.

research examples continue on page 456

RESEARCH EXAMPLES *Continued*

3. As noted in Example 3, we purposely selected good-quality studies to feature in this textbook. In the questions below, we offer some "pretend" scenarios in which the researcher for the study made different methodologic decisions than the ones she in fact did make. Write a paragraph or two critiquing these "pretend" decisions, pointing out how these alternatives would have affected the quality of the study.

a. Pretend that Knobf had used structured questionnaires rather than unstructured interviews to gather her data.

b. Pretend that Knobf had used a convenience sample.

c. Pretend that Knobf had interviewed 10 women.

SUGGESTED READINGS

Methodologic References

Beck, C. T. (1990). The research critique: General criteria for evaluating a research report. *Journal of Obstetric, Gynecologic, and Neonatal Nursing, 19,* 18–22.

Beck, C. T. (1993). Qualitative research: The evaluation of its credibility, fittingness, and auditability. *Western Journal of Nursing Research, 15,* 263–266.

Burns, N. (1989). Standards for qualitative research. *Nursing Science Quarterly, 2,* 254–260.

Cesario, S., Morin, K., & Santa-Donato, A. (2002). Evaluating the level of evidence of qualitative research. *Journal of Obstetrics, Gynecologic, & Neonatal Nursing, 31,* 708–714.

Kearney, M. H. (2001). Levels and applications of qualitative research evidence. *Research in Nursing & Health,* 145–153.

Paterson, B. L., Thorne, S. E., Canam, C., & Jillings, C. (2001). *Meta-study of qualitative health research.* Thousand Oaks, CA: Sage Publications.

Studies Cited in Chapter 17

Cheek, J., & Ballantyne, A. (2001). Moving them on and in: The process of searching for and selecting an aged care facility. *Qualitative Health Research, 11,* 221–237.

Harrison, T., Stuifbergen, A., Adachi, E., & Becker, H. (2004). Marriage, impairment, and acceptance in persons with multiple sclerosis. *Western Journal of Nursing Research, 26,* 266–285.

Medves, J. M., & O'Brien, B. (2004). The effect of bather and location of first bath on maintaining thermal stability in newborns. *Journal of Obstetric, Gynecologic, & Neonatal Nursing, 33,* 175–182.

Provencher, H. L., Perreault, M., St.-Onge, M., & Rousseau, M. (2003). Predictors of psychological distress in family caregivers of persons with psychiatric disabilities. *Journal of Psychiatric and Mental Health Nursing, 10,* 592–607.

Schultz, A. A., Andrews, A. L., Goran, S. F., Mathew, T., & Sturdevant, N. (2003). Comparison of acupressure bands and droperidol for reducing post-operative nausea and vomiting in gynecologic surgery patients. *Applied Nursing Research, 16,* 256–265.

Stark, M. A. (2003). Restoring attention in pregnancy: The natural environment. *Clinical Nursing Research, 12,* 246–265.

Zalon, M. L. (2004). Correlates of recovery among older adults after major abdominal surgery. *Nursing Research, 53,* 99–106.

Using Research in Evidence-Based Nursing Practice

STUDENT OBJECTIVES

On completion of this chapter, you will be able to:

▶ Distinguish research utilization (RU) and evidence-based practice (EBP) and discuss their
   current status within nursing
▶ Identify barriers to utilizing nursing research and strategies for improving RU and EBP
▶ Identify several models that have relevance for RU and EBP and describe the general
   steps in an RU or EBP project
▶ Discuss the role that integrative reviews play in EBP and describe basic steps in undertak-
   ing such a review
▶ Critique an integrative review
▶ Define new terms in the chapter

M ost nurse researchers would like to have their findings incorporated into nursing protocols and curricula, and most nurses working in clinical settings are aware of the benefits of research-based practice. There is a growing interest in basing specific nursing
actions on solid evidence confirming that the actions are clinically appropriate, cost-effective,
and beneficial for clients. In this chapter, we discuss various aspects of using nursing research to
support an evidence-based practice.

RESEARCH UTILIZATION AND
EVIDENCE-BASED PRACTICE

The term **research utilization** is sometimes used synonymously with **evidence-based practice**.
While there is an overlap between the two concepts, they are, in fact, distinct. Evidence-based
practice (EBP), the broader of the two terms, involves making clinical decisions on the basis of
the best possible evidence. The best evidence usually comes from rigorous research, but EBP
also uses other sources of credible information. A basic feature of EBP is that it de-emphasizes
decision-making based on custom, authority opinion, or ritual. Rather, the emphasis is on identifying the best available research evidence and *integrating* it with clinical expertise, patient
input, and existing resources.

Broadly speaking, research utilization (RU) refers to the use of the findings from a disciplined study or set of studies in a practical application that is unrelated to the original research.
In projects that have had research utilization as a goal, the emphasis is on translating empirically
derived knowledge into real-world applications. Figure 18-1 provides a basic schema of how RU
and EBP are interrelated. This section further explores and distinguishes the two concepts.

The Utilization of Nursing Research

During the 1980s and early 1990s, RU became an important buzz word, and several changes in
nursing education and nursing research were prompted by the desire to develop a knowledge base
for nursing practice. Nursing schools increasingly began to include courses on research methods

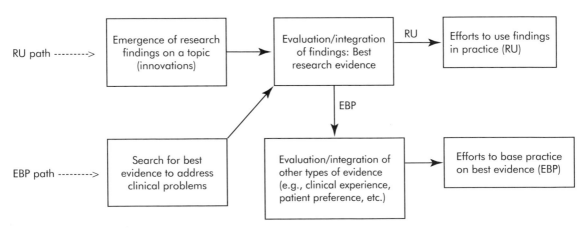

FIGURE 18.1 Research utilization (RU) and evidence-based practice (EBP).

so that students would become intelligent research consumers, and researchers shifted their focus toward clinical nursing problems. These changes, coupled with the completion of several large research utilization projects, played a role in sensitizing the nursing community to the desirability of using research as a basis for practice; the changes were not enough, however, to lead to widespread integration of research findings into the delivery of nursing care. Research utilization, as the nursing community has come to recognize, is a complex and nonlinear phenomenon that poses professional challenges.

THE RESEARCH UTILIZATION CONTINUUM

As Figure 18-1 indicates, the start-point of research utilization is new knowledge and new ideas that emerge from systematic research. When studies are undertaken, knowledge on a topic accumulates over time. In turn, knowledge works its way into use—to varying degrees and at differing rates.

Theorists who have studied the phenomenon of knowledge development and the diffusion of ideas recognize a continuum in terms of the specificity of the use to which research findings are put. At one end of the continuum is **instrumental utilization** (Caplan & Rich, 1975), which refers to discrete, clearly identifiable attempts to base specific actions on research findings. For example, a series of studies in the 1960s and 1970s demonstrated that the optimal placement time of a glass thermometer for accurate oral temperature determination is 9 minutes. When nurses specifically altered their behavior from shorter placement times to the empirically based recommendation of 9 minutes, this constituted an instance of research utilization at this end of the continuum.

Research findings can, however, be used in a more diffuse manner—in a way that promotes cumulative awareness, understanding, or enlightenment. Caplan and Rich (1975) refer to this end of the utilization continuum as **conceptual utilization**. Thus, a practicing nurse may read a qualitative research report describing *courage* among individuals with long-term health problems as a dynamic process that includes efforts to fully accept reality and to develop problem-solving skills. The nurse may be reluctant to alter his or her own behavior or suggest an intervention based on the results, but the study may make the nurse more observant in working with patients with long-term illnesses; it may also lead to informal efforts to promote problem-solving skills. Conceptual utilization, then, refers to situations in which users are influenced in their thinking about an issue based on their knowledge of studies but do not put this knowledge to any specific, documentable use.

The middle ground of this continuum involves the partial impact of research findings on nursing activities. This middle ground frequently is the result of a slow evolutionary process that does not reflect a conscious decision to use an innovative procedure but rather reflects what Weiss (1980) has termed knowledge creep and decision accretion. *Knowledge creep* refers to an evolving "percolation" of research ideas and findings. *Decision accretion* refers to the manner in which momentum for a decision builds over a period of time based on accumulated information gained through readings, informal discussions, meetings, and so on. Increasingly, however, nurses *are* making conscious decisions to use research in their clinical practice, and the EBP movement has contributed to this change.

Estabrooks (1999) studied research utilization by collecting survey data from 600 nurses in Canada. She found evidence to support three distinct types of research utilization: (1) *indirect research utilization*, involving changes in nurses' thinking and therefore analogous to conceptual utilization; (2) *direct research utilization*, involving the direct use of findings in giving patient care and therefore analogous to instrumental utilization; and (3) *persuasive utilization*, involving the use of findings to persuade others (typically those in decision-making positions) to make changes in policies or practices relevant to nursing care.

These varying ways of thinking about research utilization clearly suggest that both qualitative and quantitative research can play key roles in guiding and improving nursing practice. Indeed, Estabrooks (2001) has argued that the process of implementing research findings into practice is essentially the same for both quantitative and qualitative research. However, Estabrooks claims that qualitative research may have a privileged position in research utilization. Clinicians do not need a strong background in statistics to understand qualitative research, and thus using qualitative results is more readily accomplished.

RESEARCH UTILIZATION IN NURSING PRACTICE

During the 1980s and 1990s, there was considerable concern that nurses had failed to use research findings as a basis for making decisions and for developing nursing interventions. This concern was based on some studies suggesting that nurses were not always aware of research results or did not incorporate results into their practice. For example, Ketefian (1975) reported on the oral temperature determination practices of 87 registered nurses. As noted, there was solid evidence that the optimal placement time with glass thermometers is 9 minutes. Ketefian's study was undertaken to learn what "happens to research findings relative to nursing practice after five or ten years of dissemination in the nursing literature" (p. 90). In Ketefian's study, only 1 out of 87 nurses reported the correct placement time, suggesting that these practicing nurses were unaware of or ignored the research findings. Other studies in the 1980s (e.g., Kirchhoff, 1982), were similarly discouraging.

Coyle and Sokop (1990) investigated practicing nurses' adoption of 14 nursing innovations that had been reported in the nursing research literature, replicating a study by Brett (1987). The 14 innovations were selected based on the studies' strong scientific merit, their significance for nursing practice, and the suitability of the findings for adoption in clinical settings. A sample of 113 nurses practicing in 10 hospitals (randomly selected from the medium-sized hospitals in North Carolina) completed questionnaires that measured the nurses' awareness and use of the study findings. The results indicated much variation across the 14 innovations, with awareness of them ranging from 34% at one extreme to 94% at the other. Coyle and Sokop used a scheme to categorize each innovation according to its stage of adoption: awareness (indicating knowledge of the innovation); persuasion (indicating the nurses' belief that nurses should use the innovation in practice); occasional use in practice; and regular use in practice. Only 1 of the 14 studies was at the regular-use stage of adoption. Six studies were in the persuasion stage, indicating

Example from Coyle and Sokop's Study

One of the innovations included in Coyle and Sokop's (1990) study was the following: "Elimination of lactose from the formulas of tube-feeding diets for adult patients minimizes diarrhea, distention, flatulence, and fullness, and reduces patient rejection of feedings," a finding reported in a 1978 study. This innovation was characterized as being in the "Awareness" stage of adoption, with 38% of respondents aware of the findings (versus 19% who always used the findings). By contrast, the following was in the "Occasional use" stage of adoption, with 48% of respondents saying they used the findings (from a 1982 study) sometimes: "A formally planned and structured preoperative education program preceding elective surgery results in improved patient outcomes."

that the nurses knew of the innovation and thought it *should* be incorporated into nursing practice but were not basing their own nursing decisions on it.

More recently, a Canadian study by Varcoe and Hilton (1995) with 183 nurses found that 9 of the 10 research-based practices investigated were used by 50% or more of the acute care nurses at least sometimes. Rutledge, Greene, Mooney, Nail, and Ropka (1996) studied the extent to which oncology staff nurses adopted eight research-based practices. They found that awareness levels were high in their sample of over 1000 nurses: Between 53% and 96% reported awareness of the eight practices, and almost 90% of aware nurses used seven of them at least some of the time. Similar results have been reported in a recent survey of nearly 1000 nurses in Scotland (Rodgers, 2000).

The results of the recent studies are more encouraging than the studies by Ketefian and Kirchhoff because they suggest that, on average, practicing nurses are aware of many innovations based on research results, are persuaded that the innovations should be used, and are beginning to use them at least on occasion.

EFFORTS TO IMPROVE UTILIZATION OF NURSING RESEARCH

The need to reduce the gap between nursing research and nursing practice has been hotly discussed and has led to numerous formal attempts to bridge the gap. In this section, we briefly describe a few of these projects.

The best-known of several early nursing research utilization projects is the **Conduct and Utilization of Research in Nursing (CURN) Project**, a 5-year development project awarded to the Michigan Nurses' Association by the Division of Nursing in the 1970s. The major objective of the project was to increase the use of research findings in the daily practice of nurses by disseminating current research findings, facilitating organizational changes needed to implement innovations, and encouraging collaborative clinical research. One CURN activity was to stimulate the conduct of research in clinical settings. The project also focused on helping nurses to use research findings in their practice. CURN project staff saw research utilization as primarily an organizational process, with the commitment of organizations that employ nurses as essential to the research utilization process (Horsley, Crane, & Bingle, 1978). The project team concluded that research utilization by practicing nurses is feasible, but only if the research is relevant to practice and if the results are broadly disseminated. The CURN project generated considerable international interest. For example, the Cross Cancer Institute in Edmonton, Alberta, used the CURN model as a framework to integrate research findings into nursing practice (Alberta Association of Registered Nurses, 1997).

During the 1980s and 1990s, utilization projects were undertaken by a growing number of hospitals and organizations, and descriptions of these projects began to appear regularly in the nursing research literature. These projects were generally institutional attempts to implement a change in nursing practice on the basis of research findings and to evaluate the effects of the innovation. However, during the 1990s, the call for research utilization began to be superseded by the push for EBP.

Evidence-Based Nursing Practice

The RU process begins with an empirically based innovation or new idea that gets scrutinized for possible adoption in practice settings. Evidence-based practice, by contrast, begins with a search for information about how best to solve specific practice problems (see Figure 18-1). Findings from rigorous research are considered the best possible source of information, but EBP also draws on other sources of evidence. The emphasis is on identifying the best available research evidence and *integrating* it with clinical expertise, patient input, and existing resources.

The evidence-based practice movement has given rise to considerable debate, with both staunch, zealous advocates and skeptics who urge caution and a balanced approach to health care practice. Supporters argue that EBP offers a solution to sustaining high health care quality in our current cost-constrained environment. Their position is that a rational approach is needed to provide the best possible care to the most people, with the most cost-effective use of resources. Critics worry that the advantages of EBP are exaggerated and that individual clinical judgments and patient inputs are being devalued. Although there is a need for close scrutiny of how the EBP journey unfolds, it seems likely that the EBP path is one that health care professions are likely to follow in the 21st century.

OVERVIEW OF THE EBP MOVEMENT

One of the cornerstones of the EBP movement is the Cochrane Collaboration, which was based on the work of British epidemiologist Archie Cochrane. Cochrane published an influential book in the early 1970s that drew attention to the dearth of solid evidence about the effects of health care. He called for efforts to make research summaries available to health care decision-makers. This eventually led to the development of the Cochrane Center in Oxford in 1992, and an international collaboration called the **Cochrane Collaboration**, with centers established in 15 locations throughout the world. The aim of the collaboration is to help people make good decisions about health care by preparing, maintaining, and disseminating systematic reviews of the effects of health care interventions.

At about the same time as the Cochrane Collaboration got underway, a group from McMaster Medical School developed a clinical learning strategy they called evidence-based medicine. Dr. David Sackett, a pioneer of evidence-based medicine at McMaster, defined evidence-based medicine as "the conscientious, explicit, and judicious use of current best evidence in making decisions about the care of individual patients. The practice of evidence-based medicine means integrating individual clinical expertise with the best available external evidence from systematic research" (Sackett, Rosenberg, Gray, Haynes, & Richardson, 1996, p. 71). The evidence-based medicine movement has shifted over time to a broader conception of using best evidence by all health care practitioners (not just doctors) in a multidisciplinary team. EBP has been considered a major paradigm shift for health care education and practice.

TYPES OF EVIDENCE AND EVIDENCE HIERARCHIES

There is no consensus about what constitutes usable evidence for EBP, but there is general agreement that findings from rigorous studies are paramount. In the initial phases of the EBP movement, there was a definite bias toward reliance on information from randomized clinical trials (RCTs). This bias, in turn, led to some resistance to EBP by nurses who felt that evidence from qualitative and non-RCT studies would be ignored.

Positions about what constitutes useful evidence have loosened, but there have nevertheless been efforts to develop **evidence hierarchies** that rank studies according to the strength of evidence they provide. Several such hierarchies have been developed, many based on the one proposed by Archie Cochrane. Most hierarchies put meta-analyses of RCT studies at the pinnacle and other types of nonresearch evidence (e.g., clinical expertise) at the base. As one example, Stetler and her colleagues (1998) developed a six-level evidence hierarchy that also assigns grades on study quality (from A to D) within each of the six levels. The levels (from strongest to weakest) are as follows: (I) Meta-analyses of RCTs; (II) Individual experimental studies; (III) Quasi-experimental studies or matched case-control studies; (IV) Nonexperimental studies (e.g., correlational studies, qualitative studies); (V) Research utilization studies, quality improvement projects, case reports; and (VI) Opinions of respected authorities and of expert committees.

To date, there have been relatively few published RCT studies (Level II) in nursing, and even fewer published meta-analyses of RCT nursing studies. Therefore, evidence from other types of research will play an important role in evidence-based nursing practice. Many clinical questions of importance to nurses can best be answered with rich descriptive and qualitative data from Level IV and V studies. Another issue is that there continue to be clinical practice questions for which there is relatively little research data.

Thus, while EBP encompasses research utilization, both research and nonresearch sources of information play a role in evidence-based practice. Nurses and other health care professionals must be able to locate evidence, evaluate it, and integrate it with clinical judgment and patient preferences to determine the most clinically effective solutions to health problems. Note that an important feature of EBP is that it does not necessarily imply practice changes: The best evidence may confirm that existing practices are effective and cost-efficient.

Barriers to Research Utilization and EBP in Nursing

In the next section of this chapter, we discuss some models for RU and EBP endeavors. First, however, we review some barriers to RU and EBP in nursing and present some strategies for addressing them. Studies done in several different countries have explored nurses' perceptions of barriers to research utilization and have yielded remarkably similar results about constraints clinical nurses face (e.g., Funk, Champagne, Wiese, & Tornquist, 1995; Hutchinson & Johnston, 2004; McCaughan, Thompson, Cullum, Sheldon, & Thompson, 2002; McCleary & Brown, 2003). These barriers can be broadly grouped into four categories—research characteristics, nurse characteristics, organizational characteristics, and characteristics of the nursing profession.

RESEARCH-RELATED BARRIERS

For some nursing problems, research knowledge is at a fairly rudimentary level. Results reported in the literature may not warrant incorporation into practice if methodologic flaws are extensive or if the number of studies is small. Thus, one impediment to research utilization is that, for some problems, an extensive base of valid and trustworthy study results has not been developed.

As we have repeatedly stressed, most studies have flaws of one type or another, and so if nurses were to wait for the perfect study before basing clinical decisions on research findings, they would have a very long wait indeed. It is precisely because of the limits of research methods that replication is essential. When repeated efforts to address a research question in different settings yield similar results, there can be greater confidence in the findings. Single studies rarely provide an adequate basis for making practice changes. Therefore, another utilization constraint is the dearth of published replications.

As a consumer, you can and should evaluate the extent to which researchers have adopted strategies to enhance research utilization. These include undertaking collaborative research with clinicians, communicating their study clearly so that practicing nurses can comprehend and evaluate them, and including suggestions for clinical applications in the discussion section of reports.

NURSE-RELATED BARRIERS

Studies have found that some clinical nurses have characteristics that constrain the use of research evidence in practice. One issue concerns nurses' research skills. Many have not had any formal instruction in research and may lack the skills to judge the merits of a study. Courses on research methods are now offered in most baccalaureate nursing programs, but the ability to critique a research report is not necessarily sufficient for effectively incorporating research results into daily decision making.

Nurses' attitudes toward research and their motivation to engage in EBP have repeatedly been identified as potential barriers. Studies have found that the more positive the attitude, the more likely is the nurse to use research in practice.

Another characteristic is one that is common to most humans: People are often resistant to change. Change requires effort, retraining, and restructuring of work habits. Change may also be perceived as threatening (e.g., changes may be perceived as affecting job security). However, there is growing evidence from international surveys that many nurses value nursing research and want to be involved in research-related activities.

CONSUMER TIP

Every nurse can play a role in using research evidence. Here are some strategies:
▶ *Read widely and critically.* Professionally accountable nurses keep abreast of new developments. You should read journals relating to your specialty, including research reports in them.
▶ *Attend professional conferences.* Many nursing conferences include presentations of studies that have clinical relevance. At a conference, you can meet researchers and explore practice implications.
▶ *Learn to expect evidence that a procedure is effective.* Every time you are told about a standard nursing procedure, you have a right to ask, Why? Nurses should develop expectations that their clinical decisions are based on sound rationales.
▶ *Become involved in a journal club.* Many organizations that employ nurses sponsor journal clubs that meet to review research articles that have potential relevance to practice.
▶ *Pursue and participate in RU/EBP projects.* Sometimes ideas for RU or EBP projects come from staff nurses (e.g., ideas may emerge within a journal club). Studies have found that nurses who are involved in research-related activities (e.g., a utilization project or data collection activities) develop more positive attitudes toward research and EBP. ■

ORGANIZATIONAL BARRIERS

Many of the impediments to using research in practice stem from the organizations that train and employ nurses. Organizations, perhaps to an even greater degree than individuals, resist change unless there is a strong organizational perception that there is something fundamentally wrong with the status quo. To challenge tradition and accepted practices, a spirit of intellectual curiosity and openness must prevail.

In many practice settings, administrators have established procedures to reward competence in nursing practice; however, few have established a system to reward nurses for critiquing studies, for using research in practice, or for discussing research findings with clients. Thus, organizations have failed to motivate or reward nurses for implementing findings with clients. Research review and use are often considered appropriate activities only when time is available, but available time is generally limited. In several studies of barriers to RU, one of the greatest reported barriers was insufficient time to implement new ideas.

Organizations may also be reluctant to expend resources for RU projects. Resources may be required for the use of outside consultants, staff release time, library materials and Internet access, evaluating the effects of an innovation, and so on. With the push toward cost containment in health care settings, resource constraints may pose a barrier to change—unless the project has cost containment as an explicit goal.

EBP will become part of organizational norms only if there is a commitment on the part of managers and administrators. Strong leadership in health care organizations is essential to making evidence-based practice happen.

BARRIERS RELATED TO THE NURSING PROFESSION

Some impediments that contribute to the gap between research and practice are more global, reflecting the state of the nursing profession or, even more broadly, the state of western society.

It has sometimes been difficult to encourage clinicians and researchers to interact and collaborate. They are generally in different settings and have different professional concerns. Relatively few systematic attempts have been made to form collaborative arrangements, and even fewer of these arrangements have been made permanent.

Another potential barrier to RU and EBP is the shortage of role models—nurses who can be emulated for their success in using or promoting the use of research in clinical practice. Fortunately, much progress has been made in nursing with regard to this issue. Several professional nursing organizations have taken a strong stance to promote the use of research in practice, and formal programs have been developed to create EBP mentors. For example, the Advanced Practice Institute at the University of Iowa gives nurse leaders a chance to develop skills in EBP and to become EBP facilitators.

Yet another potential barrier is the historical "baggage" that has defined nursing in such a way that practicing nurses may not typically perceive themselves as independent professionals capable of recommending changes based on research results. If practicing nurses believe that their role is to await direction from the medical community, and if they believe they have no power to be self-directed, then they will have difficulty in initiating innovations based on research findings. However, with the growing understanding of the value of EBP and the development of more multidisciplinary efforts to improve patient care, this barrier is also less salient now than it was two decades ago.

Finally, some of the burden for changes in the profession must rest with nursing educators. As Funk and colleagues (1995) noted, "The valuing of nursing research as the *sine qua non* on which practice is based must be conveyed throughout baccalaureate, associate degree, and diploma programs. This is not the teaching of the conduct of research, but rather the valuing of it as a way of knowing and as the foundation on which practice is based" (p. 400).

THE PROCESS OF USING RESEARCH IN NURSING PRACTICE

In the years ahead, many of you are likely to be engaged in individual and institutional efforts to use research as a basis for clinical decisions. This section describes how that might be accomplished. We begin with a description of some RU and EBP models developed by nurses.

Models for Evidence-Based Nursing Practice

A number of different models of research utilization have been developed by nurse researchers in the United States, Canada, the United Kingdom, and other countries during the past few decades. These models offer guidelines for designing and implementing RU and EBP projects in practice settings. Some models focus on the use of research from the perspective of an individual clinician, some focus on utilization from an organizational perspective, whereas others have multiple perspectives. Models that have proposed steps for how RU or EBP can be accomplished include the:

Stetler Model of Research Utilization (Stetler, 1994, 2001);
Iowa Model of Research in Practice (Titler et al., 1994, 2001);
Ottawa Model of Research Use (Logan & Graham, 1998);
Evidence-Based Multidisciplinary Practice Model (Goode & Piedalue, 1999);
Model for Change to Evidence-Based Practice (Rosswurm & Larrabee, 1999); and
Center for Advanced Nursing Practice Model (Soukup, 2000).

The most prominent of these models have been the Stetler, Iowa, and Ottawa Models. The first two models were originally developed in an environment that emphasized research utilization and have been updated to incorporate EBP processes.

THE STETLER MODEL

This model was first developed in 1976 with Marram and refined in 1994. The **Stetler Model** (1994) was designed with the assumption that research utilization could be undertaken not only by organizations, but also by individual clinicians and managers. It was a model designed to promote and facilitate critical thinking about the application of research findings in practice. The updated and refined model is based on many of the same assumptions and strategies as the original, but provides "an enhanced approach to the overall application of research in the service setting" (Stetler, 2001, p. 273). Stetler's model, presented graphically in Figure 18-2, involves five sequential phases that are designed to "facilitate critical thinking about the pragmatic application of research findings" (Stetler, 2001, p. 275):

1. *Preparation.* In this phase, nurses would: define the underlying purpose of the project; search for and select sources of research evidence; consider external factors that can influence potential application and internal factors that can diminish objectivity; and affirm the clinical significance of solving the perceived problem.
2. *Validation.* The second phase involves a utilization-focused critique of each source of evidence, focusing primarily on whether it is sufficiently sound for potential application in practice. The process stops at this point if the evidence sources are rejected.
3. *Comparative evaluation and decision making.* This phase involves a synthesis of findings and the application of four criteria that, taken together, are used to determine the desirability and feasibility of applying findings from validated sources to nursing practice. These criteria (fit of setting, feasibility, current practice, and substantiating evidence) are summarized in Box 18-1. The end result of the comparative evaluation is to make a decision about using the study findings. If the decision is negative, no further steps are necessary.
4. *Translation/application.* This phase involves confirming how the findings will be used (e.g., formally or informally), spelling out the operational details of the application, and then

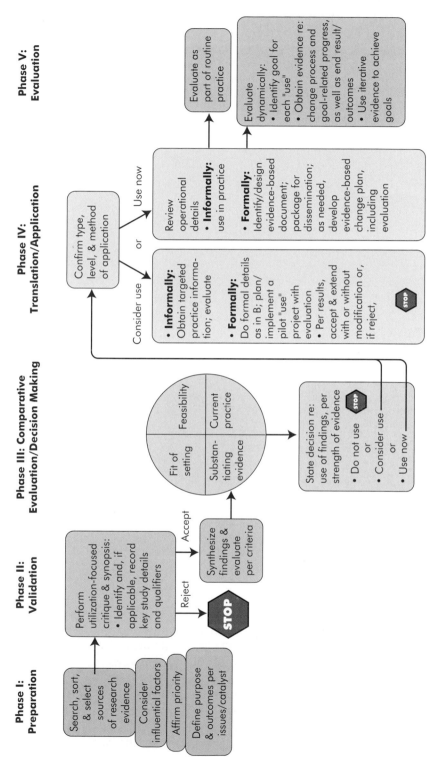

FIGURE 18.2 Stetler Model of Research Utilization to facilitate evidence-based practice. (Adapted from Stetler, C. B. [1994]. Refinement of the Stetler/Marram model for application of research findings into practice. *Nursing Outlook, 42,* 15–25.)

BOX 18.1   **Criteria for Comparative Evaluation Phase of Stetler's Model**

1. Fit of Setting

Similarity of characteristics of sample to your client population
Similarity of study's environment to the one in which you work

2. Feasibility

Potential risks of implementation to patients, staff, and the organization
Readiness for change among those who would be involved in a change in practice
Resource requirements and availability

3. Current Practice

Congruency of the study with your theoretical basis for current practice behavior

4. Substantiating Evidence

Availability of confirming evidence from other studies
Availability of confirming evidence from a meta-analysis or integrative review

---

Adapted from Stetler, C. B. (1994). Refinement of the Stetler/Marram model for application of research findings into practice. *Nursing Outlook, 42*, 15–25.

implementing the plan. The latter might involve the development of a guideline, detailed procedure, or plan of action, possibly including a proposal for formal organizational change.

5. *Evaluation.* In the final phase, the application would be evaluated. Informal use of the innovation versus formal use would lead to different evaluative strategies.

Although the Stetler Model was designed as a tool for individual practitioners, it has also been the basis of formal RU and EBP projects by groups of nurses.

 Example of an application of the Stetler Model

Bauer, Bushey, and Amaros (2002) applied the five phases of the Stetler Model to pressure ulcer prevention and care by nurses in home health care environments.

THE IOWA MODEL

Efforts to use research evidence to improve nursing practice are often addressed by groups of nurses interested in a critical practice issue. Formal RU/EBP projects typically have followed systematic procedures using a model such as the Iowa Model of Research in Practice (Titler et al., 1994). This model, like the Stetler Model, was revised recently and renamed the **Iowa Model of Evidence-Based Practice to Promote Quality Care** (Titler et al., 2001). The current version of the Iowa Model, shown in Figure 18-3, acknowledges that a formal RU/EBP project begins with a *trigger*—an impetus to explore possible changes to practice. The start-point can be either (a) a *knowledge-focused trigger* that emerges from awareness of innovative research findings (and thus follows a more traditional RU path, as in the top panel of Figure 18-3) or (b) a *problem-focused trigger* that has its roots in a clinical or organizational problem (and thus follows a path

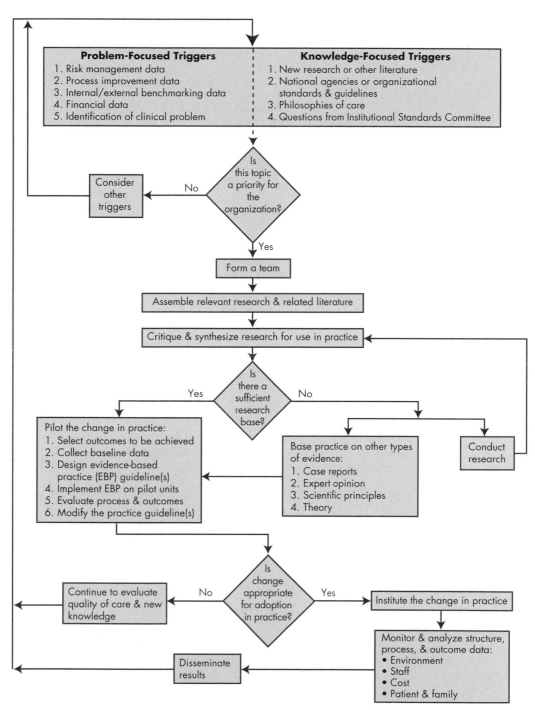

FIGURE 18.3 Iowa Model of Evidence-Based Practice to Promote Quality Care (Adapted from Titler, et al. [2001]. The Iowa Model of Evidence-Based Practice to Promote Quality Care. *Critical Care Nursing Clinics of North America, 13,* 497–509.)

that more closely resembles an EBP intent). The model outlines a series of activities with three critical decision points:

1. Deciding whether the problem is a sufficient priority for the organization exploring possible changes; if yes, a team is formed to proceed with the project, and if no, a new trigger would be identified;
2. Deciding whether there is a sufficient research base; if yes, the innovation is piloted in the practice setting, and if no, the team would either search for other sources of evidence or conduct its own research; and
3. Deciding whether the change is appropriate for adoption in practice; if yes, a change would be instituted and monitored, and if no, the team would continue to evaluate quality of care and search for new knowledge.

Example of an application of the Iowa Model

Montgomery, Hanrahan, Kottman, Otto, Barrett, and Hermiston (1999) used the Iowa Model to develop a guideline for intravenous infiltration in pediatric patients.

THE OTTAWA MODEL OF RESEARCH USE

The **Ottawa Model of Research Use (OMRU)**, developed by Logan & Graham (1998) consists of six key components interrelated through the process of evaluation. The six components deal with "the practice environment, the potential research adopter (administrators and clinical staff), the evidence-based innovation (the research intended for use in practice), strategies for transferring the innovation into practice, adoption/use of the evidence, and health and other outcomes" (Logan, Harrison, Graham, Dunn, & Bissonnette, 1999, p. 39). Systematic assessment, monitoring, and evaluation (AME) are central to the OMRU and are applied to each of the six components before, during, and after any effort to transfer research findings. The data gathered through AME serves several purposes:

▶ to determine potential barriers to and supports for research use associated with the practice environment;
▶ to offer direction for choosing and tailoring transfer strategies to surmount the recognized barriers and enhance strategies that were deemed supportive; and
▶ to evaluate the evidence-based innovation used and the influence it had on the outcomes of interest.

Example of an application of the Ottawa Model

Graham and Logan (2004) used the Ottawa Model to guide the implementation of clinical practice guidelines for skin care in a surgical program of a tertiary care hospital.

Activities in a Research Utilization or EBP Project

Using research to improve nursing practice involves a series of activities, decisions, and assessments. In this section, we discuss some of the major activities that are typical in an RU/EBP project. The Stetler, Iowa, and other models are used as a basis for discussing major activities to support RU and EBP.

SELECTING A TOPIC OR PROBLEM

The Iowa Model acknowledges that there are two types of stimulus for an EBP or RU endeavor—identification of a clinical practice problem in need of solution or through reading about an innovation in the literature. Problem-focused triggers may arise in the normal course of clinical practice or in the context of quality improvement efforts. This approach is likely to have staff support if the problem is one that numerous nurses have encountered and is likely to have considerable clinical relevance because a specific clinical situation generated interest in the problem in the first place.

Gennaro (2001) advises nurses following this approach to begin by clarifying the practice problem that needs to be solved and framing it as a question. The goal can be to find the most effective way to anticipate a problem (how to diagnose it) or the best way to solve a problem (how to intervene). Clinical practice questions may well take the form of, "What is the best way to . . . "—for example, "What is the best way to encourage women to do breast self examinations regularly?" or "What is the best way to manage hospitalized children's pain?"

A second catalyst for an RU/EBP project is the research literature, i.e., the knowledge-focused triggers identified in the Iowa model. For example, a utilization project could emerge as a result of discussions within a *journal club*. In this approach, a preliminary assessment needs to be made of the clinical relevance of the research. The central issue here is whether a problem of significance to nurses will be solved by making some change or introducing a new intervention. Five questions relating to clinical relevance (shown in Box 18-2) can be applied to a research report or set of related reports. If the answer is yes to any of these questions, the next step in the process can be pursued, but if it were determined that the research base is not clinically relevant, it would be necessary to start all over.

With both types of triggers, it is important to ensure that there is a general consensus about the importance of the problem and the need for improving practice. Titler and colleagues

---

BOX 18.2   Criteria for Evaluating the Clinical Relevance of a Body of Research

1. Does the research have the potential to help solve a problem that is currently being faced by practitioners?
2. Does the research have the potential to help with clinical decision making with respect to (a) making appropriate observations, (b) identifying client risks or complications, or (c) selecting an appropriate intervention?
3. Are clinically relevant theoretical propositions tested by the research?
4. If the research involves an intervention, does the intervention have potential for implementation in clinical practice? Do nurses have control over the implementation of such interventions?
5. Can the measures used in the study be used in clinical practice?

Adapted from Tanner, C. A. (1987). Evaluating research for use in practice: Guidelines for the clinician. *Heart & Lung, 16,* 424–430.

(2001) include as the first decision point in their revised Iowa model the determination of whether the topic is a priority for the organization considering practice changes. They advise that the following issues be taken into account when finalizing a topic for an EBP project: the topic's fit with the organization's strategic plan; the magnitude of the problem; the number of people invested in the problem; support of nurse leaders and of those in other disciplines; costs; and possible barriers to change.

CONSUMER TIP

The method of selecting a topic does not appear to have any bearing on the success of an RU/EBP project. What is important, however, is that the nursing staff who will implement an innovation are involved in the topic selection and that key stakeholders are "on board." ■

ASSEMBLING AND EVALUATING EVIDENCE

Once a clinical practice question has been selected and a team has been formed to work on the project, the next step is to search for and assemble research evidence (and other relevant evidence) on the topic. Chapter 7 provided information about locating research information and Chapter 17 discussed research critiques, but some additional issues are relevant.

In doing a literature review as background for a new study, the central goal is to discover where the gaps are and how best to advance knowledge. For EBP or RU projects, which typically have as end products prescriptive practice protocols or clinical guidelines, literature reviews are typically much more rigorous and formalized. The emphasis is on gathering comprehensive information on the topic, weighing pieces of evidence, and integrating information to draw conclusions about the evidence base. *Integrative reviews*, including meta-analyses and metasyntheses, thus play a crucial role in developing an evidence-based practice. If practitioners are to glean best practices from research findings, they must take into account as much of the evidence as possible, organized and synthesized in a rigorous manner.

High-quality integrative reviews represent a critical tool for RU/EBP, and if the assembled project team has the skills to complete one, this is clearly advantageous. It is, however, unlikely that every clinical organization will be able to assemble the skills needed to undertake a high-quality critical review of the research literature on a chosen topic. Fortunately, many researchers and organizations have taken on the responsibility of preparing integrative reviews and making them available for EBP.

Cochrane reviews are an especially important resource. These reports, which are based mainly on meta-analyses, describe the background and objectives of the review, the methods used to search for, select, and evaluate studies, the main results, and, importantly, the reviewers' conclusions. Cochrane reviews are checked and updated regularly.

Example of a Cochrane review

One Cochrane review (Rice & Stead, 2004) critically appraised the evidence about nursing interventions for smoking cessation. Data from 20 studies that compared a nursing intervention to a control or to usual care found that the interventions significantly increased the odds of quitting smoking.

Another important resource for those wishing to use available integrative reviews is the Agency for Healthcare Research and Quality (AHRQ). This agency awarded 12 5-year contracts in 1997 to establish Evidence-based Practice Centers at institutions in the United States and Canada (e.g., at Johns Hopkins University, McMaster University) and new 5-year contracts were awarded in 2002. Each center issues *evidence reports* that are based on rigorous integrative reviews of relevant scientific literature; dozens of these reports are now available to help "improve the quality, effectiveness, and appropriateness of clinical care" (AHRQ website, www.ahrq.gov).

Example of evidence reports from EBP Centers funded by AHRQ

The titles of two evidence reports recently published by EBP Centers are: *Literacy and Health Outcomes* (Evidence Report No. 87, 2004) and *Vaginal Birth After Cesarean—VBAC* (Evidence Report No. 71, 2003).

If an integrative review has been prepared by experts, it is possible that a formal evidence-based clinical guideline has been developed and can be used directly in an RU/EBP project. AHRQ, for example, has developed such guidelines on pain management, continence, and other problems of relevance to nurses. AHRQ no longer develops guidelines but helps to support the National Guideline Clearinghouse (www.guidelines.gov), which provides a comprehensive database of such guidelines. Nursing organizations (e.g., the Association of Women's Health, Obstetrics, and Neonatal Nurses) have also developed clinical practice guidelines on several topics.

In some cases, it may be possible to base an RU/EBP project on an existing published integrative review. However, it is always wise to make sure that the review is as up-to-date as possible and that new findings published after the review are taken into consideration. Moreover, even a published integrative review needs to be critiqued and the validity of its conclusions assessed. Of course, there are many clinical questions for which integrative reviews and clinical guidelines are not available, which might mean that the RU/EBP team would need to prepare its own integrative review or synthesis. Some information about conducting and critiquing integrative reviews is presented later in this chapter.

An integrative review or synthesis of research evidence is used by the RU/EBP team to draw conclusions about the sufficiency of the research base for guiding clinical practice. Adequacy of research evidence depends on such factors as the consistency of findings across studies, the quality and rigor of the studies, the strength of any observed effect, the transferability of the findings to clinical settings, and cost-effectiveness.

Conclusions about a body of evidence can lead to different decisions for further action. First, if the research base is small—or if there is a large base with ambiguous conclusions—the team could opt to pursue one of three courses. The first is to go back to the beginning to pursue a new topic. A second option (preferable in the EBP environment) is to assemble other types of nonresearch evidence (e.g., through consultation with experts, surveys of clients, and so on) and assess whether that evidence suggests a practice change. Finally, another possibility is to pursue an original clinical study to directly address the practice question, thereby gathering new evidence and contributing to the base of practice knowledge. This last course of action may well be impractical for many, and would clearly result in years of delay before any further conclusions could be drawn.

A solid research base also could point in different directions. For example, the evidence might support existing practices (which might lead to an analysis of why the clinical practice question emerged and what might make existing practices work more effectively). Another possibility is that there would be clearcut, compelling evidence that a clinical change is warranted, which would lead to the activities described next.

ASSESSING IMPLEMENTATION POTENTIAL

Some models of RU/EBP move directly from the conclusion that evidence supports a change in practice to the pilot testing of the innovation. Others include steps to first evaluate the appropriateness of the innovation within the specific organizational context; in some cases, such an assessment (or aspects of it) may be warranted even before embarking on efforts to assemble best evidence. Other models suggest evaluating issues of fit *after* the practice change has been implemented. We think a preliminary assessment of the **implementation potential** of an innovation is often sensible, although there may be situations with little need for such a formal assessment.

In determining the implementation potential of an innovation in a particular setting, several issues should be considered, particularly the transferability of the innovation, the feasibility of implementing it, and the cost–benefit ratio. Box 18-3 presents some assessment questions for these categories.

▶ *Transferability.* The main question relating to transferability is whether it makes good sense to implement the innovation in the new practice setting. If there is some aspect of the practice setting that is fundamentally incongruent with the innovation in terms of its philosophy, types of clients it serves, personnel, or financial or administrative structure, it may not be sensible to try to adopt the innovation, even if it has been shown to be clinically effective in other contexts.

▶ *Feasibility.* The feasibility questions in Box 18-3 address various practical concerns about the availability of staff and resources, the organizational climate, the need for and availability of external assistance, and the potential for clinical evaluation. An important issue here is whether nurses will have (or share) control over the innovation. When nurses do not have full control over the new procedure, it is important to recognize the interdependent nature of the project and to proceed as early as possible to establish necessary cooperative arrangements.

▶ *Cost–Benefit Ratio.* A critical part of any decision to proceed with an RU/EBP project is a careful assessment of the costs and benefits of the innovation. The *cost–benefit assessment* should encompass likely costs and benefits to various groups, including clients, staff, and the overall organization. Clearly, the most important factor is the client. If the degree of risk in introducing a new procedure is high, then potential benefits must be great and the knowledge base must be extremely sound. A cost–benefit assessment should consider the opposite side of the coin as well: the costs and benefits of *not* implementing the innovation. It is sometimes easy to forget that the status quo bears its own risks and that failure to change, especially when such change is based on rigorous evidence, is costly to clients, organizations, and the nursing community.

If the implementation assessment suggests that there might be problems in testing the innovation within that particular practice setting, the team can either identify a new problem and begin the process anew or consider adopting a plan to improve the implementation potential (e.g., seeking external resources if costs were the inhibiting factor).

BOX 18.3　Criteria for Evaluating the Implementation Potential of an Innovation Under Scrutiny

Transferability of the Findings

1. Will the innovation "fit" in the proposed setting?
2. How similar are the target populations in the research and in your setting?
3. Is the philosophy of care underlying the innovation fundamentally different from the philosophy prevailing in your setting? How entrenched is the prevailing philosophy?
4. Is there a sufficiently large number of clients in your setting who could benefit from the innovation?
5. Will the innovation take too long to implement and evaluate?

Feasibility

1. Will nurses have the freedom to carry out the innovation? Will they have the freedom to terminate the innovation if it is considered undesirable?
2. Will the implementation of the innovation interfere inordinately with current staff functions?
3. Does the administration support the innovation? Is the organizational climate conducive to research utilization?
4. Is there a fair degree of consensus among the staff and among the administrators that the innovation could be beneficial and should be tested? Are there major pockets of resistance or uncooperativeness that could undermine efforts to implement and evaluate the innovation?
5. To what extent will the implementation of the innovation cause friction within your organization? Does the utilization project have the support and cooperation of departments outside the nursing department?
6. Are the skills needed to carry out the utilization project (both the implementation and the clinical evaluation) available in the nursing staff? If not, how difficult will it be to collaborate with or to secure the assistance of others with the necessary skills?
7. Does your organization have the equipment and facilities necessary for the innovation? If not, is there a way to obtain the needed resources?
8. If nursing staff need to be released from other practice activities to learn about and implement the innovation, what is the likelihood that this will happen?
9. Are appropriate measuring tools available for a clinical evaluation of the innovation?

Cost/Benefit Ratio of the Innovation

1. What are the risks to which clients would be exposed during the implementation of the innovation and what are the potential benefits to clients?
2. What are the risks of maintaining current practices (i.e., the risks of *not* trying the innovation)?
3. What are the material costs of implementing the innovation? What are the costs in the short term during utilization, and what are the costs in the long run, if the change is to be institutionalized?
4. What are the material costs of *not* implementing the innovation (i.e., could the new procedure result in some efficiencies that could lower the cost of providing service)?
5. What are the potential nonmaterial costs and benefits of implementing the innovation to the organization (e.g., in terms of lower staff morale, staff turnover, absenteeism)?

DEVELOPING, IMPLEMENTING, AND EVALUATING THE INNOVATION

If the implementation criteria are met, the team can then proceed to design the protocol for the innovation. Building on the Iowa Model, this phase of the project would involve the following activities:

▶ Developing an evaluation plan (e.g., identifying outcomes to be achieved, determining how many clients to involve, deciding when and how often to take measurements and so on);

▶ Collecting baseline data relating to those outcomes, to develop a counterfactual against which the outcomes of the innovation would be assessed;

▶ Developing a written EBP guideline based on the synthesis of the evidence, preferably a guideline that is clear and user-friendly and that uses such devices as flow charts and decision trees;

▶ Training relevant staff in the use of the new guideline and, if necessary, "marketing" the innovation to users so that it is given a fair test;

▶ Trying the guideline out in some units or with a sample of clients; and

▶ Evaluating the pilot project, in terms of both process (e.g., How was the innovation received? To what extent were the guidelines actually followed? What implementation problems were encountered?) and outcomes (in terms of client outcomes and cost effectiveness).

Evaluation data should be gathered over a sufficiently long period (typically 6–12 months) to allow for a true test of a "mature" innovation. The end result of this process is a decision about whether to adopt the innovation, to modify it for ongoing use, or to revert to prior practices.

CONSUMER TIP

Research can be incorporated into nursing practice even without undertaking a formal RU/EBP project. Increasingly, research-based nursing protocols are being published in the literature and are essentially ready for adoption—although it is wise to undertake an implementation assessment to determine whether the adoption of a new protocol is sensible. If the publication of the protocol is not recent, it is also prudent to ensure that current research and theory on the topic remain consistent with the protocol.

■

Example of an Evidence-Based Nursing Project

Many EBP and research utilization projects are underway in practice settings, and some that have been described in the nursing literature offer rich information about planning and implementing such an endeavor. The Association of Women's Health, Obstetric, and Neonatal Nurses (AWHONN) has conducted several major RU/EBP projects as part of its Research-Based Practice program. Each project has resulted in the development and testing of evidence-based nursing protocols. For example, one project is focusing on a smoking cessation counseling strategy for pregnant women in clinical settings (Maloni, Albrecht, Thomas, Halleran, & Jones, 2003), and another is focusing on the management of cyclic perimenstrual pain and discomfort (Collins-Sharp, Taylor, Thomas, Killeen, & Dawood, in press). One AWHONN project that has been implemented and fully evaluated is described here.

An interdisciplinary team, under the leadership of neonatal clinical nurse specialist Carolyn H. Lund, undertook a 4-year project designed to develop and evaluate an evidence-based clinical practice guideline for assessment and routine care of neonatal skin (Lund, et al., 2001a, 2001b). The project also sought to educate nurses about the scientific basis for the recommended skin care practices and designed procedures to facilitate using the guideline in practice.

The project consisted of four 1-year phases. Phase 1 (Planning) involved forming the project team, synthesizing scientific and other evidence relating to neonatal skin care (Lund, Kuller, Lane, Lott, & Raines, 1999), developing the evidence-based guideline, and developing data collection instruments. Ten areas of neonatal skin care were included in the practice guidelines: bathing, emollients, adhesives, skin disinfectants, control of transepidermal water loss, diaper dermatitis, cord and circumcision care, skin assessment, and prevention and treatment of skin breakdown. The quality of the scientific evidence in each of these areas determined the strength of each recommendation.

The second phase involved the implementation of the guidelines. Clinical sites (nurseries in the United States and Canada) were recruited through various means (e.g., bulletins published in *AWHONN Lifelines* and *JOGNN*) and invited to participate in an EBP project. More than 75 nurseries expressed an interest in participating, and ultimately 51 sites prepared preguideline and postguideline assessments. Each participating institution had a site coordinator who underwent training in the use of the guidelines.

Site coordinators provided information about their hospital's current skin care practices and took a knowledge test about neonatal skin care. The site coordinators also completed assessments of the skin condition of some 1371 infants (about 30 per site) prior to the implementation of the guidelines, and these assessments served as a baseline for evaluating the effectiveness of the new procedures. Skin assessments were done twice a week using an observational rating scale that evaluated dryness, erythema, and breakdown/excoriation.

Phase III of the project (Evaluation) involved an assessment of the outcomes. The evaluation addressed three broad questions: (1) Will nurses change clinical practices after receiving education and implementing a clinical practice guideline? (2) Will patient outcomes be positively affected by the use of the guideline in neonatal intensive care units (NICUs), special-care units, and well-baby nursery settings? and (3) How does the caregiving environment influence skin integrity? Several specific hypotheses were tested (e.g., that the frequency of bathing would decrease, and that infant skin condition would improve). The results indicated that the guidelines were, in fact, integrated into care and that nurses changed their practices. For example, there was a significant and substantial decrease in the frequency of bathing in the NICU from preguideline to postguideline implementation and a significant increase in emollient use. There was also evidence that skin condition was improved, as reflected by less visible dryness, redness, and skin breakdown in all neonatal settings. Site coordinators reported a few problems during the project (e.g., organizational barriers to changing products), but they mostly described the benefits of having an evidence-based practice guideline and of having participated in a multisite EBP project. All site coordinators except one reported that their units would continue using the guidelines after project completion, and the one exception indicated partial use of the guidelines.

Finally, in Phase 4 of the project (Dissemination), the team made efforts to publish results, to make presentations at conferences, and to continue to advance evidence-based neonatal skin care through programmatic activities and educational products. The project team concluded that the results "support a wider dissemination of the project's practice guideline for neonatal skin care" (Lund et al., 2001b, p. 41).

INTEGRATIVE REVIEWS

Evidence-based practice relies on meticulous integration and critical evaluation of research evidence on a topic. This section is not specifically designed to teach you how to do an integrative review, because the conduct of such reviews requires a fair amount of methodologic sophistication. However, it is important for you to have some skills in critiquing and appraising integrative reviews so that you can decide how much confidence to place in the reviewers' conclusions. To critique integrative reviews, you will need to learn a bit about how they are done.

Steps in Doing an Integrative Review

An integrative review is in itself a systematic inquiry that follows many of the same rules as those described in this book for primary studies. In other words, those doing an integrative review develop research questions or hypotheses; devise a sampling plan and data collection strategy; collect relevant data; and analyze and interpret those data.

It should be noted that integrative reviews are sometimes done by individuals, but it is preferable to have at least two reviewers. Multiple reviewers not only help in sharing the work load, but also in minimizing subjectivity. Reviewers should have both substantive and clinical knowledge of the problem, and sufficiently strong methodologic skills to evaluate study quality.

RESEARCH QUESTIONS AND HYPOTHESES IN INTEGRATIVE REVIEWS

An integrative review begins with a problem statement and a research question or hypothesis. In critiquing an integrative review, you should determine whether the problem statement and questions are clearly worded and sufficiently specific, whether the variables or phenomena under study are adequately defined, and whether the population of interest has been stated. And, of course, it is also important to evaluate the clinical relevance of the research question or its importance to some other aspect of nursing. Whether the integrative review is a traditional narrative review, a meta-analysis, or a metasynthesis, the reviewers should clearly communicate their purpose and their rationale for undertaking the review.

Example of a research question from a metasynthesis

Carroll (2004) conducted a metasynthesis that was designed to answer the following question: "What characterizes nonvocal ventilated patients' perceptions of being understood, across qualitative studies? The goal was to provide an enlarged interpretation and understanding and to build cumulative knowledge of the communication experiences in this population" (p. 86).

Example of a research question from a meta-analysis

Hill-Westmoreland, Soeken, and Spellbring (2002) conducted a meta-analysis that addressed the following question: "What are the effects of fall prevention programs on the proportion of falls in the elderly? Falls were conceptually defined as coming to rest on the ground, floor, or other lower level, unintentionally" (p. 2).

Questions for a integrative review can be narrow, focusing, for example, on a particular type of intervention, or more inclusive, examining a range of alternative interventions or practices. Forbes (2003) described an integrative review guided by the question, "What strategies, within the scope of nursing, are effective in managing the behavioral symptoms associated with Alzheimer's disease?" (p. 182). She noted that "in retrospect, selecting specific interventions would have made the review more manageable" (p. 182). The broader the question, the more complex (and costly) the integrative review becomes. In some cases, the broader the question, the less appropriate it is to integrate studies—just as in primary research, there must be an identifiable independent and dependent variable (for quantitative studies) or phenomenon (in qualitative studies).

SAMPLING IN INTEGRATIVE REVIEWS

In an integrative review, the "sample" involves primary studies that have addressed the same or a similar research question. In most cases, the reviewers try first to identify the full population of relevant studies, only some of which (a sample) may actually be used in the review.

Reviewers must make a number of up-front decisions regarding the sample, which they should share in their written review so that readers can evaluate the rigor and generalizability of their conclusions. Sampling decisions include the following:

- What are the exclusion and/or inclusion criteria for the search?
- Will both published and unpublished reports be assembled?
- What databases and other retrieval mechanisms will be used to locate the sample?
- What key words or search terms will be used to identify relevant studies?

Example of sampling decisions for an integrative review

Nelson (2002) conducted a metasynthesis on mothering other-than-normal children. She explained that, "I made a deliberate decision to include studies that used various qualitative methodologies and represented a wide variety of children because I was unable to locate a sufficient number of studies using the same qualitative methodology and focusing on one group of children. I believed that the potential significance of synthesizing qualitative knowledge in the broad area of mothering other-than-normal children outweighed the limitations of the endeavor and was philosophically consistent with the qualitative paradigm" (p. 517).

The inclusion and exclusion criteria typically cover substantive, methodologic, and practical elements. Substantively, the criteria must stipulate what specific variables (or phenomena) were studied. For example, if the review is integrating material about the effectiveness of a nursing intervention, what outcomes (dependent variables) must the researchers have studied? Another substantive issue concerns the study population. For example, will certain age groups of study participants (e.g., children, the elderly) be excluded? Methodologically, the criteria

Example of eligibility criteria for an integrative review

Forbes (2003), in the previously mentioned meta-analysis of interventions for Alzheimer's disease patients, stipulated five criteria. The study must have: (1) been published or conducted between January 1985 and May 1997; (2) evaluated a nonpharmacologic intervention for individuals aged 65 or older with Alzheimer's disease; (3) involved an intervention within the scope of nursing practice; (4) measured at least one outcome of a stipulated type (e.g., wandering, agitation); and (5) incorporated a control group or changes over time.

might specify that (for example) only studies that used an experimental design would be included. From a practical standpoint, the criteria might exclude, for example, reports written in a language other than English, or reports published before a certain date.

There is some disagreement about whether reviewers should limit their sample to studies published in peer-reviewed journals, or should cast as wide a net as possible and include *grey literature*—that is, studies with a more limited distribution, such as dissertations, unpublished reports, nonrefereed publications, and so on. Some people use only published reports in peer reviewed journals as a proxy for study rigor. Corn, Valentine, Cooper, and Rantz (2003) conducted a study on this matter, however, and concluded that the exclusion of grey literature can lead to certain types of biases, such as overestimating effects.

In searching for a comprehensive sample of research reports, reviewers usually need to use techniques more exhaustive than simply doing a computerized literature search of a key database, and this is especially true if the sample is to include grey literature. Five search methods described in pathbreaking work by Cooper (1984) include the *ancestry approach* ("footnote chasing" of cited studies); the *descendancy approach* (searching forward in citation indexes for subsequent references to key studies), online searches (including Internet searches); informal contacts at research conferences, and the more traditional searches of bibliographic databases.

Example of a search strategy for an integrative review

Beck (2001), in an update of an earlier meta-analysis on the predictors of postpartum depression, used all five of Cooper's search methods. She noted that, "The following on-line databases were searched for the 10-year period between 1990–2000: CINAHL, Medline, Psych Info, Eric, Popline, Social Work Abstracts, Dissertation Abstracts, and JRED. Examples of search terms included postpartum depression, postnatal depression, puerperal depression, predictors, and risk factors" (p. 276).

When a potential pool of studies has been identified, reviewers then screen them for appropriateness. Typically, many located studies are discarded because they turn out not to be relevant or do not, in fact, meet the eligibility criteria. Yet another reason for excluding studies from the initial pool (particularly for meta-analyses) is that some provide insufficient information to perform the necessary analyses. All decisions relating to exclusions (preferably made by at least two reviewers to ensure objectivity) should be well documented and justified.

EVALUATING PRIMARY STUDIES FOR INTEGRATIVE REVIEWS

In any integrative review, the evidence must be evaluated to determine how much confidence to place in the findings. Strong studies clearly need to be given more weight than weaker ones in coming to conclusions about the current state of knowledge. There are different strategies for

Example of excluding low-quality studies in an integrative review

Peacock and Forbes (2003) did a systematic review of interventions for caregivers of persons with dementia. A total of 36 relevant studies were rated using various methodologic criteria, and then the scores were used to categorize the studies as strong, moderate, weak, or poor. Only the 11 studies in the strong category were included in the review.

doing this, however. Some reviewers use methodologic quality as an exclusion criterion—for example, including only studies of a certain type or with a high rating for quality. Others, however, include studies regardless of quality but incorporate information about quality into the analysis.

In narrative integrative reviews, the reviewers typically record their assessments about the key limitations and strengths of studies as narrative notes. For example, in one narrative review on quality of life among lung transplant patients, study limitations (e.g., "psychometrics of tools not addressed") and strengths (e.g., "two study sites") were noted in a summary table (Lanuza, Lefaiver, & Farcas, 2000, p. 185). Study quality must then be taken into consideration in weighing the evidence and drawing conclusions from it.

For metasyntheses, Paterson, Thorne, Canam, and Jillings (2001) have developed the Primary Research Appraisal Tool to use as a systematic means of reviewing and evaluating qualitative studies. This protocol covers such aspects of a qualitative study as the sampling procedure, data gathering strategy, data analysis, researcher credentials, and researcher reflexivity. At the end of the process, the reviewer makes a decision to include the qualitative study in the metasynthesis or to reject it.

In meta-analyses, the evaluation usually involves a quantitative rating of the scientific merit of each study. The Agency for Healthcare Research and Quality (AHRQ, 2002) has published a guide that describes and evaluates various systems and instruments to rate the strength of evidence in quantitative studies. Based on a comprehensive review of the literature, the authors identified 121 systems, including tools for evaluating randomized clinical trials, non-experimental research, diagnostic test studies, and systematic reviews. The report offers some guidance to reviewers about which systems meet certain standards: 19 systems out of the 121 reviewed fully address essential quality domains. The report concluded, however, that other factors, such as appropriateness and ease of use, need to be considered by those wanting to adopt a formal quality-evaluation system.

Example of quality assessment tool

One of the 19 systems that the AHRQ report considered to be of especially high quality was developed by a British team working at the Royal College of Nursing Institute at the University of Oxford (Sindhu, Carpenter, & Seers, 1997). The instrument, developed by an expert panel of researchers for assessing reports of randomized clinical trials, consists of 53 items on 15 dimensions (e.g., appropriateness of controls, measurement of outcomes, blinding of treatments). Those using the instrument assign scores for each dimension and then total the points, which can range from 0 to 100.

Quality assessments in integrative reviews should involve ratings by two or more qualified individuals. If there are disagreements between the two raters, there should be a discussion until a consensus has been reached or, if necessary, a third rater should be asked to help resolve the difference. Indexes of interrater reliability are often calculated to demonstrate to readers that rater agreement was adequate.

EXTRACTING AND RECORDING DATA FOR INTEGRATIVE REVIEWS

Once the sample of primary studies has been finalized and the studies have been individually evaluated, the next step is to extract and record relevant information about study characteristics, methods, and findings. Reviewers often use a written protocol or data collection form to record information. The goal of this task is to produce a *data set*, and procedures similar to those used in creating a data set with raw data from individual study participants also apply. Examples of the type of methodologic information that reviewers record for each study include type of research design, extraneous variables controlled, length of follow-up, sampling design, sample size, measurement information, and type of statistical analysis. Characteristics of the study participants are usually registered as well (e.g., age, gender, ethnicity, marital status, education). The data set usually also includes information about the data source (e.g., year of publication, type of publication, country where the study took place). For a meta-analysis, all information would be numerically coded for statistical analysis.

Finally, and most important, information about the results must be extracted and recorded. In a narrative review, results can be noted with a verbal summary or classified with simple codes (e.g., nonsignificant group difference, moderate and significant difference, strong and significant difference). In a metasynthesis, the results information to be recorded includes the key metaphors, themes, concepts, or phrases from each study. In a meta-analysis, as we subsequently discuss, the information to be recorded might include group means and standard deviations, indices of relative risk, power estimates, and, most important, the **effect size**, that is, the index summarizing the magnitude of the relationship between the independent and dependent variables.

As with ratings of quality, extraction and coding of information ideally should be completed by two or more people, at least for a portion of the studies in the sample. This allows for an assessment of interrater agreement, which should be sufficiently high to persuade readers of the review that the recorded information is accurate.

Example of interrater agreement

In Beck's (2001) meta-analysis, one fourth of the included studies (i.e., 20 out of 84) were independently coded by Beck and a research assistant. Initial interrater agreement ranging from 85% to 100% was attained.

ANALYZING DATA IN INTEGRATIVE REVIEWS

In narrative integrative reviews, reviewers interpret the pattern of findings, draw conclusions about the evidence the findings yield, and derive implications for policy, practice, and further research. There are various methods of qualitatively analyzing the data for narrative reviews, although many reviewers appear to rely primarily on judgments without making clear the rules of inference they used. Stetler and her colleagues (1998) have argued that the analysis and synthesis in narrative integrative reviews should be a group process and that a whole review team should meet to discuss their conclusions after reviewing a packet of synopsized studies and tables.

In a metasynthesis, data analysis involves identifying the key metaphors in each qualitative study and then translating them into a synthesis that transforms individual findings into a new conceptualization. Noblit and Hare (1988) provide one such data analytic approach for a metasynthesis. Their method consists of making a list of key metaphors from each study and determining their relation to each other. Are the metaphors, for example, directly comparable (reciprocal)? In opposition to each other (refutational)? Next the studies' metaphors are translated into each other.

Noblit and Hare noted that "translations are especially unique syntheses because they protect the particular, respect holism, and enable comparison. An adequate translation maintains the central metaphors and/or concepts of each account in their relation to other key metaphors or concepts in that account" (p. 28). This synthesis of qualitative studies creates a whole that is more than the sum of the parts of the individual studies.

Example of data analysis in a metasynthesis

Beck (2002) used Noblit and Hare's approach in her metasynthesis of 18 qualitative studies on postpartum depression. As part of the analysis, key metaphors were listed for each study and organized under four overarching themes, one being "spiraling downward." For instance in one study included in the metasynthesis, the key metaphors listed under this theme included "total isolation; façade of normalcy; obsessive thoughts; pervasive guilt; panic/overanxious/feels trapped; completely overwhelmed by infant demands; anger" (p. 459).

Meta-analysts analyze their data quantitatively using objective, standardized procedures that minimize the risk of biased conclusions. The essence of a meta-analysis is the calculation of a common metric—an *effect size*—for every study. The effect size represents the magnitude of the impact of an intervention on an outcome, or the degree of association between two variables. Formulas for effect size differ depending on the nature of the statistical test used in the original analysis. The simplest formula to understand is the effect size for the difference between two means (e.g., an experimental group versus a control group). In this situation, the effect size in a study equals the mean for one group, minus the mean for the second group, divided by the overall standard deviation. Effect sizes for individual studies are then pooled and averaged to yield estimates of population effects. Effect sizes yield information about not only the *existence* of a relationship between variables, but also about the *magnitude*. Meta-analysts can, for example, draw conclusions about how big an effect an intervention has (with a specified probability that the results are accurate), and this in turn can yield estimates of the intervention's cost effectiveness.

Meta analysts can also examine whether there are **moderator effects** (or **subgroup effects**), that is, whether the relationship between an independent variable and a dependent variable is *moderated* by a third variable. For example, effect sizes can be computed separately for key subgroups (e.g., men versus women, children versus adolescents) to determine if effects or relationships differ for segments of a population.

CONSUMER TIP

It is not possible to provide explicit guidance on whether an effect size is "large" because it depends on the nature of the variables in the study. However, it might help to know that effect sizes for comparing two group means are in standard deviation units. Thus, an effect size of 1.0 in an experimental–control group comparison would mean that the experimental group's average score was a full standard deviation higher (or lower) than that for the control group. This would be considered a very large effect size. An effect size of .50 would be considered a moderate effect.

Example of subgroup analysis in a meta-analysis

Smith, Appleton, Adams, Southcott, and Ruffin (2004) did a Cochrane review on the effectiveness of home care by outreach nurses for patients with chronic obstructive pulmonary disease. The meta-analysis indicated that such outreach programs were not effective in reducing one negative outcome of interest, mortality. However, a subgroup analysis indicated that the interventions *were* effective for patients with less severe disease.

Some meta-analysts exclude studies that fail to meet a specified level of quality. Many believe, however, that it is preferable to retain methodologically weak studies in the data set, and then to "downweight" them in analyzing the findings. Quality ratings can be used in various ways. For example, weights proportional to the quality rating can be assigned so that the more rigorous studies "count" more in developing estimates of effects. Another approach is to conduct **sensitivity analyses**. This involves doing the statistical analyses twice, first including low-quality studies and then excluding them to see if including them changes the conclusions, or comparing the effect sizes for low-quality versus higher-quality studies.

Example of a sensitivity analysis

Devine (2003) conducted a meta-analysis of 25 studies that examined the effect of psychoeducational interventions on pain in adults with cancer. When analyzed across all studies, there was a significant, beneficial effect on pain. Study quality was quite varied, however. When Devine limited her analysis to studies with the best methodologic quality, the effect on pain continued to be significant.

EVALUATING THE BODY OF EVIDENCE

The emphasis on evidence-based practice has led to the development of systems for not only appraising and rating individual studies, but also for evaluating the strength of a body of evidence. The report by AHQR (2002) identified seven such systems as being especially useful, four of which were specifically created for use in developing practice guidelines or recommendations, and three of which were designed more broadly to facilitate EBP. As an example, one system was developed by the Institute of Clinical Systems Improvement (ICSI), a collaboration of 17 medical groups in Minnesota (Greer, Mosser, Logan, & Halaas, 2000). ICSI has used their system to develop numerous practice guidelines and technology assessment reports. An example of an ICSI guideline developed in 2004 is "The Assessment and Management of Acute Pain."

The AQHR report identified three domains that were considered important in any system designed to grade the strength of a body of evidence on a topic: (1) *Quality*—the aggregate of quality ratings for individual studies, predicated on the extent to which bias was minimized; (2) *Quantity*—the magnitude of effect, number of studies, and sample size; and (3) *Consistency*—the extent to which similar findings are reported using similar and different study designs. The ICSI system addresses all three domains.

Meta-analysts do not typically apply a formal system such as the one developed by ICSI to the body of evidence under review. However, their conclusions should include comments about the three domains of quality, quantity, and consistency.

THE WRITTEN INTEGRATIVE REVIEW

Reports for integrative reviews typically follow much the same format as for a research report for a primary study. That is, there is typically an introduction, method section, results section, and discussion. An abstract summarizing the major features of the review project is important. The method section should be thorough: Readers of the review need to be able to assess the validity of the findings by understanding and critiquing the procedures the reviewers used.

A well-written and thorough conclusion or discussion section is especially crucial in integrative reviews. The discussion should include an overall summary of the findings, the reviewers' assessment about the strength and limitations of the body of evidence, what further research should be undertaken to extend and improve the evidence base, and what the implications of the review are for clinicians and patients.

Example of a discussion in an integrative review

Evans, Wood, and Lambert (2002) conducted an integrative review of the literature on physical restraint minimization in acute and residential care settings. Here is an excerpt from their discussion: "Evidence suggests that physical restraint can be safely reduced in residential care settings through a combination of education and clinical consultation. There is little information on restraint minimization in acute care settings. The major finding of this review is the need for further investigation into all aspects of restraint minimization" (p. 616).

The review should also discuss the consistency of findings across studies and provide an interpretation of why there might be inconsistency. Did the samples, research designs, or data collection strategies in the studies differ in important ways? Or do differences reflect substantive differences, such as variation in the interventions or outcomes themselves?

Dissemination efforts for integrative reviews are even more important than for primary studies. Ideally, the review should be made available in a variety of formats and to a wide audience.

Critiquing Integrative Reviews

Like primary studies, integrative reviews should be thoroughly critiqued before the findings are deemed trustworthy and relevant to clinicians. Box 18-4 offers guidelines for evaluating integrative reviews.

Although these guidelines are fairly broad, not all questions apply equally well to all types of integrative reviews. For example, the question on subgroup analyses under the "Data Analysis" questions is relevant primarily for integrative reviews of quantitative studies. Moreover, the list of questions in Box 18-4 is not necessarily comprehensive. Supplementary questions might be needed for particular types of review.

In drawing conclusions about an integrative review, one issue is to evaluate whether the reviewer did a good job in pulling together and summarizing the evidence, as suggested by the questions in Box 18-4. Another aspect, however, is drawing inferences about how you might use the evidence in your own practice. It is not the reviewer's job, for example, to consider such issues as barriers to making use of the evidence, acceptability of an innovation, costs and benefits of change in various settings, and so on. These are issues for practicing nurses seeking to maximize the effectiveness of their actions and decisions.

BOX 18.4	Guidelines for Critiquing Integrative Reviews

The Problem. Does the review clearly state the research problem and/or research questions? Is the topic of the review important for the nursing profession? Is the scope of the review appropriate? Are concepts, variables, or phenomena adequately defined?

Search Strategy. Does the review clearly describe the criteria for selecting primary studies, and are those criteria reasonable? Are the databases the reviewers used identified, and are they appropriate? Are key words identified, and are they appropriate? Did the reviewers use adequate supplementary efforts to identify relevant studies, including nonpublished studies?

The Sample. Did the search strategy yield an adequate sample of studies? Did the studies include an adequate sample of participants? If an original report was lacking key information, did the reviewers attempt to contact the original researchers for additional information—or did the study have to be excluded? If studies were excluded for reasons other than insufficient information, did the reviewers provide a rationale for the decision? Did the reviewers retrieve primary source materials (i.e., the actual study reports), or did they draw their data from secondary sources?

Quality Appraisal. Did the reviewers determine the methodologic comparability of the studies in the review? Did the reviewers use appropriate procedures for appraising the quality of individual studies? Were formal criteria used in the appraisal, and were those criteria explicit? Were the criteria appropriate for the type of studies in the sample? Did two or more raters do the appraisals, and was interrater reliability reported?

The Data Set. Were two or more coders used to extract and record information for analysis? Was adequate information extracted about substantive, methodologic, and administrative aspects of the study? Was sufficient information extracted to permit subgroup analysis (if appropriate)? In a meta-analysis, was it possible to compute effect sizes for a sufficient number of studies in the sample?

Data Analysis. Do the reviewers explain their method of pooling and integrating their data? In a meta-synthesis, do the reviewers describe the techniques they used to compare the findings of each study, and do they explain their method of interpreting their data? Was the analysis of data objective and thorough? Were appropriate procedures used to address differences in methodologic quality among studies in the sample? Were appropriate subgroup analyses undertaken—or was the absence of subgroup analyses justified?

Conclusions. Did the reviewers draw reasonable conclusions about the quality, quantity, and consistency of evidence? In a metasynthesis, did the synthesis achieve a fuller understanding of the phenomenon to advance knowledge? Are limitations of the review noted? Are implications for nursing practice and further research clearly stated?

CHAPTER REVIEW

Key new terms introduced in the chapter, together with a summary of major points, are presented in this section. In addition, Chapter 18 of the *Study Guide to Accompany Essentials of Nursing Research*, 6th edition offers various exercises and study suggestions for reinforcing the concepts presented in this chapter. For additional review, see the Student Self-Study Review Questions section of the Student Resource CD-ROM provided with this book.

KEY NEW TERMS

Cochrane Collaboration
Conceptual utilization

Conduct and Utilization of Research
   in Nursing (CURN) Project

Effect size
Evidence hierarchy
Implementation potential
Instrumental utilization
Iowa Model of Evidence-Based
   Practice to Provide Quality Care

Moderator effect
Ottawa Model of Research
   Use (OMRU)
Sensitivity analyses
Stetler Model
Subgroup effect

S U M M A R Y   P O I N T S

▷ **Research utilization** (RU) and **evidence-based practice** (EBP) are overlapping concepts that concern efforts to use research as a basis for clinical decisions. RU starts with a research-based innovation that gets evaluated for possible use in practice. EBP starts with a search for the best possible evidence for a clinical problem, with emphasis on research-based evidence.

▷ Research utilization exists on a continuum, with direct utilization of some specific innovation at one end (**instrumental utilization**) and more diffuse situations in which users are influenced in their thinking about an issue based on some research (**conceptual utilization**) at the other end.

▷ Several major utilization projects have been implemented (e.g., the **Conduct and Utilization of Research in Nursing—or CURN—project**), which have demonstrated that research utilization can be increased but have also shed light on barriers to utilization.

▷ EBP, which de-emphasizes clinical decision making based on custom or ritual, integrates the best available research evidence with other sources of data, including clinical expertise and patient preferences.

▷ In nursing, EBP and RU efforts often face a variety of barriers, including methodologically weak or unreplicated studies, nurses' limited training in research and EBP, resistance to change, lack of organizational support, resource constraints, and limited communication and collaboration between practitioners and researchers.

▷ Many models of RU and EBP have been developed, including models for individual clinicians (e.g., the **Stetler Model**) and models for organizations or groups of clinicians (e.g., the **Iowa Model of Evidence-Based Practice to Promote Quality Care**, the **Ottawa Model of Research Use**).

▷ Most models of utilization involve the following steps: selecting a topic or problem; assembling and evaluating evidence; assessing the **implementation potential** of an evidence-based innovation; evaluating outcomes; and deciding whether to adopt or modify the innovation or revert to prior practices.

▷ Assessing implementation potential includes the dimensions of transferability of findings, feasibility of using the findings in the new setting, and the cost–benefit ratio of a new practice.

▷ EBP relies on rigorous integration of research evidence on a topic through **integrative reviews**, which are rigorous, systematic inquiries with many similarities to original primary studies.

▷ Integrative reviews can involve either qualitative, narrative approaches to integration (including metasynthesis of qualitative studies), or quantitative (meta-analytic) methods.

▷ Integrative reviews typically involve the following activities: developing a question or hypothesis; assembling a review team; searching for and selecting a sample of studies to be included in the review; doing quality assessments of the studies; extracting and recording data from the sampled studies; analyzing the data; and writing up the review.

▷ Quality assessments (which may involve formal quantitative ratings) are sometimes used to exclude weak studies from integrative reviews, but can also be used in **sensitivity analyses** to determine if including or excluding weaker studies changes conclusions.

▷ Meta-analysis involves the computation of an effect size index (which quantifies the magnitude of relationship between the independent and dependent variables) for every study in the sample, and averaging across studies. Meta-analysts can also test for **moderator** (or **subgroup**) **effects**, that is, whether relationships are moderated by the effects of another variable.

RESEARCH EXAMPLES | **Critical Thinking Activities**

 EXAMPLE 1: A Meta-Analytic Integrative Review

Aspects of a meta-analysis, featuring terms and concepts discussed in this chapter, are presented below, followed by some questions to guide critical thinking. (The full research report is available in *Nursing Research, 51,* 119–124).

Study

"Reducing venipuncture and intravenous insertion pain with eutectic mixture of local anesthetic" (Fetzer, 2002)

Purpose

The purpose of the study was to identify and synthesize research on the effectiveness of an eutectic mixture of local anesthetics (EMLA) on venipuncture (VE) and intravenous (IV) insertion pain. The study also explored whether the effect is moderated by various other factors (e.g., patients' age, duration of application, research design, date of the research).

Eligibility Criteria

A primary study was included in the sample if (1) the design was a true experiment or repeated measures; (2) EMLA was administered as the experimental intervention; (3) the control group received a placebo cream without active compounds (i.e., not with a different anesthetic treatment); (4) the procedure involved needle puncture of the skin and underlying vein; (5) pain was measured by self-report; (6) adequate information was available to compute an effect size; (7) the report was in English; and (8) the report was published between 1980 and 2000.

Search Strategy

Fetzer used a variety of search procedures, including online databases (CINAHL, Medline); online journals; citations in bibliographies (the ancestry method); Dissertation Abstracts; and networking at conferences. The key words used in searches were EMLA, eutectic mixture local anesthesia, lidocaine and prilocaine cream, dermal anesthesia, VE pain, and IV insertion pain.

┌───

RESEARCH EXAMPLES *Continued*

Sample

Twenty-two reports met the inclusion criteria, but three had to be eliminated (e.g., one was a duplicate of another study), yielding 19 reports for the meta-analysis. There were seven studies on VE pain, with data based on 542 subjects in the United States, Canada, and Europe. There were 13 studies on IV pain, with over 600 subjects from the United States, Canada, Europe, and Asia.

Quality Assessments

A quality index for each study was calculated using a scoring system adapted from Beck. Scores could range, theoretically, from 6 to 26. The actual range of scores for the 19 studies was 13 to 20.

Data Extraction and Coding

A formal protocol was used to extract information about the study. The variables included substantive ones (e.g., health status of subjects; age and gender of subjects; EMLA application time; puncture site); methodologic ones (sample size; sampling method; research design; pain measurement method); and miscellaneous factors (e.g., country and date of study). Each study was independently coded by two nurse researchers. Rate of agreement on variables ranged from 97% to 100%, and discrepancies were resolved.

Data Analysis

Computer software was used to calculate effect sizes, which were computed three ways: unweighted, weighted by sample size, and weighted by quality rating. The effect size was found to be smallest when weighted by sample size, and these were the results reported.

Key Findings

▎ The beneficial effect of EMLA on pain was substantial across studies for both VE and IV. The mean effect size was 1.05 for VE pain and 1.04 for IV pain.
▎ The effect sizes for VE and IV pain were not moderated by any substantive variable; that is, effects were similarly beneficial for patients of different ages, with different health statuses, and so on.

Discussion

Fetzer concluded that EMLA cream has a large effect on both VE and IV insertion pain, and noted that there were no moderator effects, indicating that the effectiveness of EMLA is not diminished in relation to patient characteristics or insertion technique. Fetzer did note, however, that caution is appropriate in interpreting the moderator findings, because the number of studies in the various subgroups was limited. Fetzer recommended the use of EMLA cream to reduce pain, especially for patients at highest risk of insertion pain and associated side effects.

research examples continue on page 490

RESEARCH EXAMPLES | *Continued*

Critical Thinking Suggestions*

*See the Student Resource CD-ROM for a discussion of these questions.

1. Answer appropriate questions from Box 18-4 regarding this study.

2. Also consider the following targeted questions, which may assist you in further assessing aspects of the study:

    a. Comment on Fetzer's decision to include studies from countries outside North America.

    b. As it turns out, all of the studies in the meta-analysis were in published journals. Comment on what this might mean.

3. If the results of this study are valid and reliable, what might be some of the uses to which the findings could be put in clinical practice?

 EXAMPLE 2: A Metasynthesis

Aspects of a metasynthesis, featuring terms and concepts discussed in this chapter, are presented below, followed by some questions to guide critical thinking. (The full research report is available in *MCN: The American Journal of Maternal Child Nursing, 28,* 93–99.)

Study

"Adolescent motherhood: A meta-synthesis of qualitative studies" (Clemmens, 2003)

Purpose

The purpose of the study was to synthesize qualitative studies on the phenomenon of adolescent motherhood.

Eligibility Criteria

A study was included if the phenomenon under investigation was the experience of adolescent motherhood and if a qualitative approach was used, regardless of research tradition. Studies were excluded if the focus was on depression in adolescent mothers or if the study findings were not organized into themes or metaphors on the experience of adolescent motherhood.

Search Strategy

Clemmens searched the following databases for studies published from 1990 through 2001 with the key words "adolescent motherhood" AND "Qualitative studies": CINAHL, Medline, PsychINFO, ERIC, Sociological Abstracts, and Dissertation Abstracts.

Sample

Of the 50 studies initially identified, 18 met the sample inclusion and exclusion criteria. The 18 studies included 7 descriptive studies, 5 interpretive/ phenomenological studies, 3 grounded theory studies, and 3 ethnographies. Thirteen were from published journal articles, and 5 were from dissertations. The combined sample of participants included 257 adolescent mothers from the United States, Canada, Australia, England, and China.

RESEARCH EXAMPLES *Continued*

Data Extraction and Analysis

Noblit and Hare's comparative approach was used to compare study findings. The original metaphors, themes, concepts, and phrases from each of the 18 studies were organized into a grid and then reciprocally translated, one into the other, resulting in the construction of an initial list of metaphors. The complexity of experiences required a second level of analysis that revealed five overarching metaphors.

Key Findings

The five overarching metaphors were:

▶ The reality of motherhood brings hardships;
▶ Living in the two worlds of adolescence and motherhood;
▶ Motherhood as positively transforming;
▶ Baby as a stabilizing influence; and
▶ Supportive context as turning point for future.

Discussion

Clemmens concluded that the metasynthesis provides nurses with a comprehensive picture of adolescent motherhood. She argued that nurses working in hospital, home care, and school settings can use the results to help develop appropriate interventions, and she offered some examples. She noted that the regularity of the themes and metaphors was important considering the diversity of racial backgrounds and cultures in the original studies.

Critical Thinking Suggestions

1. Answer appropriate questions from Box 18-4 regarding this study.
2. Also consider the following targeted questions, which may assist you in further assessing aspects of the study:
  a. Comment on Clemmens's decision to include studies from countries outside of North America.
  b. Comment on Clemmens's decision to include studies from various qualitative research traditions.
3. If the results of this study are trustworthy, what are some of the uses to which the findings might be put in clinical practice?

SUGGESTED READINGS

Methodologic and Nonempirical References

Agency for Healthcare Research and Quality. (2002). *Systems to rate the strength of scientific evidence.* Washington, DC: AHRQ.

Alberta Association of Registered Nurses. (1997). Nursing research dissemination and utilization. Retrieved October 8, 2004, from http://www.nurses.ab.ca/publications/papers.html

Beck, C. T. (1997). Use of meta-analysis as a teaching strategy in nursing research courses. *Journal of Nursing Education, 36*, 87–90.

Caplan, N., & Rich, R. F. (1975). *The use of social science knowledge in policy decisions at the national level.* Ann Arbor, MI: Institute for Social Research, University of Michigan.

Cooper, H. (1984). *The integrative research review: A social science approach.* Beverly Hills, CA: Sage Publications.

Dobbins, M., Ciliska, D., Cockerill, R., Barnsley, J., & DiCenso, A. (2002). A framework for the dissemination and utilization of research for health-care policy and practice. *The Online Journal of Knowledge Synthesis for Nursing, 9*(7), 1–15.

Estabrooks, C. E. (2001). Research utilization and qualitative research. In J. M. Morse, J. M. Swanson, & A. J. Kuzel (Eds.), *The nature of qualitative evidence.* Thousand Oaks, CA: Sage Publications.

Gennaro, S. (2001). Making evidence-based practice a reality in your institution. *Maternal Child Nursing, 26*, 236–244.

Goode, C., & Piedalue, F. (1999). Evidence based clinical practice. *Journal of Nursing Administration, 29*(6), 15–21.

Greer, N., Mosse, M., Logan, G., & Hallas, G. W. (2000). A practical approach to evidence grading. *Joint Commission Journal on Quality Improvement, 26*, 700–712.

Logan, J., & Graham, I. (1998). Toward a comprehensive interdisciplinary model of health care research use. *Science Communication, 20*, 227–246.

Logan, J., Harrison, M. B., Graham, I. D., Dunn, K., & Bissonnette, J. (1999). Evidence-based pressure-ulcer practice: The Ottawa Model of Research Use. *Canadian Journal of Nursing Research, 31*, 37–52.

Noblit, G., & Hare, R. D. (1988). *Meta-ethnography: Synthesizing qualitative studies.* Newbury Park, CA: Sage Publications.

Paterson, B. L., Thorne, S. E., Canam, C., & Jillings, C. (2001). *Meta-study of qualitative health research.* Thousand Oaks, CA: Sage Publications.

Rosenfeld, P., Duthie, E., Bier, J., Bower-Ferres, S., Fulmer, T., Iervolino, L., McClure, M., McGivern, D., & Roncoli, M. (2000). Engaging staff nurses in evidence-based research to identify nursing practice problems and solutions. *Applied Nursing Research, 13*, 197–203.

Rosswurm, M. A., & Larrabee, J. H. (1999). A model for change to evidence-based practice. *Image: Journal of Nursing Scholarship, 31*, 317–322.

Sackett, D. L., Rosenberg, W., Gray, J. A., Haynes, R., & Richardson, W. (1996). Evidence based medicine: What it is and what it isn't. *British Medical Journal, 312*, 71–72.

Sindhu, F., Carpenter, L., & Seers, K. (1997). Development of a tool to rate the quality assessment of randomized controlled trials using a Delphi technique. *Journal of Advanced Nursing, 25*, 1262–1268.

Soukup, Sr. M. (2000). The Center for Advanced Nursing Practice Evidence-Based Practice Model: Promoting the scholarship of practice. *Nursing Clinics of North America, 35*, 301–309.

Stetler, C. B. (1994). Refinement of the Stetler/Marram Model for application of research findings into practice. *Nursing Outlook, 42*, 15–25.

Stetler, C. B. (2001). Updating the Stetler Model of Research Utilization to facilitate evidence-based practice. *Nursing Outlook, 49*, 272–279.

Stetler, C. B., Morsi, D., Rucki, S., Broughton, S., Corrigan, B., Fitzgerald, J., et al. (1998). Utilization-focused integrative reviews in a nursing service. *Applied Nursing Research, 11*, 195–206.

Titler, M. G., Kleiber, C., Steelman, V., Goode, C., Rakel, B., Barry-Walker, J., et al. (1994). Infusing research into practice to promote quality care. *Nursing Research, 43*, 307–313.

Titler, M. G., Kleiber, C., Steelman, V., Rakel, B., Budreau, G., Everett, L., et al. (2001). The Iowa Model of Evidence-Based Practice to Promote Quality Care. *Critical Care Nursing Clinics of North America, 13*, 497–509.

Weiss, C. (1980). Knowledge creep and decision accretion. *Knowledge: Creation, Diffusion, Utilization, 1*, 381–404.

Studies Cited in Chapter 18

Bauer, N., Bushey, F., & Amaros, D. (2002). Diffusion of responsibility and pressure ulcers. *World Council of Enterostomal Therapist Journal, 22*(3), 9–18.

Beck, C. T. (2001). Predictors of postpartum depression: An update. *Nursing Research, 50*, 275–285.

Beck, C. T. (2002). Postpartum depression: A metasynthesis. *Qualitative Health Research, 12*, 453–472.

Brett, J. L. L. (1987). Use of nursing practice research findings. *Nursing Research, 36*, 344–349.

Carroll, S. M. (2004). Nonvocal ventilated patients' perceptions of being understood. *Western Journal of Nursing Research, 26*, 85–103.

Clemmens, D. (2003). Adolescent motherhood: A meta-synthesis of qualitative studies. *MCN: The American Journal of Maternal/Child Nursing, 28*, 93–99.

Collins-Sharp, B. A., Taylor, D. L., Thomas, K. K., Killeen, M. B., & Dawood, M. Y. (in press). Cyclic perimenstrual pain and discomfort: The scientific basis for practice. *Journal of Obstetric, Gynecologic, & Neonatal Nursing.*

Corn, V. S., Valentine, J. C., Cooper, H. M., & Rantz, M. J. (2003). Grey literature in meta-analyses. *Nursing Research, 52*, 256–261.

Coyle, L. A., & Sokop, A. G. (1990). Innovation adoption behavior among nurses. *Nursing Research, 39*, 176–180.

Devine, E. C. (2003). Meta-analysis of the effect of psychoeducational interventions on pain in adults with cancer. *Oncology Nursing Forum, 30*, 75–89.

Estabrooks, C. A. (1999). The conceptual structure of research utilization. *Research in Nursing & Health, 22*, 203–216.

Evans, D., Wood, J., & Lambert, L. (2002). A review of physical restraint minimization in the acute and residential care settings. *Journal of Advanced Nursing, 40*, 616–625.

Fetzer, S. J. (2002). Reducing venipuncture and intravenous insertion pain with eutectic mixture of local anesthetic. *Nursing Research, 51*, 119–124.

Forbes, D. A. (2003). An example of the use of systematic reviews to answer an effectiveness question. *Western Journal of Nursing Research, 25*, 179–192.

Funk, S. G., Champagne, M. T., Wiese, R. A., & Tornquist, E. M. (1991). Barriers to using research findings in practice: The clinician's perspective. *Applied Nursing Research, 4*, 90–95.

Funk, S. G., Tornquist, E. M., & Champagne, M. T. (1995). Barriers and facilitators of research utilization: An integrative review. *Nursing Clinics of North America, 30*, 395–407.

Graham, K., & Logan, J. (2004). Using the Ottawa Model of Research Use to implement a skin care program. *Journal of Nursing Care Quality, 19*, 18–24.

Hill-Westmoreland, E. E., Soeken, K., & Spellbring, A. M. (2002). A meta-analysis of fall prevention programs for the elderly: How effective are they? *Nursing Research, 51*, 1–8.

Horsley, J. A., Crane, J., & Bingle, J. D. (1978). Research utilization as an organizational process. *Journal of Nursing Administration, 8*, 4–6.

Hutchinson, A. M., & Johnston, L. (2004). Bridging the divide: A survey of nurses' opinions regarding barriers to, and facilitators of, research utilization in the practice setting. *Journal of Clinical Nursing, 13*, 304–315.

Ketefian, S. (1975). Application of selected nursing research findings into nursing practice. *Nursing Research, 24*, 89–92.

Kirchhoff, K. T. (1982). A diffusion survey of coronary precautions. *Nursing Research, 31*, 196–201.

Lanuza, D. M., Lefaiver, C. A., & Farcas, G. A. (2000). Research on the quality of life of lung transplant candidates and recipients: An integrative review. *Heart & Lung, 29*, 180–195.

Lund, C. H., Kuller, J., Lane, A. T., Lott, J. W., & Raines, D. A. (1999). Neonatal skin care: The scientific basis for practice. *Journal of Obstetric, Gynecologic, & Neonatal Nursing, 28*, 241–254.

Lund, C. H., Kuller, J., Lane, A. T., Lott, J. W., Raines, D. A., & Thomas, K. K. (2001a). Neonatal skin care: Evaluation of the AWHONN/NANN research-based practice project on knowledge and skin care practices. *Journal of Obstetric, Gynecologic, & Neonatal Nursing, 30*, 30–40.

Lund, C. H., Osborne, J. W., Kuller, J., Lane, A. T., Lott, J. W., & Raines, D. A. (2001b). Neonatal skin care: Clinical outcomes of the AWHONN/NANN evidence-based clinical practice guideline. *Journal of Obstetric, Gynecologic, & Neonatal Nursing, 30*, 41–51.

Maloni, J. A., Albrecht, S. A., Thomas, K. K., Halleran, J., & Jones, R. (2003). Implementing evidence-based practice: Reducing risk for low birth weight through pregnancy smoking cessation. *Journal of Obstetric, Gynecologic, & Neonatal Nursing, 32*, 676–682.

McCaughan, D., Thompson, C., Cullum, N., Sheldon, T. A., & Thompson, D. R. (2002). Acute care nurses' perceptions of barriers to using research information in clinical decision-making. *Journal of Advanced Nursing, 39*, 46–60.

McCleary, L., & Brown, G. T. (2003). Barriers to paediatric nurses' research utilization. *Journal of Advanced Nursing, 42*, 364–372.

Montgomery, L., Hanrahan, K., Kottman, K., Otto, A., Barrett, T., & Hermington, B. (1999). Guideline for i.v. infiltration in pediatric patients. *Pediatric Nursing, 25*, 167–169.

Nelson, A. M. (2002). A metasynthesis: Mothering other-than-normal children. *Qualitative Health Research, 12*, 515–530.

Peacock, S. C., & Forbes, D. A. (2003). Interventions for caregivers of persons with dementia: A systematic review. *Canadian Journal of Nursing Research, 35*, 88–107.

Rice, V., & Stead, L. (2004). Nursing interventions for smoking cessation. *Cochrane Database of Systematic Reviews,* (1), No. CD001188.

Rodgers, S. E. (2000). The extent of nursing research utilization in general medical and surgical wards. *Journal of Advanced Nursing, 32*, 182–193.

Rutledge, D. N., Greene, P., Mooney, K., Nail, L. M., & Ropka, M. (1996). Use of research-based practices by oncology staff nurses. *Oncology Nursing Forum, 23*, 1235–1244.

Smith, B., Appleton, S., Adams, R., Soutcott, A., & Ruffin, R. (2004). Home care by outreach nursing for chronic obstructive pulmonary disease. *The Cochrane Library,* (1).

Varcoe, C., & Hilton, A. (1995). Factors affecting acute-care nurses' use of research findings. *Canadian Journal of Nursing Research, 27*(4), 51–71.

World Wide Websites
- AHCPR/AHRQ Clinical Practice Guidelines
  http://www.ahrq.gov and http://www.guidelines.gov.

- The Cochrane Collaboration
  http://www.cochrane.org/
- Registered Nurses Association of Ontario Best Practice Guidelines
  http://www.rnao.org/bestpractices
- University of Alberta University of Alberta's "Evidence-Based Medicine Tool Kit"
  http://www.med.ualberta.ca/ebm/ebm.htm
- University of Iowa's Evidence Based Practice Center
  http://www.uihealthcare.com/depts/nursing/rqom/evidencebasedpractice/toolkit.html
- University of Sheffield (United Kingdom), "Netting the Evidence"
  http://www.shef.ac.uk/scharr/ir/netting/

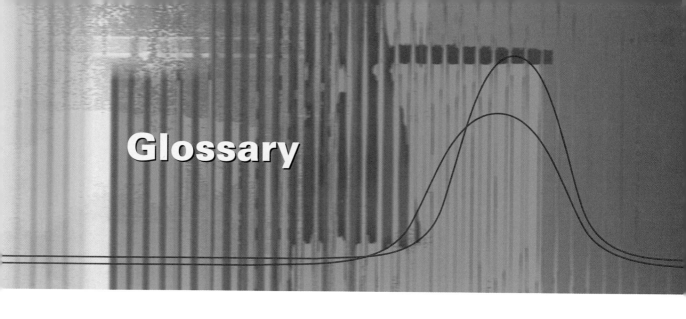

Glossary

Note: Entries preceded by an asterisk (*) are terms that were not explained in this book, but they are included here because you might come across them in the research literature. For further explanation of these terms, please refer to Polit and Beck (2004), *Nursing Research: Principles and Methods* (7th ed.), Philadelphia, PA: Lippincott Williams & Wilkins.

abstract A brief description of a completed or proposed study, usually located at the beginning of the report or proposal.

accessible population The population of people available for a particular study; often a nonrandom subset of the target population.

acquiescence response set A bias in self-report instruments, especially in psychosocial scales, created when study participants characteristically agree with statements ("yea-say") independent of their content.

after-only design An experimental design in which data are collected from subjects only after an experimental intervention has been introduced.

alpha (α) (1) In tests of statistical significance, the level designating the probability of committing a Type I error; (2) in estimates of internal consistency, a reliability coefficient, as in Cronbach's alpha.

analysis The process of organizing and synthesizing data so as to answer research questions and test hypotheses.

analysis of covariance (ANCOVA) A statistical procedure used to test mean differences among groups on a dependent variable, while controlling for one or more extraneous variables (covariates).

analysis of variance (ANOVA) A statistical procedure for testing mean differences among three or more groups by comparing variability between groups to variability within groups.

anonymity Protection of participants in a study such that even the researcher cannot link individuals with the information provided.

applied research Research designed to find a solution to an immediate practical problem.

assent The affirmative agreement of a vulnerable subject (e.g., a child) to participate in a study.

associative relationship An association between two variables that cannot be described as causal (i.e., one variable *causing* the other).

assumption A basic principle that is accepted as being true based on logic or reason, but without proof or verification.

asymmetric distribution A distribution of data values that is skewed, i.e., has two halves that are not mirror images of each other.

attrition The loss of participants over the course of a study, which can create bias and undermine internal validity by changing the composition of the sample.

audit trail The systematic documentation of material that allows an independent auditor of a qualitative study to draw conclusions about the trustworthiness of the data.

auditability The extent to which an external reviewer or reader can follow a qualitative researcher's steps and decisions and draw conclusions about the analysis and interpretation of the data.

auto-ethnography Ethnographic studies in which researchers study their own culture or group.

axial coding The second level of coding in a grounded theory study using the Strauss and Corbin approach, involving the process of categorizing, recategorizing, and condensing all first-level codes by connecting a category and its subcategories.

*back-translation The translation of a translated text back into the original language, so that a comparison of the original and back-translated version can be made.

baseline data Data collected prior to an intervention, including pretreatment data from a measure of the dependent variable.

basic research Research designed to extend the base of knowledge in a discipline for the sake of knowledge production or theory construction, rather than for solving an immediate problem.

basic social process (BSP) The central social process emerging through an analysis of grounded theory data.

before–after design An experimental design in which data are collected from research subjects both before and after the introduction of an experimental intervention.

beneficence A fundamental ethical principle that seeks to prevent harm and exploitation of, and maximize benefits for, study participants.

beta (β) (1) In multiple regression, the standardized coefficients indicating the relative weights of the independent variables in the regression equation; (2) in statistical testing, the probability of a Type II error.

between-subjects design A research design in which there are separate groups of people being compared (e.g., smokers and nonsmokers).

bias Any influence that produces a distortion in the results of a study.

bimodal distribution A distribution of data values with two peaks (high frequencies).

bivariate statistics Statistics derived from analyzing two variables simultaneously to assess the empirical relationship between them.

blind review The review of a manuscript or proposal such that neither the author nor the reviewer is identified to the other party.

blinding The masking or withholding of information (e.g., from research subjects, research personnel, or reviewers) to reduce the possibility of certain biases.

bracketing In phenomenological inquiries, the process of identifying and holding in abeyance any preconceived beliefs and opinions about the phenomena under study.

bricolage The tendency in qualitative research to assemble a complex array of data from a variety of sources.

*canonical analysis A statistical procedure for examining the relationship between two or more independent variables *and* two or more dependent variables.

carry-over effect The influence that one treatment can have on subsequent treatments.

case-control design A nonexperimental research design involving the comparison of a "case" (i.e., a person with the condition under scrutiny, such as lung cancer) and a matched control (a similar person without the condition).

case study A research method involving a thorough, in-depth analysis of an individual, group, institution, or other social unit.

categorical variable A variable with discrete values (e.g., gender) rather than values along a continuum (e.g., weight).

category system In observational studies, the prespecified plan for organizing and recording the behaviors and events under observation; in qualitative studies, the system used to sort and organize narrative data.

causal modeling The development and statistical testing of an explanatory model of hypothesized causal relationships among phenomena.

causal (cause-and-effect) relationship A relationship between two variables such that the presence or absence of one variable (the "cause") determines the presence or absence, or value, of the other (the "effect").

cell (1) The intersection of a row and column in a table with two or more dimensions; (2) in an experimental design, the representation of an experimental condition in a schematic diagram.

central (core) category The main category or pattern of behavior of the research in a Strauss and Corbin grounded theory analysis.

central tendency A statistical index of the "typicalness" of a set of scores, derived from the center of the score distribution; indices of central tendency include the mode, median, and mean.

chi-squared test A nonparametric test of statistical significance used to assess whether a relationship exists between two nominal-level variables. Symbolized as χ^2.

clinical research Research designed to generate knowledge to guide clinical practice in nursing and other health care fields.

clinical trial A study designed to assess the safety and effectiveness of a new clinical treatment, sometimes involving several phases, one of which (Phase III) is a randomized clinical trial using an experimental design.

closed-ended question A question that offers respondents a set of mutually exclusive and jointly exhaustive response options, from which the one most closely approximating the "right" answer must be chosen.

*cluster analysis A multivariate statistical procedure used to cluster people or things based on patterns of association.

*cluster randomization The random assignment of intact groups of subjects—rather than individual subjects—to treatment conditions.

cluster sampling A form of sampling in which large groupings ("clusters") are selected first (e.g., nursing schools), with successive subsampling of smaller units (e.g., nursing students).

code of ethics The fundamental ethical principles established by a discipline or institution to guide researchers' conduct with human (or animal) subjects.

coding The process of transforming raw data into standardized form for data processing and analysis; in quantitative research, the process of attaching numbers to categories; in qualitative research, the process of identifying recurring themes or concepts within the data.

coefficient alpha (Cronbach's alpha) A reliability index that estimates the internal consistency or homogeneity of a measure composed of several items or subparts.

coercion In a research context, the explicit or implicit use of threats (or excessive rewards) to gain people's cooperation in a study.

comparison group A group of subjects whose scores on a dependent variable are used to evaluate the outcomes of the group of primary interest (e.g., nonsmokers as a comparison group for smokers); term often used in lieu of control group when the study design is not a true experiment.

concealment A tactic involving the collection of research data without participants' knowledge or consent, to obtain an accurate view of naturalistic behavior when the known presence of an observer would distort the behavior.

concept An abstraction based on observations of—or inferences from—behaviors or characteristics (e.g., stress, pain).

conceptual definition The abstract or theoretical meaning of the concept being studied.

conceptual file A manual method of organizing qualitative data, by creating file folders for each category in the coding scheme and inserting relevant excerpts from the data.

conceptual model Interrelated concepts or abstractions assembled together in a rational scheme by virtue of their relevance to a common theme; sometimes called *conceptual framework*.

conceptual utilization The use of research findings in a general, conceptual way to broaden one's thinking about an issue, without putting the knowledge to any specific, documentable use.

concurrent validity The degree to which scores on an instrument are correlated with some external criterion, measured at the same time.

*confidence interval (CI) The range of values within which a population parameter is estimated to lie.

*confidence level The estimated probability that a population parameter lies within a given confidence interval.

confidentiality Protection of study participants such that individual identities are not linked to information provided and are never publicly divulged.

confirmability A criterion for evaluating the quality of qualitative research, referring to the objectivity or neutrality of the data or the analysis and interpretation.

*confirmatory factor analysis A factor analysis, based on maximum likelihood estimation, designed to confirm a hypothesized measurement model.

consent form A written agreement signed by a study participant and a researcher concerning the terms and conditions of voluntary participation in a study.

constant comparison A procedure used in a grounded theory analysis wherein newly collected data are compared in an ongoing fashion with data obtained earlier, to refine theoretically relevant categories.

constitutive pattern In hermeneutic analysis, a pattern that expresses the relationships among relational themes and is present in all the interviews or texts.

construct An abstraction or concept that is deliberately invented (constructed) by researchers for a scientific purpose (e.g., health locus of control).

construct validity The degree to which an instrument measures the construct under investigation.

consumer An individual who reads, reviews, and critiques research findings and who attempts to use and apply the findings in his or her practice.

*contamination The inadvertent, undesirable influence of one experimental treatment condition on another treatment condition.

content analysis The process of organizing and integrating narrative, qualitative information according to emerging themes and concepts.

content validity The degree to which the items in an instrument adequately represent the universe of content for the concept being measured.

content validity index (CVI) An indicator of the degree to which an instrument is content valid, based on average ratings of a panel of experts.

contingency table A two-dimensional table that permits a crosstabulation of the frequencies of two categorical variables.

continuous variable A variable that can take on an infinite range of values along a specified continuum (e.g., height).

control The process of holding constant extraneous influences on the dependent variable under investigation.

control group Subjects in an experiment who do not receive the experimental treatment and whose performance provides a baseline against which the effects of the treatment can be measured (see also *comparison group*).

convenience sampling Selection of the most readily available persons as participants in a study; also called *accidental sampling*.

*convergent validity An approach to construct validation that involves assessing the degree to which two methods of measuring a construct are similar (i.e., converge).

core variable (category) In a grounded theory study, the central phenomenon that is used to integrate all categories of the data.

correlation An association or connection between variables, such that variation in one variable is related to variation in another.

correlation coefficient An index summarizing the degree of relationship between variables, typically ranging from $+1.00$ (for a perfect positive relationship) through 0.0 (for no relationship) to -1.00 (for a perfect negative relationship).

correlation matrix A two-dimensional display showing the correlation coefficients between all pairs of a set of study variables.

correlational research Research that explores the interrelationships among variables of interest without any active intervention by the researcher.

cost–benefit analysis An evaluation of the monetary costs of a program or intervention relative to the monetary gains attributable to it.

counterbalancing The process of systematically varying the order of presentation of stimuli or treatments to control for ordering effects, as in a crossover design.

counterfactual The condition or group used as a basis of comparison in a study.

covariate A variable that is statistically controlled (held constant) in ANCOVA, typically an extraneous influence on the dependent variable or a preintervention measure of the dependent variable.

covert data collection The collection of information in a study without participants' knowledge.

*Cramér's *V* An index describing the magnitude of the relationship between nominal-level data, used when the contingency table to which it is applied is larger than 2×2.

credibility A criterion for evaluating data quality in qualitative studies, referring to confidence in the truth of the data.

criterion sampling A sampling approach in qualitative research that involves selecting cases that meet a predetermined criterion of importance.

criterion-related validity The degree to which scores on an instrument are correlated with some external criterion.

critical ethnography An ethnography that focuses on raising consciousness in the group or culture under study in the hope of effecting social change.

critical incident technique A method of obtaining data from study participants by in-depth exploration of specific incidents and behaviors related to the topic under study.

*critical region The area in the sampling distribution representing values that are "improbable" if the null hypothesis is true.

critical theory A view of the world that involves a critique of society, with the goal of envisioning new possibilities and effecting social change.

critique An objective, critical, and balanced appraisal of a research report's various dimensions (e.g., conceptual, methodologic, ethical).

Cronbach's alpha A widely used reliability index that estimates the internal consistency or homogeneity of a measure composed of several subparts; also called *coefficient alpha*.

crossover design An experimental design in which one group of subjects is exposed to more than one condition or treatment in random order; sometimes called a *repeated measures design*.

cross-sectional design A study design in which data are collected at one point in time; sometimes used to infer change over time when data are collected from different age or developmental groups.

crosstabulation A determination of the number of cases occurring when two variables are considered simultaneously (e.g., gender—male/female—crosstabulated with smoking status—smoker/nonsmoker). The results are typically presented in a table with rows and columns divided according to the values of the variables.

data The pieces of information obtained in the course of a study (singular is *datum*).

data analysis The systematic organization and synthesis of research data and, in most quantitative studies, the testing of research hypotheses using those data.

data collection The gathering of information to address a research problem.

data collection protocols The formal procedures researchers develop to guide the collection of data in a standardized fashion.

data saturation See *saturation*.

data set The total collection of data on all variables for all study participants.

data source triangulation The use of multiple data sources for the purpose of validating conclusions.

debriefing Communication with study participants after participation is complete regarding various aspects of the study.

deception The deliberate withholding of information, or the provision of false information, to study participants, usually to reduce potential biases.

deductive reasoning The process of developing specific predictions from general principles (see also *inductive reasoning*).

degrees of freedom (*df*) A concept used in statistical testing, referring to the number of sample values free to vary (e.g., with a given sample mean, all but one value would be free to vary).

*Delphi technique A method of obtaining written judgments from a panel of experts about an issue of concern; experts are questioned individually in several rounds, with a summary of the panel's views circulated between rounds, to achieve some consensus.

dependability A criterion for evaluating data quality in qualitative data, referring to the stability of data over time and over conditions.

dependent variable The variable hypothesized to depend on or be caused by another variable (the *independent variable*); the outcome variable of interest.

descriptive phenomenology A type of phenomenology, developed by Husserl, that emphasizes the careful description of ordinary conscious experience of everyday life.

descriptive research Research that has as its main objective the accurate portrayal of the characteristics of persons, situations, or groups, and/or the frequency with which certain phenomena occur.

descriptive statistics Statistics used to describe and summarize data (e.g., means, standard deviations).

descriptive theory A broad characterization that thoroughly accounts for a single phenomenon.

determinism The belief that phenomena are not haphazard or random, but rather have antecedent causes; an assumption in the positivist paradigm.

*deviation score A score computed by subtracting the mean of a set of scores from an individual score.

dichotomous variable A variable having only two values or categories (e.g., gender).

directional hypothesis A hypothesis that makes a specific prediction about the direction and nature of the relationship between two variables.

discourse analysis A qualitative tradition, from sociolinguistics, that seeks to understand the rules, mechanisms, and structure of conversations.

*discrete variable A variable with a finite number of values between two points.

discriminant function analysis A statistical procedure used to predict group membership or status on a categorical (nominal level) variable on the basis of two or more independent variables.

*discriminant validity An approach to construct validation that involves assessing the degree to which a single method of measuring two constructs yields different results (i.e., discriminates the two).

disproportionate sample A sample in which the researcher samples differing proportions of study participants from different population strata to ensure adequate representation from smaller strata.

domain In ethnographic analysis, a unit or broad category of cultural knowledge.

double-blind experiment An experiment in which neither the subjects nor those who administer the treatment know who is in the experimental or control group.

*dummy variable Dichotomous variables created for use in many multivariate statistical analyses, typically using codes of 0 and 1 (e.g., female = 1, male = 0).

ecological psychology A qualitative tradition that focuses on the environment's influence on human behavior and attempts to identify principles that explain the interdependence of humans and their environmental context.

editing analysis style An approach to the analysis of qualitative data, in which researchers read through texts in search of meaningful segments and develop a categorization scheme that is used to sort and organize the data.

effect size A statistical expression of the magnitude of the relationship between two variables, or the magnitude of the difference between two groups, with regard to some attribute of interest.

*eigenvalue In factor analysis, the value equal to the sum of the squared weights for each factor.

element The most basic unit of a population from which a sample is drawn—typically humans in nursing research.

eligibility criteria The criteria used to designate the specific attributes of the target population, and by which people are selected for participation in a study.

emergent design A design that unfolds in the course of a qualitative study as the researcher makes ongoing design decisions reflecting what has already been learned.

*emergent fit A concept in grounded theory that involves comparing new data and new categories with existing conceptualizations (e.g., from the literature).

emic perspective A term used by ethnographers to refer to the way members of a culture view their own world; the "insider's view."

empirical evidence Evidence rooted in objective reality and gathered using one's senses as the basis for generating knowledge.

*endogenous variable In path analysis, a variable whose variation is determined by other variables within the model.

error of measurement The deviation between true scores and obtained scores of a measured characteristic.

*error term The mathematic expression (typically in a regression analysis) that represents all unknown or immeasurable attributes that can affect the dependent variable.

estimation procedures Statistical procedures that have as their goal the estimation of population parameters based on sample statistics.

*eta squared In ANOVA, a statistic calculated to indicate the proportion of variance in the dependent variable explained by the independent variables, analogous to R in multiple regression.

ethics A system of moral values that is concerned with the degree to which research procedures adhere to professional, legal, and social obligations to the study participants.

ethnography A branch of human inquiry, associated with anthropology, that focuses on the culture of a group of people, with an effort to understand their world view.

ethnomethodology A branch of human inquiry, associated with sociology, that focuses on the way in which people make sense of their everyday activities and come to behave in socially acceptable ways.

ethnonursing research The study of human cultures, with a focus on a group's beliefs and practices relating to nursing care and related health behaviors.

etic perspective A term used by ethnographers to refer to the "outsider's" view of the experiences of a cultural group.

evaluation research Research that investigates how well a program, practice, or policy is working.

event sampling In observational studies, a sampling plan that involves the selection of integral behaviors or events.

evidence hierarchy A ranked arrangement of the validity and dependability of evidence based on the rigor of the design that produced it.

evidence-based practice A practice that involves making clinical decisions on the best available evidence, with an emphasis on evidence from disciplined research.

ex post facto research Nonexperimental research conducted after variations in the independent variable have occurred in the natural course of events and, therefore, any causal explanations are inferred "after the fact."

exclusion criteria The criteria that specify characteristics that a population does *not* have.

*exogenous variable In path analysis, a variable whose determinants lie outside the model.

experiment A study in which the researcher controls (manipulates) the independent variable and—in a true experiment—randomly assigns subjects to different conditions.

experimental group Subjects in a study who receive the experimental treatment or intervention.

experimental intervention (experimental treatment) See *intervention*; *treatment*.

*exploratory factor analysis A factor analysis undertaken to determine the underlying dimensionality of a set of variables.

exploratory research A study that explores the dimensions of a phenomenon or that develops or refines hypotheses about relationships between phenomena.

external validity The degree to which study results can be generalized to settings or samples other than the one studied.

extraneous variable A variable that confounds the relationship between the independent and dependent variables and that needs to be controlled either through research design or statistical procedures.

extreme case sampling A sampling approach used by qualitative researchers that involves the purposeful selection of the most extreme or unusual cases.

extreme response set A bias in self-report instruments, especially in psychosocial scales, created when participants select extreme response alternatives (e.g., "strongly agree"), independent of the item's content.

F-ratio The statistic obtained in several statistical tests (e.g., ANOVA) in which variation attributable to different sources (e.g., between groups and within groups) is compared.

face validity The extent to which a measuring instrument looks as though it is measuring what it purports to measure.

factor analysis A statistical procedure for reducing a large set of variables into a smaller set of variables with common characteristics or underlying dimensions.

*factor extraction The first phase of a factor analysis, which involves the extraction of as much variance as possible through the successive creation of linear combinations of the variables in the analysis.

*factor loading In factor analysis, the weight associated with a variable on a given factor.

*factor rotation The second phase of factor analysis, during which the reference axes for the factors are moved such that variables more clearly align with a single factor.

*factor score A person's score on a latent variable (factor).

factorial design An experimental design in which two or more independent variables are simultaneously manipulated, permitting a separate analysis of the main effects of the independent variables, plus the interaction effects of those variables.

feasibility study A small-scale test to determine the feasibility of a larger study (see also *pilot study*).

feminist research Research that seeks to understand, typically through qualitative approaches, how gender and a gendered social order shapes women's lives and their consciousness.

field diary A daily record of events and conversations in the field; also called a *log*.

field notes The notes taken by researchers describing the unstructured observations they have made in the field and their interpretation of those observations.

field research Research in which the data are collected "in the field" from individuals in their normal roles, with the aim of understanding the practices, behaviors, and beliefs of individuals or groups as they normally function in real life.

fieldwork The activities undertaken by researchers (usually qualitative researchers) to collect data out in the field (i.e., in natural settings outside the research environment).

findings The results of the analysis of research data.

*Fisher's exact test A statistical procedure used to test the significance of the difference in proportions, used when the sample size is small or cells in the contingency table have no observations.

fit In grounded theory analysis, the process of identifying characteristics of one piece of data and comparing them with the characteristics of another datum to determine similarity.

fittingness In an assessment of the transferability of findings from a qualitative study, the degree of congruence between the research sample and another group or setting of interest.

fixed alternative question A question that offers respondents a set of prespecified responses, from which the respondent must choose the alternative that most closely approximates the correct response.

focus group interview An interview with a group of individuals assembled to answer questions on a given topic.

focused interview A loosely structured interview in which an interviewer guides the respondent through a set of questions using a topic guide; also called a *semistructured interview*.

follow-up study A study undertaken to determine the outcomes of individuals with a specified condition or who have received a specified treatment.

forced-choice question A question that requires respondents to choose between two statements that represent polar positions or characteristics.

formal grounded theory A theory developed at a highly abstract level of theory by integrating several substantive grounded theories.

framework The conceptual underpinnings of a study; often called a *theoretical framework* in studies based on a theory, or a *conceptual framework* in studies rooted in a specific conceptual model.

frequency distribution A systematic array of numerical values from the lowest to the highest, together with a count of the number of times each value was obtained.

frequency polygon Graphic display of a frequency distribution in which dots connected by a straight line indicate the number of times score values occur in a data set.

*Friedman test A nonparametric analog of ANOVA, used with paired-groups or repeated-measures situations.

full disclosure The communication of complete information to potential study participants about the nature of the study, the right to refuse participation, and the likely risks and benefits that would be incurred.

functional relationship A relationship between two variables in which it cannot be assumed that one variable caused the other, but it can be said that one variable changes values in relation to changes in the other variable.

gaining entrée The process of gaining access to study participants in qualitative field studies through the cooperation of key actors in the selected community or site.

generalizability The degree to which the research methods justify the inference that the findings are true for a broader group than study participants; in particular, the inference that the findings can be generalized from the sample to the population.

*"going native" A pitfall in qualitative research wherein a researcher becomes too emotionally involved with participants and therefore loses the ability to observe objectively.

grand theory A broad theory aimed at describing large segments of the physical, social, or behavioral world; also called a *macrotheory*.

grand tour question A broad question asked in an unstructured interview to gain a general overview of a phenomenon, the basis for more focused questions.

*graphic rating scale A scale in which respondents are asked to rate something (e.g., a concept or an issue) along an ordered bipolar continuum (e.g., "excellent" to "very poor").

grounded theory An approach to collecting and analyzing qualitative data that aims to develop theories and theoretical propositions grounded in real-world observations.

Hawthorne effect The effect on the dependent variable resulting from subjects' awareness that they are participants under study.

hermeneutic circle In hermeneutics, the qualitative circle signifies a methodologic process in which, to reach understanding, there is continual movement between the parts and the whole of the text that are being analyzed.

hermeneutics A qualitative research tradition, drawing on interpretive phenomenology, that focuses on the lived experiences of humans and on how they interpret those experiences.

heterogeneity The degree to which objects are dissimilar (i.e., characterized by high variability) with respect to some attribute.

*hierarchical multiple regression A multiple regression analysis in which predictor variables are entered into the equation in steps that are prespecified by the analyst.

historical research Systematic studies designed to discover facts and relationships about past events.

history threat The occurrence of events external to an intervention (or other independent variable) but occurring concurrent with it, which can affect the dependent variable and threaten the study's internal validity.

homogeneity (1) In terms of the reliability of an instrument, the degree to which its subparts are internally consistent (i.e., are measuring the same critical attribute); (2) more generally, the degree to which objects are similar (i.e., characterized by low variability).

homogenous sampling A sampling approach used by qualitative researchers involving the deliberate selection of cases with limited variation.

hypothesis A prediction, usually a statement of predicted relationships between variables.

hypothesis testing A statistical procedure that involves the comparison of empirically observed sample findings with theoretically expected findings that would be observed if the null hypothesis were true.

impact analysis An evaluation of the effects of a program or intervention on outcomes of interest, net of other factors influencing those outcomes.

implementation analysis In an evaluation, a description of the process by which a program or intervention was implemented in practice.

implementation potential The extent to which an innovation is amenable to implementation in a new setting, an assessment of which is usually made in an evidence-based practice (or research utilization) project.

implied consent Consent to participate in a study that a researcher assumes has been given based on certain actions of the participant (such as returning a completed questionnaire).

IMRAD format The organization of a research report into four sections: the Introduction, Methods, Research, and Discussion sections.

*incidence rate The rate of new "cases" with a specified condition, determined by dividing the number of new cases over a given period of time by the number at risk of becoming a new case (i.e., free of the condition at the outset of the time period).

independent variable The variable that is believed to cause or influence the dependent variable; in experimental research, the manipulated (treatment) variable.

inductive reasoning The process of reasoning from specific observations to more general rules (see also *deductive reasoning*).

inferential statistics Statistics that permit inferences on whether relationships observed in a sample are likely to occur in the population.

informant A term used to refer to an individual who provides information to researchers about a phenomenon under study (usually in qualitative studies).

informed consent An ethical principle that requires researchers to obtain the voluntary participation of subjects, after informing them of possible risks and benefits.

inquiry audit An independent scrutiny of qualitative data and relevant supporting documents by an external reviewer to determine dependability and confirmability.

insider research Research on a group or culture—usually in an ethnography—by a member of the group or culture.

Institutional Review Board (IRB) A group of individuals from an institution who convene to review proposed and ongoing studies with respect to ethical considerations.

instrument The device used to collect data (e.g., questionnaire, test, observation schedule, etc.).

instrumental utilization Clearly identifiable attempts to base some specific action or intervention on the results of research findings.

integrative review A review of research that amasses comprehensive information on a topic, weighs pieces of evidence, and integrates information to draw conclusions about the state of knowledge.

*intention to treat A principle for analyzing data that involves the assumption that each person received the treatment to which he or she was assigned; contrary to *on-protocol analysis.*

interaction effect The effect of two or more independent variables acting in combination (interactively) on a dependent variable rather than as unconnected factors.

intercoder reliability The degree to which two coders, operating independently, agree in their coding decisions.

internal consistency The degree to which the subparts of an instrument are all measuring the same attribute or dimension, as a measure of the instrument's reliability.

internal validity The degree to which it can be inferred that the experimental treatment (or independent variable), rather than extraneous factors, is responsible for observed effects.

interpretation The process of making sense of the results of a study and examining their implications.

interpretive phenomenology An approach to phenomenology in which interpreting and understanding—and not just describing—human experience is stressed; also called *hermeneutics.*

interrater (interobserver) reliability The degree to which two raters or observers, operating independently, assign the same ratings or values for an attribute being measured or observed.

*interrupted time series design See *time series design.*

*interval estimation A statistical estimation approach in which the researcher establishes a range of values that are likely, within a given level of confidence, to contain the true population parameter.

interval measurement A level of measurement in which an attribute of a variable is rank ordered on a scale that has equal distances between points on that scale (e.g., Fahrenheit degrees).

intervention An experimental treatment or manipulation.

intervention protocol In experimental research, the specification of exactly what the treatment and the alternative condition (the counterfactual) will be, and how treatments are to be administered.

*intervention research A systematic research approach distinguished not so much by a particular research methodology as by a distinctive *process* of planning, developing, implementing, testing, and disseminating interventions.

interview A method of data collection in which one person (an interviewer) asks questions of another person (a respondent); interviews are conducted either face-to-face or by telephone.

interview schedule The formal instrument, used in structured self-report studies, that specifies the wording of all questions to be asked of respondents.

intuiting The second step in descriptive phenomenology, which occurs when researchers remain open to the meaning attributed to the phenomenon by those who experienced it.

inverse relationship A relationship characterized by the tendency of high values on one variable to be associated with low values on the second variable; also called a *negative relationship.*

investigator triangulation The use of two or more researchers to analyze and interpret a data set to enhance the validity of the findings.

item A single question on a test or questionnaire, or a single statement on an attitude or other scale (e.g., a final examination might consist of 100 items).

*item analysis A type of analysis used to assess whether items are tapping the same construct and are sufficiently discriminating.

journal article A report appearing in professional journals such as *Nursing Research.*

journal club A group that meets (often in clinical settings) to discuss and critique research reports appearing in journals, sometimes to assess the potential use of the findings in practice.

judgmental sampling A type of nonprobability sampling method in which the researcher selects study participants based on personal judgment about who will be most representative or informative; also called *purposive sampling.*

*Kendall's tau A correlation coefficient used to indicate the magnitude of a relationship between ordinal-level variables.

key informant A person well-versed in the phenomenon of research interest and who is willing to share the information and insight with the researcher.

keyword An important concept or term used to search for references on a topic (e.g., in an electronic bibliographic database).

known-groups technique A technique for estimating the construct validity of an instrument through an analysis of the degree to which the instrument separates groups predicted to differ based on known characteristics or theory.

*Kruskal-Wallis test A nonparametric test used to test the difference between three or more independent groups, based on ranked scores.

*latent variable An unmeasured variable that represents an underlying, abstract construct (usually in the context of a LISREL analysis).

*least-squares estimation A commonly used method of statistical estimation in which the solution minimizes the sums of squares of error terms; also called OLS (*ordinary least squares*).

level of measurement A system of classifying measurements according to the nature of the quantitative information and the type of mathematical operations to which they are amenable; the four levels are nominal, ordinal, interval, and ratio.

level of significance The risk of making a Type I error in a statistical analysis, established by the researcher beforehand (e.g., the .05 level).

life history A narrative self-report about a person's life experiences vis-à-vis a theme of interest.

*life table analysis A statistical procedure used when the dependent variable represents a time interval between an initial event (e.g., onset of a disease) and an end event (e.g., death); also called *survival analysis*.

Likert scale A composite measure of attitudes involving the summation of scores on a set of items that are rated by respondents for their degree of agreement or disagreement.

*linear regression An analysis for predicting the value of a dependent variable by determining a straight-line fit to the data that minimizes the sum of squared deviations from the line.

LISREL The widely used acronym for linear structural relation analysis, typically used for testing causal models.

literature review A critical summary of research on a topic of interest, often prepared to put a research problem in context.

log In participant observation studies, the observer's daily record of events and conversations that took place.

logical positivism The philosophy underlying the traditional scientific approach; see also *positivist paradigm*.

logistic regression A multivariate regression procedure that analyzes relationships between multiple independent variables and categorical dependent variables; also called *logit analysis*.

logit The natural log of the odds, used as the dependent variable in logistic regression; short for logistic probability unit.

longitudinal study A study designed to collect data at more than one point in time, in contrast to a cross-sectional study.

macrotheory A broad theory aimed at describing large segments of the physical, social, or behavioral world; also called a *grand theory*.

main effects In a study with multiple independent variables, the effects of a single independent variable on the dependent variable.

*manifest variable An observed, measured variable that serves as an indicator of an underlying construct (i.e., a latent variable), usually in the context of a LISREL analysis.

manipulation An intervention or treatment introduced as the independent variable in an experimental or quasi-experimental study, to assess its impact on the dependent variable.

*manipulation check In experimental studies, a test to determine whether the manipulation was implemented as intended.

*Mann-Whitney *U*-test A nonparametric statistic used to test the difference between two independent groups, based on ranked scores.

MANOVA See *multivariate analysis of variance*.

matching The pairing of subjects in one group with those in another group, based on their similarity on one or more dimension, to enhance the overall similarity of comparison groups.

maturation threat A threat to the internal validity of a study that results when changes to the outcome measure (dependent variable) occur as a result of the passage of time.

*maximum likelihood estimation An estimation approach (sometimes used in lieu of the least-squares approach) in which the estimators are ones that estimate the parameters most likely to have generated the observed measurements.

maximum variation sampling A sampling approach used by qualitative researchers involving the purposeful selection of cases with a wide range of variation.

*McNemar test A statistical test for comparing differences in proportions when values are derived from paired (nonindependent) groups.

mean A descriptive statistic that is a measure of central tendency, computed by summing all scores and dividing by the number of subjects.

measurement The assignment of numbers to objects according to specified rules to characterize quantities of an attribute.

*measurement model In LISREL, the model that stipulates the hypothesized relationships among the manifest and latent variables.

median A descriptive statistic that is a measure of central tendency, representing the exact middle value in a score distribution; the value above and below which 50% of the scores lie.

*median test A nonparametric test involving the comparison of median values of two independent groups to determine if the groups are from populations with different medians.

mediating variable A variable that mediates or acts like a "go-between" in a chain linking two other variables (e.g., coping skills mediate the relationship between stressful events and anxiety).

member check A method of validating the credibility of qualitative data through debriefings and discussions with informants.

meta-analysis A technique for quantitatively integrating the findings from multiple studies on a given topic.

meta-matrix A device sometimes used in mixed-method studies that permits researchers to recognize important patterns and themes across data sources and to develop hypotheses.

metasynthesis The theories, grand narratives, generalizations, or interpretive translations produced from the integration or comparison of findings from multiple qualitative studies.

method triangulation The use of multiple methods of data collection about the same phenomenon to enhance the validity of the findings.

methodologic notes In observational field studies, the researcher's notes about the methods used in collecting data.

methodologic research Research designed to develop or refine methods of obtaining, organizing, or analyzing data.

methods (research) The steps, procedures, and strategies for gathering and analyzing data in a research investigation.

middle-range theory A theory that focuses on only a piece of reality or human experience involving a selected number of concepts (e.g., theories of stress).

minimal risk Anticipated risks that are no greater than those ordinarily encountered in daily life or during the performance of routine tests or procedures.

***missing values** Values missing from a data set for some study participants, due, for example, to refusals, researcher error, or skip patterns in an instrument.

modality A characteristic of a frequency distribution describing the number of peaks (i.e., values with high frequencies).

mode A descriptive statistic that is a measure of central tendency; the score or value that occurs most frequently in a distribution of scores.

model A symbolic representation of concepts or variables and interrelationships among them.

moderator effect The effect that a third variable (a *moderator variable*) has on the relationship between the independent and dependent variables.

mortality threat A threat to the internal validity of a study, referring to the differential loss of participants (attrition) from different groups.

multimethod (mixed-method) research Generally, research in which multiple approaches are used to address a problem; often used to designate studies in which both qualitative and quantitative data are collected and analyzed.

multimodal distribution A distribution of values with more than one peak (high frequency).

multiple comparison procedures Statistical tests, normally applied after an ANOVA indicates statistically significant group differences, that compare different pairs of groups; also called *post hoc tests*.

multiple correlation coefficient An index (symbolized as *R*) that summarizes the degree of relationship between two or more independent variables and a dependent variable.

multiple regression analysis A statistical procedure for understanding the simultaneous effects of two or more independent (predictor) variables on a dependent variable.

multistage sampling A sampling strategy that proceeds through a set of stages from larger to smaller sampling units (e.g., from states, to nursing schools, to faculty members).

***multitrait–multimethod matrix method** A method of establishing the construct validity of an instrument that involves the use of multiple measures for a set of subjects; the target instrument is valid to the extent that there is a strong relationship between it and other measures purporting to measure the same attribute (convergence) and a weak relationship between it and other measures purporting to measure a different attribute (discriminability).

multivariate analysis of variance (MANOVA) A statistical procedure used to test the significance of differences between the means of two or more groups on two or more dependent variables, considered simultaneously.

multivariate statistics Statistical procedures designed to analyze the relationships among three or more variables; commonly used multivariate statistics include multiple regression, analysis of covariance, and factor analysis.

N The symbol designating the total number of subjects (e.g., "the total *N* was 500").

n The symbol designating the number of subjects in a subgroup of a study (e.g., "each of the four groups had an *n* of 125, for a total *N* of 500").

***narrative analysis** A type of qualitative approach that focuses on the story as the object of the inquiry.

***natural experiment** A nonexperimental study that takes advantage of some naturally occurring event (e.g., an earthquake) that is presumed to have implications for people's behavior or condition, typically by comparing people exposed to the event with those not exposed.

naturalistic paradigm An alternative to the positivist paradigm that holds that there are multiple interpretations of reality, and that the goal of research is to understand how individuals construct reality within their context; often associated with qualitative research.

naturalistic setting A setting for the collection of research data that is natural to those being studied (e.g., homes, places of work, and so on).

***needs assessment** A study designed to describe the needs of a group, a community, or an organization, usually as a guide to policy planning and resource allocation.

negative case analysis A method of refining a hypothesis or theory in a qualitative study that involves the inclusion of cases that appear to disconfirm earlier hypotheses.

negative relationship A relationship between two variables in which there is a tendency for higher values on one variable to be associated with lower values on the other (e.g., as temperature increases, people's productivity may decrease); also called an *inverse relationship*.

negative results Research results that fail to support the researcher's hypotheses.

negatively skewed distribution An asymmetric distribution of data values with a disproportionately high number of cases having high values—when displayed graphically, the tail points to the left.

net effect The effect of an independent variable on a dependent variable after controlling for the effect of one or more covariates through multiple regression or ANCOVA.

network sampling The sampling of participants based on referrals from others already in the sample; also called *snowball sampling* and *nominated sampling*.

*nocebo effect Adverse side effect experienced by those receiving a placebo treatment.

nominal measurement The lowest level of measurement involving the assignment of characteristics into categories (e.g., males, category 1; females, category 2).

nominated sampling A sampling method in which researchers ask early informants to make referrals to other study participants; also called *snowball sampling* and *network sampling*.

nondirectional hypothesis A research hypothesis that does not stipulate in advance the expected direction of the relationship between variables.

nonequivalent control group design A quasi-experimental design involving a comparison group that was not developed on the basis of random assignment, but from whom preintervention data usually are obtained to assess the initial equivalence of the groups.

nonexperimental research Studies in which the researcher collects data without introducing an intervention.

nonparametric statistical tests A class of inferential statistical tests that do not involve rigorous assumptions about the distribution of critical variables; most often used with nominal or ordinal data.

nonprobability sampling The selection of sampling units (e.g., participants) from a population using nonrandom procedures, as in convenience, judgmental, and quota sampling.

*nonrecursive model A causal model that predicts reciprocal effects (i.e., a variable can be both the cause of and an effect of another variable).

nonresponse bias A bias that can result when a nonrandom subset of people invited to participate in a study fail to participate.

nonsignificant result The result of a statistical test indicating that group differences or a relationship between variables could have occurred as a result of chance at a given level of significance; sometimes abbreviated as *NS*.

normal distribution A theoretical distribution that is bell-shaped, symmetrical, and not too peaked or flat; also called a *normal curve*.

*norms Test-performance standards, based on test score information from a large, representative sample.

null hypothesis A hypothesis stating no relationship between the variables under study; used primarily in statistical testing as the hypothesis to be rejected.

nursing research Systematic inquiry designed to develop knowledge about issues of importance to the nursing profession.

objectivity The extent to which two independent researchers would arrive at similar judgments or conclusions (i.e., judgments not biased by personal values or beliefs).

*oblique rotation In factor analysis, a rotation of factors such that the reference axes are allowed to move to acute or oblique angles, and hence the factors are allowed to be correlated.

observational notes An observer's in-depth descriptions about events and conversations observed in naturalistic settings.

observational research Studies in which data are collected by observing and recording behaviors or activities of interest; medical researchers sometimes use this term to refer to nonexperimental research.

observed (obtained) score The actual score or numerical value assigned to a person on a measure.

odds The ratio of two probabilities, namely, the probability of an event occurring to the probability that it will not occur.

odds ratio (OR) The ratio of one odds to another odds; used in logistic regression as a measure of association and as an estimate of relative risk.

*on-protocol analysis An analysis approach that includes data only from those members of a treatment group who actually received the treatment; contrary to an *intention-to-treat* analysis.

*one-tailed test A test of statistical significance in which only values at one extreme (tail) of a distribution are considered in determining significance; used when the researcher can predict the direction of a relationship (see *directional hypothesis*).

open-ended question A question in an interview or questionnaire that does not restrict respondents' answers to preestablished alternatives.

open coding The first level of coding in a grounded theory study, referring to the basic descriptive coding of the content of the narrative data.

operational definition The definition of a concept or variable in terms of the procedures by which it is to be measured.

operationalization The process of translating research concepts into measurable phenomena.

*oral history An unstructured self-report technique used to gather personal recollections of events and their perceived causes and consequences.

ordinal measurement A level of measurement that rank orders phenomena along some dimension.

ordinary least squares (OLS) regression Regression analysis that uses the least-squares criterion for estimating the parameters in the regression equation.

*orthogonal rotation In factor analysis, a rotation of factors such that the reference axes are kept at a right angle, and hence the factors remain uncorrelated.

outcome analysis An evaluation of what happens with regard to outcomes of interest after implementing a program or intervention, without using an experimental design to assess net effects; see also *impact analysis*.

outcome variable The measure that captures the outcome of an intervention, i.e., the dependent variable.

outcomes research Research designed to document the effectiveness of health care services and the end results of patient care.

p value In statistical testing, the probability that the obtained results are due to chance alone; the probability of committing a Type I error.

pair matching See *matching*.

panel study A type of longitudinal study in which data are collected from the same people (a *panel*) at two or more points in time, often in the context of a survey.

paradigm A way of looking at natural phenomena that encompasses a set of philosophical assumptions and that guides one's approach to inquiry.

paradigm case In a hermeneutic analysis following the precepts of Benner, a strong examplar of the phenomenon under study, often used early in the analysis to gain understanding of the phenomenon.

parameter A characteristic of a population (e.g., the mean age of all Japanese citizens).

parametric statistical tests A class of inferential statistical tests that involve (a) assumptions about the distribution of the variables, (b) the estimation of a parameter, and (c) the use of interval or ratio measures.

participant See *study participant*.

participant observation An approach to collecting observational data in which researchers immerse themselves in the world of study participants and participate in that world insofar as possible.

participatory action research A research approach with an ideological perspective based on the premise that the use and production of knowledge can be used to exert power.

path analysis A regression-based procedure for testing causal models, typically using nonexperimental data.

*path coefficient The weight representing the impact of one variable on another in a path analytic causal model.

*path diagram A graphic representation of the hypothesized linkages and causal flow among variables in a causal relationship.

Pearson's *r* A widely used correlation coefficient designating the magnitude of the relationship between two variables measured on at least an interval scale; also called the *product-moment correlation*.

peer debriefing Sessions with peers to review and explore various aspects of a study—typically in a qualitative study.

peer reviewer A person who reviews and critiques a research report or proposal, who himself or herself is a researcher (usually working on similar types of research problems as those under review), and who makes a recommendation about publishing or funding the research.

perfect relationship A correlation between two variables such that the values of one variable permit perfect prediction of the values of the other; designated as 1.00 or −1.00.

persistent observation In qualitative research, the researcher's intense focus on the aspects of a situation that are relevant to the phenomena being studied.

personal interview A face-to-face interview between an interviewer and a respondent.

personal notes In field studies, written comments about the observer's own feelings during the research process.

phenomenology A qualitative research tradition, with roots in philosophy and psychology, that focuses on the lived experience of humans.

phenomenon The abstract concept under study, most often used by qualitative researchers in lieu of the term "variable."

*phi coefficient A statistical index describing the magnitude of the relationship between two dichotomous variables.

pilot study A small scale version, or trial run, done in preparation for a major study.

placebo A sham or pseudo intervention, often used as a control condition.

placebo effect Changes in the dependent variable attributable to the placebo condition.

*point estimation A statistical estimation procedure in which the researcher uses information from a sample to estimate the single value (statistic) that best represents the value of the population parameter.

*point prevalence rate The number of people with a condition or disease divided by the total number at risk, multiplied by the number of people for whom the rate is being established (e.g., per 1000 population).

population The entire set of individuals or objects having some common characteristics (e.g., all RNs in South Africa); sometimes called a *universe*.

positive relationship A relationship between two variables in which there is a tendency for high values on one variable to be associated with high values on the other (e.g., as physical activity increases, pulse rate also increases).

positive results Research results that are consistent with the researcher's hypotheses.

positively skewed distribution An asymmetric distribution of values with a disproportionately high number of cases having low values—when displayed graphically, the tail points to the right.

positivist paradigm The traditional paradigm underlying the scientific approach, which assumes that there is a fixed, orderly reality that can be objectively studied; often associated with quantitative research.

post hoc **test** A test for comparing all possible pairs of groups following a significant test of overall group differences (e.g., in an ANOVA).

poster session A session at a professional conference in which several researchers simultaneously present visual displays summarizing their studies.

postpositivist paradigm A modification of the traditional positivist paradigm that acknowledges the impossibility of total objectivity; postpositivists appreciate the impediments to knowing reality with certainty and therefore seek *probabilistic* evidence.

posttest The collection of data after introducing an experimental intervention.

posttest-only design An experimental design in which data are collected from subjects only after the experimental intervention has been introduced; also called an *after-only design*.

power A research design's ability to detect relationships that exist among variables.

power analysis A procedure for estimating either the likelihood of committing a Type II error or sample size requirements.

prediction The use of empirical evidence to make forecasts about how variables will behave in a new setting and with different individuals.

predictive validity The degree to which an instrument can predict some criterion observed at a future time.

predictor variables In a regression analysis (and other multivariate analyses), the independent variables entered into the analysis to predict the dependent variable.

preexperimental design A research design that does not include mechanisms to compensate for the absence of either randomization or a control group.

pretest (1) The collection of data prior to the experimental intervention; sometimes called *baseline data*; (2) the trial administration of a newly developed instrument to identify flaws or assess time requirements.

pretest-posttest design An experimental design in which data are collected from research subjects both before and after introducing the experimental intervention; also called a *before–after design*.

*prevalence study A study undertaken to determine the point prevalence rate of some condition (e.g., a disease or behavior, such as smoking) at a particular point in time.

primary source First-hand reports of facts, findings, or events; in research, the primary source is the original research report prepared by the investigator who conducted the study.

*principal investigator (PI) The person who is the lead researcher and who has primary responsibility for overseeing the project.

probability sampling The random selection of elements (e.g., participants) from a population, as in simple random sampling, cluster sampling, and systematic sampling.

*probing Eliciting more useful or detailed information from a respondent in an interview than was volunteered in the first reply.

problem statement An expression of a dilemma or disturbing situation that needs investigation.

process analysis An evaluation focusing on the process by which a program or intervention gets implemented and used in practice.

process consent In a qualitative study, an ongoing, transactional process of negotiating consent with study participants, allowing them to play a collaborative role in the decision making regarding their continued participation.

product moment correlation coefficient (*r*) A widely used correlation coefficient, designating the magnitude of the relationship between two variables measured on at least an interval scale; also called *Pearson's r*.

*projective technique A method of measuring psychological attributes (values, attitudes, personality) by providing respondents with unstructured stimuli to which to respond.

prolonged engagement In qualitative research, the investment of sufficient time during data collection to have an in-depth understanding of the group under study, thereby enhancing data credibility.

proportionate sample A sample that results when the researcher samples from different strata of the population in proportion to their representation in the population.

proposal A document specifying the researcher's proposed study plans; it communicates the research problem, its significance, planned procedures for solving the problem, and, when funding is sought, how much the study will cost.

prospective design A study design that begins with observations of presumed causes (e.g., smoking) and then goes forward in time to observe presumed effects (e.g., lung cancer).

psychometric assessment An evaluation of the quality of an instrument, based primarily on evidence of its reliability and validity.

purposive (purposeful) sampling A nonprobability sampling method in which the researcher selects participants based on personal judgment about who will be most representative or informative; also called *judgmental sampling*.

Q sort A data collection method in which participants sort statements into a number of piles (usually nine or 11) along a bipolar dimension (e.g., most useful/least useful).

qualitative analysis The organization and interpretation of non-numerical data for the purpose of discovering important underlying dimensions and patterns of relationships.

qualitative data Information collected in narrative (non-numerical) form, such as the transcript of an unstructured interview.

qualitative outcome analysis (QOA) An approach to address the gap between qualitative research and clinical practice, involving the identification and evaluation of clinical interventions based on qualitative findings.

qualitative research The investigation of phenomena, typically in an in-depth and holistic fashion, through the collection of rich narrative materials using a flexible research design.

quantitative analysis The manipulation of numerical data through statistical procedures for the purpose of describing phenomena or assessing the magnitude and reliability of relationships among them.

quantitative data Information collected in a quantified (numerical) form.

quantitative research The investigation of phenomena that lend themselves to precise measurement and quantification, often involving a rigorous and controlled design.

quasi-experiment A study involving an intervention in which subjects are not randomly assigned to treatment conditions, but the researcher exercises certain controls to enhance the study's internal validity.

quasi-statistics An "accounting" system used to assess the validity of conclusions derived from qualitative analysis.

questionnaire A method of gathering self-report information from respondents through self-administration of questions in a paper-and-pencil format.

quota sampling The nonrandom selection of participants in which the researcher prespecifies characteristics of the sample to increase its representativeness.

r The symbol for a bivariate correlation coefficient, summarizing the magnitude and direction of a relationship between two variables.

R The symbol for a multiple correlation coefficient, indicating the magnitude (but not direction) of the relationship between the dependent variable and multiple independent variables, taken together.

R² The squared multiple correlation coefficient, indicating the proportion of variance in the dependent variable accounted for or explained by a group of independent variables.

random assignment The assignment of subjects to treatment conditions in a random manner (i.e., in a manner determined by chance alone); also called *randomization*.

random number table A table displaying hundreds of digits (from 0 to 9) set up so that each number is equally likely to follow any other.

random sampling The selection of a sample such that each member of a population has an equal probability of being included.

randomization The assignment of subjects to treatment conditions in a random manner (i.e., in a manner determined by chance alone); also called *random assignment*.

randomized block design An experimental design involving two or more factors (independent variables), only one of which is experimentally manipulated.

randomized clinical trial (RCT) A full experimental test of a new treatment, involving random assignment to treatment groups and, typically, a large and diverse sample (also known as a Phase III clinical trial).

randomness An important concept in quantitative research, involving having certain features of the study established by chance rather than by design or personal preference.

range A measure of variability, computed by subtracting the lowest value from the highest value in a distribution of scores.

rating scale A scale that requires ratings of an object or concept along a continuum.

ratio measurement A level of measurement with equal distances between scores and a true meaningful zero point (e.g., weight).

raw data Data in the form in which they were collected, without being coded or analyzed.

reactivity A measurement distortion arising from the study participant's awareness of being observed, or, more generally, from the effect of the measurement procedure itself.

readability The ease with which research materials (e.g., a questionnaire) can be read by people with varying reading skills, often empirically determined through readability formulas.

receiver operating characteristic curve (ROC curve) A method used in developing and refining screening instruments that plots sensitivity and specificity to determine the best cutoff point for "caseness."

recursive model A path model in which the causal flow is unidirectional, without any feedback loops; opposite of a nonrecursive model.

refereed journal A journal in which decisions about the acceptance of manuscripts are made based on recommendations from peer reviewers.

reflective notes Notes that document a qualitative researcher's personal experiences, reflections, and progress in the field.

reflexive journal A journal maintained by qualitative researchers during data collection and data analysis to document their self-analysis of both how they affected the research and how the research affected them.

reflexivity In qualitative studies, critical self-reflection about one's own biases, preferences, and preconceptions.

regression analysis A statistical procedure for predicting values of a dependent variable based on the values of one or more independent variables.

relationship A bond or a connection between two or more variables.

relative risk An estimate of risk of "caseness" in one group compared to another, computed by dividing the rate for one group by the rate for another.

reliability The degree of consistency or dependability with which an instrument measures the attribute it is designed to measure.

reliability coefficient A quantitative index, usually ranging in value from .00 to 1.00, that provides an estimate of how reliable an instrument is.

repeated-measures design An experimental design in which one group of subjects is exposed to more than one condition or treatment in random order; also called a *crossover design*.

replication The deliberate repetition of research procedures in a second investigation for the purpose of determining if earlier results can be repeated.

representative sample A sample whose characteristics are comparable to those of the population from which it is drawn.

research Systematic inquiry that uses orderly, disciplined methods to answer questions or solve problems.

research control See *control*.

research design The overall plan for addressing a research question, including specifications for enhancing the study's integrity.

research hypothesis The actual hypothesis a researcher wants to test (as opposed to the *null hypothesis*), stating the anticipated relationship between two or more variables.

research methods The techniques used to structure a study and to gather and analyze information in a systematic fashion.

research misconduct Fabrication, falsification, plagiarism, or other practices that seriously deviate from those that are commonly accepted within the scientific community for proposing, conducting, or reporting research.

research problem A situation involving an enigmatic, perplexing, or conflictful condition that can be investigated through disciplined inquiry.

research proposal See *proposal*.

research question A statement of the specific query the researcher wants to answer to address a research problem.

research report A document summarizing the main features of a study, including the research question, the methods used to address it, the findings, and the interpretation of the findings.

research utilization The use of some aspect of a study in an application unrelated to the original research.

researcher credibility The faith that can be put in a researcher, based on his or her training, qualifications, and experience.

*residuals In multiple regression, the error term or unexplained variance.

respondent In a self-report study, the study participant responding to questions posed by the researcher.

response rate The rate of participation in a study, calculated by dividing the number of persons participating by the number of persons sampled.

response set bias The measurement error introduced by the tendency of some individuals to respond to items in characteristic ways (e.g., always agreeing), independently of the items' content.

results The answers to research questions, obtained through an analysis of the collected data; in a quantitative study, the information obtained through statistical tests.

retrospective design A study design that begins with the manifestation of the dependent variable in the present (e.g., lung cancer) and then searches for the presumed cause occurring in the past (e.g., cigarette smoking).

risk–benefit ratio The relative costs and benefits, to an individual subject and to society at large, of participation in a study; also, the relative costs and benefits of implementing an innovation.

rival hypothesis An alternative explanation, competing with the researcher's hypothesis, to account for the results of a study.

sample A subset of a population, selected to participate in a study.

sample size The total number of study participants participating in a study.

sampling The process of selecting a portion of the population to represent the entire population.

sampling bias Distortions that arise when a sample is not representative of the population from which it was drawn.

sampling distribution A theoretical distribution of a statistic (e.g., a mean), using values computed from an infinite number of samples as the data points.

sampling error The fluctuation of the value of a statistic from one sample to another drawn from the same population.

sampling frame A list of all the elements in the population from which the sample is drawn.

sampling plan The formal plan specifying a sampling method, a sample size, and procedures for recruiting subjects.

saturation The collection of data in a qualitative study to the point where closure is attained because new data yield redundant information.

scale A composite measure of an attribute, involving the combination of several items that have a logical and empirical relationship to each other, resulting in the assignment of a score to place people on a continuum with respect to the attribute.

*scatter plot A graphic representation of the relationship between two variables.

scientific merit The degree to which a study is methodologically and conceptually sound.

scientific method A set of orderly, systematic, controlled procedures for acquiring dependable, empirical—and typically quantitative—information; the methodologic approach associated with the positivist paradigm.

screening instrument An instrument used to determine whether potential subjects for a study meet eligibility criteria, or for determining whether a person has a specified condition.

secondary analysis Research in which data collected by one researcher are reanalyzed, usually by another investigator, to answer new research questions.

secondary source Second-hand accounts of events or facts; in a research context, a description of a study or studies prepared by someone other than the original researcher.

selection threat (self-selection) A threat to the internal validity of the study resulting from preexisting differences between groups under study; the differences affect the dependent variable in ways extraneous to the effect of the independent variable.

selective coding A level of coding in a grounded theory study that begins after the core category is discovered and involves systematically integrating relationships between the core category and other categories and validating those relationships.

self-determination A person's ability to voluntarily decide whether or not to participate in a study.

self-report A method of collecting data that involves a direct report of information by the person who is being studied (e.g., by interview or questionnaire).

semantic differential A technique that asks respondents to rate a concept of interest on a series of bipolar rating scales.

semistructured interview An interview in which the researcher has listed topics to cover rather than specific questions to ask.

sensitivity The ability of screening instruments to correctly identify a "case" (i.e., to correctly diagnose a condition).

sensitivity analysis In a meta-analysis, a method to determine whether conclusions are sensitive to the quality of the studies included.

*sequential clinical trial A clinical trial in which data are continuously analyzed and "stop rules" are used to decide when the evidence about the intervention's efficacy is sufficiently strong to stop the experiment.

setting The physical location and conditions in which data collection takes place in a study.

*sign test A nonparametric test for comparing two paired groups based on the relative ranking of values between the pairs.

significance level The probability that an observed relationship could be caused by chance (i.e., as a result of sampling error); significance at the .05 level indicates the probability that a relationship of the observed magnitude would be found by chance only 5 times out of 100.

simple random sampling The most basic type of probability sampling, wherein a sampling frame is created by enumerating all members of a population and then selecting a sample from the sampling frame through completely random procedures.

*simultaneous multiple regression A multiple regression analysis in which all predictor variables are entered into the equation simultaneously; sometimes called *direct* or *standard* multiple regression.

*single-subject experiment A study that tests the effectiveness of an intervention with one subject, typically using a time series design.

site The overall location where a study is undertaken.

skewed distribution The asymmetric distribution of data values around a central point.

snowball sampling The selection of participants through referrals from earlier participants; also called *network sampling* or *nominated sampling*.

social desirability response set A bias in self-report instruments created when participants have a tendency to misrepresent their opinions in the direction of answers consistent with prevailing social norms.

Spearman's rank-order correlation (Spearman's rho) A correlation coefficient indicating the magnitude of a relationship between variables measured on the ordinal scale.

specificity The ability of a screening instrument to correctly identify noncases.

split-half technique A method for estimating internal consistency reliability by correlating scores on half of the instrument with scores on the other half.

standard deviation The most frequently used statistic for measuring the degree of variability in a set of scores.

standard error The standard deviation of a theoretical sampling distribution, such as a sampling distribution of means.

*standard scores Scores expressed in terms of standard deviations from the mean, with raw scores transformed to have a mean of zero and a standard deviation of one; also called *z* scores.

statement of purpose A declarative statement of the overall goals of a study.

statistic An estimate of a parameter, calculated from sample data.

statistical analysis The organization and analysis of quantitative data using statistical procedures.

statistical conclusion validity The degree to which conclusions about relationships and differences from a statistical analysis of the data are legitimate.

statistical control The use of statistical procedures to control extraneous influences on the dependent variable.

statistical inference The process of inferring attributes about the population based on data from a sample, using laws of probability.

statistical power The ability of the research design and analysis to detect true relationships among variables.

statistical significance A term indicating that the results from an analysis of sample data are unlikely to have been caused by chance, at some specified level of probability.

statistical test An analytic tool that estimates the probability that obtained results from a sample reflect true population values.

*stepwise multiple regression A multiple regression analysis in which predictor variables are entered into the equation in steps, in the order in which the increment to R^2 is greatest.

stipend A monetary payment to study participants to serve as an incentive for participation and/or to compensate for time and expenses.

strata Subdivisions of the population according to some characteristic (e.g., males and females); singular is *stratum*.

stratified random sampling The random selection of study participants from two or more strata of the population independently.

***structural equations** Equations representing the magnitude and nature of hypothesized relations among sets of variables in a theory.

structured data collection An approach to collecting information from participants, either through self-report or observations, in which the researcher determines response categories in advance.

study participant An individual who participates and provides information in a study.

subgroup effect The differential effect of the independent variable on the dependent variable for various subsets of the sample.

subject An individual who participates and provides data in a study; term used primarily in quantitative research.

substantive theory In grounded theory, a theory that is grounded in data from a single study on a specific substantive area (e.g., postpartum depression); in contrast to *formal theory*.

summated rating scale A composite scale with multiple items, each of which is scored; item scores are added together to yield a total score that distributes people along a continuum (e.g., a Likert scale).

survey research Nonexperimental research in which information regarding the activities, beliefs, preferences, and attitudes of people is gathered via direct questioning.

***survival analysis** A statistical procedure used when the dependent variable represents a time interval between an initial event (e.g., onset of a disease) and an end event (e.g., death); also called *life table analysis*.

symmetric distribution A distribution of values with two halves that are mirror images of each other; a distribution that is not skewed.

systematic sampling The selection of a sample such that every kth (e.g., every tenth) person (or element) in a sampling frame is chosen.

_t_-test A parametric statistical test for analyzing the difference between two means.

table of random numbers See *random number table*.

tacit knowledge Information about a culture that is so deeply embedded that members do not talk about it or may not even be consciously aware of it.

target population The entire population in which the researcher is interested and to which he or she would like to generalize study results.

taxonomy In an ethnographic analysis, a system of classifying and organizing terms and concepts, developed to illuminate the internal organization of a domain and the relationship among the subcategories of the domain.

template analysis style An approach to qualitative analysis in which a preliminary template or coding scheme is used to sort the data.

test statistic A statistic used to test for the statistical significance of relationships between variables; the sampling distributions of test statistics are known for circumstances in which the null hypothesis is true; e.g., Pearson's r.

test–retest reliability Assessment of the stability of an instrument by correlating the scores obtained on repeated administrations.

theme A recurring regularity emerging from an analysis of qualitative data.

theoretical notes In field studies, notes detailing the researcher's interpretations of observed behavior.

theoretical sampling In qualitative studies, the selection of sample members based on emerging findings as the study progresses to ensure adequate representation of important themes.

theory An abstract generalization that presents a systematic explanation about the relationships among phenomena.

theory triangulation The use of competing theories or hypotheses in the analysis and interpretation of data.

thick description A rich and thorough description of the research context in a qualitative study.

think-aloud method A qualitative method used to collect data about cognitive processes (e.g., decision making), involving the use of audio recordings to capture people's reflections on problems as they are being solved.

time sampling In observational research, the selection of time periods during which observations will take place.

time series design A quasi-experimental design involving the collection of data over an extended time period, with multiple data collection points both prior to and after an intervention.

topic guide A list of broad question areas to be covered in a semistructured interview or focus group interview.

transferability The extent to which findings can be transferred to other settings or groups—often used in qualitative research and analogous to generalizability in quantitative research.

treatment The experimental intervention under study; the condition being manipulated.

treatment group The group receiving the intervention being tested; the experimental group.

trend study A longitudinal study in which different samples from a population are studied over time with respect to some phenomenon (e.g., annual Gallup polls on abortion attitudes).

triangulation The use of multiple methods to collect and interpret data about a phenomenon so as to converge on an accurate representation of reality.

true score A hypothetical score that would be obtained if a measure were infallible.

trustworthiness The degree of confidence qualitative researchers have in their data, assessed using the criteria of credibility, transferability, dependability, and confirmability.

Type I error An error created by rejecting the null hypothesis when it is true (i.e., the researcher concludes that a relationship exists when in fact it does not—a false positive).

Type II error An error created by accepting the null hypothesis when it is false (i.e., the researcher concludes that *no* relationship exists when in fact it does—a false negative).

*two-tailed tests Statistical tests in which both ends of the sampling distribution are used to determine improbable values.

typical case sampling An approach to sampling in qualitative research involving the selection of participants who highlight what is typical or average.

unimodal distribution A distribution of values with one peak (high frequency).

unit of analysis The basic unit or focus of an analysis; typically the individual study participant.

univariate statistics Statistical procedures for analyzing a single variable for purposes of description.

unstructured interview An oral self-report in which the researcher asks a respondent questions without having a predetermined plan regarding the content or flow of information to be gathered.

unstructured observation The collection of descriptive information through direct observation that is not guided by a formal, prespecified plan for observing, enumerating, or recording the information.

validity The degree to which an instrument measures what it is intended to measure.

validity coefficient A quantitative index, usually ranging in value from .00 to 1.00, that provides an estimate of how valid an instrument is.

variability The degree to which values on a set of scores are dispersed.

variable An attribute of a person or object that varies, that is, takes on different values (e.g., body temperature, age, heart rate).

variance A measure of variability equal to the standard deviation squared.

vignette A brief description of an event, person, or situation about which respondents are asked to describe their reactions.

visual analog scale A scaling procedure used to measure certain clinical symptoms (e.g., pain, fatigue) by having people indicate on a straight line the intensity of the symptom.

vulnerable subjects Special groups of people whose rights in research studies need special protection because of their inability to provide meaningful informed consent or because their circumstances place them at higher-than-average risk of adverse effects (e.g., children, unconscious patients).

weighting A correction procedure used to arrive at population values when a disproportionate sampling design has been used.

*Wilcoxon signed ranks test A nonparametric statistical test for comparing two paired groups based on the relative ranking of values between the pairs.

*Wilk's lambda An index used in discriminant function analysis to indicate the proportion of variance in the dependent variable unaccounted for by predictors; $\lambda = 1 - R^2$.

within-subjects design A research design in which a single group of subjects is compared under different conditions or at different points in time (e.g., before and after surgery).

*z score A standard score, expressed in terms of standard deviations from the mean.

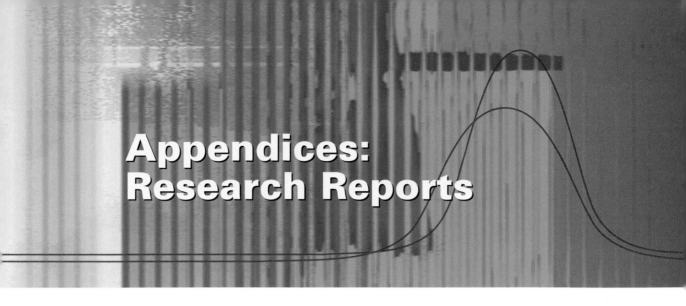

Appendices: Research Reports

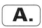

Sense of Coherence and Quality of Life in Women With and Without Irritable Bowel Syndrome

Sandra Adams Motzer, Vicky Hertig, Monica Jarrett, Margaret M. Heitkemper

▶ **Background:** Despite ongoing physical and psychological distress, little is known about sense of coherence (SOC) and holistic quality of life (QOL) in women with irritable bowel syndrome (IBS).

▶ **Objectives:** The purposes of this study were to (a) describe and compare SOC and holistic QOL of women with and without IBS, and (b) examine the relationships among SOC, holistic QOL, and gastrointestinal (GI) and psychological distress symptoms.

▶ **Method:** A two-group comparison design was used to test the study hypotheses that women with IBS would have lower SOC and holistic QOL than control women without IBS, and that SOC and holistic QOL would be inversely related to GI and psychological distress. A total of 324 women were studied ($n = 235$ with IBS, $n = 89$ controls). Measures included the 13-item SOC Questionnaire, Modified Flanagan QOL Scale, Bowel Disease Questionnaire, and Symptom-Checklist-90-R.

▶ **Results:** Both SOC and holistic QOL were lower in women with IBS ($p < .001$). Correlations between SOC and global distress, depression, anxiety, and somatization without GI symptoms were moderately and inversely related ($r = -.64, -.64, -.53,$ and $-.31,$ respectively; $p < .001$) in the total sample. Relationships between holistic QOL and psychological distress indicators were universally of lower magnitude ($r = -.56$ to $-.27, p < .001$). The only GI symptom indicator significantly related to SOC and holistic QOL was alternating constipation and diarrhea ($\tau = -.21$ and $-.17,$ respectively; $p < .001$).

Reprinted with permission from *Nursing Research* 2003; 52[5]: 329–337.

▶ **Discussion:** Women with IBS have a reduced SOC and holistic QOL when compared to women without IBS. It remains to be determined whether interventions targeted at enhancing SOC and holistic QOL can impact the psychological distress associated with IBS.

▶ **Key Words:** irritable bowel syndrome, psychological distress, quality of life, sense of coherence.

Irritable bowel syndrome (IBS) is a chronic, functional bowel disorder characterized by abdominal discomfort or pain relieved by defecation and/or associated with a change in stool frequency or appearance (Thompson, 1999). In the United States as well as other industrialized countries, IBS predominantly affects women (American College of Gastroenterology Functional Gastrointestinal Disorders Task Force, 2002; Kay & Jorgensen, 1996), often beginning in individuals in their early adolescent or adult years. Health-related quality of life (QOL) is reduced in patients with IBS (International Foundation for Functional Gastrointestinal Disorders, 2002) possibly due to several factors including:

▶ the chronic and relapsing nature of IBS symptoms
▶ the lack of treatment strategies that are consistently effective for all symptoms
▶ the concurrence of other symptoms (e.g., psychological distress)

Recent surveys of women with IBS have validated the disorder impacts on multiple aspects of the individual's life. Two-thirds of persons with IBS describe their gastrointestinal (GI) symptoms as extreme or bothersome in regards to interference with daily comfort, work, or leisure activities (International Foundation for Functional Gastrointestinal Disorders, 2002). In addition, many women feel that their healthcare providers do not take their symptoms seriously or provide adequate information regarding the condition (Heitkemper et al., 2002). To date, the exact etiology of IBS remains elusive. There is neither known organic pathology nor consistently effective medical treatment for the multiple symptoms often experienced by patients with IBS (American College of Gastroenterology Functional Gastrointestinal Disorders Task Force, 2002; Brandt et al., 2002). In addition, its diagnosis remains one of exclusion (Cash, Schoenfeld, & Chey, 2002).

Psychological distress symptoms commonly reported by persons with IBS include anxiety, depression, and somatization (Jarrett et al., 1998; Whitehead, Bosmajian, Zonderman, Costa, & Shuster, 1988). Levels of anxiety and depression are significantly greater among persons with an IBS diagnosis or IBS symptoms compared to apparently healthy persons without IBS (Jarrett et al.; Jones et al., 2001; Kumar, Pfeffer, & Wingate, 1990). In addition, patients with IBS frequently report somatic complaints (Whorwell, McCallum, Creed, & Roberts, 1986) including:

▶ headache
▶ back pain
▶ fatigue
▶ poor sleep
▶ urinary symptoms
▶ dyspareunia
▶ bad breath/unpleasant taste in mouth
▶ heart palpitations
▶ muscle soreness and stiffness (Zaman, Chavez, Krueger, Talley, & Lembo, 2001).

Persons (50%) with comorbid somatic conditions, (e.g., fibromyalgia, chronic fatigue syndrome, temporomandibular joint disorder, chronic pelvic pain) also report having IBS (Whitehead, Palsson, & Jones, 2002).

Another factor that may contribute to the reduction in health-related QOL in patients with IBS is reduced sense of coherence (SOC). This is associated with resilience in individuals with other chronic health problems. The SOC is defined as a global orientation that expresses the extent to which one has a pervasive, enduring, though dynamic feeling of confidence that life is comprehensible, manageable, and meaningful (Antonovsky, 1987).

It is the key construct of Antonovsky's (1979; 1987) salutogenic theory, which focuses on why some persons remain healthy despite otherwise stressful conditions. The salutogenic theory and the SOC emerged from interviews of 51 Holocaust survivors who were thought to be doing well in their everyday lives. Subsequently, Antonovsky developed the 29-item SOC questionnaire (SOCQ). An expert panel assessed its content validity, and known-groups technique across Israeli, US, Canadian, and Nordic samples provided evidence of construct validity. Antonovsky posited that a strong SOC allows persons to successfully cope with life stressors. Stress has been identified as a symptom-precipitation factor for persons with IBS. Although same-day psychological distress predicted same-day GI symptom distress levels in women with an IBS diagnosis ($n = 32$) or IBS symptoms ($n = 30$), it remains unclear whether psychological distress precipitated the GI symptoms or whether the GI symptoms precipitated the psychological distress (Jarrett et al., 1998).

Strauss and colleagues (1984) and Corbin and Strauss (1988) believed that chronic illness potentially causes multiple problems of daily living for persons with the illness and their families, resulting in the need to accommodate to the demands of the illness, often on a daily basis. Within Strauss' (1984) framework, problems of living with a chronic health disturbance might include:

- predicting and controlling symptoms
- adjusting to changes in symptoms
- pursuing a diagnosis
- covering healthcare costs
- confronting attendant psychological, marital, and familial problems.

These problems are applicable to IBS as well as other chronic health conditions, such as chronic heart disease or fibromyalgia. Predicting and controlling symptoms may be especially problematic for the 25% of persons with IBS who experience alternating constipation and diarrhea (International Foundation for Functional Gastrointestinal Disorders, 2002). Each of these problems of daily living could be considered as stressors. Thus, a strong SOC might lessen the impact of the stressor on well-being, or stressors themselves might weaken SOC.

Motzer and colleagues (Dantas, Motzer, & Ciol, 2002; Motzer & Stewart, 1996) previously examined SOC in survivors of cardiac arrest and patients after coronary artery bypass graft surgery. Using Antonovsky's (1987) questionnaire, SOC was found to be higher than expected in a sample of persons ($N = 149$) with coronary heart disease surviving a cardiac arrest (Motzer & Stewart, 1996), but not higher than anticipated in a sample of persons ($N = 84$) with coronary heart disease following bypass graft surgery (Dantas et al., 2002).

To date only two studies have examined SOC in patients with IBS. Sperber and colleagues (1999) have demonstrated that SOC was lower in IBS participants ($n = 54$) and

IBS-fibromyalgia participants ($n = 25$) compared to age- and sex-matched control participants ($n = 72$) ($p < .001$). No differences were found in SOC between IBS-only subjects compared to IBS-fibromyalgia subjects. The levels of SOC in Sperber's IBS group were equivalent to normative levels seen in undergraduate student groups (Antonovsky, 1987). Although Sperber's participants were matched for sex, specific sex differences in SOC were not described in their predominantly female sample (77% female IBS/fibromyalgia vs. 75% female controls). In an earlier study (Motzer, Jarrett, Heitkemper, & Tsuji, 2002), SOC was examined in a small cohort of women with IBS ($n = 12$) and women controls without IBS ($n = 9$). Although control women had higher SOC scores than IBS women, the differences were not significant, likely due to the small sample size.

Quality of life is an important variable used in descriptive, predictive, and experimental health-related research. Gill and Feinstein (1994) posited that QOL is a uniquely personal perception, and that its measurement can only be determined through patient self-report. Anderson and Burckhardt (1999) concurred, arguing for the importance of a holistic approach in evaluating QOL that specifically asks the respondent to rate satisfaction with life domains, including but not limited to the domain of health. The focus of health-related QOL assessment is narrowly defined around health and illness variables (Gill & Feinstein, 1994; Ware, 1995) such as physiological dysfunction, symptoms, and functional capacity (Anderson & Burckhardt, 1999). Although these variables are important to assess, they more aptly reflect health status and not QOL (Gill & Feinstein, 1994). Holistic QOL has not been reported in persons with IBS, but many investigators have examined disease-specific, health-related QOL (Gralnek, Hays, Kilbourne, Naliboff, & Mayer, 2000; Groll et al., 2002; Hahn, Kirchdoerfer, Fullerton, & Mayer, 1997; Hahn, Yan, & Strassels, 1999) using a variety of measures (e.g., Medical Outcomes Study Short-Form-36 [SF-36], IBS-36, and the IBS QOL Questionnaire). For example, Gralnek's group found lower self-report health-related QOL using the SF-36 (Ware & Sherbourne, 1992) in persons with IBS compared to normal controls. Those IBS participants ($N = 877$) were predominantly female (62%) and ranged from 19 to 84 years of age (45.6 ± 13.4). Likewise, Hahn and colleagues (1999), also using the SF-36, found that persons with IBS ($N = 630$) had poorer health-related QOL than published norms. The majority of their respondents were women over the age of 45 years.

Flanagan (1982) conceptualized QOL holistically. Based on interviews with a random sample ($N = 3000$) of apparently healthy (30-, 50-, or 70-year-old) American men and women, Flanagan defined QOL as

▶ satisfaction with physical and material well being
▶ relations with other people
▶ social, community, and civic activities
▶ personal development and fulfillment
▶ recreation.

Subsequently, Flanagan developed a 15-item QOL scale from those interviews. After testing its reliability and validity in four chronic illness groups, Burckhardt, Woods, Schultz, and Ziebarth (1989) modified the definition and the scale by adding a domain of independence, or being able to do for oneself. It seems likely that accommodating to the demands of a chronic illness (e.g., predicting, controlling, and adjusting to changes in symptoms) would affect holistic QOL because the areas of life involved in this accommodation are congruent with these QOL domains.

Using the Modified Flanagan QOL scale (MQOLS) (Burckhardt et al., 1989; Flanagan, 1982), Motzer and colleagues (Dantas et al., 2002; Motzer & Stewart, 1996) examined holistic QOL in two samples of persons with chronic heart disease, and found them mostly satisfied with their QOL. For the cardiac arrest survivors, SOC contributed an additional (15%) of explained variance in QOL after social status, social support, self-esteem, and health-related variables had been entered into the model (Motzer & Stewart, 1996).

Little is known about SOC and holistic QOL in young-to-middle-aged women with IBS. It can be hypothesized that women with IBS in general have lower levels of SOC and holistic QOL relative to women without IBS, and that both SOC and holistic QOL are related inversely to symptom severity. Therefore, the purposes of this study were to:

▶ describe and compare SOC and holistic QOL of women 18 to 49 years of age
▶ examine the relationships among SOC, holistic QOL, and GI and psychological distress symptoms.

It was hypothesized that the relationships between SOC and holistic QOL with abdominal pain, global psychological distress, depression, anxiety, and somatization would be moderately strong and negative in all women.

METHOD

Sample

The sample was combined from four studies that used similar eligibility criteria, recruitment sites and protocols, and self-report measures. Data were collected between the years 1996 and 2002. Each of these studies examined the relationship of menstrual cycle phase with specific outcome variables, such as symptom experiences, immune function indicators, and catecholamine levels, which are not reported here. After Human Subjects Committee review and approval, women ($N = 342$) were recruited (aged 18 to 49 years) into the studies. No subject participated in more than one study. A total of 38 women dropped out before study completion; however, 20 completed some or all of the self-report measures. Thus, 324 women are included in this report ($n = 235$ with IBS, $n = 89$ controls without IBS).

All control women and the majority of women with IBS self-referred into the study from community advertisements ($n = 264$, 81% of entire sample). For this self-referred IBS group, determination of IBS diagnosis was made by self-report of healthcare provider diagnosis. A small number of women with IBS ($n = 60$, 26% of IBS sample, 19% of total sample) were recruited from a large health maintenance organization using direct mailings to all potentially eligible women enrollees who had a healthcare provider determined diagnosis of IBS. To be eligible, women in the IBS group had to be diagnosed with IBS and have current GI symptoms indicative of IBS (Thompson, 1999). Comorbid GI disorders were exclusion criteria. For the control women to be eligible, they could not have a diagnosis of IBS, regular GI symptoms, or any other GI disorder. After telephone screening to establish eligibility, women met with a study investigator, provided written informed consent, and completed self-report measures. After all data were collected, each woman received payment for her participation.

Measures

Demographic data were obtained for age, ethnicity, marital/partnered status, living situation, educational level, occupation, personal and family income, and health insurance. These data were used descriptively.

The SOC was measured for most subjects ($n = 252$) using the 13-item version of the SOC Questionnaire (SOCQ). For this short-form version, Antonovsky (1987) chose 13 of the original SOCQ 29 items, which was also validated using known-groups technique. For the remaining subjects ($n = 66$), the 29-item version was used. Content and construct validity are well documented for both versions (Antonovsky, 1993). Each version uses a 7-point response format, where 7 represented the strongest SOC and 1 represented the weakest SOC. Examples of SOCQ items follow.

▶ Has it happened in the past that you were surprised by the behavior of people you thought you knew? (1 = always happened, 7 = never happened)
▶ Do you have the feeling that you are being treated unfairly? (1 = very often, 7 = very seldom or never)
▶ Until now your life has had: (1 = no clear goals or purpose at all, 7 = very clear goals and purpose).

For the 29-item version, Cronbach alphas of .84 to .94 were reported in 13 samples ($N = 2,824$) from Israel, the US, and Norway (Antonovsky, 1987; Dantas et al., 2002; Sagy, Antonovsky, & Adler, 1990). Previously, Motzer and Stewart (1996) reported a Cronbach alpha of .87 for the 13-item version in persons surviving cardiac arrest ($N = 147$). Here, for the respondents ($n = 66$) completing the 29-item version, a score for the 13 items on the short form also was calculated. The validity of that approach was examined by correlating the two scales, and a very strong and positive relationship was found ($r = .96$, p <.001). Thus, we concluded that approach was acceptable. Therefore, the 13-item score was used for all participants. Items are summed, and then an item mean is calculated. The potential summated range is 13–91, and the potential item average range is 1–7, with higher scores indicating a stronger SOC. In this sample, Cronbach alphas for the long and short versions were .92 and .88, respectively.

Holistic QOL was measured using the 16-item MQOLS (Burckhardt et al., 1989; Flanagan, 1982). Respondents rated satisfaction with specific areas using the 7-point Delighted-Terrible scale (Andrews & Crandall, 1976), where 7 represented "delighted" and 1 represented "terrible." Examples of MQOLS items are satisfaction with:

▶ material comforts (home, food, financial security)
▶ close relations with spouse or significant other
▶ participation in active recreation.

For the modified version, Burckhardt and colleagues reported Cronbach alphas of .82 to .92, and test-retest reliabilities of .76 (6-week interval) to .78 and .84 (two 3-week intervals). The items are summed, and an item mean is calculated, with potential ranges (16–112) for the summated scale and the item average (1–7). Higher scores indicate higher QOL. In this sample, the Cronbach alpha was .79.

The Bowel Disease Questionnaire (BDQ) (Talley, Phillips, Melton, Wiltgen, & Zinsmeister, 1989) is a self-report questionnaire designed to identify bowel disease. This 97-item questionnaire covers GI symptoms, GI screening, and includes a 17-item psychosomatic checklist. Test-retest kappa statistic ranged from .52 to 1.0 ($M = .78$) for all questions based on a sample of 361. When used with a clinical sample of 399 participants, the questionnaire discriminated functional GI disease from organic disease, somatoform disorder, and health states (Talley, Phillips, Wiltgen, Zinsmeister, & Melton, 1990). In this study items were used specific to physical distress and its impact on daily activities. In particular, we evaluated the occurrence and severity of stomach or belly (gut) pain, predominant bowel patterns (normal, diarrhea alone, constipation alone, or alternating constipation and diarrhea), and interruption in activities attributed to stomach or bowel problems or to other illnesses. These data were used for descriptive and correlational purposes.

Symptom Checklist-90-R (SCL-90-R) (Derogatis, 1977) is a 90-item self-report inventory of psychopathology originally developed from the Minnesota Multiphasic Personality Inventory. The Global Severity Index (GSI) (a summation of all 90 items), and the subscales depression, anxiety, and somatization were used. Given that women in the IBS group experienced GI symptoms and women in the control group did not, the somatization subscale was modified to exclude items related to GI somatization (i.e., nausea or upset stomach). Symptom distress is rated from not-at-all (0) to extremely (4). The GSI and the subscales are mean scores. Internal consistency reliabilities of the subscales range from .77 to .90, and 1-week test-retest reliabilities range from .78 to .90 (Derogatis, 1977). The Cronbach alphas for this sample were .97 for the GSI, and .89, .85, .83, and .82 for the subscales depression, anxiety, somatization, and somatization without GI symptoms, respectively.

A response tendency of social desirability is of methodological concern in studies using self-report measures. The 20-item version (Strahan & Gerbasis, 1972) of the original Marlowe-Crowne Social Desirability index (SDI) examined its influence. This summated scale has a true-false response format (more socially desirable responses = 1, less socially desirable responses = 0). Correlations were made between the SDI and the other self-report scales. In this sample, Cronbach alpha was .73.

Analysis

Independent samples t tests were used to examine differences in SOC, holistic QOL, psychological distress, and the response (tendency of social desirability between women with and without IBS. Pearson's r or Kendall's tau was used to evaluate relationships between variables. Bonferroni corrections for multiple comparisons were performed for each analysis.

RESULTS

On average, women in the IBS and control groups were the same age. There were fewer minority IBS women than minority control women. Otherwise there were no group differences in demographic variables or in a response tendency toward social desirability. The demographic characteristics of the sample are displayed in Table 1.

Virtually all women with IBS experienced abdominal pain in the past year, but nearly one-half of control women also reported abdominal pain in the past year (Table 2). However, severity of abdominal pain differed between groups, with most control women who had pain reporting only mild-to-moderate pain, whereas more than one-third of the IBS women reported severe-to-very-severe abdominal pain. Bowel patterns also differed between groups. Nearly all control women (but far fewer IBS women) reported having a normal bowel pattern. In the IBS

TABLE 1	Demographic Characteristics of the Sample ($N = 324$)	
DEMOGRAPHIC CHARACTERISTICS	**IBS ($n = 235$) FREQUENCY (%)**	**CONTROL ($n = 89$) FREQUENCY (%)**
Age (years, M, SD)	32.7 (7.6)	32.4 (7.2)
Ethnicity		
Asian/Pacific Islander	9 (3.8)	16 (18)
African American	7 (3.0)	5 (5.6)
Hispanic or Latino	10 (4.3)	3 (3.4)
Native American/Alaskan Native	2 (0.9)	1 (1.1)
White	206 (87.7)	64 (71.9)
Married/Partnered	103 (43.8)[a]	37 (41.6)
Living with roommate, family, spouse, or partner	186 (79)	73 (82)
Bachelor's or graduate degrees	145 (61.7)	67 (75.2)
Occupation		
Professional, technical, managerial	119 (50.6)	42 (47.2)
Clerical, sales/service, other	79 (33.6)	15 (16.9)
Student	37 (15.7)	32 (36.0)
Personal annual income $\leq$ $30,000	147 (65.6)[b]	65 (74.7)[c]
Family annual income $\leq$ $50,000	119 (58.9)[d]	36 (54.5)[e]
Currently have health insurance	229 (97.4)[f]	83 (93.3)[g]
SDI (M, SD)	9.87 (3.73)[a]	10.23 (3.72)[c]

Note. IBS = irritable bowel syndrome; SDI = Social Desirability Index (potential range is 0–20, where higher scores = higher social desirability).
[a]$n = 230$
[b]$n = 224$
[c]$n = 87$
[d]$n = 202$
[e]$n = 66$
[f]$n = 234$
[g]$n = 88$

group, the most frequent abnormal bowel pattern was alternating constipation and diarrhea. Many more women with IBS than control women reported that GI symptoms and other illnesses interrupted their usual activities.

As hypothesized, SOC and holistic QOL were significantly lower in women with IBS compared to control women (Table 3). All 16 MQOL items were lower for women with IBS compared to control women, but only three of those items were significantly lower. They included satisfaction with:

▶ health: being physically fit and vigorous ($p < .001$)
▶ relationships with parents, siblings, and other relatives: communicating, visiting, helping ($p = .002$)
▶ learning: attending school and improving knowledge ($p = .001$).

On average, women with IBS ranked satisfaction with health lowest (4.1 ± 1.3 on this 7-point scale) of the MQOLS items. On the SCL-90-R, the GSI and the subscales somatization

TABLE 2 Self-Report Gastrointestinal Symptoms (Bowel Disease Questionnaire) in the Past Year in Women with and Without IBS

SYMPTOMS	IBS (*n* = 235) FREQUENCY (%)	CONTROL (*n* = 89) FREQUENCY (%)
Experienced abdominal pain	228 (99)	40 (46)
Severity of abdominal pain		
Mild	18 (7.9)	15 (39.5)
Moderate	120 (52.6)	21 (55.3)
Severe	68 (29.8)	2 (5.3)
Very severe	22 (9.6)	0
Bowel patterns		
Normal	31 (13.5)	84 (95.5)
Constipated	36 (15.3)	1 (1)
(Less than 3 bowel movements/week)	42 (18.3)	1 (1)
Diarrhea	44 (19.2)	0
Alternating constipation and diarrhea	118 (50.2)	3 (3)
Activities interrupted due to stomach pains	172 (75)	6 (7)
Activities interrupted due to bowel problems	166 (72)	3 (3)
Activities interrupted due to other illnesses	119 (51)	30 (34)

Note IBS = irritable bowel syndrome.

TABLE 3 Differences in Self-Report Scores for the IBS and Control Groups

VARIABLE	IBS MEAN (*SD*)	CONTROL MEAN (*SD*)	*p* VALUE
SOCQ, 13-item	*n* = 224	*n* = 86	
Summated score, potential range is 13–91	61.58 (13.00)	67.36 (12.33)	<.001
Item average score, potential range is 1–7	4.74 (1.00)	5.19 (0.95)	
SOCQ, 29-item	*n* = 32	*n* = 34	
Summated score, potential range is 29–203	131.75 (21.73)	148.94 (21.38)	.002
Item average score, potential range is 1–7	4.55 (0.75)	5.15 (0.73)	
MQOLS	*n* = 225	*n* = 88	
Summated score, potential range is 16–112	79.60 (12.18)	84.89 (10.68)	<.001
Item average score, potential range is 1–7	4.98 (0.76)	5.31 (0.67)	
SCL-90-R	*n* = 230	*n* = 88	
Global Severity Index	0.64 (0.45)	0.32 (0.33)	<.001
Somatization	0.75 (0.55)	0.32 (0.37)	<.001
Somatization without GI symptoms	0.68 (0.56)	0.32 (0.37)	<.001
Depression	0.90 (0.66)	0.46 (0.48)	<.001
Anxiety	0.58 (0.58)	0.27 (0.44)	<.001

Note. IBS = irritable bowel syndrome; SOCQ = Sense of Coherence Questionnaire (7 = *strongest* and 1 = *weakest*); MQOLS = Modified Flanagan Quality of Life Scale (7 = *delighted*, 1 = *terrible*); SCL-90-R = Symptom Checklist-90-R (0 = *not-at-all* and 4 = *extremely*); GI = gastrointestinal. All comparisons between groups remained statistically significant at the $p < 05$ level after correcting for 8 comparisons.

(with and without GI symptoms), depression, and anxiety differed significantly between groups, with the IBS group having the highest levels of psychological distress.

Relationships among SOC and holistic QOL with other self-report measures are displayed for the total sample in Table 4. As hypothesized, correlations between SOC and indicators of psychological distress were moderately and inversely related. Of the psychological distress indicators of primary interest, the GSI, and the depression and anxiety subscales were moderately related to SOC. The other psychological distress variable of primary interest, the somatization subscale without GI symptoms, was less strongly related to SOC. Relationships between holistic QOL and the psychological distress indicators also were negative but were lower magnitude universally. The experience of alternating constipation and diarrhea was inversely and weakly related to both SOC and holistic QOL, whereas having a normal bowel pattern was positively related to both SOC and holistic QOL. Severity of abdominal pain was weakly and inversely related to holistic QOL but not to SOC. Social desirability was weakly related to both SOC and holistic QOL. Relationships between social desirability and the self-report GI symptoms and psychological distress variables also were examined but were not significant after Bonferroni corrections for multiple comparisons.

TABLE 4   Correlation Coefficients for Sense of Coherence (13-item SOCQ) and Holistic Quality of Life (MQOLS) with Gastrointestinal Symptoms (BDQ) and Psychological Distress (SCL-90-R)

Variable	r WITH SOCQ-13			r WITH MQOLS		
	n	r	p	n	r	p
SOCQ-13	310	1.00	—	309	.67	<.001
MQOLS	309	.66	<.001	313	1.00	—
Severity of abdominal pain	257	−.08	NS	259	−.22	<.001
Constipation (τ)	307	−.07	NS	310	−.05	NS
Diarrhea (τ)	307	.01	NS	310	.01	NS
Alternating constipation/diarrhea (τ)	307	−.21	<.001	310	−.17	<.001
Normal bowel pattern (τ)	307	.25	<.001	310	.20	<.001
SCL-90-R GSI	307	−.64	<.001	310	−.51	<.001
SCL-90-R Somatization without GI	307	−.31	<.001	310	−.27	<.001
SCL-90-R Depression	307	−.64	<.001	310	−.56	<.001
SCL-90-R Anxiety	307	−.53	<.001	310	−.37	<.001
SDI	309	.20	.001	312	.21	<.001

Note. All correlations were Pearson *r* unless noted as Kendall's tau (τ). SOCQ-13 = Sense of Coherence Questionnaire, 13-item version; MQOLS = Modified Flanagan Quality of Life Scale; BDQ = Bowel Disease Questionnaire; SCL-90-R = Symptom Checklist-90-R; GSI = Global Severity Index; GI = gastrointestinal; SDI = Social Desirability Index; NS = not significant. The variables constipation, diarrhea, alternating constipation/diarrhea, and normal bowel pattern were dichotomous and mutually exclusive.

DISCUSSION

Our data support that women 18–49 years of age with IBS had a lower SOC than women without IBS. The average levels of SOC in the IBS group and the control group are roughly equivalent to Antonovsky's (1987) lowest normative level (undergraduate students) and middle normative level (healthcare workers), respectively. These data are also consistent with the IBS group and control group SOC scores of Sperber and colleagues (1999) ($M = 59.6$ and $M = 65.7$, respectively).

SOC scores for this sample, however, do differ from scores obtained from cardiac arrest survivors (13-item version) (Motzer & Stewart, 1996) and post coronary artery bypass graft patients (29-item version) (Dantas et al., 2002). Both of these groups had higher item average levels of SOC but comparable variability ($M = 5.3 \pm 1.0$, $M = 5.0 \pm 0.9$, respectively). A major difference between these samples may be that the cardiac arrest group survived a truly life-threatening event (i.e., the cardiac arrest) in addition to the ongoing management of their chronic health disturbance (i.e., coronary heart disease, which potentially is also life threatening). Thus, they may have been able to derive more meaning from survival of cardiac arrest and/or the experience of having potentially life-threatening heart disease than could persons with a chronic but non-life threatening health disturbance like IBS. However, age and gender could contribute to these differences as well.

The weak relationship of the SDI with both the SOCQ and the MQOLS suggests that respondents' SOC and holistic QOL scores may have been reported in a more socially acceptable way than the other measures. However, SDI scores did not differ by group. Therefore, it is believed that the group differences in SOC and holistic QOL are valid differences.

Antonovsky posited that SOC is crystallized near the age of 30 (Antonovsky, 1987). The IBS and control groups in this study were younger ($M = 32$ years) than (a) the IBS and control subjects ($M = 47$ years) (Sperber et al., 1999), (b) cardiac arrest survivors ($M = 63$ years) (Motzer & Stewart, 1996), and (c) postcoronary artery bypass graft patients ($M = 66.5$ years) (Dantas et al., 2002). Although SOC may still have been developing in our younger population, resulting in lower levels than in these older study groups, the SOC values were not markedly different than those noted by Sperber with a somewhat older IBS population. Thus, it is unlikely that the lower scores could be attributable to age differences. All of our subjects, and the majority (76%) of Sperber's subjects were women; whereas women composed only 27% of the cardiac arrest sample (Motzer & Stewart, 1996) and 20% of the postcoronary artery bypass graft sample (Dantas et al., 2002). It is unclear if there is an effect of sex on SOC; however, normative SOC data do not support sex-related differences in SOC.

Holistic QOL is significantly lower for women aged 18–49 with IBS compared to control women; key differences were:

▶ satisfaction with health
▶ relationships with family
▶ learning

Levels of holistic QOL, for women with IBS were comparable to persons following coronary artery bypass graft surgery (Dantas et al., 2002) but lower than the holistic QOL reported by cardiac arrest survivors' (Motzer & Stewart, 1996). Holistic QOL was comparable between the cardiac arrest survivors and control women in this study. In this study, on average, control women reported being mostly satisfied-to-pleased with their QOL, while women with

IBS reported being mostly satisfied with their QOL. Thus, persons with a chronic health disturbance can experience a satisfactory overall QOL despite ongoing physical and psychological distress, supporting the positions of several researchers (Anderson & Burckhardt, 1999; Gill & Feinstein, 1994). More women with IBS experienced interruptions in usual activities. These functional GI problems, symptoms, and interruption with life activities are the types of areas assessed in disease-specific, health-related QOL instruments such as the SF-36 or IBS-36 (Groll et al., 2002), but not in holistic QOL instruments.

Sense of coherence was strongly and positively associated with holistic QOL in the total sample of women with and without IBS. However, the strength of this association was less than the relationship Motzer and Stewart (1996) previously reported in cardiac arrest survivors ($r = .73$). At that time, they evaluated potential conceptual and measurement overlaps between the two constructs, and concluded that SOC and holistic QOL were distinct. To determine whether these relationships were similar in separate groups (IBS and controls) a posthoc analysis was performed. The strength of this association held both for women with ($r = .63$) and without IBS ($r = .70$), supporting the link between SOC and holistic QOL in both healthy persons as well as persons with a chronic health disturbance.

More women with IBS than control women experienced both physical and psychological symptom distress. This finding supports our previous work (Jarrett et al., 1998; Motzer et al., 2002) as well as the work of others (e.g., Whitehead et al., 1988). Psychological distress variables were moderately and negatively related to SOC in the total sample. In the posthoc analysis of the IBS and control groups, after controlling for multiple correlations, only somatization without GI symptoms in relationship to both SOC and holistic QOL appeared different between groups: with SOC, $r = -.46$ ($p < .001$) for control and $r = -.24$ ($p < .001$) for IBS; and with holistic QOL, $r = -.38$ ($p < .001$) for control and $r = -.19$ ($p = .004$) for IBS. In the total sample, severity of abdominal pain and having alternating constipation/ diarrhea were inversely and weakly related to holistic QOL, and having a normal bowel pattern was weakly and positively related to holistic QOL. In this total sample, SOC was weakly related to bowel pattern (inversely to alternating constipation/diarrhea, and positively to normal pattern) but surprisingly not related to severity of abdominal pain. None of these correlations held in the posthoc analysis of either the IBS or control groups. Whether the lack of relationship between SOC and abdominal pain reflects a true lack of association or a poor choice of physical distress markers remains unclear. A concurrent daily measure of abdominal pain may have clarified the relationship.

In summary, on average, women with IBS have weaker SOC and lower holistic QOL than do control women. They also experience more psychological distress than control women. It remains to be determined whether interventions targeted at enhancing SOC and holistic QOL can impact the psychological distress associated with IBS.

REFERENCES

American College of Gastroenterology Functional Gastrointestinal Disorders Task Force. (2002). Evidence-based position statement on the management of irritable bowel syndrome in North America. *American Journal of Gastroenterology, 97*(11 Suppl), S1–5.

Anderson, K. L., & Burckhardt, C. S. (1999). Conceptualization and measurement of quality of life as an outcome variable for health care intervention and research. *Journal of Advanced Nursing, 29*(2), 298–306.

Andrews, R. M., & Crandall, R. (1976). *Social Indicators of Well-Being: The Development and Measurement of Perceptual Indicators*. New York: Plenum Press.

Antonovsky, A. (1979). *Health, Stress, and Coping*. San Francisco: Jossey-Bass.

Antonovsky, A. (1987). *Unraveling the Mystery of Health*. San Francisco: Jossey-Bass.

Antonovsky, A. (1993). The structure and properties of the sense of coherence scale. *Social Science in Medicine, 36*(6), 725–733.

Brandt, L. J., Bjorkman, D., Fennerty, M. B., Locke, G. R., Olden, K., Peterson, W., et al. (2002). Systematic review on the management of irritable bowel syndrome in North America. *American Journal of Gastroenterology, 97*(11 Suppl), S7–26.

Burckhardt, C. S., Woods, S. L., Schultz, A. A., & Ziebarth, D. M. (1989). Quality of life in adults with chronic illness: A psychometric study. *Research in Nursing and Health, 12,* 347–354.

Cash, B. D., Schoenfeld, P., & Chey, W. D. (2002). The utility of diagnostic tests in irritable bowel syndrome patients: A systematic review. *American Journal of Gastroenterology, 97*(11), 2812–2819.

Corbin, J. M., & Strauss, A. (1988). *Unending Work and Care. Managing Chronic Illness at Home.* San Francisco: Jossey-Bass.

Dantas, R. A. S., Motzer, S. A., & Ciol, M. A. (2002). The relationship between quality of life, sense of coherence and self-esteem in persons after coronary artery bypass graft surgery. *International Journal of Nursing Studies, 39*(7), 745–755.

Derogatis, L. (1977). *SCL-90. Administrative Scoring and Procedures Manual II.* (2nd ed.). Baltimore: Clinical Psychometric Research.

Flanagan, J. C. (1982). Measurement of quality of life. Current state of the art. *Archives of Physical Medicine & Rehabilitation, 63,* 56–59.

Gill, T. M., & Feinstein, A. R. (1994). A critical appraisal of the quality of quality-of-life measurements. *Journal of the American Medical Association, 272*(8), 619–626.

Gralnek, I. M., Hays, R. D., Kilbourne, A., Naliboff, B., & Mayer, E. A. (2000). The impact of irritable bowel syndrome on health-related quality of life. *Gastroenterology, 119*(3), 654–660.

Groll, D., Vanner, S. J., Depew, W. T., DaCosta, L. R., Simon, J. B., Groll, A., et al. (2002). The IBS-36: A new quality of life measure for irritable bowel syndrome. *American Journal of Gastroenterology, 97*(4), 962–971.

Hahn, B. A., Kirchdoerfer, L. J., Fullerton, S., & Mayer, E. (1997). Evaluation of a new quality of life questionnaire for patients with irritable bowel syndrome. *Alimentary Pharmacology & Therapeutics, 11*(3), 547–552.

Hahn, B. A., Yan, S., & Strassels, S. (1999). Impact of irritable bowel syndrome on quality of life and resource use in the United States and United Kingdom. *Digestion, 60*(1), 77–81.

Heitkemper, M., Elta, G., Carter, E., Ameen, V., Olden, K., & Chang, L. (2002). Women with irritable bowel syndrome: Differences in patients' and physicians' perceptions. *Gastroenterology Nursing, 25*(5), 192–200.

Heitkemper, M. M., & Jarrett, M. (1992). Pattern of gastrointestinal and somatic symptoms across the menstrual cycle. *Gastroenterology, 102,* 505–513.

International Foundation for Functional Gastrointestinal Disorders. (2002). *IBS in the Real World. IBS Research Findings by IFFGD.* Retrieved December 31, 2002 from http://www.iffgd.org/Research/IBS2002Survey.html

Jarrett, M., Heitkemper, M., Cain, K. C., Tuftin, M., Walker, E. A., Bond, E. F., et al. (1998). The relationship between psychological distress and gastrointestinal symptoms in women. *Nursing Research, 47*(3), 154–161.

Jones, K. R., Palsson, O. S., Levy, R. L., Feld, A. D., Longstreth, G. F., Bradshaw, B. H., et al. (2001). Comorbid disorders and symptoms in irritable bowel syndrome (IBS) compared to other gastroenterology patients. *Gastroenterology, 120*(Suppl 1), A66.

Kay, L., & Jorgensen, T. (1996). Re-defining abdominal syndromes: Results from a population-based study. *Scandinavian Journal of Gastroenterology, 31,* 469–475.

Kumar, D., Pfeffer, J., & Wingate, D. L. (1990). Role of psychological factors in the irritable bowel syndrome. *Digestion, 45*(2), 80–87.

Motzer, S. A., Jarrett, M., Heitkemper, M. M., & Tsuji, J. (2002). Natural killer cell function and psychologic distress in women with and without irritable bowel syndrome. *Biological Research for Nursing, 4*(1), 31–42.

Motzer, S. U., & Stewart, B. J. (1996). Sense of coherence as a predictor of quality of life in persons with coronary heart disease surviving cardiac arrest. *Research in Nursing and Health, 19*(4), 287–298.

Sagy, S., Antonovsky, A., & Adler, I. (1990). Explaining life satisfaction in later life: The sense of coherence model and activity theory. *Behavior, Health, and Aging, 1*(1), 11–25.

Sperber, A. D., Carmel, S., Atzmon, Y., Weisberg, I., Shalit, Y., Neumann, L., et al. (1999). The sense of coherence index and the irritable bowel syndrome. *Scandinavian Journal of Gastroenterology, 3,* 259–263.

Strahan, R., & Gerbasis, K. C. (1972). Short, homogeneous versions of the Marlowe-Crowne Social Desirability Scale. *Journal of Clinical Psychology, 28,* 191–193.

Strauss, A. L., Corbin, J., Fagerhaugh, S., Glaser, B. G., Maines, D., Suczek, B., et al. (1984). *Chronic illness and the quality of life.* St. Louis: C. V. Mosby.

Talley, N. J., Phillips, S. F., Melton, L. J., Wiltgen, C., & Zinsmeister, A. R. (1989). A patient questionnaire to identify bowel disease. *Annals of Internal Medicine, 111,* 671–674.

Talley, N. J., Phillips, S. F., Wiltgen, C. M., Zinsmeister, A. R., & Melton, L. J., III. (1990). Assessment of functional gastrointestinal disease: The Bowel Disease Questionnaire. *Mayo Clinic Proceedings, 65,* 1456–1479.

Thompson, W. G., Longstreth, G. F., Drossman, D. A., Heaton, K. W., Irvine, E. J., & Muller-Lisner, S. A. (1999). Functional bowel disorders and functional abdominal pain. *Gut, 45* (Suppl 2), II43–II47.

Ware, J. E., Jr. (1995). The status of health assessment 1994. *Annual Review of Public Health, 16,* 327–354.

Ware, J. E., Jr., & Sherbourne, C. D. (1992). The MOS 36-item short-form health survey (SF-36). I. Conceptual framework and item selection. *Medical Care, 30*(6), 473–483.

Whitehead, W. E., Bosmajian, L., Zonderman, A., Costa, P., & Shuster, M. (1988). Symptoms of psychologic distress associated with irritable bowel syndrome. *Gastroenterology, 95,* 709–714.

Whitehead, W. E., Palsson, O., & Jones, K. R. (2002). Systematic review of the comorbidity of irritable bowel syndrome with other disorders: What are the causes and implications? *Gastroenterology, 122*(4), 1140–1156.

Whorwell, P. J., McCallum, M., Creed, F. H., & Roberts, C. T. (1986). Non-colonic features of irritable bowel syndrome. *Gut, 27*(1), 37–40.

Zaman, M. S., Chavez, N. F., Krueger, R., Talley, N. J., & Lembo, T. (2001). Extraintestinal symptoms in patients with irritable bowel syndrome (IBS). *Gastroenterology, 120*(Suppl 1), A636.

Sandra Adams Motzer, PhD, RN, FAHA, is Assistant Professor;

Vicky Hertig, PhC, RN, is Doctoral Candidate;

Monica Jarrett, PhD, RN, is Associate Professor; and

Margaret M. Heitkemper, PhD, RN, FAAN, is Professor and Chair, Biobehavioral Nursing and Health Systems, University of Washington, Seattle.

Accepted for publication May 28, 2003.

This study was supported by grants from the National Institute of Nursing Research and the Office of Research on Women's Health, R55 NR04913 (Motzer), R01 NR04913 (Motzer), R01 NR04101 (Heitkemper), and R01 NR04142 (Heitkemper).

The authors thank the Center for Women's Health Research at the University of Washington School of Nursing (P30 NR04001) for their support.

Corresponding author: Sandra Adams Motzer, PhD, RN, FAHA, Department of Biobehavioral Nursing and Health Systems, Box 357266, University of Washington, Seattle, WA 98195-7266 (e-mail: underhil@u.washington.edu).

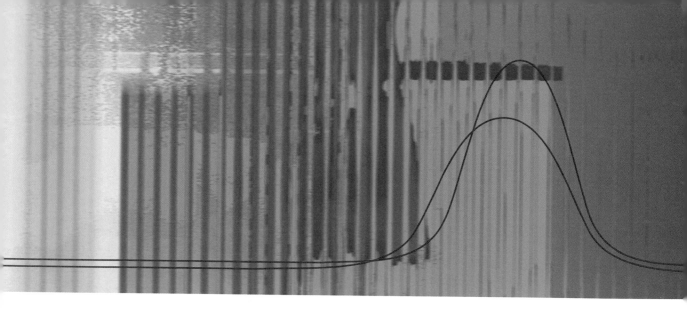

B.

Birth Trauma: In the Eye of the Beholder

Cheryl Tatano Beck

▸ **Background:** The reported prevalence of posttraumatic stress disorder after childbirth ranges from 1.5% to 6%.

▸ **Objective:** To describe the meaning of women's birth trauma experiences.

▸ **Methods:** Descriptive phenomenology was the qualitative research design used to investigate mothers' experiences of traumatic births. Women were recruited through the Internet, primarily through Trauma and Birth Stress (TABS), a charitable trust located in New Zealand. The purposive sample consisted of 40 mothers: 23 in New Zealand, 8 in the United States, 6 in Australia, and 3 in the United Kingdom. Each woman was asked to describe the experience of her traumatic birth and to send it over the Internet to the researcher. Colaizzi's method was used to analyze the 40 mothers' stories.

▸ **Results:** Four themes emerged that described the essence of women's experiences of birth trauma: To care for me: Was that too much too ask? To communicate with me: Why was this neglected? To provide safe care: You betrayed my trust and I felt powerless, and The end justifies the means: At whose expense? At what price?

▸ **Conclusions:** Birth trauma lies in the eye of the beholder. Mothers perceived that their traumatic births often were viewed as routine by clinicians.

▸ **Key Words:** birth trauma, phenomenology, PTSD, qualitative research

Reprinted with permission from *Nursing Research* 2004; 53[1]: 28–35.

I n her 1878 novel *Molly Bawn*, Margaret Wolfe Hungerford, an Irish-born 19th century romance novelist, first penned the phrase "beauty is in the eye of the beholder." Beauty is not the only quality or phenomenon that lies in the eye of the beholder; birth trauma also does. What a mother perceives as birth trauma may be seen quite differently through the eyes of obstetric care providers, who may view it as a routine delivery and just another day at the hospital. The reported prevalence of posttraumatic stress disorder (PTSD) after childbirth ranges from 1.5% (Ayers & Pickering, 2001) to 5.6% (Creedy, Shochet, & Horsfall, 2000). Although there is a reported prevalence of PTSD after childbirth, little research has aimed at an understanding of this phenomenon from the women's experience. This phenomenologic study investigated the meaning of women's birth trauma experiences.

LITERATURE REVIEW

A review of the literature on birth trauma showed limited research on the trauma itself rather than its aftermath, PTSD. This literature review focused on the studies that investigated traumatic births and their risk factors as well as research on the components of physical-emotional-mental birth trauma that can lead to the development of PTSD. Birth trauma is an event occurring during the labor and delivery process that involves actual or threatened serious injury or death to the mother or her infant. The birthing woman experiences intense fear, helplessness, loss of control, and horror.

Three studies were found that discussed elements of birth trauma, although their main focus was on identifying the prevalence of diagnosed PTSD resulting from childbirth.

In the United Kingdom, women ($N = 500$) volunteered to participate in research on psychological stress related to obstetric or gynecologic procedures. Advertisement in newspapers and magazines was the method of recruitment. A small number of women ($n = 102$) in this sample described their experiences of obstetric or gynecologic procedures as "terrifying" and "still affecting them now" (Menage, 1993). These women completed the PTSD Interview questionnaire (Watson, Juba, Manifold, Kucala, & Anderson, 1991). Of the 102 women, 30 met the *Diagnostic and Statistical Manual* (DSM-III-R) criteria for a diagnosis of PTSD. These women with a diagnosis of PTSD resulting from birth trauma reported that during the procedures, they felt powerless, lacked information about the procedures, experienced physical pain, perceived unsympathetic attitudes of the healthcare providers, and lacked a clearly understood consent on their part for the procedures. As compared with the nontrauma group, the women with trauma had experienced significantly more infant death and a higher number of invasive procedures.

In a cross-sectional study of all the women who had given birth over a 1-year period in an obstetric department in Sweden, Wijma, Soderquist, and Wijma (1997) reported that 28 of 1,640 women (1.7%) met the criteria for PTSD. Factors related to the women's experience of PTSD after childbirth included a history of psychiatric counseling, a negative cognitive appraisal of the past delivery, nulliparity, and a negative contact with the delivery staff.

Creedy, Shochet, and Horsfall (2000) conducted a prospective, longitudinal study in Australia. Recruited into the study during their third trimester, the women completed various questionnaires including the State Trait Anxiety Inventory (Spielberger, Gorsuch, & Lushene, 1983). Eligibility criteria for inclusion in the sample required that participants be older than 18 years, in the third trimester of pregnancy, at low risk for obstetric complications, and able to understand English. Telephone interviews with the women ($n = 499$) 4 to 6 weeks post-partum explored their perceptions of the labor and delivery care and the presence of trauma symptoms. The DSM-IV diagnostic criteria for acute posttraumatic stress disorder were met by 28 mothers (5.6%). These stressful birth events included extreme pain, fear of the mother for her life or that of her infant, and a perception of a real or actual lack of obstetric care. Two variables were associated significantly ($p < .0001$) with acute trauma symptoms: a high degree of obstetric intervention and dissatisfaction with the care received during labor and delivery.

The following three studies focused on traumatic births and posttraumatic stress symptoms. No formal diagnosis of PTSD was included as part of the research.

In Sweden, Ryding, Wijma, and Wijma (1998) interviewed women ($N = 53$) approximately 2 days after emergency cesarean delivery to determine whether this trauma met the stressor criterion of PTSD. Other sample criteria besides the experience of an emergency cesarean included use of the Swedish language and delivery of a live infant who had not been transferred to another hospital for special care. In this study, 29 mothers (55%) reported experiencing intense fear of death or injury to themselves or to their baby during the delivery process, which fulfilled the stressor criterion of DSM-IV. The most common fear was related to concerns that the baby would die or be injured. The mothers who feared for their own lives had experienced a painful labor. The findings showed that 8% of the women were angry because they felt that the delivery staff had treated them very badly. These mothers felt violated and helpless during the care provided by the delivery staff.

Czarnocka and Slade (2000) assessed the prevalence and potential predictors of posttraumatic stress symptoms with a sample of women ($N = 264$) in the United Kingdom. Eligibility criteria specified women who (a) were older than 18 years, (b) had delivered a healthy infant, (c) spoke English, and (d) had no immediate plans of moving out of the area. At 6 weeks postpartum, the mothers completed the Post-Traumatic Stress Disorder Questionnaire (PTSD-Q) and Interview (Watson et al., 1991). In this assessment, 3% of the sample ($n = 8$) reported symptoms on the PTSD-Q indicating clinically significant levels of the three posttraumatic stress dimensions: intrusions, avoidance, and hyperarousal. Regression analysis showed the following significant predictors of posttraumatic stress symptoms related to childbirth: low levels of perceived support from labor and delivery staff and partner and low perceived control during labor.

One study conducted in the United States investigated the prevalence and predictors of psychological trauma experienced by women during childbirth (Soet, Brack, & Dilorio, 2003). Women were recruited from childbirth education classes. In late pregnancy, the women ($N = 103$) completed questionnaires measuring such concepts as locus of control and social support. Approximately 4 weeks after delivery, a follow-up interview was conducted by telephone. The mother's experience of birth trauma was measured using the Traumatic Event Scale (TES) (Wijma et al., 1997). In these interviews, 35 women (34%) reported traumatic births. Significant predictors of birth trauma included cesarean delivery, medical intervention, long painful labor, feelings of powerlessness, inadequate information, negative interaction with medical personnel, and differences between expectations and the actual event of childbirth.

The literature review found only one qualitative study that had investigated traumatic births. Women who perceived having traumatic deliveries were recruited by health visitors when they brought their infant for the 8-month well baby checkup. Allen (1998) interviewed women ($N = 20$) in the United Kingdom 10 months after their delivery who perceived that they had experienced distressing labor. Grounded theory analysis showed that the core category related to a traumatic birth experience was the mothers' feelings of not being in control of events or of their own behavior. Causal factors leading to the perception of a traumatic birth were the belief that the baby would be harmed, past experiences in labor, and pain during labor. The mothers tried to gain control by seeking reassurance and knowledge provided by staff and partners.

Seng (2002) acknowledged the complexities of conducting research on PTSD and childbearing. A conceptual framework for research was developed to study the effects of past and current abuse and posttraumatic stress on childbearing women. Seng's framework emphasized PTSD as a potential mediator in the relation between trauma and adverse childbearing outcomes. By both behavioral and neuroendocrine pathways PTSD can be a possible mechanism for adverse maternal and infant outcomes using Seng's conceptual framework, studies can be designed where treatment for PTSD and decreasing high life event stress can potentially decrease association between PTSD and negative childbearing outcomes.

The literature review found a limited number of studies on birth trauma. These quantitative studies focused on identifying predictors of PTSD that related to childbirth. None of the studies investigated the long-term effects of birth trauma for women. Current PTSD knowledge does not address the meaning of a traumatic birth for women. The purpose of the current phenomenologic study was to investigate the following research question: What is the essential structure of women's experiences of birth trauma?

METHODS

Research Design

Descriptive phenomenology was the qualitative research design chosen for the study of mothers' experiences of traumatic births. Husserl's (1970) descriptive (eidetic) phenomenology was the philosophical underpinning for this study. In phenomenology, the nature of a phenomenon (i.e., what makes something what it is without which it could not be what it is) is investigated (Husserl, 1962). Phenomena as they are experienced consciously are described without theories about causes and as free as possible from unexamined preconceptions and presuppositions (Spiegelberg, 1975). One assumption of descriptive phenomenology is that for any human experience there are distinct essential structures that make up that phenomenon regardless of the particular person who experiences it. These essential structures are discovered by studying the particulars encountered in the lived experience.

An understanding of these essential structures requires phenomenologic reduction (Husserl, 1960), in which researchers attempt to put aside temporarily any presuppositions they may hold about the phenomena they are studying, allowing phenomena to come directly into view without distortion by the researchers' preconceptions. "Bracketing" is the term used by Husserl (1960) to describe this process of peeling away the layers of interpretation so the phenomena can be seen as they are. Bracketing does not eliminate perspective, but brings the experience into clearer focus.

Procedure

After approval had been obtained from the university's institutional review board, women were recruited via the Internet primarily through Trauma and Birth Stress (TABS), a charitable trust located in New Zealand. Trauma and Birth Stress was founded by five mothers who had experienced birth trauma. This self-help organization supports women who have experienced birth trauma and educates about birth trauma and the resulting PTSD.

Members of TABS were informed of the study by a packet sent to each of them by regular postal mail from the chairperson of TABS. Two letters were included in the packet. The first letter was written by the chairperson as an introduction to the study. The researcher wrote the second letter, explaining her role and describing the research program. An announcement recruiting women also was placed in the TABS newsletter. Women interested in participating had two options: e-mail or regular postal mail. In addition to recruitment through TABS, a few mothers learned of the study from the researcher's university Web site. Finally, two women from Australia joined the study after hearing a joint presentation on PTSD after childbirth by the chairperson of TABS, a psychiatrist, and the researcher.

A purposive sample was used to gain perspectives from the participants who had experienced the phenomenon investigated in the study. The sample criteria required that the mother had experienced birth trauma, was willing to articulate her experience, and could read and write English. Ability to use the Internet was not a sample criterion. The mothers who chose the Internet as the means of participation e-mailed the researcher concerning their interest. The researcher then sent the interested women two attachments: an informed consent form and directions for participating in the study. After reading both documents, the women had the opportunity of e-mailing the researcher with any further questions about the study. They electronically signed the informed consent form and returned it to the researcher by attachment. The mothers who chose to participate in the study by regular postal mail contacted the chairperson of TABS, who then sent them the informed consent form. Each mother was asked to describe her experience of traumatic birth in as much detail as she could remember and wished to share.

Of the 40 mothers, 38 participated in the study through the Internet. They sent their birth trauma stories as attachments to the researcher. The remaining two women wrote their experiences of birth trauma and sent them by regular postal mail to the researcher. After the researcher read each mother's birth trauma story, she e-mailed the woman if she had any questions or needed clarification concerning what had been written. Two participants also sent the researcher boxes of journals they had written chronicling their traumatic birth experiences and the PTSD that followed. Data collection extended over an 18-month period.

Data Analysis

The study used Colaizzi's (1978) method of data analysis, which consists of the following seven steps:

1. Read all the participants' descriptions of the phenomenon under study.
2. Extract significant statements that pertain directly to the phenomenon.
3. Formulate meanings for these significant statements.
4. Categorize the formulated meanings into clusters of themes.
5. Integrate the findings into an exhaustive description of the phenomenon being studied.
6. Validate the exhaustive description by returning to some of the participants to ask them how it compares with their experiences.
7. Incorporate any changes offered by the participants into the final description of the essence of the phenomenon.

A portion of the audit trail for the data analysis can be found in Table 1, which includes selected examples of significant statements and corresponding formulated meanings. With

TABLE 1   **Selected Examples of Significant Statements and Their Formulated Meanings for Two Themes**

THEME NO.	SIGNIFICANT STATEMENTS	FORMULATED MEANINGS
1. To care for me: Was that too much to ask?	When you returned to my labor room and I was vomiting and shaking and no longer handling the contractions, you never reassured me or explained what was happening.	The woman felt uninformed and lacked reassurance about her labor process.
	Lying indecently and asking why the curtain behind me was open and could they close it. I felt exposed to the outside world!	The mother felt stripped of her dignity as her privacy was not respected.
2. To communicate with me: Why was this neglected?	While waiting for a scan for retained placenta fragments, I read my chart and learned for the first time my congenitally deformed baby was born alive. I thought he had been born dead and that they had brought him back to life. I went into a real inner panic and made me think, "what else don't I know or haven't they told me."	The mother panicked and became distrustful of her health care providers once she learned that information about her baby had been withheld from her.
	The midwife never told me or my support people where she was going, what she was doing, how long she would be, or what to do if I needed help.	During labor the woman felt abandoned by her primary clinician.

regard to the clustering of the formulated meanings around the four themes, the largest number of formulated meanings clustered around themes 1 and 2, followed by themes 3 and 4.

Colaizzi's (1978) process for thematic analysis was used. Once the formulated meanings were organized into clusters of themes, these clusters were referred back to the women's original birth trauma stories for their validation. At this stage of thematic analysis, the researcher must not be tempted to ignore data or themes that do not fit (Colaizzi).

The four themes were validated by nine mothers who had participated in the study. This group of mothers, who met with the researcher while she was in New Zealand, felt that none of the results needed to be changed. In addition, four mothers who had participated in the study and one father reviewed this article before it was submitted for publication. All agreed that the results captured the essence of their birth trauma experiences. The rationale for not including all the participants for validation of the results was that once some of the women had written their story, they did not want to revisit it again.

RESULTS

Sample

The purposive sample consisted of 40 mothers who perceived that they had experienced birth trauma. The length of time since their traumatic deliveries ranged from 5 weeks to 14 years. The mothers lived in New Zealand ($n = 23$), the United States ($n = 8$), Australia ($n = 6$), and the United Kingdom ($n = 3$). According to the diagnoses, 32 of the women (80%) had PTSD attributable to birth trauma, whereas 8 women (20%) had experienced PTSD symptoms, but had not yet gone for mental healthcare after delivery. The mean age of the sample at the time the women participated in the study was 34 years (range, 25–44 years). Of the 40 women, 34 were married, 3 were divorced, and 3 were single. Of the 15 women who shared their education level, 1 had graduated from medical school, 4 had completed graduate school, 8 had graduated from college, 1 had a partial college education, and 1 had graduated from high school. Sixteen of the women were primiparas, whereas 24 were multiparas. Eighteen of the women (45%) had undergone cesarean deliveries, whereas 22 (55%) had delivered vaginally. Almost an equal number of birth traumas in this sample had occurred during cesarean and vaginal deliveries. Labor had been induced for 17 of the mothers. Two mothers delivered twins and one mother had triplets. Three mothers in the sample were bipolar, and one had experienced prenatal depression with this most recent pregnancy.

Themes

The study results clearly show that birth trauma is in the eye of the beholder. The birth traumas identified by the women in the sample are presented in Table 2. The concept of birth trauma involves traumatic experiences that may occur during any phase of childbearing. During any phase, the trauma may be classified as a negative outcome including a stillbirth, an obstetric complication (e.g., an emergency cesarean), or psychological distress (fear of an epidural).

THEME 1. TO CARE FOR ME: WAS THAT TOO MUCH TO ASK?

I am amazed that 31/2 hours in the labor and delivery room could cause such utter destruction in my life. It truly was like being the victim of a violent crime or rape.

What could have happened to this woman and others to turn the delivery process into a rape scene? Perceived lack of a caring approach during such a vulnerable time was one of the core components in this scenario for a traumatic birth. The mothers reported that feeling abandoned

---

TABLE 2   List of Birth Traumas

▷ Stillbirth/infant death	▷ Forceps/vacuum extraction/skull fracture
▷ Emergency cesarean delivery/fetal distress	▷ Severe toxemia
▷ Cardiac arrest	▷ Premature birth
▷ Inadequate medical care	▷ Separation from infant in NICU
▷ Fear of epidural	▷ Prolonged, painful labor
▷ Congenital anomalies	▷ Rapid delivery
▷ Inadequate pain relief	▷ Degrading experience
▷ Postpartum hemorrhage/manual removal of placenta	

and alone, stripped of their dignity, lack of interest in them as unique persons, and lack of support and reassurance all contributed to their birth trauma. One mother said she "felt betrayed by a system that is supposedly there to care for me."

The women who participated in this study reported that their expectations for their labor and delivery care were shattered. One mother painfully stated:

The labor care has hurt deep in my soul and I have no words to describe the hurt. I was treated like a nothing, just someone to get data from. The nurse took my pulse, temperature, blood pressure, and weight without talking to me as a person. She then asked about teeth, colds and smoking without acknowledging me as a person. She left me, tears rolling down my face.

A multipara who had an induced labor said:

I felt like just a vessel into which you poured hormones hoping for the quick release of another baby.

The adjectives used by the mothers in this study to describe the care they had received during the delivery process included "mechanical," "arrogant," "cold," "technical," and "lack of empathy." For example, within 24 hours of giving birth, one mother had to say goodbye forever to her beloved newborn daughter. As her baby was dying in the neonatal intensive care unit (NICU), her husband took lots of photos until the film ran out. She and her husband asked for more film and ignored the disapproving looks of the staff members. They wondered:

Was this too much to ask for—for us it was our only opportunity to do this before our daughter died.

The mothers reported that being stripped of their dignity also played a part in birth trauma. As one young Puerto Rican mother recounted:

They had me in all kinds of positions (including all fours) to hear the heartbeat with a stethoscope, and about 20 students came in the room without my permission. All I heard them saying was that I was now 7½ dilated. By the way, while I was on all fours, I was trying to cover my bottom by holding the gown, and a nurse took my hands from the gown. So, I felt raped, and my dignity was taken from me.

During the delivery process, some women were shaken to the core by feeling abandoned and alone, as illustrated by the following quote:

I had a major bleed and started shaking involuntarily all over. Even my jaw shook and I couldn't stop. I heard the specialist say he was having trouble stopping the bleeding. I was very frightened, and then it hit me. I might not make it! I can still recall the sick dread of real fear. I needed urgent reassurance, but none was offered.

THEME 2. TO COMMUNICATE WITH ME: WHY WAS THIS NEGLECTED?

At times, the mothers perceived that the labor and delivery staff failed to communicate with their patients. During a traumatic birth, women often felt invisible. Clinicians spoke to each other as if the woman were not present. One woman who was having her first baby recalled:

After an hour trying to deliver the baby with a vacuum extractor, the obstetrician said it was too late for an emergency cesarean. The baby was truly stuck. By now the doctors are acting like I'm not there. The attending physician was saying, "We may have lost this bloody baby." The hospital staff discussed my baby's possible death in front of me and argued in front of me just as if I weren't there.

The following segment of a mother's story dramatically illustrates how someone merely communicating with her and explaining what was happening could have prevented her birth trauma:

The doctor turned on this machine that sounded like a swimming pool pump. He proceeded and hurriedly showed me the piece that was to be inserted into me. It was chrome metal and extremely large in circumference. Next thing he begins to pull on this hose, which was the extension of the suction. He gritted his teeth and pulled. I felt sick. On the end of this machine was our baby's head. He used every ounce of his male strength to pull the baby out. I was horrified, I started to imagine, and any minute now a head will come out, ripped off of its body. I was really in shock. He had his foot up on the bed, using it as leverage to pull. All of a sudden, the loud sucking machine made an even louder noise, and it broke suction. The doctor fell back and nearly landed on his bum. Blood came spurting out of me, all over him. That was it for me. I thought he'd ripped the head off. He then swore and said hurriedly, "Get the forceps." I can still remember the feeling of him ripping the baby out of me. It was the most awful unnatural devastating feeling ever. Well, finally out came this baby. I was, by this stage, still stuck in my own private horror movie, visualizing my baby being born dead with half of its head missing. The pediatrician was standing beside the doctor, and I assumed that he would take the dead baby away. But, much to my horror and surprise, the doctor pulled out this blood red baby and threw it onto my tummy. I screamed, "Get him off of me!" I cried my eyes out!

Clinicians also at times failed to communicate among themselves, which influenced the women's perceptions of their deliveries as traumatic. For example, labor was induced for one woman who had experienced a previous serious vasovagal reaction before pregnancy and it came time for her to receive an epidural. She was terrified because the midwife did not tell the anesthetist about her history. As this mother shared,

I remember my husband trying to tell the anesthetist that I was fearful of a vasovagal attack. The midwife should have been doing that. My husband kept saying, "My wife, my wife." He could not remember what to say. I was terrified for my life. My soul was in agony because the medical people did not know the situation. I was terrified to the core of my being. I called out, "I'm scared, I'm scared." Not scared of the needle, scared for

THEME 3. TO PROVIDE SAFE CARE: YOU BETRAYED MY TRUST AND I FELT POWERLESS

Women began their labors confident that the delivery staff would ... them as they ...
entrusted their lives and that of their unborn baby into the ... the dangerous ...
women perceived that they received unsafe care, which ... they
their own safety and that of their infants, but felt pow... ld know wh... and loss of
one mother vehemently recounted: st mistake. T...
                                                           eelings of p...

I remember believing that the labor an...
would be there should things go w...
weren't! I strongly believe my...
control of what people did t...

One brief scenario vividly illustrates this third theme. Shortly before becoming pregnant the second time, one mother had surgery to repair a hiatal hernia. During this pregnancy, gestational diabetes developed, and at 28 weeks a scan detected a mass in the brain of her fetus. Her desired birth plan was to have a cesarean delivery to save her baby the distress of a vaginal birth. The doctor "pressured" her into a trial of labor because her first delivery had been so straightforward and rapid. The doctor assured her that if she got into any difficulties she could "easily convert to cesarean." As this mother explained,

> I went into the delivery room assured that my baby and I would be in safe hands. I got into difficulties at 9 p.m. with severe abdominal pain and felt something was terribly wrong. I was in what I describe as "white pain," a terrible ripping pain. I told the staff something was wrong and I begged for a cesarean. I was refused without an examination. An epidural was administered without an examination. I was pushing for hours to no avail, flat on my back, numb from the waist down and feeling that my vague pushes were killing my unborn daughter. I started to die inside. The whole of my genital area was swollen to resemble a baboon. My daughter was posterior, brow presenting, and I continued in second stage labor actively pushing for over 6 hours. My daughter was distressed and her heartbeat kept disappearing. An episiotomy was cut without so much as eye contact with me. My daughter was born flat, resuscitated with Apgars of 2 and 6, and taken to the NICU. After being stitched up, I went to see my baby, and I didn't recognize her, felt no bond, nothing. She wasn't my baby; my baby had died. In my mind, my efforts to give birth had killed her. After delivery I was incontinent. The familiar stomach pain returned. My hiatus hernia repair had now failed. I later had repair surgery to reattach a part of my labia majora. I had an anal sphincter repair and my pelvic floor was refashioned at the same time. I'm waiting for a repeat hiatus hernia repair, and I am still going to physiotherapy to improve the incontinence. During labor, I had expected pain, and I had expected a powerful experience. I expected that, if necessary, medical staff would intervene to keep us safe. Why didn't anyone use their professional judgment? That was what I expected from them. I have posttraumatic stress disorder.

THEME 4. THE END JUSTIFIES THE MEANS: AT WHOSE EXPENSE? AT WHAT PRICE?

Mothers believed that the bottom line in considering a delivery a successful and fulfilling experience was the outcome of the baby. If the baby was born alive with good Apgar scores, that was what mattered to the labor and delivery staff and even to the mother's family and friends. The safe arrival of a live, healthy infant symbolized the achievement of clinical efficiency and of professional and fiscal goals. Mothers perceived that their traumatic deliveries giving over and pushed into the background as the healthy newborn took center stage.

Why, 18 years o damper on this celebration by focusing on the mother's traumatic experience

The needle had been hospitalized with chronic sciatica 20 years earlier when she was ove and had an epidural steroid injection for treatment. As the woman recalled,
ral.

> back and created a frightful situation where I could not
> ensation I vowed on the spot never ever to have another

Submitting to her most dreaded epidural and saying goodbye to her dreams of a vaginal delivery, this woman experienced an out-of-body experience as she lay on the delivery table hemorrhaging. She wrote,

> *I would have done anything to have this baby and did everything, even stuff I didn't want to. All I get told when dealing with the residual emotional effects is, "You should be happy with the outcome."*

After an hour of pushing, one primipara was offered forceps. The epidural was topped up, but not given enough time to work properly, nor was it checked. The mother felt the cut, the forceps going in, and her body tearing as the doctor pulled the baby out. She screamed loud and long. She shared that she

> *was congratulated for how "quickly and easily" the baby came out and that he scored a perfect 10! The worst thing was that nobody acknowledged that I had a bad time. Everyone was so pleased it had gone so well! I felt as if I had been raped!*

Women, who perceived that they had experienced traumatic births viewed the site of their labor and delivery as a battlefield. While engaged in battle, their protective layers were stripped away, leaving them exposed to the onslaught of birth trauma. Stripped from these women were their individuality, dignity, control, communication, caring, trust, and support and reassurance.

DISCUSSION

The birth traumas experienced by the mothers in this study have been identified previously such as emergency cesarean deliveries (Ballard, Stanley, & Brockington, 1995; Soet et al., 2003), long, painful labors with inadequate pain relief (Ballard et al., 1995; Fones, 1996; Soet et al., 2003), epidurals (Ballard et al., 1995; Fones, 1996), forceps deliveries (Fones, 1996), fetal or newborn deaths (Ballard et al., 1995; Turton, Hughes, Evans, & Fainman, 2001), premature infants and infants in the NICU (DeMier, Hynan, Harris, & Manniello, 1996; Holditch-Davis, Bartlett, Blickman, & Miles, 2003), degrading experiences (Menage, 1993), and perceptions of unsafe care during childbirth (Creedy, et al., 2000). Creedy et al. (2000) reported that the perception of unsafe care had a significant additive effect on birth trauma symptoms for women who also had a high level of obstetric intervention during their labor and delivery.

Parts of the four themes that describe the essence of a traumatic birth have been reported in previous studies, but nowhere has the totality of the experience been reported. Aspects of theme 1 (To care for me: Was that too much to ask?) have been mentioned by Ballard et al. (1995), Menage (1993), and Wijma et al. (1997). Theme 2 (To communicate with me: Why was this neglected?) appears in the research of Ballard et al. (1995), Creedy et al. (2000), Menage (1993), and Soet et al. (2003). The mothers' feelings of powerlessness and loss of control (theme 3) have been echoed previously by Allen (1998), Czarnocka and Slade (2000), Menage (1993), and Soet et al. (2003). Maes, Delmeire, Mylle, and Altramura (2001) reported that loss of control is a significant component of the traumatic event for many mothers who experience PTSD. Theme 4 (The end justifies the means: At whose expense? At what price?) has not been specifically addressed in any previous research. Whereas some of the mothers in this study felt as if they had been raped, the clinicians appeared to the women as oblivious to their plight. The mothers perceived that the clinicians focused only on the successful outcomes of clinical efficiency and live healthy infants.

In reviewing this manuscript before it was submitted for publication, two mothers made a special point to emphasize the importance of this fourth theme. The one mother wrote:

> *For me the most telling statement remains, "The end justifies the means: At whose expense? At what price?" For me, this sums up my situation and many others I know of.*

The other mother said:

> *This I believe is the actual contributing factor toward PTSD occurring. As no one is comfortable enough in themselves to be honest with the mother and the partner too I might add. So let's just breathe a sigh of relief and focus on the fact that the baby arrived.*

Besides providing safe care, what is it that clinicians can do to help prevent traumatic births? At a woman's admission to labor and delivery, it is important that clinicians take a careful history from her regarding any particular fears she may have about giving birth, such as needle phobia. If a woman has had previous deliveries, this admission history should include questions on whether previous deliveries were perceived as traumatic. Identification of any possible contributing factors to birth trauma can alert clinicians so that special care can be taken regarding these factors.

During labor and delivery, clinicians should strive to enhance a woman's sense of control by offering her options when possible. Many events during the delivery process are, however, out of the control of both the obstetric care providers and the mothers. Obstetric care providers need to discuss with the women the means of delivery, and not just the outcome. When hopes for the best laid birth plans are dashed, women's unmet expectations regarding their anticipated birth process need to be addressed by clinicians. Mothers' perceptions of birth trauma can be based not only on the event, but also on their unmet expectations regarding the event.

Church and Scanlan (2002) alert clinicians to have a proactive role in preventing PTSD after childbirth by vigilantly watching mothers during the postpartum period for recognition of early trauma-related symptoms: a dazed appearance, withdrawal, or temporary amnesia. Knowing that birth trauma lies in the eye of the beholder, they should treat every woman as though she were a survivor of a previous traumatic experience (Crompton, 2003).

REFERENCES

Allen, S. (1998). A qualitative analysis of the process, mediating variables, and impact of traumatic childbirth. *Journal of Reproductive and Infant Psychology, 16*, 107–131.

Ayers, S., & Pickering, A. (2001). Do women get posttraumatic stress disorder as a result of childbirth? A prospective study of incidence. *Birth, 28*, 111–118.

Ballard, C. G., Stanley, A. K., & Brockington, I. F. (1995). Post-traumatic stress disorder (PTSD) after childbirth. *British Journal of Psychiatry, 166*, 525–528.

Church, S., & Scanlan, M. (2002). Posttraumatic stress disorder after childbirth: Do midwives play a preventative role? *The Practicing Midwife, 5*, 10–13.

Colaizzi, P. F. (1978). Psychological research as the phenomenologist views it. In R. Valle & M. King (Eds.), *Existential phenomenological alternatives for psychology* (pp. 48–71). New York: Oxford University Press.

Creedy, D. K., Shochet, I. M., & Horsfall, J. (2000). Childbirth and the development of acute trauma symptoms: Incidence and contributing factors. *Birth, 27*, 104–111.

Crompton, J. (2003). Posttraumatic stress disorder and childbirth. *Childbirth Educators New Zealand Education Effects,* summer, 25–31.

Czarnocka, J., & Slade, P. (2000). Prevalence and predictors of posttraumatic stress symptoms following childbirth. *British Journal of Clinical Psychology, 39,* 35–51.

DeMier, R. L., Hynan, M. T., Harris, H. B., & Manniello, R. L. (1996). Perinatal stressors as predictors of symptoms of posttraumatic stress in mothers of infants at high risk. *Journal of Perinatology, 16,* 276–280.

Fones, C. (1996). Posttraumatic stress disorder occurring after painful childbirth. *Journal of Nervous and Mental Disease, 184,* 195–196.

Holditch-Davis, D., Bartlett, T. R., Blickman, A. L., & Miles, M. S. (2003). Posttraumatic stress symptoms in mothers of premature infants. *Journal of Obstetric, Gynecologic, and Neonatal Nursing, 32,* 161–171.

Hungerford, M. W. (1878). *Molly Bawn,* London: Smith, Elder and Company.

Husserl, E. (1960). *Cartesian meditations* (Trans. D. Cairns). The Hague: Martineus Nijhoff.

Husserl, E. (1962). Ideas: *General introduction to pure phenomenology.* New York: MacMillan.

Husserl, E. (1970). *The crisis of European sciences and transcendental phenomenology* (Trans. D. Carr). Evanston, IL: Northwestern University Press.

Maes, M., Delmeire, I., Mylle, J., & Altramura, C. (2001). Risk and preventive factors of posttraumatic stress disorder (PTSD). *Journal of Affective Disorders, 63,* 113–121.

Menage, J. (1993). Posttraumatic stress disorder in women who have undergone obstetric or gynecological procedures. *Journal of Reproduction and Infant Psychology, 11,* 221–228.

Ryding, E. L., Wijma, K., & Wijma, B. (1998). Experiences of emergency Cesarean section: A phenomenological study of 53 women. *Birth, 25,* 246–251.

Seng, J. S. (2002). A conceptual framework for research on lifetime violence, posttraumatic stress, and childbearing. *Journal of Midwifery and Women's Health, 47,* 337–346.

Soet, J. E., Brack, G. A., & Dilorio, C. (2003). Prevalence and predictors of women's experience of psychological trauma during childbirth. *Birth, 30,* 36–46.

Spielberger, C., Gorsuch, R., & Lushene, R. (1983). *Manual for the state-trait anxiety inventory.* Palo Alto, CA: Consulting Psychological Press.

Spiegelberg, H. (1975). *Doing phenomenology: Essays on and in phenomenology.* The Hague: Martinus Nijhoff.

Turton, P., Hughes, P., Evans, C. D., & Fainman, D. (2001). Incidence, correlates, and predictors of posttraumatic stress disorder in the pregnancy after stillbirth. *British Journal of Psychiatry, 178,* 556–560.

Watson, C. G., Juba, M. P., Manifold, V., Kucala, T., & Anderson, E. D. (1991). The PTSD interview: Rationale, description, reliability, and concurrent validity of a DSM-III-based technique. *Journal of Clinical Psychology, 47,* 179–189.

Wijma, K., Soderquist, J., & Wijma, B. (1997) Posttraumatic stress disorder after childbirth: A cross-sectional study. *Journal of Anxiety Disorders, 11,* 587–597.

Cheryl Tatano Beck, DNSc, CNM, FAAN, is Professor of Nursing, University of Connecticut School of Nursing, Storrs.

Accepted for publication September 18, 2003.

The author thanks Sue Watson, the Chairperson of Trauma and Birth Stress (TABS), a charitable trust in New Zealand, for her unwavering support and enthusiastic assistance with this research project. Without her help, this research study would never have come to fruition. To all the courageous women who shared their most personal and powerful stories of birth trauma, the author is forever indebted.

Corresponding author: Cheryl Tatano Beck, DNSc, CNM, FAAN, University of Connecticut, School of Nursing, 231 Glen-brook Road, Storrs, CT 06269-2026 (e-mail: Cheryl.beck@uconn.edu).

INDEX